Register Now for On[...]
to Your Boo[...]

SPRINGER PUBLISHING
CONNECT™

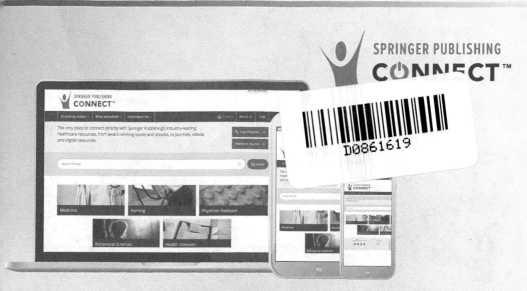

Your print purchase of *Neonatal Nursing Care Handbook, Third Edition,* **includes online access to the contents of your book**—increasing accessibility, portability, and searchability!

Access today at:
http://connect.springerpub.com/content/book/978-0-8261-3564-3
or scan the QR code at the right with your smartphone. Log in or register, then click "Redeem a voucher" and use the code below.

G1UV3EU2

Having trouble redeeming a voucher code?
Go to https://connect.springerpub.com/redeeming-voucher-code

If you are experiencing problems accessing the digital component of this product, please contact our customer service department at cs@springerpub.com

Scan here for quick access.

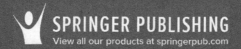

SPRINGER PUBLISHING
View all our products at springerpub.com

NEONATAL NURSING CARE HANDBOOK

Carole Kenner, PhD, RN, FAAN, FNAP, ANEF, is the Carol Kuser Loser Dean and Professor at the School of Nursing, Health, and Exercise Science at The College of New Jersey. She received her bachelor's in nursing from the University of Cincinnati and her master's and doctorate in nursing from Indiana University. She specialized in neonatal/perinatal nursing for her master's and obtained a minor in higher education for her doctorate. She has authored more than 100 journal articles and 40 textbooks. Her career is dedicated to nursing education and to the health of neonates and their families, as well as to educational and professional development of healthcare practices in neonatology. Her dedication includes providing a healthcare standard for educating neonatal nurses nationally and internationally. Her passion led her to begin the journal *Newborn and Infant Nursing Reviews*, for which she served as editor and then associate editor. She worked with the National Coalition on Health Professional Education in Genetics (NCHPEG) and the American Nurses Association to develop genetic competencies. Dr. Kenner helped develop the End-of-Life Nursing Education Consortium (ELNEC) Neonatal/Pediatric modules. She served as the co-chair of the Oklahoma Attorney General's Task Force on End of Life/Palliative Care. She also helped develop program recommendations for perinatal/neonatal palliative care as part of a family-centered/developmental care project sponsored by the National Perinatal Association. She serves on the Consensus Committee of Neonatal Intensive Care Design Standards, which sets recommendations for NICU designs, and serves on the March of Dimes Nursing Advisory Committee. Dr. Kenner is a fellow of the American Academy of Nursing (FAAN), a fellow in the National Academies of Practice, a fellow in the Academy of Nursing Education, past president of the National Association of Neonatal Nurses (NANN), and founding president of the Council of International Neonatal Nurses, Inc. (COINN), the first international organization representing neonatal nursing-setting standards globally. She is the 2011 recipient of the Audrey Hepburn Award for Contributions to the Health and Welfare of Children Internationally.

Marina V. Boykova, PhD, RN, is an associate professor of nursing in the School of Nursing and Allied Health Professions, Holy Family University, Philadelphia, Pennsylvania. She has a diploma in nursing practice, School of Nursing #3, Saint Petersburg, Russia; a certificate in theory and practice of nurse education, Medical College #1, Saint Petersburg, Russia; a certificate in theory and practice of nurse education, Chester, United Kingdom; a BSc with honours in professional practice (nursing), University of Liverpool, Chester, United Kingdom; a diploma of higher education in nursing, Novgorod University of Y. Mudrogo, Novgorod, Russia; an MSc in health promotion (distinction), University of Liverpool, Chester, United Kingdom; and a PhD in nursing, University of Oklahoma, Oklahoma City, Oklahoma. She is a member of Sigma Theta Tau International. She serves as a nonexecutive director for the Council of International Neonatal Nurses, Inc. (COINN). Her clinical background is neonatal intensive care nursing. Her research interests center on transition from hospital to home and to primary care for parents of preterm infants. Dr. Boykova has published in this area as well as neonatal care topics. She coauthored a policy brief on reducing preterm births for the American Academy of Nursing.

NEONATAL NURSING CARE HANDBOOK

An Evidence-Based Approach to Conditions and Procedures

Third Edition

Carole Kenner, PhD, RN, FAAN, FNAP, ANEF

Marina V. Boykova, PhD, RN

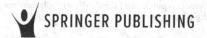

SPRINGER PUBLISHING

Springer Publishing Company, LLC
11 West 42nd Street, New York, NY 10036
www.springerpub.com
connect.springerpub.com/

Acquisitions Editor: Rachel X. Landes
Compositor: Amnet Systems

ISBN: 978-0-8261-3548-3
ebook ISBN: 978-0-8261-3564-3
DOI: 10.1891/9780826135643

21 22 23 24 25 / 5 4 3 2 1

The author and the publisher of this Work have made every effort to use sources believed to be reliable to provide
information that is accurate and compatible with the standards generally accepted at the time of publication. Because
medical science is continually advancing, our knowledge base continues to expand. Therefore, as new information
becomes available, changes in procedures become necessary. We recommend that the reader always consult current
research and specific institutional policies before performing any clinical procedure or delivering any medication.
The author and publisher shall not be liable for any special, consequential, or exemplary damages resulting, in whole
or in part, from the readers' use of, or reliance on, the information contained in this book. The publisher has no
responsibility for the persistence or accuracy of URLs for external or third-party Internet websites referred to in this
publication and does not guarantee that any content on such websites is, or will remain, accurate or appropriate.

Library of Congress Cataloging-in-Publication Data
Names: Kenner, Carole, editor. | Boykova, Marina V., editor.
Title: Neonatal nursing care handbook : an evidence-based approach to
   conditions and procedures / [edited by] Carole Kenner, Marina V.
   Boykova.
Other titles: Neonatal nursing pocket guide.
Description: Third edition. | New York, NY : Springer Publishing Company,
   LLC [2022] | Preceded by Neonatal nursing pocket guide / [edited by]
   Carole Kenner, Judy Wright Lott. c2004. Second edition. [2016] |
   Includes bibliographical references and index.
Identifiers: LCCN 2021027885 (print) | LCCN 2021027886 (ebook) | ISBN
   9780826135483 (paperback) | ISBN 9780826135643 (ebook)
Subjects: MESH: Neonatal Nursing—methods | Evidence-Based Nursing |
   Infant, Newborn, Diseases—nursing | Handbook
Classification: LCC RJ254 (print) | LCC RJ254 (ebook) | NLM WY 49 | DDC
   618.92/01—dc23
LC record available at https://lccn.loc.gov/2021027885
LC ebook record available at https://lccn.loc.gov/2021027886

Carole Kenner: https://orcid.org/0000-0002-1573-5240
Marina V. Boykova: https://orcid.org/0000-0002-9065-3704

Printed in the United States of America.

Contents

Section I: Systems Assessment and Management of Disorders

Section II: Special Care Considerations in Neonatal Nursing

Section III: Common Procedures, Diagnostic Tests, Lab Values, and Drugs

Contributors

Leslie B. Altimier, DNP, RNC, NE-BC Director of Clinical Innovation and Research, Philips Healthcare, Cambridge, Massachusetts

Gail A. Bagwell, DNP, APRN, CNS President, National Association of Neonatal Nurses, Clinical Nurse Specialist, Nationwide Children's Hospital, Division of Neonatology, Columbus, Ohio

Susan Tucker Blackburn, PhD, RN, FAAN Professor Emerita, School of Nursing, University of Washington, Seattle, Washington

Marina V. Boykova, PhD, RN Associate Professor, School of Nursing and Allied Health Professions, Holy Family University, Philadelphia, Pennsylvania

Caitlin Bradley, PhD, RN, NNP-BC Neonatal Nurse Practitioner, Neonatal Intensive Care Unit, Boston Children's Hospital, Boston, Massachusetts

Julie Briere, MSN, RN, NNP, CCRN Neonatal Nurse Practitioner, Neonatal Intensive Care Unit, Boston Children's Hospital, Boston, Massachusetts

Beth Brown, MSN, RNC Clinical Nurse Educator, Special Care Nursery (SCN), Premier Health, Dayton, Ohio

Denise Casey, MS, RN, CCRN, CPNP Advanced Practice Nurse II, Neonatal Intensive Care Unit, Boston Children's Hospital, Boston, Massachusetts

Christine Catts, DNP, NNP-BC Instructor, College of Nursing, Thomas Jefferson University, Philadelphia, Pennsylvania

Mary Coughlin, MS, NNP, RNC-E Certified Trauma-Informed Professional, President and Founder, Caring Essentials Collaborative, LLC, Boston, Massachusetts

Michele DeGrazia, PhD, RN, NNP-BC, FAAN Director of Nursing Research, Neonatal Intensive Care Unit, Boston Children's Hospital, Boston, Massachusetts

Eileen C. DeWitt, MS, RN, NNP-BC Neonatal Nurse Practitioner II, Neonatal Intensive Care Unit, Boston Children's Hospital, Boston, Massachusetts

Tara DeWolfe, PT, DPT, CNT   Certified Trauma-Informed Professional, Certified to Reliability in NIDCAP, Faculty, Caring Essentials Collaborative Quantum Caring Institute, Pediatric Physical Therapist and Developmental Specialist, Way to Grow Pediatric Therapy, Peoria, Illinois

Deb Discenza, MA   Founder, Chief Executive Officer, and Publisher, Preemieworld, LLC, Springfield, Virginia

Georgia R. Ditzenberger, PhD, NNP-BC   Neonatal Nurse Practitioner, Salem Health Hospital, Neonatal Intensive Care Unit, Salem, Oregon

Noel L. H. Dwyer, MBA, RN, CCRN   Staff Nurse II, Neonatal Intensive Care Unit, Boston Children's Hospital, Boston, Massachusetts

Wakako M. Eklund, DNP, APRN, NNP-BC   Neonatal Nurse Practitioner, Advance Neonatal Solutions, LLC, Pediatrix Medical Group of Tennessee, Nashville, Tennessee; Affiliate Associate Professor, School of Nursing, Bouve College of Health Sciences, Northeastern University, Boston, Massachusetts

Avery Forget, MSN, RN, CCRN   Staff Nurse II, Infection Prevention Liaison, Neonatal Intensive Care Unit, Boston Children's Hospital, Boston, Massachusetts

Kristy Fuller, OTR/L, CNT   Certified Trauma-Informed Professional, Certified to Reliability in NIDCAP, Faculty, Caring Essentials Collaborative Quantum Caring Institute, President, Infant Feeding Strategies, LLC, Bettendorf, Iowa

Tricia Grandinetti, BSN, RN, CCRN   Staff Nurse II, Neonatal Intensive Care Unit, Boston Children's Hospital, Boston, Massachusetts

Mona Liza Hamlin, MSN, IBCLC   Nurse Manager, Perinatal Resources and Community Programs, Milk Bank, Center for Womens' and Childrens' Health, ChristianaCare, Newark, Delaware

Carole Kenner, PhD, RN, FAAN, FNAP, ANEF   CEO, Council of International Neonatal Nurses, Inc. (COINN), Carol Kuser Loser Dean and Professor, School of Nursing, Health, and Exercise Science, College of New Jersey, Ewing, New Jersey

Michelle LaBrecque, MSN, RN, CCRN   Advanced Practice Nurse II, Neonatal Intensive Care Unit, Boston Children's Hospital, Boston, Massachusetts

Lisa A. Lubbers, MSN, RN, NNP-BC   Neonatal Nurse Practitioner, Avera McKennan Hospital, Sioux Falls, South Dakota; Clinical Instructor, Department of Pediatrics, University of South Dakota Sanford School of Medicine, Vermillion, South Dakota

Carolyn Lund, MS, RN, FAAN Neonatal Clinical Nurse Specialist, Benioff Children's Hospital, Oakland, California; Associate Clinical Professor, School of Nursing, University of California, San Francisco, San Francisco, California

Mary-Jeanne Manning, MSN, RN, PNP-BC, CCRN Advanced Practice Nurse II, Medical Surgical Intensive Care Unit, Boston Children's Hospital, Boston, Massachusetts

Jacqueline M. McGrath, PhD, RN, FNAP, FAAN Thelma and Joe Crow Endowed Professor, Vice Dean for Faculty Excellence, School of Nursing, University of Texas Health Science Center San Antonio, San Antonio, Texas

Samual L. Mooneyham, MSN, RN Registered Nurse for Frederick Mandell, MD (Pediatrician), Brookline, Massachusetts; Registered Nurse, Boston Endoscopy Center, Wellesley, Massachusetts

Susan M. Orlando, DNS, APRN, NNP-BC, CNS Associate Clinical Professor, Program Director, Neonatal Nurse Practitioner Program, Louisiana State University Health Sciences Center School of Nursing, New Orleans, Louisiana

Leslie A. Parker, PhD, APRN, NNP-BC, FAAN, FAANP Associate Professor, College of Nursing, University of Florida, Gainesville, Florida

Ann Gibbons Phalen, PhD, CRNP, NNP-BC Dean, Frances M. Maguire School of Nursing and Health Professions, Gwynedd Mercy University, Gwynedd Valley, Pennsylvania

Raylene M. Phillips, MD, FAAP, FABM, IBCLC Neonatologist, Loma Linda University Children's Hospital, Loma Linda, California

Shahirose Sadrudin Premji, PhD, MScN, BSc, BScN, RN, FAAN Director and Professor, School of Nursing, Faculty of Health, York University, Toronto, Ontario, Canada

Jana L. Pressler, PhD, RN Professor Emerita, College of Nursing, University of Nebraska Medical Center–Lincoln, Lincoln, Nebraska

Katie L. Roy, DNP, RN, CPNP-AC, FNP-BC Pediatric/Family Nurse Practitioner, Medical Surgical Intensive Care Unit, Boston Children's Hospital, Boston, Massachusetts

Michele Kacmarcik Savin, DNP, APRN, NNP-BC Assistant Professor, Thomas Jefferson College of Nursing, Neonatal Nurse Practitioner Program Director, Thomas Jefferson University, Philadelphia, Pennsylvania

Ethan Schuler, DNP, RN, CPNP-PC/AC Pediatric Nurse Practitioner II, Medical Surgical Intensive Care Unit, Boston Children's Hospital, Boston, Massachusetts

Elizabeth L. Sharpe, DNP, APRN, NNP-BC, VA-BC, FAAN Associate Professor Clinical Nursing, College of Nursing, The Ohio State University, Columbus, Ohio

Beth Shields, PharmD, BCPPS   Associate Director, Operations, Rush University Medical Center, Chicago, Illinois

Stephanie R. Sykes, DNP, APRN-CNP, NNP-BC   Assistant Professor of Clinical Practice, College of Nursing, The Ohio State University, Columbus, Ohio

Jodi A. Ulloa, DNP, APRN-CNP, NNP-BC   Assistant Professor of Clinical Practice, Neonatal Nurse Practitioner Program, College of Nursing, The Ohio State University, Columbus, Ohio

Dorothy Vittner, PhD, RN, FAAN   Assistant Professor, Egan School of Nursing and Health Studies, Fairfield University, Fairfield, Connecticut; Connecticut Children's, Neonatal Intensive Care Unit, Hartford, Connecticut

Ksenia Zukowsky, PhD, APRN, NNP-BC   Associate Professor and Chair, Graduate Programs, College of Nursing, Thomas Jefferson University, Philadelphia, Pennsylvania

Past Contributors

Donna Armstrong, MSN, CAGS, RN, CCRN

Carrie-Ellen Briere, BSN, RN, CLC

Monica A. Carleton, BSN, RN

Anita Catlin, DNSc, FNAP, FAAN

Xiaomei Cong, PhD, RN

Patricia Fleck, PhD, RN, NNP-BC

Maura Heckmann, DNP, MSN, CPNP, RN

Judy Wright Lott, PhD, NNP-BC, RN, FAAN

Ruth Lucas, PhD, RN-IPO, CLS

Stephanie Packard, BSN, RN, CCRN

Melissa Roberts, MSN, RN, CPNP

Ann Schwoebel, RNC-NIC, CRNP

Tamara Wallace, DNP, RN, NNP-BC

Charlotte Wool, PhD, RN

Foreword

The health of newborns in all countries must be at the forefront of all activities (teaching, research, and service) if neonatal nursing is to embrace health for all and end preventable deaths of newborns globally by 2030. It is within this ethos of reducing neonatal mortality to at least 12 per 1,000 live births that the *Neonatal Nursing Care Handbook: An Evidence-Based Approach to Conditions and Procedures, Third Edition,* has been updated to serve a global cadre of neonatal nurses!

The neonatal handbook goes beyond providing an explanation of common conditions and procedures that are widely implemented in practice. The handbook now provides information on trauma-informed care, recognizing the role of toxic stress in the trajectory of health across the life span of the newborn, the mother, and the family. The COVID-19 pandemic, though a worldwide experience, will have varied emotional and mental consequences and risk of toxic stress. Trauma-informed care enables provision of safe and supportive care while also ensuring personal wellness.

There is an appreciation that learners and clinicians in some countries are not able to readily access knowledge or evidence to inform practice. This neonatal handbook has therefore been written with the intent of making evidence easily accessible to learners in the classroom or clinical setting, as well as to practitioners in clinical care who want to improve the quality of care. The revised handbook provides updates on new ventilatory techniques and palliative and bereavement care. The neonatal handbook employs a systems approach, detailing management of disorders related to each system. Many of the special care considerations can be applied universally, for instance, developmental care and breastfeeding. A separate section covers procedures and diagnostic tests.

The editors, Drs. Carole Kenner and Marina V. Boykova, have been mindful that resources may vary significantly in some countries where the handbook will be utilized. The neonatal handbook is therefore available, keeping at the forefront the principles of evidence-based nursing practice while appreciating that clinical decisions will be guided by the best evidence shared in the neonatal handbook, the resources available in the practice setting, the clinical practice skills of the neonatal nurse, and the parents' preference with respect to care provided to their newborn. Evidence-informed practice improves patient outcomes, and sharing knowledge about best practices (i.e., current state of evidence) is an important step in this regard. The gift of knowledge will ensure the health and well-being of newborns in all countries.

Dr. Shahirose Sadrudin Premji, PhD, MScN, BSc, BScN, RN, FAAN
Director and Professor, School of Nursing, Faculty of Health
York University
Toronto, Ontario, Canada

Preface

This handbook is a quick reference for nurses who care for the small and sick newborn. It addresses the most common conditions and procedures. The material is offered in an easy-to-use format and is meant to be a quick reference, not a comprehensive one. It can be used by anyone providing care to this population. A systems approach is used in Section I. Section II highlights special care considerations, and Section III presents the common procedures, diagnostic tests, and lab values. The appendices house additional material on weights and temperatures, common abbreviations, and web resources. In this third edition, all chapters have been updated to reflect new evidence for neonatal nursing care. Additions include oral/nasogastric tube feedings, bottle feedings, high-frequency ventilation, and new ventilation techniques. There is a new section on neonatal abstinence syndrome and neonatal opioid withdrawal. This book can be used internationally to provide evidence-based practice for consistent high-quality care in order to improve neonatal outcomes.

For more comprehensive information, please see the sixth edition of *Comprehensive Neonatal Nursing* (2020), written by Carole Kenner, Leslie B. Altimier, and Marina V. Boykova and published by Springer Publishing Company. We hope you find this book useful.

Carole Kenner
Marina V. Boykova

Acknowledgments

I want to express my appreciation to all the neonatal nurses and the families throughout the years who have given me feedback on what content is needed to include. This book is dedicated to the memory of my parents who encouraged me to write and contribute to improving outcomes for neonates and their families.

Carole Kenner

For my mom, whose love and support were endless.

Marina V. Boykova

Together we would like to express our appreciation for the assistance from Elizabeth Nieginski from Springer Publishing Company for all her support and guidance throughout the project's process. Thank you too to Rachel Landes from Springer Publishing Company who answered our myriad of questions. Thank you to all our contributors who provided their expertise and demonstrated the compassion and commitment to educating and supporting the next generation of neonatal nurses as well as those neonatal nursing health professionals who have been around for a while. Finally, we want to thank the professionals across the globe who take care of babies and their families.

Carole and Marina

I

Systems Assessment and Management of Disorders

1

1

Respiratory System

LISA A. LUBBERS AND WAKAKO M. EKLUND

OVERVIEW

Neonatal respiratory compromise can be pulmonary in nature or related to other neonatal comorbidities, including congenital heart defects, congenital malformations, metabolic abnormalities, and disorders of the central nervous system (CNS). Regardless of origin, these infants often present in a similar fashion with respiratory distress that includes increased rate and effort of breathing, cyanosis, and oxygen requirement. Ninety percent of all respiratory distress in neonates is caused by respiratory distress syndrome (RDS), aspiration, transient tachypnea, air leaks, and congenital pneumonia (Fraser, 2021).

"Respiratory distress" is a global term that refers to disorders of the respiratory system that begin at or shortly following birth. Although most common in those infants born prior to term, respiratory distress can result from any neonatal condition that leads to progressive atelectasis, hypoventilation, and/or hypoxia. Diseases that affect the respiratory system in the early neonatal period may extend well into infancy or childhood.

If lung compliance is decreased, there is also a decrease in tidal volume, which is the amount of air that enters or exits the lungs with every inhalation or exhalation. For the neonate to achieve sufficient minute ventilation (tidal volume x respiratory rate per minute), the respiratory rate will increase (tachypnea) when tidal volume is small. Hypoxemia will also trigger an increased respiratory rate to compensate. Increased work of breathing is the result of mismatched pulmonary mechanics, including increased airway resistance, diminished lung compliance, or both (Reuter et al., 2014).

Complex mechanisms and structures bring about normal pulmonary development and function in the neonate. Both anatomic and physiologic processes occur to facilitate the maturation of the respiratory system. This process occurs along an orderly sequence of events from the fourth week of gestation through the eighth year of life.

RESPIRATORY SYSTEM DEVELOPMENT

Anatomic Development of the Respiratory System

Outgrowth of the laryngotracheal groove found in the floor of the caudal end of the anterior foregut starts the complex process of respiratory system development. By the end of the fourth week, this groove has protruded and developed into a pouch-like structure, laryngotracheal diverticulum. The diverticulum lengthens and enlarges to form a globular lung bud from which the tracheobronchial tree originates. Initially, the right and left lung buds appear as lateral outpouchings of foregut on each side of the tracheal primordium. By the end of the fifth week of development, the tracheoesophageal septum has developed from the longitudinal growth and fusion of the tracheoesophageal folds. This septum separates the cranial portion of the foregut into a ventral part, laryngotracheal tube, and a dorsal part, which is the origin of the oropharynx and esophagus. Separation of the single foregut tube into trachea and esophagus occurs through a complex process requiring multiple signaling pathways and transcription factors.

Development of the Larynx

The larynx develops from the endoderm of the cranial end of the laryngotracheal tube. Cartilages develop from mesenchyme derived from neural crest cells. The mesenchyme grows rapidly, eventually producing the slit-like laryngeal inlet by the end of the sixth week. Temporary occlusion of the laryngeal lumen occurs thereafter with recanalization by the 10th week, during which time the laryngeal ventricles, vocal cords, and vestibular folds develop. The epiglottis arises from the caudal part of the hypopharyngeal prominence. Laryngeal muscles developed from myoblasts in the fourth and sixth pairs of pharyngeal arches are innervated by the vagus nerves (cranial nerve X). Of note, the larynx is situated high in the neck of the neonate, which allows the epiglottis to come in contact with the soft palate. This location provides almost complete separation between the respiratory and digestive tract to facilitate feeding later on. However, this also makes the neonate an obligatory nose breather. The larynx structurally descends over the first 2 years of life.

Development of the Trachea

During separation from the foregut, the laryngotracheal diverticulum forms the beginning of the trachea and primary bronchial buds. Splanchnic mesenchyme gives rise to the cartilage, connective tissue, and muscles of the trachea. This development goes through the 12th week of gestation.

Development of the Bronchi and Lungs

The respiratory bud that developed during the fourth week divides into two bronchial buds. The bronchial buds grow laterally into the pericardio-peritoneal canals forming the beginning of the pleural cavities. The buds and splanchnic mesenchyme evolve into the bronchi and their branches in the lungs. At the beginning of the fifth week, the connection of the bud to the trachea enlarges and forms the main bronchi. The right main bronchus is slightly larger than the left. The main bronchi subdivides, eventually forming three lobes on the right and two on the left. Progressive branching continues until the end of the seventh week, and 10 segmental bronchi in the right and eight or nine in the left form. By 24 weeks, about 17 orders of branches have formed, and bronchioles have developed. Additionally, seven more orders of branches develop after birth.

The splanchnic mesenchyme develops into cartilaginous plates, bronchial smooth muscle, connective tissue, and capillaries. As the lungs continue to develop, a layer of visceral pleura forms from the same splanchnic mesenchyme. Eventually, the lungs and pleural cavities grow caudally into the mesenchyme of the body wall and lie close to the heart.

Physiologic Development of the Respiratory System

Five overlapping microscopic stages comprise the maturation periods of the lungs: pseudoglandular, canalicular, saccular, surfactant, and alveolar (Moore et al., 2020).

Pseudoglandular: Weeks 5 to 17. At this point, the lungs are similar to exocrine glands. By 16 weeks, all major elements have formed except those involving gas exchange. Fetuses born during this time are unable to survive due to the lack of respiratory function to enable gas exchange.

Canalicular: Weeks 16 to 25. Lumen of the bronchi and terminal bronchioles becomes larger, and the lung tissue itself becomes very vascular. The production of surfactant begins around 20 to 22 weeks in small amounts, but it does not reach adequate amounts until later in gestation. Lamellar bodies store surfactant. Having adequately developed pulmonary vasculature that allows gas exchange and having the ability to produce surfactant are the two critical keys to neonatal survival for the extremely premature infants. By week 24, each terminal bronchiole has formed respiratory bronchioles, which further divide into early alveolar ducts. Respiration is possible near the end of this stage, because early alveoli have formed and the tissue is well vascularized. However, supplemental surfactant is necessary at this early stage.

Saccular: Weeks 24 to late in fetal development. More alveoli develop and the epithelium becomes very thin with capillaries protruding into the sacs to further facilitate gas exchange. Differentiation of type I and II pneumocytes occurs. Establishment of a blood-air barrier permits adequate gas exchange across type I pneumocytes if the fetus were born at this gestation. Surfactant (a complex mixture of phospholipids and proteins) is also being secreted by type II pneumocytes at this time; however, not in adequate amounts.

Surfactant: As stated earlier, these five microscopic stages overlap, and surfactant production begins around 20 to 22 weeks and does not reach adequate levels until later in gestation. Surfactant forms a thin film over the insides of alveolar sacs.

- Counteracts surface tension at the air–alveolar interface, thus preventing air sac collapse, which leads to atelectasis, decreases opening pressure of the alveoli, enhances alveolar fluid clearance, and provides a level of protection for the fragile epithelial cell surface (Gardner et al., 2021).
- Phosphatidylglycerol (PG), which is the second most common phospholipid in surfactant, usually appears at about 36 weeks' gestation and continues to increase until term.

- It is stored, recycled, and secreted in the neonatal lung; however, under certain conditions, the metabolism and/or effectiveness of surfactant will be altered. These include maternal conditions such as diabetes, infection, hypertension, drug use, and placental insufficiency, as well as infant conditions such as acidemia, hypoxia, need for mechanical ventilation, hypercapnia, twin gestation, sepsis, and prematurity (Gardner et al., 2021).
- Adequate amounts of surfactant to prevent atelectasis are generally not achieved until at least 32 weeks.

Alveolar: The alveolar stage is the late gestational period up to 8 years of age. By 34 weeks, each bronchiole ends with an alveolar sac. These sacs will eventually become alveolar ducts. By 38 weeks, the alveolar capillary membrane across which gas exchange occurs is very thin. Three adaptive changes must occur during transition from fetal life to extrauterine life: (1) parallel pulmonary and systemic circulations, (2) lungs transform from secretory organs to gas-exchanging organs, and (3) production of surfactant in the alveolar sacs. Much of lung development after birth results from multiplication of alveoli and capillaries. Approximately 150 million alveoli (half of the adult number) are present in the lungs at full term (Moore et al., 2020).

At birth, the lungs are partially filled with a fluid continually produced by the lungs. Aeration of the lungs requires rapid replacement of fluid with air in the alveoli. The fluid is cleared through the mouth and nose via compression of the thorax, moves into the pulmonary capillaries, arteries, and veins, and then travels into the lymphatics.

This transition to extrauterine life begins as the infant takes the first breath of air, usually in response to tactile stimulation upon birth. This first breath of the term infant requires an opening pressure of 60 to 80 cm of water with subsequent breaths requiring less as the surface tension of the liquid-filled airways and alveoli is stabilized.

Oxygen passively diffuses across the alveolar–capillary membrane, due to the difference in oxygen pressure, which is higher in the alveoli than in the capillary blood supply. Oxygen dissolves in the plasma and then binds to the hemoglobin and circulates systemically. Oxygen is deposited throughout the tissues in much the same passive manner. The oxygen pressure is higher in the arterial blood supply than in the tissues; therefore, the oxygen moves from the hemoglobin to the tissues.

RESPIRATORY SYSTEM ASSESSMENT

A thorough and systematic review of the prenatal and birth history will provide the clinician with information regarding specific risk factors that will impact neonatal care and resuscitation requirements. Certain maternal conditions greatly influence the development and subsequent function of the neonatal respiratory system. Maternal history is typically separated into three separate time frames: antepartum (during pregnancy), intrapartum (labor and delivery), and postpartum (following delivery). Maternal conditions, both chronic and acute, affect the fetal well-being, both in the short term and potentially the long term. Maternal serologies including blood type, history of infection, ultrasound findings including estimated fetal weight, and gestation should be identified prior to delivery whenever possible.

An overall review of the infant's vital signs (heart rate, respiratory rate, temperature, and blood pressure) and general appearance during the adaptation to the extrauterine environment are the beginning of the infant assessment. Numerous specific visual clinical observations will provide information before a stethoscope is even placed on the infant's chest.

■ Respiratory rate: Respiratory rates in an infant can be highly variable. Deviation from normal respiratory rates of approximately 40 to 60 breaths per minute can be due to numerous reasons, including pulmonary dysfunction, metabolic derangements, central nervous system (CNS) dysfunction, periodic breathing pattern related to prematurity, and blood gas abnormalities. Low respiratory rates can result in decreased minute ventilation, and high rates may be a result of low tidal volumes. Infants can adjust their respiratory rate to minimize the work of breathing. Visually counting the respiratory rate removes the error associated with interference or artifact from the EKG leads. Periodic breathing is a cycle of very shallow breaths or even apnea lasting 5 to 10 seconds interspersed with adequate respirations. This is common in premature infants related to the immature CNS. Bradypnea is a respiratory rate below 30 breaths per minute. Apnea is the cessation of respirations lasting longer than 20 seconds, and it can be a sign of impending respiratory failure requiring prompt initiation of assisted respirations.

■ Retractions: Neonates have a very compliant chest wall resulting in very visible retractions in the suprasternal, substernal, subcostal, and intercostal areas. Negative intrapleural pressure generated by the diaphragm and respiratory accessory muscles causes retractions.

■ Nasal flaring: Infants are almost exclusively nose breathers. Therefore, nasal resistance contributes to overall total airway resistance. Nasal flaring results from dilation of the muscles, thereby reducing nasal resistance and the overall work of breathing.

■ Grunting: Exhaling through a partially closed glottis results in a grunting noise. This is a compensatory method to maintain functional residual capacity (FRC) to maintain alveolar distention and promote gas exchange. This may be heard audibly without a stethoscope. Grunting can be intermittent or continuous in nature. Grunting must be differentiated from gasping, which is a sign of impending respiratory failure during which immediate intervention with positive pressure ventilation is indicated.

■ Cyanosis: The visible discoloration most easily noted on central mucous membranes can be purple or blue in appearance. Clinical cyanosis is visible at varying levels of oxygen saturation based on hemoglobin. Infants with anemia can exhibit low PaO_2 without obvious visible cyanosis. Conversely, patients with polycythemia may have clinical cyanosis but normal PaO_2. Cyanosis is a classic sign of hypoxemia.

■ General appearance: Symmetry of the chest, barrel chest or pigeon chest appearance, and scaphoid appearance of the abdomen can provide clues to pathology causing respiratory symptoms (and connect to) such as diaphragmatic hernia.

■ Pallor, mottling, or poor color of the infant may indicate hypotension or acidosis.

■ Tachycardia, bradycardia, blood pressure changes, and perfusion are important signs of cardiac compromise from congenital heart disease (CHD) or ongoing respiratory compromise and failure.

■ Diminished muscle tone and poor activity are critical signs of profound hypoxia and acidosis.

■ Auscultation of the chest is difficult due to the small size of the neonate and referred breath sounds. It includes.

● Comparing and contrasting bilateral lung sounds

● Quality and volume of air exchange

● Adventitious breath sounds (crackles, rales, and decreased air entry)

● Absence or asymmetric volume of air exchange

■ Percussion and palpation of the neonatal chest have little diagnosis value.

Generalized Nursing Care

Nursing care of the neonate exhibiting respiratory distress is multifaceted and should be geared toward maintaining homeostasis within the body. Acquiring the nursing skills to adequately assess and care for the sick neonate requires a strong nursing education as foundation and additional mentoring by experienced neonatal nurses. Nurses must be efficient, gentle, and also acutely aware of maintaining a supportive environment for their young patients. In the case of neonates, sometimes a hands-off approach may be more supportive to the infant versus overstimulation.

■ Maintaining a neutral thermal environment: Supporting the temperature regulation of the neonate by providing heat and/or humidity and eliminating heat loss or gain from evaporative, radiant, conductive, and convective sources. Avoiding hypothermia or hyperthermia allows the infant to conserve metabolic expenditure. Radiant warmers and incubators can be used to assist in temperature support.

■ Any infant exhibiting respiratory distress should have close nursing support of glucose homeostasis. During the critical phase of respiratory management, this is accomplished by glucose and protein intravenous (IV) support. Nurses require skills in obtaining and maintaining IV access, ensuring appropriate rates of infusions, and checking blood sugar levels at appropriate intervals in accordance with the policy or guidance based on the provider order.

■ Maintaining the ordered respiratory support is a key nursing skill. A variety of respiratory support devices (nasal cannula [NC], continuous positive airway pressure [CPAP] apparatus, conventional ventilator, and high-frequency ventilator) must be maintained by nurses in collaboration with respiratory therapists, medical team providers, and parents to achieve optimal success. Recognizing when clinical changes are occurring with the neonate and understanding what those changes may indicate are crucial. Using a variety of tools such as suctioning, positioning, blood gas monitoring, and end-tidal CO_2 trending helps nurses optimize respiratory support. Maintaining an infant on CPAP is very labor-intensive for nursing staff. Generally CPAP devices have three interface options: mask, prong, and cannula. The mask must be situated such that it sits on the bridge of the nose, covers the nostrils, and rests on the philtrum. Improperly fitted/positioned masks may occlude the nares, sit on the lip, or cover the eyes. This results in an ineffective seal, pressure to the skin and eyes, and risk of skin irritation or breakdown. CPAP prongs must be sized such that they allow for the most air flow through them without putting undo pressure to the inside of the nostrils. The seal is imperative to achieve the desired CPAP. Use of a cannula-type device is being undertaken by some neonatal intensive care units and does not require a seal.

■ Monitoring intake and output to avoid over- or underhydration is important depending on other clinical issues such as gestational age.

■ Monitoring oxygen saturations and titrating oxygen as needed helps to achieve the ordered target range for the specific infant and disease process.

■ Obtaining blood gases and other labs as needed via arterial, venous, or capillary sampling and understanding the results of these tests is a key skill.

■ Vigilant nursing observation and assessment is needed to notice subtle changes in the infant's condition, such as sudden increase in work of breathing or oxygen requirement.

■ Assisting with positioning of the infant helps achieve optimal radiographic images.

■ Assessing and managing pain and agitation is performed using nonpharmacologic and/or pharmacologic measures.

In summary, generalized nursing care of the neonate exhibiting respiratory distress is complex and multifaceted. It requires continuous ongoing assessment by astute nurses.

Brief Overview of Blood Gas Analysis

The goal of blood gas analysis in the neonate is to determine the type and degree of disorder and presence of any compensation. Indications include all forms of respiratory distress, metabolic conditions, sepsis, and neurologic concerns. Cord gases may provide the clinician with a specific quantity in which to determine the degree of asphyxia experienced prior to birth (see Figure 1.1). Oxygen moves from the oxygen-rich alveolar–capillary membrane through passive measures to the blood, where the oxygen level is lower. This passive mechanism is the partial pressure of oxygen. The oxygen dissolves into the plasma and binds to the hemoglobin. This measure is reflected in the PaO_2 value.

Carbon dioxide moves rapidly across the cell membrane in response to ventilation. The movement from tissues is more efficient than oxygenation. The $PaCO_2$ reflects ventilation status.

Blood gas results must be evaluated based on the type of sample (capillary, venous, arterial). Arterial samples provide valid data pertaining to acid–base

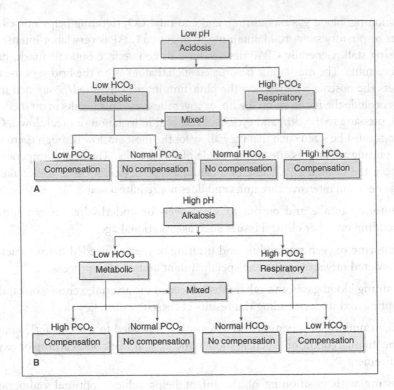

FIGURE 1.1 Acid–base balance: diagnostic approach. (A) Low pH. (B) High pH.

Source: Gentle, S., Travers, C., & Carlo, W. A. (2020). Respiratory system. In C. Kenner, L. B. Altimier, & M. V. Boykova (Eds.), *Comprehensive neonatal nursing care* (6th ed., pp 127–146). Springer Publishing Company.

balance and oxygenation, whereas capillary samples are not useful for evaluating accurate PO_2. Arterial samples are always preferred but not necessarily easily obtained since they require an advanced skill to perform arterial puncture when infants do not have an arterial line, such as a peripheral or umbilical artery line. Capillary specimens may not be accurate in the setting of hypotension, hypothermia, or shock where perfusion is not optimal. Warming the heel for 3 to 5 minutes prior to sampling optimizes conditions so the best quality sample may be obtained. Bicarbonate and base excess/deficit are calculated numbers based on measured pH and pCO_2. Blood gas results for pH and bicarbonate are slightly lower than normal values in the first 48 hours of life (Karlsen, 2013).

The acid–base balance depends on the interaction between bicarbonate ions and carbon dioxide. Acidosis or low pH is not well tolerated by the neonate and can increase vasoconstriction in sensitive pulmonary vasculature, increasing the state of hypoxemia (see Figure 1.1; also see the MedCalc Acid–Base Calculator at www.medcalc.com/acidbase.html).

Common neonatal respiratory conditions are listed and described in the following text. Common diagnoses with a decision-making algorithm for the infant who presents with respiratory disease are included (see Figure 1.2). Specific care and treatment of these conditions are described under each topical heading.

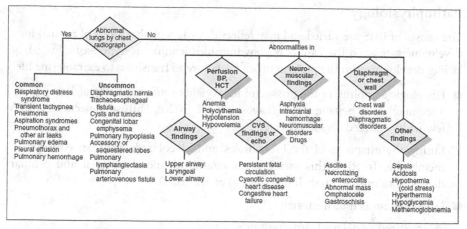

FIGURE 1.2 Diagnostic algorithm for the neonate with acute respiratory distress.

Source: Gentle, S., Travers, C., & Carlo, W. A. (2020). Respiratory system. In C. Kenner, L. B. Altimier, & M. V. Boykova (Eds.), *Comprehensive neonatal nursing care* (6th ed., pp 127–146). Springer Publishing Company.

REFERENCES

Fraser, D. (2021). Respiratory distress. In M. T. Verklan, M. Walden, & S. Forest (Eds.), *Core curriculum for neonatal intensive care nursing* (6th ed., pp. 394–424). Elsevier.

Gardner, S. L., Enzman-Hines, M., & Nyp, M. (2021). Respiratory diseases. In S. L. Gardner, B. S. Carter, M. Enzman-Hines, & S. Niermeyer (Eds.), *Merenstein & Gardner's handbook of neonatal intensive care: An interprofessional approach* (9th ed., pp. 729–1245). Elsevier.

Gentle, S., Travers, C., & Carlo, W. A. (2020). Respiratory system. In C. Kenner, L. B. Altimier, & M. V. Boykova (Eds.), *Comprehensive neonatal nursing care* (6th ed., pp 127–146). Springer Publishing Company.

Karlsen, K. (2013). *The S.T.A.B.L.E. program pre-transport/post-resuscitation stabilization care of sick infants' guidelines for neonatal healthcare providers* (6th ed.). S.T.A.B.L.E., Inc.

Moore, K. L., Persaud, T. V. N., & Torchia, M. G. (2020). Respiratory system. In K. L. Moore, T. V. N. Persaud, & M. G. Torchia (Eds.), *The developing human* (11th ed., pp. 181–192). Elsevier.

Reuter, S., Moser, C., & Baack, M. (2014). Respiratory distress in the newborn. *Pediatrics in Review, 35*(10), 417–428. https://doi.org/10.1542/pir.35-10-417

RESPIRATORY DISTRESS SYNDROME

Incidence

■ Inverse relationship to gestational age: Nearly all infants born at 22 to 24 weeks and decreasing as birthweight increases down to ~10% at 34 weeks and less than 1% at 37 weeks (Lagoski et al., 2020).

■ European descent, late preterm delivery (35–36 weeks), and elective delivery in the absence of labor are well-known risk factors.

■ Higher occurrence with maternal history of gestational or chronic diabetes (infant of a diabetic mother [IDM] or gestational diabetes mellitus [GDM]), chorioamnionitis, or perinatal asphyxia.

■ Slight male predominance.

Pathophysiology

The causes of RDS are varied and may reflect disorders of alterations of normal lung development (e.g., in the case of oligohydramnios leading to hypoplastic lungs), or lack of development in the preterm infant, or failure to transition to extrauterine life.

■ Histologic sampling of lung tissue of RDS yields uniform ruddy airless appearance much like hepatic tissue (Lagoski et al., 2020). Diffuse atelectasis with a few widely dilated alveoli is evident.

■ Lining the airspaces of the bronchioles and alveolar ducts is an eosiniphilic membrane. In RDS, this membrane contains fibrinous material and cellular debris from injured epithelium (Lagoski et al., 2020).

■ Development is multifactorial:

● Impaired or delayed surfactant production

● Exposure to high oxygen concentrations

● Effects of volutrauma

These factors trigger a proinflammatory response involving cytokines and chemokines causing more damage to the alveolar lining, which results in decreased surfactant synthesis and function (Lagoski et al., 2020).

The inflammatory cascade is often initiated secondary to the pulmonary cellular injury or globally in the case of perinatal/neonatal asphyxia. Inflammation causes increased metabolic workload on the neonate, including increased oxygen requirement, and can contribute to cell damage and death of the affected and surrounding tissues (Newnam et al., 2013).

Diagnosis

The RDS diagnosis is based on history, physical findings, blood gas analysis, x-rays, and exclusion of other causes such as infection or cardiac causes. Distress is usually present at birth or shortly thereafter. Progressive respiratory difficulty typically coincides with increasing atelectasis of the alveoli and may take place over the first few minutes of life or several hours following birth. Infants with poor or deficient respiratory effort can progress to respiratory failure rapidly, if effective intervention is not provided in a timely manner.

Blood Gas Analysis

■ Respiratory acidosis; increased CO_2 levels as the atelectasis progresses.

■ Increased acidosis (respiratory and metabolic) ensues as the hypoxemia progresses. The pH decreases, the CO_2 level increases, PaO_2 level decreases, and bicarbonate decreases.

■ If aerobic respiration is compromised or cardiac function is impeded, the lactic acid builds up and increases systemically, predisposing the infant to a state of progressive systemic acidosis (lowering of pH and bicarbonate levels).

Radiographic Findings

■ The anteroposterior (AP) view is usually sufficient for initial examination.

■ Diffuse reticulogranular appearance caused by atelectasis and possibly pulmonary edema often described as ground glass is observed (see Table 1.1, Figure 1.3).

■ Air bronchograms representative of aerated bronchioles superimposed on a background of nonaerated alveoli are notable (see Table 1.1, Figure 1.3).

■ It is usually symmetric and homogeneous in appearance.

■ In severe cases, the view may have complete opacification throughout the lung field.

■ Heart size is generally normal or slightly enlarged. Cardiomegaly can be a sign of development of congestive heart failure.

Treatment

■ Respiratory support includes:

● Surfactant administration—a number of modalities have been studied to deliver surfactant including via endotracheal tube (ETT), via laryngeal mask airway, and brief tracheal catheterization with a thin catheter (Dargaville, 2019).

● Nasal CPAP, "sigh" synchronized intermittent airway pressure (SiPAP), or noninvasive positive pressure ventilation (NIPPV) may be used.

 * Stabilize alveoli, maintain lung recruitment, and decrease work of breathing, which may reduce apnea of prematurity (AOP).

 * In recent years, strategies have focused on trying to avoid invasive ventilation for extremely low birth weights (ELBWs). However, the frequency of need for supplemental oxygen at 36 weeks has not decreased and pulmonary function during childhood has not significantly improved (Doyle et al., 2017).

● Mechanical ventilation pressure-controlled, volume-controlled, and high-frequency ventilation techniques may be employed.

● Supplemental oxygen delivery—maintenance of distending pressure facilitates the alveolar expansion.

 * Low-flow NC humidified gas at less than 1 L per minute

 * High-flow NC humidified and warmed gas delivered at 1 L per minute or greater (Wilkinson et al., 2016)

● Surveillance and management of comorbidities

 * Patent ductus arteriosus (PDA)

 * Sepsis

 * AOP

TABLE 1.1 Chest Radiographic Images of Varying Pathology

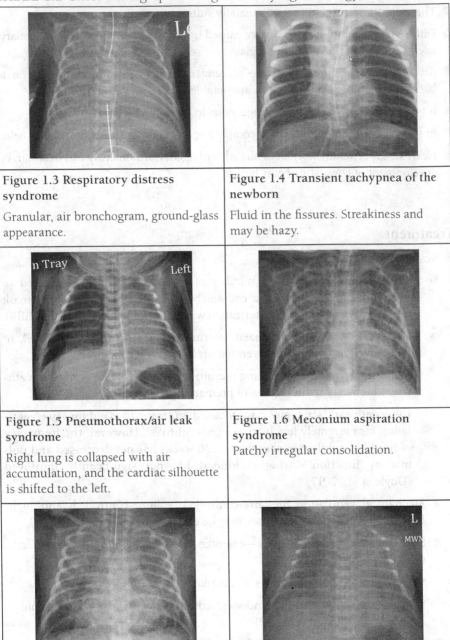

Figure 1.3 Respiratory distress syndrome Granular, air bronchogram, ground-glass appearance.	**Figure 1.4 Transient tachypnea of the newborn** Fluid in the fissures. Streakiness and may be hazy.
Figure 1.5 Pneumothorax/air leak syndrome Right lung is collapsed with air accumulation, and the cardiac silhouette is shifted to the left.	**Figure 1.6 Meconium aspiration syndrome** Patchy irregular consolidation.
Figure 1.7 Meconium aspiration syndrome	**Figure 1.8 Pneumonia** Bilateral consolidation, often similar to RDS.

RDS, respiratory distress syndrome.

Source: Images courtesy of Avera McKennan Hospital and University Health Center.

■ Pharmacologic management includes:
  ● Caffeine administration to prevent or reduce frequencies of apnea
  ● Broad-spectrum antibiotics as clinically indicated when high suspicion exists for possible sepsis following the culture

■ Nursing support by highly skilled caregivers provides optimal outcomes.

Prognosis

Survival rates for the preterm infant with RDS are based on gestational age, birth weight, degree of RDS, timely initiation of treatment and support, and underlying comorbidities, such as hypoplastic lung disease or diaphragmatic hernia. Prolonged use of mechanical ventilation, although lifesaving, has negative consequences for the pulmonary structures. The airway and alveolar pressure created with positive pressure can cause overdistention and scarring of the lung parenchyma, leading to long-term pulmonary sequelae often termed as bronchopulmonary dysplasia (BPD) or chronic lung disease (CLD). BPD/CLD is generally thought of as mild, moderate, or severe depending on the duration of supplemental oxygen and/or respiratory support. Pulmonary morbidities and adverse neurodevelopmental outcomes were more prevalent as the severity of BPD/CLD increased (Reuter et al., 2014). Additionally, systemic oxygen toxicity can lead to or complicate retinopathy of prematurity (ROP).

REFERENCES

Dargaville, P. A. (2019). Newer strategies for surfactant delivery. In E. Bancalari, M. Keszler, P. G. Davis, & R. A. Polin (Eds.), *The newborn lung: Neonatology questions and controversies* (3rd ed., pp. 221–238). Elsevier.

Doyle, L. W., Ranganathan, S., & Cheong, J. L. Y. (2017). Ventilation in preterm infants and lung function at 8 years. *New England Journal of Medicine, 377,* 1601–1602. https://doi .org/10.1056/NEJMc1711170

Lagoski, M., Hamvas, A., & Wamback, J. A. (2020). Respiratory distress syndrome in the neonate. In R. J. Martin, A. A. Fanaroff, & M. C. Walsh (Eds.), *Fanaroff and Martin's neonatal-perinatal medicine* (11th ed., pp. 1159–1177). Elsevier.

Newnam, K. M., Gephart, S. M., & Wright, L. (2013). Common complications of dysregulated inflammation in the neonate. *Newborn & Infant Nursing Reviews, 13,* 154–160. https:// doi.org/10.1053/j.nainr.2013.09.006

Reuter, S., Moser, C., & Baack, M. (2014). Respiratory distress in the newborn. *Pediatrics in Review, 35*(10), 417–428. https://doi.org/10.1542/pir.35-10-417

Wilkinson, D., Andersen, C., O'Donnell, C. P., De Paoli, A. G., & Manley, B. J. (2016). High flow nasal cannula for respiratory support in preterm infants. *Cochrane Database of Systematic Reviews, 22*(2), CD006405. https://doi.org/10.1002/14651858.CD006405.pub3

TRANSIENT TACHYPNEA OF THE NEWBORN

Incidence

■ Transient tachypnea of the newborn (TTN) occurs in 5.7 per 1,000 live births in term and late preterm infants (Crowley, 2020).

■ Risk factors: Delivery without labor, large for gestational age, maternal diabetes, maternal asthma, multiple gestation, and male gender (Crowley, 2020).

Pathophysiology

■ TTN is a decrease in lung compliance caused by pulmonary edema secondary to retained lung fluid. The fetal lung fluid has a high-chloride concentration, higher than plasma, interstitial fluid, or the amniotic fluid. During labor, chemical release of catecholamines occurs that results in the reduction of active chloride and fluid transport into the fetal lung and the reabsorption of fetal lung fluid via a protein gradient and sodium channels. The fluid is transported to the lymphatic system, with an estimated two-thirds of the fetal lung volume removed prior to birth. Increased oxygen tension following infant birth increases the epithelium's capacity to transport sodium, further reducing the fetal lung fluid.

■ Mechanisms for failure to clear retained fluid are not clearly understood:

● Mechanical force of birth canal squeeze is now believed to be a minor contributor

● Immaturity of the epithelial sodium channel may exist in a preterm infant.

● Hormonal changes associated with spontaneous labor are missing.

As described in the "Respiratory Distress Syndrome" section, as lung compliance decreases, the tidal volume will decrease. In order for the neonate to achieve sufficient minute ventilation, the respiratory rate will increase (tachypnea). Hypoxemia also will trigger an increased respiratory rate to compensate.

The delayed clearance of the lung fluid by the lymphatics will cause an accumulation of fluid in the peribronchiolar lymphatics and cause bronchiolar collapse. Air trapping is the consequence of this bronchiolar collapse, which causes hyperinflation of the alveoli. Hypoxemia and hypercarbia result from inadequate perfusion at the gas exchange interface. This increased work of breathing is the result of mismatched pulmonary mechanics, including increased airway resistance, diminished lung compliance, or both (Reuter et al., 2014).

The differential diagnoses include both common and uncommon conditions including those with origins in other neonatal systems.

Diagnosis

The diagnosis of TTN is based on history, timing of the clinical presentation, gestational age, physical findings, blood gas analysis, and x-ray findings.

Physical Exam Findings

■ Moderate-to-profound tachypnea (>60 breaths per minute)

■ May have retractions (subcostal, substernal, intercostal, and/or supraclavicular)

■ May present with nasal flaring

■ May have oxygen requirement to maintain systemic oxygenation at PaO_2 at 50 to 70 mmHg

■ Paradoxical or seesaw respirations

Diagnostic Procedures/Tests

■ Blood gas results will typically show mild respiratory acidosis (see previously mentioned blood gas analysis).

■ Radiology findings will include diffuse haziness and streakiness in both peripheral lung fields. Fluid-filled interlobar fissures with mild hyperinflation may be visible (see Table 1.1, Figure 1.4).

Treatment

■ As noted previously, this diagnosis is one of exclusion, so other disorders should be ruled out.

■ Blood gases should be serially monitored (see the "Brief Overview of Blood Gas Analysis" section).

■ If history indicates risk factors for infection, broad-spectrum antibiotic therapy should be considered until blood culture results are negative for 36 to 48 hours.

■ Supportive care includes:

● Oxygen delivery by NC or nasal CPAP

● Continuous oxygen saturation monitoring and cardiopulmonary monitoring

● Thermoregulation to avoid increased metabolic load

● Adequate fluid intake (mild fluid losses through increased respiratory rate)

● Adequate nutrition (usually by gavage tube if resting rate [RR] >60 bpm to prevent aspiration)

● Serial monitoring and management of blood glucose levels within acceptable range

■ Fluid restriction and/or the use of diuretics has not been supported in the treatment of TTN (Crowley, 2020; Stroustrup et al., 2012).

Prognosis

TTN is usually self-limiting with excellent prognosis. The need for respiratory support is usually transient and improves steadily over several hours to days. A few infants will demonstrate high pulmonary artery (PA) pressures and symptoms of persistent pulmonary hypertension of the newborn (PPHN), which can complicate or prolong the infant's clinical course and outcome (see the "Persistent Pulmonary Hypertension of the Newborn" section).

REFERENCES

Crowley, M. A. (2020). Neonatal respiratory disorders. In R. J. Martin, A. A. Fanaroff, & M. C. Walsh (Eds.), *Fanaraoff and Martin's neonatal-perinatal medicine* (11th ed., pp. 1203–1230). Elsevier.

Reuter, S., Moser, C., & Baack, M. (2014). Respiratory distress in the newborn. *Pediatrics in Review, 35*(10), 417–428. https://doi.org/10.1542/pir.35-10-417

Stroustrup, A., Trasande, L., & Holzman, I. R. (2012). Randomized controlled trial of restrictive fluid management in transient tachypnea of the newborn. *Journal of Pediatrics, 160*(1), 38–42. https://doi.org/10.1016/j.jpeds.2011.06.027

APNEA AND APNEA OF PREMATURITY

Incidence

■ Apnea in full-term neonates occurs in less than 2% of infants and is typically related to other organic causes (sepsis, obstruction, or neurologic or metabolic influences).

■ Present in nearly all infants less than 1,000 grams at birth.

■ It is inversely correlated with body weight (Patrinos, 2020).

■ It is not accompanied by cyanosis or changes in heart rate initially. Bradycardia and hypoxia will ensue if apnea is not corrected rapidly.

■ Normal neurologic development reduces the episodes of periodic breathing and apnea around term gestation.

Pathophysiology

Neonates exhibit an irregular breathing pattern. Apnea represents one of the most common respiratory complications in the preterm infant. It is typically defined as cessation of respiratory effort for longer than 20 seconds in length. Most apnea occurs in the preterm infant, classified as AOP, and occurs independent of other organic causes. This is not to be confused with periodic breathing, which is recurrent sequences of pauses in respiratory effort for 10 to 15 seconds followed by a brief "catch up" phase of tachypnea.

AOP is typically classified into one of four types: central apnea, obstructive apnea, mixed apnea, or idiopathic apnea.

1. Central apnea is the absence of respiratory effort and airflow into the respiratory system with no apparent obstruction, and it accounts for approximately 15% of apnea. While the causes of central apnea in the preterm infant are not fully understood, contributing factors are chest wall afferent neuromuscular immaturity, chest wall instability, diaphragmatic fatigue, and the immature response to hypoxia and hypercapnia. Most AOP is in this classification (Martin, 2017).

2. Obstructive apnea is the absence of airflow with continued respiratory effort; it is thought to contribute to up to 30% of apneic events. This is usually caused by

the blockage of the airway at the pharynx or larynx, which can be obstructed due to poor head and neck position of the neonate. Other causes of obstruction may be congenital anomalies of the airway and are described in a later section.

3. Mixed apnea is a combination of obstructive and central apnea.

4. Idiopathic apnea is diagnosed when the baby has apnea that does not result from the other three types of apnea. The cause is unknown.

Apnea in the premature infant is believed to be due to the immature central respiratory center secondary to poor CNS myelination, decreased number of synapses, and dendritic arborization.

In the term infant, the chemoreceptors that are located centrally within the medulla and peripherally in the carotid and aortic bodies transmit important information regarding the pH and oxygen levels to the respiratory center in the brain via pathways along the vagus and glossopharyngeal nerves. Increased respiratory rate is triggered when these levels are low. In the preterm infant, these pathways are not well established and/or not responsive to systemic hypoxemia (Martin, 2017). This explanation supports the cessation of AOP secondary to the normal maturation of the preterm brain and plasticity/development of neuropathways. However, apneic events may also be a classic first sign of systemic stress in the preterm infant. Other pathologic causes should be considered prior to the assumption that events are caused by AOP. Apnea in the term newborn is always an abnormal finding and should be systematically investigated for other causes. A thorough history and physical assessment are crucial.

Diagnosis

The diagnosis of apnea for the preterm or term infant is based on history, physical findings, x-rays, and blood gas results.

Physical Exam Findings

■ Prolonged pauses in the respiratory pattern longer than 20 seconds in length

■ Bradycardia or pallor that will ensue if a spontaneous or assisted respiratory pattern does not occur

Treatment

■ Prompt and gentle tactile stimulation is often sufficient to have the infant respond with spontaneous respiratory effort and avert further therapy.

■ Maintain neck in neutral position with assistance of positioning aids, such as a small neck roll. (Educate the family.)

■ Coordinate optimization of respiratory status and blood gases in collaboration with the medical staff members.

■ Maintain oxygen saturations within targeted range by adjusting the oxygen concentration.

■ Apneic events with profound associated bradycardia with or without cyanosis require more aggressive diagnostic and therapeutic interventions and investigation, including:

- Close clinical observation and physiologic monitoring, including pulse oximeter reading and blood gas analysis on regular intervals (see the "Brief Overview of Blood Gas Analysis" section).

- AP chest x-ray for evaluation of lung structures, including atelectasis, ventilation, and presence of air leaks. Also consider lateral decubitus film if concerned for air leaks.

- Sepsis evaluation to include blood culture (urine and cerebral spinal fluid as well if indicated), complete blood count (CBC), C-reactive protein (CRP), and vital signs ensuring the infant is normothermic and perfusion is adequate. Antibiotic therapy is initiated as suggested by the clinical condition of the infant, CBC with differential, and blood gas findings for at least 36 to 48 hours.

- Increased respiratory support, including nasal cannula (NC) for stimulation with or without supplemental oxygen, has been shown to be beneficial.

- Nasal CPAP to provide support of FRC and reduce atelectasis in the preterm neonate may be required. A high-flow NC may also offer adequate support for infants who are flow dependent.

- Intubation and provision of mechanical ventilation to support the infant's respiratory status will be required when other methods prove ineffective.

■ Optimize oxygen-carrying capacity by avoiding or managing anemia.

■ Xanthine therapy (caffeine, aminophylline) appear to exert a positive influence on respiratory neural output. Caffeine has a much longer half-life and can be dosed daily without the need for serial studies to evaluate the serum level.

- Adverse effects include tachycardia, increased diuresis, and gastrointestinal symptoms (increased emesis or clinical gastroesophageal reflux symptoms).

- Caffeine appears to have fewer side effects or toxicity concerns.

■ Doxapram is a potent respiratory stimulant used only for apnea refractory to xanthine therapy (Fraser, 2021).

■ Automated control of inspired oxygen and supplementation of inspired air with very low concentration of supplemental CO_2 to increase respiratory drive are novel treatments being studied (Martin, 2017).

■ Mechanosensory stimulation using kinesthetic approaches may hold future promise (Shah et al., 2019).

Prognosis

The overall prognosis for preterm neonates with AOP is excellent, and infants will typically cease symptoms by 39- to 41-week corrected age. The prognosis for term infants who demonstrate symptoms of apnea is based on the organic cause of the episodes. See the section that follows on pulmonary air leaks.

REFERENCES

Fraser, D. (2021). Respiratory distress. In M. T. Verklan, M. Walden, & S. Forest (Eds.), *Core curriculum for neonatal intensive care nursing* (6th ed., pp. 394–424). Elsevier.

Martin, R. J. (2017). Control of ventilation. In J. P. Goldsmith, E. H. Karotkin, M. Keszler, & G. K. Suresh (Eds.), *Assisted ventilation of the neonate* (6th ed., pp. 31–35). Elsevier.

Patrinos, M. E. (2020). Neonatal apnea and the foundation of respiratory control. In R. J. Martin, A. A. Fanaroff, & M. C. Walsh (Eds.), *Fanaraoff and Martin's neonatal-perinatal medicine* (11th ed., pp. 1231–1243). Elsevier.

Shah, V. P., Di Fiore, J. M., & Martin, R. J. (2019). Respiratory control and apnea in premature infants. In E. Bancalari, M. Keszler, P. G. Davis, & R. A. Polin (Eds.), *The newborn lung: Neonatology questions and controversies* (3rd ed., pp 239–249). Elsevier.

AIR LEAK SYNDROME

Air leak syndrome includes pneumothorax, pneumomediastinum, pneumopericardium, pneumoperitoneum, and subcutaneous emphysema.

Incidence

■ Air leaks occur in 1% to 2% of term newborns.

■ Incidence increases to 16% to 36% in those infants requiring delivery room resuscitation, nasal CPAP, bag-mask ventilation, or mechanical ventilation (Fraser, 2021).

Pathophysiology

Air leak syndrome is an overdistention of the alveolar sac that causes rupture. This rupture can occur spontaneously or by mechanical means during assisted ventilation or in resuscitation with positive pressure ventilation. When the air dissects from the alveolus, it can accumulate in five primary locations: the mediastinum, the pleural space, the space surrounding the heart, the peritoneal cavity, or subcutaneously.

In the healthy term infant, the required opening airway pressure during the first spontaneous breath is 60 to 80 cm of water, with subsequent breaths requiring less as the surface tension of the liquid-filled airways and alveoli is stabilized. If secretions or other mechanical obstructions prevent even air distribution, some areas of the newborn's lung will remain collapsed. The infant will generate additional pressure to open these collapsed areas, and spontaneous rupture of the open airways can occur.

Air leaks typically occur when a neonate has some underlying respiratory pathology. The preterm infant with RDS is at risk due to the noncompliant lung parenchyma. This "stiff" and nonresponsive lung status is at risk for air leak syndrome.

In the infant with meconium aspiration syndrome (MAS), the obstructive nature of the meconium may cause a ball-valve trapping of air, allowing air to flow into small airways and alveoli but not escape. This will cause hyperventilation and rupture in some cases. Positive pressure or respiratory care that is required to support ventilation and oxygen exceeds the capacity of the alveoli and rupture may result.

Diagnosis

Based on history, physical findings, x rays, and blood gas results, physical exam findings include:

■ A sudden deterioration may occur if the air leak is large (decreased saturation, increase in oxygen requirement, increased work of breathing, hemodynamic instability)

■ Decreased breath sounds on the affected side or bilaterally

■ Muffled heart sounds

■ Bradycardia if cardiac tamponade is present

■ Hypotension, due to the tension caused by the pneumothorax disallowing full cardiac filling and emptying

■ Perfusion changes (mottled or pale coloring with prolonged capillary refill time)

Typical findings of diagnostic procedures/tests for *air leak syndrome* are:

■ AP and/or lateral decubitus chest x-rays

● In pulmonary interstitial emphysema (PIE), the affected alveoli may be bilateral or unilateral with microcystic areas throughout. This pattern has been described as a "shotgun" pattern. The lung fields are often hyperinflated with a flattened diaphragm.

● A partial or complete pneumothorax will be a collapse of the lung field bilaterally or unilaterally (affected side). Without air inflation, the lung field is darkened without pulmonary markings. Other structures may be shifted to the right or left (heart, trachea; see Table 1.1, Figure 1.5).

● In pneumomediastinum, the patient may develop a "sail sign" indicating the elevation of the thymus by surrounding air.

● In pneumopericardium, a halo of air around the heart will be visible.

Treatment

■ For pneumothorax:

● Supportive care is needed, sometimes urgently.

● If asymptomatic, no treatment may be needed as the air may spontaneously reabsorb.

● If symptomatic, the treatment is removal of air with thoracentesis (needle aspiration) and/or chest tube placement until resolution.

- Thoracostomy (chest) tube is placed in the anterior chest on the affected side(s) and connected to a negative pressure system.
- Administration of oxygen may be beneficial in the absorption of the air leak for term infants (oxygen toxicity caution).

■ For pneumomediastinum:
  - Supportive care is needed.
  - Monitor for worsening clinical condition or pneumothorax.

■ For pneumopericardium:
  - This life-threatening condition requires immediate intervention.
  - Emergency treatment includes placement of the chest tube or long catheter into the pericardial sac with constant light negative pressure or pericardial window performed by a cardiologist or general or cardiac surgeon (may be completed with ultrasound guidance).

■ For PIE:
  - Supportive care is needed.
  - If unilateral, the infant may be placed affected side down to aid in decompression of the hyperventilated areas.
  - Attempt must be made to minimize pressures through mechanical or noninvasive respiratory management.
  - High-frequency ventilation may optimize clinical status.
  - Selective intubation of unaffected mainstem bronchus may improve condition.

Prognosis

The overall prognosis will depend on the overall pathology of the lung as well as systematic influences. The newborn with spontaneous pneumothorax may resolve fully without intervention. The mortality rate with pneumopericardium, significant PIE, and/or pneumothorax in the extremely low birth weight (ELBW) or newborn with pulmonary hypoplasia is high.

REFERENCE

Fraser, D. (2021). Respiratory distress. In M. T. Verklan, M. Walden, & S. Forest (Eds.), *Core curriculum for neonatal intensive care nursing* (6th ed., pp. 394–424). Elsevier.

MECONIUM ASPIRATION SYNDROME

Incidence

■ Meconium-stained amniotic fluid (MSAF) occurs in 8% to 29% of all term and near-term deliveries (Fraser, 2021).

■ Increases in occurrence are noted with increasing gestational age.

■ Overall incidence of MAS is 3% to 12% (Vain & Batton, 2017).

■ Equal incidence occurs in males and females.

■ Cesarean delivery is associated with a higher incidence of MAS.

■ Associated mortality is 5% to 37%.

Pathophysiology

MAS has been described as the most common type of neonatal aspiration and is typically characterized by early and significant respiratory distress in the meconium-stained infant. During stress or perinatal asphyxia, intestinal peristalsis is stimulated and rectal tone is decreased. Meconium, containing a mixture of epithelial cells and bile salts, is then passed into the amniotic fluid. Fetal stress will often lead to primary or secondary apnea, where the infant makes gasping respiratory efforts while aspirating the meconium-containing amniotic fluid prior to delivery. Controversy surrounds whether the contact between vulnerable pulmonary structures and irritating bile salts or the stressed state of the fetus ultimately leads to significant respiratory distress. Meconium passage in utero has been correlated with a stressed state or asphyxia event prior to or during labor.

Following aspiration of the meconium-containing amniotic fluid, a partial airway obstruction can occur. As pulmonary structures are obstructed (atelectasis), others are hyperinflated through a ball-valve effect, resulting in ventilation–perfusion mismatch and hypoxemia. Air leaks such as pneumothorax or pneumomediastinum are a potential complication.

The neonatal inflammatory cascade will be triggered by the chemical pneumonitis. The lung compliance is altered, causing increased pulmonary vascular resistance (PVR) and increased hypoxemia. Meconium decreases the levels or inactivates the surfactant proteins, SP-A and SP-B, and phospholipids thus increasing respiratory distress, hypoxemia, acidosis, and/or risk for PPHN.

Diagnosis

The diagnosis of MAS is based on history, physical findings, and radiographic findings.

Physical Exam Findings

■ Yellow-green–stained skin and nail beds or presence of meconium in the amniotic fluid at birth

■ Respiratory distress ranging from mild and transient to severe

■ Rales and rhonchi on auscultation

■ No specific laboratory data for diagnosis

Diagnostic Procedures/Tests

■ Chest x-ray may be specific for hyperexpanded areas mixed with patchy atelectasis or cotton-like appearance (see Table 1.1, Figures 1.6 and 1.7).

■ Blood gas results are specific for acidosis (both metabolic and respiratory) with low PaO_2

Treatment

■ In the delivery room:

- If the infant is vigorous with good respiratory effort and tone, the initial steps of care (drying, stimulating, providing warmth) with gentle bulb suctioning are indicated.

- A nonvigorous infant with depressed respirations and/or poor tone should undergo the initial steps; if not breathing or heart rate is less than 100, positive pressure ventilation should begin.

- Routine intubation for tracheal suction is not suggested. The infant should be cared for following neonatal resuscitation guidelines with positive pressure ventilation if no response to initial steps and progress to alternative airway as indicated (Weiner & Zaichkin, 2016).

■ Provide assisted ventilation and/or supplemental oxygen as needed; also consider high-frequency ventilation.

■ Consider inhaled nitric oxygen (iNO) if the infant demonstrates symptoms of PPHN affecting the oxygenation. Inhaled nitric oxide causes selective vasodilation of the pulmonary vasculature, thus potentially improving oxygen uptake.

■ Use surfactant replacement as indicated in some cases. Although the mechanism is unclear, this intervention reduces ventilation–perfusion mismatch and probably reduces the risk of ventilator-associated lung injury (Greenberg et al., 2019).

■ Use of corticosteroids has variable success and is generally not recommended routinely (Vain & Batton, 2017).

■ Monitor for signs/symptoms of pneumothorax and intervene in a timely manner if suspected.

■ Consider performing CBC with differential and blood culture and consider broad-spectrum antibiotic coverage while blood culture is monitored.

Prognosis

The overall prognosis for term neonates with mild MAS is excellent with supportive care. If the clinical picture is complicated with PPHN or severe asphyxia, mortality rates are higher.

REFERENCES

Fraser, D. (2021). Respiratory distress. In M. T. Verklan, M. Walden, & S. Forest (Eds.), *Core curriculum for neonatal intensive care nursing* (6th ed., pp. 394–424). Elsevier.

Greenberg, J. M., Haberman, B., Narendran, V., Nathan, A. T., & Schibler, K. (2019). Neonatal morbidities of prenatal and perinatal origin. In R. Resnik, C. J. Lockwood, T. R. Moore, M. F. Greene, J. A. Copel, & R. M. Silver (Eds.), *Creasy and Resnik's maternal-fetal medicine: Principles and practice* (8th ed., pp. 1309–1333). Elsevier.

Vain, N. E., & Batton, D. G. (2017). Meconium "aspiration" (or respiratory distress associated with meconium-stained amniotic fluid?). *Seminars in Fetal & Neonatal Medicine, 22*(4), 214–219. https://doi.org/10.1016/j.siny.2017.04.002

Weiner, G. M., & Zaichkin, J. (Eds.). (2016). *Textbook of neonatal resuscitation* (7th ed.). American Academy of Pediatrics.

PNEUMONIA

Incidence

■ The true incidence and impact on neonatal care is difficult to pinpoint due to the overlapping nature of the symptoms (Zaidi et al., 2016)

■ Neonatal pneumonia can have early (within the first 7 days of life) or late (after the first 7 days of life) onset

■ Early pneumonia

● Congenital pneumonia

* Subset of early neonatal pneumonia

* Presents immediately after delivery

* Acquired from aspiration of infected amniotic fluid, ascending infection through ruptured or intact membranes, or spread through placenta (Crowley, 2020)

● Aspiration pneumonia

■ Late pneumonia includes ventilator-associated pneumonia (VAP) and is usually nosocomial.

Pathophysiology

Bacterial, viral, and fungal agents can cause pneumonia (see Table 1.2).

An immature tracheobronchial ciliary system inhibits optimal removal of debris, mucus, and pathogens (Fraser, 2021). Inflammation will cause the alveoli to become edematous and fluid filled, complicating air exchange. Macrophages, in response to the invading organisms, will invade the pulmonary parenchyma.

Infants born to mothers with chorioamnionitis or prolonged rupture of membranes (>18 hours) are at a higher risk for congenital or prenatally acquired pneumonia. Systemic fetal infection can be caused by organisms that cross the placenta

TABLE 1.2 Common Organisms Associated With Neonatal Pneumonia

BACTERIAL	VIRAL	OTHER
Group B Streptococcus	Cytomegalovirus	Candida and other fungi
Escherichia coli	Adenovirus	Ureaplasma
Klebsiella	Rhinovirus	Chlamydia
Staphylococcus aureus	Respiratory syncytial virus	Syphilis
Listeria monocytogenes	Parainfluenza	Pneumocystis jiroveci
Enterobacter	Enterovirus	Tuberculosis
Haemophilus influenzae	Rubella	
Streptococcus pneumonia		
Pseudomonas		
Bacteroides		
Other		

Source: Adapted from Battista, M. A., & Carlo, W. A. (1992). Differential diagnosis of acute respiratory distress in the neonate. *Tufts University School of Medicine and Floating Hospital for Children Reports on Neonatal Respiratory Disease, 2*(3), 1–4, 9–11.

and enter the fetal circulation prior to delivery. Infants will often show symptoms of illness at birth or shortly thereafter.

Diagnosis

The diagnosis of pneumonia is based on history, physical findings, x-rays, and lab values.

Maternal history should be reviewed for significant findings to include:

■ Maternal serologies
■ History of maternal illness suspicious of infection, such as maternal fever and/or abdominal pain
■ Evidence of chorioamnionitis
■ Antenatal antibiotic therapy
■ Gestational age

General History

■ Postnatal history (intubation, prematurity, recent exposures to illness)

Physical Exam Findings

■ Often unable to clinically distinguish from other respiratory or sepsis causes

■ Symptoms of respiratory distress (cyanosis, hypoxemia, hypercapnia, grunting, retractions, and tachypnea)

■ Diminished breath sounds with or without rales

Diagnostic Procedures/Tests

■ Lab testing
  ● A CBC may be specific for neutropenia, leukopenia, or left shift (abnormal ratio of immature to total neutrophils)

■ Polymerase chain reactions (PCRs) looking for viral etiologies
  ● Samples of blood for viral and bacterial culture should be obtained and monitored during treatment. Results are often negative unless systemic bacterial/viral sepsis is present.
  ● Tracheal aspirate culture in an intubated infant
  ● Blood gas analysis
  ● Cerebrospinal fluid when stable as meningitis often occurs concurrently
  ● Evaluation for coagulopathy

■ Radiographic findings are variable (see Table 1.1, Figure 1.8)
  ● Unilateral or bilateral infiltrates
  ● Diffuse interstitial pattern
  ● Pleural effusions
  ● Similar in appearance to neonates with RDS

Treatment

■ Neutral thermal environment/thermoregulation

■ Monitor glucose levels and correct hypoglycemia or hyperglycemia as appropriate

■ Maintain optimal hemodynamics by monitoring blood pressure and perfusion
  ● Treat anemia with adding ferrous sulfate or by transfusions
  ● Treat hypotension using volume infusion or vasoactive agents, such as dopamine or dobutamine
  ● Close monitoring of intake/output

■ Supportive respiratory management
  ● Supplemental oxygen

- Assisted ventilation using NC, humidified and warmed high-flow nasal cannula (HFNC), nasal CPAP, and/or NIPPV
- Intubation and mechanical ventilation as indicated
- Monitor blood gases and adjust therapy as indicated
- Consider surfactant replacement as warranted
- Inhaled nitric oxide and/or extracorporeal membrane oxygenation (ECMO) for severe cases (timely transfer of infants to tertiary care centers where these treatments are available must be considered when symptoms warrant)

■ Pharmacologic management includes:

- Broad-spectrum antibiotics
- Antiviral therapies
- Vasopressors as indicated

Prognosis

The overall morbidity and mortality rates for neonatal pneumonia are significant and depend on the severity of illness and causative agent.

REFERENCES

Crowley, M. A. (2020). Neonatal respiratory disorders. In R. J. Martin, A. A. Fanaroff, & M. C. Walsh (Eds.), *Fanaroff and Martin's neonatal-perinatal medicine* (11th ed., pp. 1203–1230). Elsevier.

Fraser, D. (2021). Respiratory distress. In M. T. Verklan, M. Walden, & S. Forest (Eds.), *Core curriculum for neonatal intensive care nursing* (6th ed., pp. 394–424). Elsevier.

Zaidi, A. K. M., Darmstadt, G. L., & Stoll, B. J. (2016). Neonatal infections: A global perspective. In C. B. Wilson, V. Nizet, Y. A. Maldonado, J. S. Remington, & J. O. Klein (Eds.), *Remington and Klein's infectious diseases of the fetus and newborn infant* (8th ed., pp. 24–53). Elsevier Saunders.

PERSISTENT PULMONARY HYPERTENSION OF THE NEWBORN

Incidence

■ The condition complicates the course of up to 10% of infants with respiratory failure (Steinhorn & Abman, 2018).

■ Typically occurs in term or near-term infants.

Pathophysiology

PPHN, formerly known as persistent fetal circulation, is a condition where high right-sided pressure at the PA is combined with right-to-left shunting through fetal pathways (foramen ovale and/or ductus arteriosus). The increased pressure at the PA is caused by an elevated pulmonary vascular resistance (PVR), which is a process of maladaptation between fetal and neonatal circulation. The pulmonary vascular bed and heart are structurally normal. This vasoconstriction may be transient or persistent and reactive or resistant to therapy.

■ In utero:

  ● PVR is high secondary to pulmonary vasoconstriction

  ● Oxygenation of fetus occurs via placenta

  ● Majority of blood bypasses fetal lungs (84%; Lakshminrusimha & Steinhorn, 2017)

  ● In fetal circulation, blood is shunted through the ductus venosus, patent foramen ovale (PFO), and patent ductus arteriosus (PDA)

■ Following birth:

  ● Umbilical cord is clamped.

  ● Lungs expand with first breaths.

  ● Oxygenation occurs via the lungs.

  ● Lungs begin to clear fluid.

  ● PVR falls.

  ● Pulmonary blood flow increases.

  ● The fetal shunts begin to close.

The PVR usually falls by about 50% in the first 24 hours of life; however, when the PVR remains high, the transition from fetal to neonatal circulation is delayed. The pulmonary vessels in the neonate are reactive and respond to hypoxia or acidosis with vasoconstrictive properties. This high PVR further restricts pulmonary blood flow, which increases this acidotic state and makes oxygenation difficult. In cases of hypothermia, pulmonary vessels also increase resistance; therefore, infants undergoing therapeutic hypothermia are at a higher risk of PPHN.

■ Pulmonary hypertension is often divided into three categories (Steinhorn, 2020):

  ● Pulmonary vasoconstriction caused by lung diseases like MAS, RDS, or pneumonia

  ● Normal lung parenchyma and remodeled pulmonary vasculature: idiopathic, chronic intrauterine hypoxia, placental insufficiency

  ● Hypoplastic vasculature like congenital diaphragmatic hernia (CDH), congenital cystic adenoid malformation

Certain newborn conditions increase the risk for PPHN and include MAS, CDH, RDS, asphyxia, sepsis, pneumonia, hypoglycemia, polycythemia, or other neonatal stressors. Conditions that increase the acidotic state in the newborn, like hypothermia, can also contribute to pulmonary vasoconstriction. Fetal stressors like systemic hypertension, maternal diabetes, maternal preeclampsis, maternal smoking, and premature closure of the ductus arteriosus increase the likelihood of PPHN (Fraser, 2021). Studies in animal models and humans suggest maternal usage of selective serotonin receptor inhibitors (SSRIs) and nonsteroidal anti-inflammatory agents may alter fetal PVR (Lakshminrusimha & Steinhorn, 2017). More research needs to be done in this area. These infants share several characteristics: elevated PVR, abnormal pulmonary vasoreactivity, diminished response to vasodilators (oxygen, medications), and increased blood levels of endothelin, a potent vasoconstrictor.

Clinical Manifestations

A complete, thorough physical examination is imperative. Hypothermia or hyperthermia may alter the metabolic load of the neonate. The hypoxic or hypotensive infant may require rapid intervention and is often associated with respiratory compromise. Clinical presentation is similar to other respiratory conditions and may be difficult to differentiate initially. See earlier section "Respiratory System Assessment." Additional assessment points:

■ Pallor, mottling, or poor color of the infant may indicate hypotension or acidosis.

■ Cyanosis or blue discoloration of the skin and mucous membranes is a classic sign of hypoxemia leading to hypoxia. This is a late and serious sign of compromise, and the infant will require immediate interventions. This is often associated with respiratory distress, leading to respiratory failure with severe metabolic acidosis.

■ Tachycardia, bradycardia, blood pressure, and perfusion are important signs of cardiac compromise from CHD or ongoing respiratory compromise and failure.

■ Diminished muscle tone and poor activity are critical signs of profound hypoxia and acidosis.

Diagnosis

The diagnosis of PPHN is based on history, physical findings, x-rays, and echocardiogram. Echocardiogram findings include right ventricular dilation, leftward bowing of the intraventricular septum, tricuspid regurgitation, and right to left or bidirectional shunting at the PFO and PDA. Estimation of PA pressures are cardinal findings.

Significant Prenatal and Delivery Findings

■ Meconium-stained fluid, maternal infection, tight nuchal cord, hypovolemia (placental abruption, accreta, previa, or cord accident), maternal sedation

■ History of hypoxia or asphyxia at delivery (low Apgar scores, required resuscitation, acidotic cord blood gases)

Physical Exam Findings
■ Near-term or term infant
■ Symptoms of respiratory distress
■ Hypoxemia with or without cyanosis
■ Low PaO_2 despite high levels of delivered supplemental oxygen

Diagnostic Procedures or Tests
■ AP chest x-ray may be abnormal or normal. Usually obtained to rule out other pathology that could contribute to the state of hypoxia.
■ Arterial blood gas is a good serial monitoring method to determine oxygenation and state of acidosis.
■ Pre- and postductal oxygen saturation monitoring will be valuable to determine differences between the preductal measurement (right upper extremity) with postductal locations (lower extremities). If SpO_2 difference of 10% to 15% or if PaO_2 measurements from right radial artery and umbilical artery are more than 15 mmHg, this is an indication of ductal shunting.
■ Echocardiogram is the gold standard and will rule out CHD and evaluate the structure and function of the heart and myocardium. The presence of bidirectional or right-to-left shunting across the foramen ovale or ductus arteriosus is confirmatory. Other signs such as flattened septum, tricuspid regurgitation, and right ventricle dilation suggest the diagnosis (Steinhorn & Abman, 2018).
■ Hyperoxia test is placing the infant in 100% FiO_2 (fraction of inspired oxygen) and monitoring the oxygen saturations (postductal) or arterial PaO_2. If the infant's oxygenation does not significantly change, this is a clear sign of CHD or PPHN.
■ Serum electrolytes are important to monitor glucose and serum CO_2 levels.
■ Lactate will measure the state of systemic acidosis.
■ CBC and blood cultures should be obtained for sepsis evaluation.
■ Oxygen index calculation evaluates the severity of the disease process and is an important component in evaluation need for escalating intervention.

Treatment
■ Minimal stimulation occurs as infants demonstrate significant alterations in PVR with even gentle handling and touch.

■ Supportive care (based on the cause of PPHN) may include antibiotic therapy, cooling protocol, thermoregulation, maintenance of fluid, and electrolyte balance.

■ A central arterial line may be placed to monitor systemic blood pressure and obtain serial arterial blood gases.

■ A central venous line may be placed to administer fluids and vasopressors as indicated.

■ Ventilation and oxygenation are supported with intubation, mechanical ventilation (conventional, high-frequency jet, high-frequency oscillatory ventilator), and supplementation oxygen (a potent vasodilator) as indicated. Oxygen targets suggest SpO_2 91% to 97% and pre-ductal PaO_2 between 60 and 80 mm Hg.

■ iNO, a selective pulmonary vasodilator, has been shown to improve oxygenation.

■ Surfactant replacement should be considered for infants with parenchymal lung disease.

■ Correct acidosis through ventilation and the administration of fluids over time. Judicious administration of sodium bicarbonate should be done only after adequate volume resuscitation and adequate ventilation. Sodium bicarbonate breaks down to water and carbon dioxide; therefore, adequate ventilation is imperative before administering. Acidosis leads to pulmonary vasoconstriction, and causing alkalosis is not optimal in these cases either (Steinhorn & Abman, 2018).

■ Close evaluation and fluid adjustments are made based on urine output; avoid pulmonary edema.

■ Optimize cardiac output and systemic hemodynamics using volume and medications.

■ Extracorporeal membrane oxygenation (ECMO) should be considered when conventional therapies are not successful, if available in the region (by making determination to transfer the infant to an appropriate center).

■ Pharmacologic intervention:

● Sedatives to maintain calm state

● Vasopressors to increase systemic blood pressure, thereby reducing PVR; this will decrease right-to-left shunting

● iNO as discussed earlier

● Sildenafil as an adjunct therapy to iNO to promote pulmonary vasodilation

● Analgesics as an adjunct to sedatives to maintain calm state and reduce metabolic need during acute phase of illness

Prognosis

The overall prognosis for term neonates with PPHN is based on the underlying cause or disease process. Residual effects from PPHN include CLD from prolonged ventilation requirement, symptoms of withdrawal secondary to long-term narcotic/sedative requirement, sensorineural hearing loss, learning disabilities, and feeding challenges.

REFERENCES

Fraser, D. (2021). Respiratory distress. In M. T. Verklan, M. Walden, & S. Forest (Eds.), *Core curriculum for neonatal intensive care nursing* (6th ed., pp. 394–424). Elsevier.

Lakshminrusimha, S., & Steinhorn, R. H. (2017). Pathophysiology of persistent pulmonary hypertension of the newborn. In R. A. Polin, S. H. Abman, D. H. Rowitch, W. E. Benitz, & W. W. Fox (Eds.), *Fetal and neonatal physiology* (5th ed., pp. 1576–1588). Elsevier.

Steinhorn, R. H. (2020). Pulmonary vascular development. In R. J. Martin, A. A. Fanaroff, & M. C. Walsh (Eds.), *Fanaraoff and Martin's neonatal-perinatal medicine* (11th ed., pp. 1306–1319). Elsevier.

Steinhorn, R. H., & Abman, S. H. (2018). Persistent pulmonary hypertension. In C. A. Gleason & S. E. Juul (Eds.), *Avery's diseases of the newborn* (10th ed., pp. 768–778). Elsevier.

PULMONARY HEMORRHAGE

Incidence

■ Occurs in 5% of low birth weight infants and 10% in ELBW infants (Crowley, 2020)

■ Eighty percent occur in first 72 hours

■ May be associated with other complications (PDA, sepsis)

■ Following surfactant administration incidence increases

Pathophysiology

Pulmonary hemorrhage is the presence of bloody fluid in the trachea or lung fields. The event can be a massive event or slow leak into the alveoli. Pulmonary hemorrhage is hypothesized to be caused by a sudden decrease in PVR resulting in increased left-to-right shunting, pulmonary edema, and rupture of pulmonary capillaries. This acute event can be life-threatening secondary to airway obstruction and/or hypovolemia. This condition will often accompany or be the complication of a comorbid condition such as disseminated intravascular coagulation (DIC), PDA, RDS, or CHD. Pulmonary hemorrhage is a known complication of surfactant administration or tracheal suctioning.

Diagnosis

The diagnosis of pulmonary hemorrhage is based on history, physical findings, and x-ray.

- Presents with sudden deterioration (vital sign changes, oxygen saturations)
- Symptoms of severe RDS
- Bright red blood or pink-tinged secretions noted in the endotracheal tube (ETT) when suctioning, if intubated
- Hypotension
- Anemia
- Shock
- X-rays demonstrate varying degrees of fluffy infiltrates to complete white out

Treatment

- Provide blood or blood products based on clotting studies
- Support respiratory requirements; additional positive end-expiratory pressure (PEEP) helps with oxygenation and acts to tamponade bleeding
- Suction/clear ETT; replacement may be indicated but risk for poor outcome
- Correct acidosis and anemia
- Assess for and treat PDA
- Treat underlying causes (sepsis)

Prognosis

The overall prognosis for term neonates with pulmonary hemorrhage is poor if massive bleeding cannot be stopped or slowed with PEEP or administration of fresh frozen plasma (FFP) and other blood products. If hemorrhage is small, the infant will recover unless the underlying cause is significant. Mortality approaches 50% in ELBW infants (Crowley, 2020).

REFERENCE

Crowley, M. A. (2020). Neonatal respiratory disorders. In R. J. Martin, A. A. Fanaroff, & M. C. Walsh (Eds.), *Fanaroff and Martin's neonatal-perinatal medicine* (11th ed., pp. 1203–1230). Elsevier.

CONGENITAL ANOMALIES THAT AFFECT THE RESPIRATORY SYSTEM

PULMONARY HYPOPLASIA

Incidence

- Occurs in 9 to 11 of 10,000 live births
- Mortality rates 71% to 95%

- Equal incidence in male/female
- Frequently associated with oligohydramnios

Pathophysiology

Pulmonary hypoplasia is a rare but often lethal condition in which the lungs are underdeveloped, usually secondary to a space-occupying mass, renal anomaly, or urinary tract anomalies with oligohydramnios. Primary pulmonary hypoplasia is rare and caused by abnormalities of transcription factors and growth factors regulating early lung development (Kallaper & Jobe, 2020). Diaphragmatic hernia and diaphragmatic eventration are also present with symptoms of RDS secondary to pulmonary hypoplasia, as the displaced bowel occupies pulmonary space that prevents adequate growth (see the following section).

Hypoplastic lungs have a decrease in lung volume/mass under conditions of restricted space to develop in utero. This decrease occurs in both number of airway generations and smaller peripheral alveoli than normal term or preterm infants. The unaffected area of the lung has a structure that is appropriate for gestational age.

Infants who are affected by oligohydramnios have lung parenchyma that are structurally and biochemically immature for gestational age, although the exact mechanism for this is still undetermined. These infants have poor epithelial maturation, a lack of elastic tissue development, and low concentrations of lung phospholipids (Chen et al., 2010). It is uncertain if this condition is secondary to a lack of exposure to fetal lung fluid, which provides lung tissue the mechanical stretching necessary for development, or if it is a lack of growth factor secretion.

Assessment

Assessment is the same as other conditions of acute respiratory distress noted in the previous sections.

Diagnosis

The diagnosis of pulmonary hypoplasia is based on history, physical findings, blood gas results, and x-rays. Respiratory findings often mimic other causes of respiratory distress.

- Hypoxemia is difficult to manage with routine approach.
- If the condition progresses, the infant will have changes in cardiac function including decreased perfusion, pallor, tachycardia (early), and bradycardia (late).
- If the condition progresses, the infant will demonstrate CNS changes including lethargy, decreased or obtunded response to stimuli, and loss of muscle tone.

Diagnostic Procedures/Tests

- Arterial blood gas (analysis as described earlier)

Radiographic Findings

■ AP view, which is usually sufficient for initial examination—generally reveals low lung volumes on the affected side or overall

■ CT of the chest (if mass is suspected)

Treatment

■ Respiratory support as indicated (may require intubation)

■ High index of suspicion for signs/symptoms of pneumothorax

■ Symptomatic management

■ Palliative support for genetic anomalies

Prognosis

The overall prognosis for term neonates with pulmonary hypoplasia is poor, with mortality rates ~70% to 90%.

REFERENCES

Chen, C. M., Wang, L. F., Chou, H. C., & Lang, Y. D. (2010). Mechanism of oligohydramnios-induced pulmonary hypoplasia. *Journal of Experimental Clinical Medicine, 2*(3), 104–110. https://doi.org/10.1016/S1878-3317(10)60017-4

Kallaper, S. G., & Jobe, A. H. (2020). Lung development and maturation. In R. J. Martin, A. A. Fanaroff, & M. C. Walsh (Eds.), *Fanaroff and Martin's neonatal-perinatal medicine* (11th ed., pp. 1124–1142). Elsevier.

CONGENITAL DIAPHRAGMATIC HERNIA

Incidence

■ One in 2,500 live births

■ Most symptomatic at birth with severe RDS

■ Left-sided defect 90% of the time

Pathophysiology

This defect is caused by the herniation of abdominal contents, primarily intestine, into the chest cavity. This defect occurs as early as 4 to 5 weeks' gestation. The dual-hit hypothesis for the pulmonary hypoplasia has emerged (Crowley, 2020). Likely pulmonary development has been affected prior to diaphragm development and before the compression from abdominal organs occurs. The first hit affects both lungs and likely is the reason both lungs have some degree of pulmonary hypoplasia. The second hit affects the growth of the ipsilateral lung from compression of herniated contents. CDH can be an isolated defect or associated with other congenital anomalies including cardiac, urogenital, chromosomal, and musculoskeletal issues (Crowley, 2020).

Antenatal measurements to predict morbidity to 28 weeks' survival have been evaluated. Lung area-to-head circumference ratio (LHR) done between 22 and 28 weeks, the presence of liver in the chest cavity, and estimated fetal lung volume on MRI have been helpful in prognosticating outcomes. The LHR ratio appears to be most helpful when compared to expected ratio at the gestation in question. The ability of these to predict survival has been inconsistent, but these data do give some information to guide families to plan treatment.

Delivery of these infants in a tertiary care center equipped to provide the whole complement of care strategies is recommended to attain the most optimal outcomes.

Assessment

■ The infant with CDH may simply appear to have RDS or present with a scaphoid abdomen.

■ Some degree of RDS may be observed, which may be mild to severe.

■ Bowel sounds may be heard in the chest.

■ Heart sounds may be shifted to the right side.

Diagnosis

The diagnosis of diaphragmatic hernia is based on history, physical findings, and x-rays. The diagnosis is frequently known before delivery but can be unknown prior to delivery.

Physical Exam Findings

■ Symptoms of respiratory distress (cyanosis, hypoxemia, hypercapnia, grunting, retractions, and tachypnea)

■ Diminished breath sounds (asymmetrical)

■ May auscultate bowel sounds in chest

Diagnostics

■ Dextrocardia may be present.

■ Radiographic findings are significant for bowel presence above the diaphragm, most frequently in the left side of the chest.

■ A CBC is performed.

■ Samples of blood for viral and bacterial culture should be obtained and monitored during treatment. Results are often negative unless systemic bacterial/viral sepsis is present.

Treatment

■ Once the diagnosis is suspected, avoid positive pressure ventilation as this can force air into the intestines, which are in the chest cavity and further compromise ventilation.

■ If diagnosis is known prenatally, the infant should be intubated immediately to provide mechanical ventilation to the lungs.

■ Proved respiratory support with ventilation and supplemental oxygen, gentle ventilation, and permissive hypercapnia are frequently used (Crowley, 2020).

■ Use a decompression tube to suction (prevent bowel from filling with air).

■ Consider iNO when symptoms of PPHN exist. However, the routine use of iNO is not supported by current data (Crowley, 2020).

■ ECMO may be considered based on oxygen index (OI) greater than 40, persistent hypoxemia, failure of management to support oxygenation, and ventilation and tissue perfusion.

■ Suggest a surgical consult—surgical repair is generally delayed until PPHN has resolved/improved.

■ Hypotension is a common problem related to impedance on cardiac function and should be managed with volume resuscitation and medications as clinically indicated.

■ Surfactant administration does not appear to be helpful.

Prognosis

The overall prognosis for term neonates with diaphragmatic hernia is poor with a high incidence of PPHN and ECMO sometimes used for management.

REFERENCE

Crowley, M. A. (2020). Neonatal respiratory disorders. In R. J. Martin, A. A. Fanaroff, & M. C. Walsh (Eds.), *Fanaroff and Martin's neonatal-perinatal medicine* (11th ed., pp. 1203–1230). Elsevier.

CHOANAL ATRESIA

Incidence

■ Occurs in one in 8,000 births (Fraser, 2021).

■ Fifty percent of cases have bilateral blockages (Gentle et al., 2020).

■ Affected infants have associated anomalies such as CHARGE syndrome (coloboma, heart defects, atresia of the choanae, retardation of growth and development, genital/urinary abnormalities, and ear abnormalities and/or hearing deficit).

■ It affects females more than males.

Pathophysiology

Infants are obligate nasal breathers, allowing them to breathe effectively during oral feedings. When nasal passages are blocked or obstructed by tissue or mucus, the infant will exhibit symptoms of RDS. Choanal atresia causes upper airway obstruction as the choanae or nasal passages do not connect to the nasopharynx. The majority of the blockages are bony occlusions with a small number being membranous.

Assessment

The degree of respiratory compromise at delivery usually determines the severity of the obstruction. If both nares are obstructed, the infant will require assistance to support oral airway patency and air exchange. If a single naris is obstructed, respiratory compromise may only be detected when the infant is feeding and the oral airway is obstructed with breast or bottle.

Diagnosis

The diagnosis of choanal atresia is based on history and physical findings.

History and Physical Exam

- Benign prenatal history and ultrasound results unless CHARGE association
- Severe respiratory distress (retractions, poor aeration)
- Cyanosis that becomes pink with crying due to breathing through oropharynx (Bean et al., 2017)
- Failure to pass a nasogastric tube (NGT) in one or both nares

Treatment

- Oral airway
- Tracheal intubation as indicated
- Maintain calm state with comfort measures
- Evaluation for CHARGE association (echocardiogram, renal ultrasound, eye exam, hearing evaluation)
- Eventual surgical correction

Prognosis

The overall prognosis for term neonates with choanal atresia is excellent. The mortality rate for surgical correction is less than 1%, and complications are rare.

REFERENCES

Bean, J., Arensman, R. M., Srinivasan, N., Maheshware, A., & Ambalavan, N. (2017). Medical and surgical interventions for respiratory distress and airway management. In J. P. Goldsmith & E. H. Karotkin (Eds.), *Assisted ventilation of the neonate* (6th ed., pp. 435–451. Elsevier Saunders.

Fraser, D. (2021). Respiratory distress. In M. T. Verklan, M. Walden, & S. Forest (Eds.), *Core curriculum for neonatal intensive care nursing* (6th ed., pp. 394–424). Elsevier.

Gentle, S., Travers, C., & Carlo, W. A. (2020). Respiratory system. In C. Kenner, L. B. Altimier, & M. V. Boykova (Eds.), *Comprehensive neonatal nursing care* (6th ed., pp. 127–146). Springer Publishing Company.

PIERRE ROBIN SEQUENCE

Incidence

■ Sixty percent of affected patients have a cleft palate.

■ It can be seen in isolation (50%–70%) or in combination with other anomalies (Stickler, 22q deletion, and Treacher Collins, primarily).

■ It occurs in one per 8,500 to 14,000 live births (Lee & Bradley, 2014).

■ Increased risk occurs in families with other children affected by Pierre Robin sequence (1%–5% chance).

■ Between 13% and 27.7% of other family members are affected with cleft lip with or without cleft palate.

■ Recent research has linked mutations in the SOX_9 gene (Keller et al., 2018).

Pathophysiology

The major feature of the Pierre Robin sequence is micrognathia or small mandible, glossoptosis, and upper airway obstruction. Hypoplastic development of the mandible can lead to airway obstruction and cyanosis. The tongue is posteriorly placed close to the oropharynx and will obstruct the airway. The mandible is formed at about the fourth week of gestation from the first pharyngeal arch and migrating neural crest cells. At about 6 weeks' gestation, the trigeminal nerve innervates the area and promotes osteogenesis, forming the major structures of the mandible. Prenatal or genetic factors disrupt the normal growth of the mandible and micrognathia occurs.

Pierre Robin sequence without other genetic syndrome may be the result from intrauterine forces acting on the mandible, which restrict its growth. Due to the poor mandibular growth, the tongue is displaced between the palatal shelves. Cases of Pierre Robin sequence have been associated with oligohydramnios with an unclear etiology. In these cases, the micrognathia results from intrauterine molding, and the mandibular growth can continue following delivery. When the Pierre Robin sequence is combined with other genetic causes, varied responses to extrauterine growth are possible without surgical intervention.

Diagnosis

The diagnosis of Pierre Robin sequence is based on history and physical findings.

Physical Exam Findings

■ Small mandible

■ Respiratory distress and cyanosis that may be relieved when the infant is placed prone

■ Tongue that appears large for mouth

Treatment

■ Prone position to allow tongue to fall forward. Positioning will resolve the airway obstruction in ~70% of cases.

■ Surgical tongue–lip adhesion, where the tongue is affixed to the lip with sutures to prevent airway obstruction from the tongue position.

■ Oral feedings in a prone or side-lying position may be tolerated. Nasogastric feedings are often required initially.

■ Mandibular distraction osteogenesis is an established technique used to treat infants with Pierre Robin sequence associated with severe airway obstruction. Mandibular distraction has shown favorable results with a 50% reduction in tracheostomy placement (Lee & Bradley, 2014).

Prognosis

Excellent survival rates are noted for these infants in the absence of lung hypoplasia. Mandibular growth contributes to resolution by 6 to 12 months of age. Prognostic outcomes in infants with comorbidities including syndromes or genetic diseases have various results based on those genetic conditions.

REFERENCES

Keller, B. A., Hirose, S., & Farmer, D. L. (2018). Surgical disorders of the chest and airways. In C. A. Gleason & S. E. Juul (Eds.), *Avery's diseases of the newborn* (10th ed., pp. 695–723). Elsevier.

Lee, J. C., & Bradley, J. P. (2014). Surgical considerations in Pierre Robin sequence. *Clinical Plastic Surgery, 41,* 211–217. https://doi.org/10.1016/j.cps.2013.12.007

CONGENITAL PULMONARY MALFORMATIONS

Congenital pulmonary malformations (CPMs) are a group of rare abnormalities that affect different parts of the neonatal lung or supporting structures, including the main or terminal airways, the parenchyma, and the supportive vasculature. These abnormalities are typically caused by aberrant embryologic lung development at various stages and can be self-limiting or cause significant respiratory distress at birth or shortly thereafter.

CPMs are currently classified as five types according to location and tissue type found in the abnormal growth (Fraser, 2021). This condition was previously known as congenital cystic adenomatoid malformation (CCAM).

Incidence

■ It occurs in one per 8,300 to 35,000 live births.

■ Males and females are affected equally.

Pathophysiology

Pathophysiology is dependent on the type of congenital pulmonary airway malformation (CPAM; Fraser, 2021). All CPAMs develop from an overgrowth of abnormal lung tissue (Keller et al., 2018).

■ Type 0: arise from tracheobronchial tree, lobulated, no alveoli involved

■ Type 1: most common, usually limited to one lobe of lung, single or a few large cysts, communicate with bronchi

■ Type 2: multiple, small cysts resembling bronchioles, 50% have other anomalies (sirenomelia, renal agenesis, extra lobar pulmonary sequestration)

■ Type 3: large, solid lesion but made up of small cysts, resembles canalicular stage of lung development

■ Type 4: similar to type 1 but larger cysts, usually in periphery of one lobe

Diagnosis

The diagnosis of CPAM is based on history, physical findings, and radiologic evaluation.

Physical Exam Findings

■ Ranges from normal respiratory exam (75%) when the mass is small to acute distress.

Typical findings of diagnostic procedures/tests for CPAM are:

■ AP chest x-ray will be specific for the location and size of the CPAM.

■ Chest (thoracic) CT scan is required to identify subtle structures of the CPAM.

Treatment

■ Some minor cases spontaneously regress without intervention.

■ Surgical intervention with excision is typically recommended based on the severity.

■ Of note: In fetal cases with CPAM and nonimmune hydrops, fetal resection or thoracoamniotic shunt have reportedly been effective.

■ Type 1 CPAM can develop malignant changes, and long-term follow-up is needed.

Prognosis

Prognosis depends on the size and location of the CPAM and necessary treatment.

REFERENCES

Fraser, D. (2021). Respiratory distress. In M. T. Verklan, M. Walden, & S. Forest (Eds.), *Core curriculum for neonatal intensive care nursing* (6th ed., pp. 394–424). Elsevier.

Keller, B. A., Hirose, S., & Farmer, D. L. (2018). Surgical disorders of the chest and airways. In C. A. Gleason & S. E. Juul (Eds.), *Avery's diseases of the newborn* (10th ed., pp. 695–723). Elsevier.

Cardiovascular System

SAMUAL L. MOONEYHAM

CARDIOVASCULAR SYSTEM DEVELOPMENT

Fetal circulation differs from extrauterine circulation because of the following in utero characteristics:

■ Pulmonary vascular resistance is higher than systemic vascular resistance.

■ Gas exchange for the fetus occurs in the placenta and bypasses the lungs.

■ Lungs are filled with fluid.

■ Fetal structures such as the foramen ovale (FO), ductus arteriosus (DA), and ductus venosus (DV) are present.

Fetal circulation is shown in Figure 2.1.

The fetal circulatory system uses the placenta to act as the organ to supply oxygen and nutrition to the fetus. It also allows for carbon dioxide and waste to be excreted. Inside the fetal heart, blood enters the right atrium (RA). After entering the RA, most of it flows through the FO into the left atrium (LA). The blood then enters into the left ventricle (LV). Blood then passes to the aorta. Through the aorta, blood is sent out to the body. After circulating there, the blood returns to the RA of the heart through the superior/inferior vena cava (IVC).

This less oxygenated blood is pumped from the right ventricle (RV) into the pulmonary artery. A small amount of the blood continues on to the lungs. Most of this blood is shunted through the DA to the descending aorta. This blood then enters the umbilical arteries and flows into the placenta. In the placenta, carbon dioxide and waste products are released into the mother's circulatory system. Oxygen and nutrients from the mother's blood are released into the fetus' blood.

TRANSITION OF EXTRAUTERINE CIRCULATION

■ Pulmonary vascular resistance decreases and systemic vascular resistance increases.

■ DA and DV closure

■ Left-to-right shunting through the FO

■ FO closure

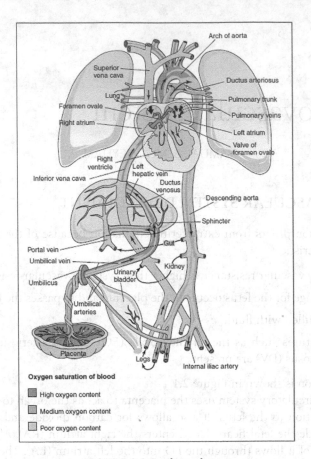

FIGURE 2.1 Fetal circulation.

Source: Adapted and modified from Ross Laboratories (1985).

Anatomy of the normal heart is shown in Figure 2.2.

At birth, the umbilical cord is clamped and the baby no longer gets oxygen and nutrients from the mother. With the first breaths of life, the lungs start to expand. As the lungs expand, the alveoli in the lungs are cleared of fluid. An increase in the baby's blood pressure and a major reduction in the pulmonary pressures reduce the need for the DA to shunt blood. These changes help the shunt close. These changes raise the pressure in the LA of the heart. They also lower the pressure in the RA. The shift in pressure stimulates the FO to close. In addition, the closure of the DA, DV, and FO completes the change of fetal circulation to newborn circulation.

IMPORTANCE OF MATERNAL AND PERINATAL HISTORY

There are several maternal conditions that can affect a newborn's cardiovascular system. See Table 2.1 for heart defects associated with maternal history.

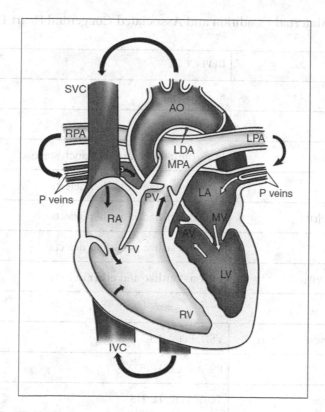

FIGURE 2.2 Normal cardiac anatomy and circulation.

AO, aorta; AV, aortic valve; IVC, inferior vena cava; LA, left atrium; LDA, ligamentum ductus arteriosus; LPA, left pulmonary artery; LV, left ventricle; MPA, main pulmonary artery; MV, mitral valve; PV, pulmonary valve; P veins, pulmonary veins; RA, right atrium; RPA, right pulmonary artery; RV, right ventricle; SVC, superior vena cava; TV, tricuspid valve.

Source: Adapted and modified from Ross Laboratories (1985).

TABLE 2.1 Maternal Condition and Associated Congenital Heart Defects

CONDITION	DEFECT
Maternal Disease	
Diabetes mellitus	Cardiomyopathy, TGA, VSD, PDA
Lupus erythematosus	Congenital heart block
Collagen disease	Congenital heart block
Congenital heart defect	Increased risk for congenital heart defect (3%–4%)

(*continued*)

TABLE 2.1 Maternal Condition and Associated Congenital Heart Defects (*continued*)

CONDITION	DEFECT
Viral Disease	
Rubella	
First trimester	PDA, pulmonary artery branch stenosis
Later	Various cardiac and other defects
Cytomegalovirus	Various cardiac and other defects
Herpesvirus	Various cardiac and other defects
Coxsackie B virus	Various cardiac and other defects
Drugs	
Amphetamines	VSD, PDA, ASD, TGA
Phenytoin	PS, AS, COA, PDA
Trimethadione	TGA, TOF, HLHS
Progesterone/estrogen	VSD, TOF, TGA
Alcohol	VSD, PDA, ASD, TOF

AS, aortic stenosis; ASD, atrial septal defect; COA, coarctation of the aorta; HLHS, hypoplastic left heart syndrome; PDA, patent ductus arteriosus; PS, pulmonary stenosis; TOF, tetralogy of Fallot; TGA, transposition of the great arteries; VSD, ventricular septal defect.

Source: Goff, D. A. (2020). Cardiovascular system. In C. Kenner, L. B. Altimier, & M. V. Boykova (Eds.), *Comprehensive neonatal nursing care* (6th ed., pp. 147–178). Springer Publishing Company.

GENERAL FOCUSED ASSESSMENT OF THE CARDIOVASCULAR SYSTEM

Complete the history by reviewing maternal, family, and other birth histories to see what risk factors could contribute to cardiovascular diseases. The initial cardiovascular assessment should include general appearance and behavior. Inspect the skin and mucous membranes of the newborn for color and temperature; these can be early signs of cardiac defects. Cyanosis is bluish color of the skin, lips, earlobes, nailbeds, and scrotum in males with significant arterial oxygen desaturation. The two types of cyanosis are central and peripheral (bluish color in hand, feet, and

TABLE 2.2 Grading of Pulses

GRADE	DESCRIPTION
0	Not palpable
+1	Difficult to palpate, thready, weak, easily obliterated with pressure
+2	Difficult to palpate, may be obliterated with pressure
+3	Easy to palpate, not easily obliterated with pressure (NORMAL)
+4	Strong, bounding, not obliterated with pressure

Source: Hockenberry, M. J., Wilson, D., & Rodgers, C. C. (2019). *Wong's nursing care of infants and children.* Elsevier.

around mouth). Peripheral cyanosis is a normal finding in newborns until around day 2 of life. Pallor and mottling can also be signs of cardiac defects. Pallor is caused by vasoconstriction and shunting blood from the skin to vital organs. Mottling can be associated with cardiogenic shock; this may be caused by a decrease in cardiac output or hypovolemia. Be aware that you might see mottling with normal newborns that are stressed or cold. Perfusion is also important; looking at capillary filling time, greater than 3 to 4 seconds is abnormal. Peripheral pulse should be assessed and measured (Vargo, 2019). See Table 2.2 for grading of pulses.

ATRIAL SEPTAL DEFECT

Incidence

■ Accounts for 5% to 10% of all congenital heart defects (CHDs).

Physiology

Atrial septal defect (ASD) is an opening in the atrial septum that develops as a result of improper septal formation early in fetal cardiac development.
There are three types of ASDs (Park & Salamat, 2021; Webb et al., 2018):

■ Ostium, commonly associated with mitral valve (MV)

■ Ostium primum, an endocardial cushion defect (ECD) associated with anomalies of one or both atrioventricular (AV) valves

■ Sinus venosus, often associated with partial anomalous pulmonary venous connection

ASD is shown in Figure 2.3.

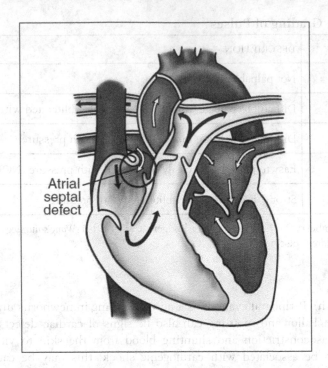

FIGURE 2.3 Atrial septal defect is a communication between the right and left atria.
Source: Adapted and modified from Ross Laboratories (1985).

Hemodynamics

ASD usually does not produce symptoms until pulmonary vascular resistance begins to decrease and right ventricular end-diastolic and right atrial pressure decline. ASDs produce some blood flow alterations. Blood shunts from left to right through the defect because the RV offers less resistance to fill it. The left-to-right shunt increases right ventricular volume and decreases pulmonary vascular resistance, so the pulmonary artery pressure is almost normal. The large pulmonary blood flow gradually leads to increased pulmonary artery pressure.

Clinical Manifestations/Diagnosis

Newborns with ASDs are usually asymptomatic, although there may be grade 2/6 to 3/6 systolic ejection murmurs (SEMs); see Table 2.3 for a grading scale of murmurs, which can best be heard at the upper left sternal border (ULSB). In a large ASD, there can be middiastolic rumble caused by the relative tricuspid stenosis audible at the lower left sternal border (LLSB; Park & Salmat, 2021; Webb et al., 2018). On a chest radiograph, the heart is enlarged, with a prominent main pulmonary artery (MPA) segment and increased pulmonary vascularity. Echocardiogram enhances detection of the ASD; it shows a right axis deviation and mild right ventricular hypertrophy. There may be an incomplete right bundle branch block (Danford et al., 2000; Park & Salamat, 2021).

TABLE 2.3 Grading Scale of Murmurs

Grade 1	Barely heard
Grade 2	Soft but easily audible
Grade 3	Moderately loud, no thrill
Grade 4	Loud, thrill present
Grade 5	Loud, audible with stethoscope barely on chest
Grade 6	Loud, audible with stethoscope near chest

Source: Goff, D. A. (2020). Cardiovascular system. In C. Kenner, L. B. Altimier, & M. V. Boykova (Eds.), *Comprehensive neonatal nursing care* (6th ed., pp. 147–178). Springer Publishing Company.

Echocardiogram shows increased tight ventricular dimension and paradoxical movement of the ventricular septum. Diagnosis can be made by two-dimensional echocardiogram, which shows the location and size of the defect. Children with ASDs are usually thin and may be easily fatigued. By late infancy, there may be a precordial bulge caused by an enlarged right side of the heart.

Management

Untreated ASD can lead to congestive heart failure (CHF), pulmonary hypertension, and atrial dysrhythmias in adulthood. Spontaneous closure of ASDs occurs in the first 5 years of age in up to 40% of children (Park & Salamat, 2021). Medical management of ASD consists of prevention or treatment of CHF. There is no need to limit activity. If there is an ASD that has right-side dilatation and significant hemodynamic changes, a noninvasive technique using a transcatheter device can be effective (Goff, 2020).

Surgical correction is reserved for infants for whom the transcatheter approach is contraindicated or unsuccessful. The surgical process is done during open heart surgery by placing a patch or with direct closure. This process requires cardiopulmonary bypass. Surgery usually occurs between 2 and 5 years but depends on the severity of the defect and the significance of left-to-right shunting. Mortality rate of surgery is less than 1%, with the highest risk for infants with CHF or increased pulmonary vascular resistance (Goff, 2020; Park & Salamat, 2021; Webb et al., 2018).

REFERENCES

Danford, D., Gumbiner, C., Martin, A., & Fletcher, S. (2000). Effects of electrocardiography and chest radiography on the accuracy of preliminary diagnosis of common congenital cardiac defects. *Pediatric Cardiology, 21*(4), 334–340. https://doi.org/10.1007/s002460010075

Goff, D. A. (2020). Cardiovascular system. In C. Kenner, L. B. Altimier, & M. V. Boykova (Eds.), *Comprehensive neonatal nursing care* (6th ed., pp. 147–178). Springer Publishing Company.

Park, M. K., & Salamat, M. (2021). *Park's pediatric cardiology for practitioner* (7th ed.). Mosby.

Webb, G., Smallhorn, J., Therrien, J., & Reddington, A. (2018). Congenital heart disease in the adult and pediatric patient. In D. P. Zipes, P. Libby, R. O. Bonow, D. L. Mann, & G. F. Tomaselli (Eds.), *Braunwald's heart disease: A textbook of cardiovascular medicine* (11th ed., pp. 1411–1467). Elsevier.

VENTRICULAR SEPTAL DEFECT

Incidence

■ Accounts for 20% to 25% of all CHDs. It is the most common defect.

Physiology

Ventricular septal defect (VSD) is a defect or opening of the ventricular septum. VSD results from imperfect ventricular division during early fetal development. It can occur anywhere on the muscular or membranous septum. This size and degree of pulmonary vascular resistance may vary. This is more important than where it is located. Small defects have a large resistance to the left-to-right shunting and shunting is not dependent on pulmonary vascular resistance. Large defects have little resistance to the left-to-right shunting and are dependent on the level of pulmonary vascular resistance (Park & Salamat, 2021; Turner et al., 1999; Webb et al., 2018). VSD is shown in Figure 2.4.

Hemodynamics

The hemodynamic considerations depend on the size of the VSD.

■ Small VSD—These produce minimal shunting and may not show any signs or symptoms. A chest radiograph and echocardiogram may appear normal. During auscultation, a loud, harsh pansystolic murmur may be heard at the third and fourth left intercostal space at the sternal border (Park & Salamat, 2021; Turner et al., 1999; Webb et al., 2018).

■ Moderate VSD—There is shunting from the LV to RV because of the high pressure of the LV and higher systemic vascular resistance. The shunting occurs during systole, when the RV contracts, moving blood to the pulmonary artery versus staying in the RV. This prevents right ventricular hypertrophy.

■ Large VSD—There is shunting from the LV to RV; the amount depends on the size of the VSD. The larger the size, the greater the amount of shunting; this creates higher pressure in the RV and pulmonary artery. When there is significantly increased pressure in the pulmonary artery, the walls of the pulmonary arterioles thicken and increased resistance may decrease the left-to-right shunting. Pulmonary vascular disease can lead to right-to-left shunting and cyanosis.

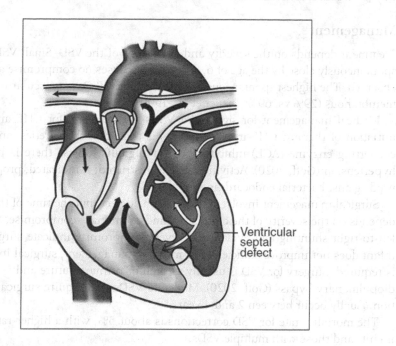

FIGURE 2.4 VSD is a communication between the right and left ventricles.

VSD, ventricular septal defect.

Source: Adapted and modified from Ross Laboratories (1985).

Clinical Manifestations/Diagnosis

Manifestations depend on the size/shunting. Smaller VSDs may be asymptomatic with no change in hemodynamics. Larger VSDs are associated with decreased exertional tolerance, recurrent pulmonary infections, poor growth, and symptoms of CHF. Pulmonary hypertension and cyanosis are seen in severe VSDs.

A systolic thrill may be palpated at the LLSB. A precordial bulge may appear with larger VSDs. Grade 2/6 to 5/6 regurgitant systolic murmurs can be heard at LLSB. During auscultation, you may hear an apical diastolic rumble and perhaps loud pulmonary heart sounds.

X-ray testing can detect moderate-to-large VSDs (Danford et al., 2000). Radiographs show cardiomegaly that involves the LA, LV, maybe the RV, and increased pulmonary vascularity. Echocardiogram may show left ventricular hypertrophy and, in severe cases, right hypertrophy. Two-dimensional echocardiogram shows the size and location of the defect as well as other defects (Park & Salamat, 2021; Webb et al., 2018). The MRI shows the volume of blood flow to the lungs.

With large VSDs not detected in the neonatal period, physical examination in the infant may show inadequate weight gain, cyanosis, and clubbing of the digits.

Management

Treatment depends on the severity and symptoms of the VSD. Small VSDs usually spontaneously close by the age of 6, as long as it causes no compromise and can be observed. The highest spontaneous closure rate with VSDs is muscular versus perimembranous (29% vs. 69%; Turner et al., 1999).

Medical management for significant VSDs is monitored for CHF and prompt initiation of therapy. CHF in older infants is treated with diuretics, angiotensin-converting enzyme (ACE) inhibitors and/or digitalis, unless there is pulmonary hypertension (Goff, 2020). Activities are not restricted; if indicated, prophylaxis is used against bacterial endocarditis.

Surgical management involves closure of the defect, but the time of this surgery depends on the severity of the circulatory and pulmonary compromise. Significant left-to-right shunting and evidence of severe compromise indicate surgery. If the infant does not improve sufficiently to medical management, surgical intervention is required. Surgery for VSD is usually a patch or primary suture and requires cardiopulmonary bypass (Goff, 2020). Moderate VSDs that require surgical intervention usually occur between 2 and 4 years.

The mortality rate for VSD corrections is about 5%, with a higher rate in small infants and those with multiple VSDs.

REFERENCES

Danford, D., Gumbiner, C., Martin, A., & Fletcher, S. (2000). Effects of electrocardiography and chest radiography on the accuracy of preliminary diagnosis of common congenital cardiac defects. *Pediatric Cardiology, 21*(4), 334–340. https://doi.org/10.1007/s002460010075

Goff, D. A. (2020). Cardiovascular system. In C. Kenner, L. B. Altimier, & M. V. Boykova (Eds.), *Comprehensive neonatal nursing care* (6th ed., pp. 147–178). Springer Publishing Company.

Park, M. K., & Salamat, M. (2021). *Park's pediatric cardiology for practitioner* (7th ed.). Mosby.

Turner, S., Hunter, S., & Wyllie, J. (1999). The natural history of ventricular septal defects. *Archives of Disease in Childhood, 81*(1), 49–52. https://doi.org/10.1136/adc.81.5.413

Webb, G., Smallhorn, J., Therrien, J., & Reddington, A. (2018). Congenital heart disease in the adult and pediatric patient. In D. P. Zipes, P. Libby, R. O. Bonow, D. L. Mann, & G. F. Tomaselli (Eds.), *Braunwald's heart disease: A textbook of cardiovascular medicine* (11th ed., pp. 1411–1467). Elsevier.

PATENT DUCTUS ARTERIOSUS

Incidence

■ Occurs in 5% to 10% of all CHDs in term newborns.

■ Higher occurrence in females (3:1)

■ More common in infants with trisomy 21 or Down syndrome

■ Infants of mothers with rubella during pregnancy (Goff, 2020)

Physiology

The DA is a wide muscular connection between the pulmonary artery and the aorta that originates from the left pulmonary artery (LPA) and enters the aorta below the subclavian artery. The purpose of the DA is to allow oxygenated blood from the placenta to bypass the nonfunctional lungs and enter the fetal circulation. The DA should close functionally by about 15 hours postbirth. Intermittent shunting of blood is quite common during the first 24 hours in response to changes in the systemic or pulmonary vascular resistance, such as infusion of fluids or handling the neonate. Increased arterial oxygen concentration after the neonate begins to breathe causes ductal closure. Decreased prostaglandin E (PGE) and increased acetylcholine and bradykinin contribute to the closure (Goff, 2020).

Pathophysiology

Failure of the DA to close, allowing shunting of blood in the term neonate after 24 hours postdelivery, is considered a patent ductus arteriosus (PDA) in the term neonate. PDA in the preterm neonate presents a different clinical problem that is discussed separately.

After birth, blood flow through the DA is reversed. Blood flows from left to right through the PDA, reentering the pulmonary system (Figure 2.5). The amount of blood that flows through the PDA and the effects of the increased flow depend on the difference between systemic and pulmonary vascular resistance and the diameter and length of the ductus. Prolonged increased pulmonary blood flow can cause increased pulmonary vascular resistance, pulmonary hypertension, and right ventricular hypertrophy (Goff, 2020).

Assessment

The severity of the PDA is determined by the diameter and length of the DA and the amount of blood shunted into the pulmonary system. A small PDA may be asymptomatic. A large PDA with significant shunting causes signs of CHF, such as tachypnea, dyspnea, and hoarse cry. Infants with uncorrected PDA may have frequent lower respiratory tract infections, coughing, and poor weight gain (Goff, 2020).

Clinical Manifestations/Diagnosis

The diagnosis of PDA is based on history, physical findings, x-rays, and echocardiogram.

Physical Exam Findings

▪ Bounding peripheral pulses
▪ Widened pulse pressure of more than 25 mmHg

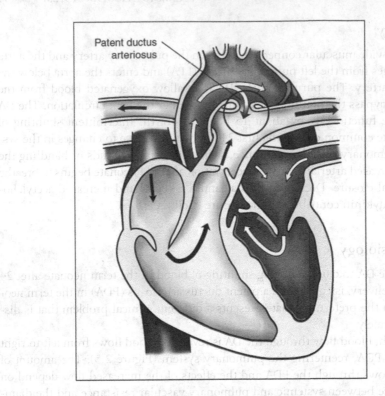

FIGURE 2.5 PDA is a communication between the pulmonary artery and the aorta.

PDA, patent ductus arteriosus.

Source: Adapted and modified from Ross Laboratories (1985).

- Hyperactive precordium
- Systolic thrill at the ULSB
- Murmur (grade 1/6–4/6) at ULSB or infraclavicular area
- Murmur heard throughout the cardiac cycle
- Definitive diagnosis made by echocardiogram

  Typical findings of diagnostic procedures/tests for PDA are illustrated in Table 2.4.

Treatment

For term infants who are feeding and gaining weight, medications to promote closure are not the treatment of choice. Fluid management and diuretics may be used (Goff, 2020). If the infant's condition is compromised then

- Cardiac catheterization and insertion of coil or device are placed into ductus to obstruct flow.
- Definitive treatment of a large PDA with significant shunting is surgical ligation (Goff, 2020).

TABLE 2.4 Diagnosis of Congenital Heart Defects

DEFECT	CHEST RADIOGRAPH	EKG	ECHOCARDIOGRAM	CATHETERIZATION	LAB TESTS
PDA	Increased pulmonary vascularity; cardiac enlargement; left aortic arch	Left atrial and ventricular enlargement; abnormal QRS axis for age	LA:AO ratio >1.3 (term); 1 (preterm); increased left atrium and ventricle (2D)	Increased O_2 saturation in pulmonary artery; increased right ventricular and pulmonary artery pressure (with pulmonary hypertension)	NA
ASD	Mild heart enlargement; prominent main pulmonary artery; increased pulmonary vascularity	Right axis deviation; incomplete right bundle branch block; right ventricular hypertrophy	Dilated right ventricle; paradoxical movement of ventricular septum	Increased O_2 in right atrium; normal right side atrium; normal right side pressure; 10%; PAPVR	NA
VSD	Enlarged heart; increased pulmonary markings	Left and right ventricular hypertrophy	Large left atrium (M-mode); presence or absence of other defects (2D)	Increased O_2 in right ventricle; increased systolic pressure in right ventricle and pulmonary artery	NA
TOF	Normal heart size; boot-shaped contour; decreased pulmonary markings; prominent aorta; right aortic arch in 13 cases	Right axis deviation; right ventricular hypertrophy	Large VDS, aortic dextroposition, and PS; size of main, right, and left pulmonary arteries (2D)	Demonstrates anatomy of right ventricular outflow region; microcytic anemia	Increased Hgb and HCT clotting time

(continued)

TABLE 2.4 Diagnosis of Congenital Heart Defects (continued)

DEFECT	CHEST RADIOGRAPH	EKG	ECHOCARDIOGRAM	CATHETERIZATION	LAB TESTS
PS	Normal heart size; normal pulmonary vascularity; enlarged pulmonary artery; right ventricle filling (lateral)	Right axis deviation; right atrial enlargement; right ventricular hypertrophy	Decreased valve leaflet motion; small changes in right ventricular wall thickness	Elevated right ventricular pressure; normal or slightly lowered pulmonary artery pressure	NA
TGA	Enlarged heart with narrow base; enlarged ventricles; increased pulmonary vascularity	Right axis deviation; right ventricular hypertrophy	Abnormal origin of great vessels	Increased right ventricular pressure; catheter can enter aorta from right ventricle; pulmonary artery can be entered only through PDA or ASD	Increased Hgb and HCT; polycythemia
COA	Cardiomegaly; postcoarctation dilation (by age 5 years); notching of ribs from collateral vessels	Left ventricular hypertrophy; inverted T waves in left precordial leads; right ventricular hypertrophy (severe)	Visualization of narrowed aorta and location of associated defects; allows evaluation of aortic valve movement, structure, and function and left ventricular size and function	Performed to determine exact location and evaluation	NA

ASD, atrial septal defect; COA, coarctation of the aorta; HCT, hematocrit test; PAPVR, partial anomalous pulmonary venous return; PDA, patent ductus arteriosus; PS, pulmonary stenosis; TOF, tetralogy of Fallot; TGA, transposition of the great arteries; VSD, ventricular septal defect.

Source: Goff, D. A. (2020). Cardiovascular system. In C. Kenner, L. B. Altimier, & M. V. Boykova (Eds.), *Comprehensive neonatal nursing care* (6th ed., pp. 147–178). Springer Publishing Company. *Data Source:* Park, M. K. (2014). *Pediatric cardiology for practitioners.* Mosby.

Prognosis

The overall prognosis for term neonates with PDA is excellent. The mortality rate for surgical ligation is less than 1%, and complications are rare (Goff, 2020). Medical closure is not effective in older infants.

REFERENCE

Goff, D. A. (2020). Cardiovascular system. In C. Kenner, L. B. Altimier, & M. V. Boykova (Eds.), *Comprehensive neonatal nursing care* (6th ed., pp. 147–178). Springer Publishing Company.

TETRALOGY OF FALLOT

Incidence

- This accounts for 10% of all CHDs.
- It is the most common cyanotic heart defect beyond infancy because repair is usually carried out after the patient becomes 1 year old.

Physiology

Tetralogy of Fallot (TOF) is developed as a lack of subpulmonary conus during fetal life. It consists of a large VSD, pulmonary stenosis (PS) or other right ventricular outflow tract obstruction, overriding aorta, and RV hypertrophy, although initially the RV may not be hypertrophied. TOF is shown in Figure 2.6.

Hemodynamics

The VSD in TOF causes pressures in the ventricles to be equal. The obstruction of the pulmonary artery causes oxygenated blood to flow into the aorta through the VSD.

Clinical Manifestations/Diagnosis

The cardinal signs of TOF are cyanosis, hypoxia, and dyspnea. Newborns may present with a loud murmur or may be cyanotic. Severe decompensation or "tet" spells are common in infants and children; they can occur in the neonatal period, too. Instinctively children will squat; this decreases systemic venous return by trapping venous blood in the legs. Chronic arterial desaturation stimulates erythropoiesis, leading to polycythemia. Increased red blood cells and microcytic anemia increase the viscosity of blood and can lead to cerebrovascular accident (stroke). Chronic hypoxemia and polycythemia cause an increased risk of hemorrhagic diathesis because reduced platelet aggregation and decreased platelet survival time cause thrombocytopenia and impaired synthesis of vitamin K–dependent clotting factors.

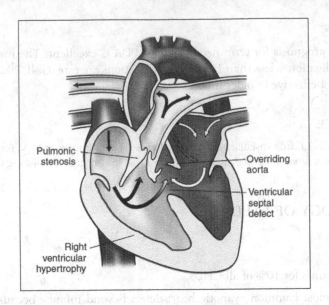

FIGURE 2.6 Tetralogy of Fallot consists of PS, ventricular septal defect, overriding aorta, and hypertrophy of the RV.

PS, pulmonary stenosis; RV, right ventricle.

Source: Adapted and modified from Ross Laboratories (1985).

TOF exhibits varying degrees of cyanosis, depending on the obstruction of blood flow to the right ventricular outflow. A very loud grade 3/6 to 5/6 SEM is heard at the middle and ULSB. In severe TOF, a PDA may be heard (Park & Salamat, 2021).

A chest radiograph may show decreased or normal heart size with decreased pulmonary vascularity. The heart may be boot shaped because of a concaved MPA segment with upturned apex. It may also show an enlarged right atrial and a right aortic arch.

An echocardiogram will show a large VSD and overriding aorta. A two-dimensional echocardiogram identifies the right ventricular outflow tract and pulmonary valve (PV).

TOF may show clubbing of fingers.

Management

The definitive treatment for TOF is surgical correction. This procedure requires cardiopulmonary bypass. Surgical correction may be delayed with medical management. Decreasing pulmonary vascular resistance may improve mild cyanosis. Medical management is used to prevent or treat hypoxemia, polycythemia, infection, and microcytic hypochromic anemia. Continuous follow-up is needed, as well as parent education and support for home management (Dipchand et al., 1999; Park & Salamat, 2021). Parents need education in recognizing early signs and symptoms of decompensation. They also need to recognize and treat hypercyanotic or "tet" spells (Goff, 2020). See Table 2.5 for recognition and treatment of "tet"

TABLE 2.5 Recognition and Treatment of Tet Spells

MANIFESTATIONS	TREATMENT	RATIONALE
Irritability, crying, hyperpnea	Knee to chest or squatting position	Traps blood in the lower extremities to decrease systemic venous return; increases pulmonary blood flow
Cyanosis	Oxygen administration	Improves arterial oxygen saturation
Diaphoresis, loss of consciousness	Morphine sulfate (0.1–0.2 mg/kg/dose)	Suppresses respiratory center to decrease hyperpnea
Seizures	Bicarbonate	Corrects acidosis and eliminates stimulation of respiratory center
Decreased murmur	Propranolol (Inderal; 0.15–0.25 mg/kg/dose)	May decrease spasm of right ventricular outflow tract or may act peripherally to stabilize

Source: Goff, D. A. (2020). Cardiovascular system. In C. Kenner, L. B. Altimier, & M. V. Boykova (Eds.), *Comprehensive neonatal nursing care* (6th ed., pp. 147–178). Springer Publishing Company.

spells. Lowering the systemic vascular resistance and a large right-to-left ventricular shunt leads to a "tet" spell. Increased activity, crying, nursing, or defecation can trigger hypoxemic episodes. A right-to-left shunt results in a decrease in PaO_2, increase in PCO_2, and decrease in pH. This stimulates the respiratory system and causes an increase in rate and depth of respiration, known as hyperpnea. This causes an increase in systemic venous return. The right ventricular outflow tract obstruction prevents the increased blood flow from entering the pulmonary artery, so it is shunted to the aorta. This further decrease in PaO_2 with severe uninterrupted hypercyanotic spells can lead to seizures, hypoxemia, loss of consciousness, and even death.

An indication for immediate surgical treatment is the presence of "tet" spells; this increases hypoxemia, increases metabolic acidosis, leads to inadequate systemic perfusion, increases cyanosis, and increases polycythemia. Systemic perfusion evaluation occurs by observing peripheral pulse intensity, urine output, capillary refill time, blood pressure, or peripheral vasoconstriction.

Surgical management is divided into palliative or corrective procedures. Palliative procedure is used to create a pathway between the systemic and pulmonary system. This also allows for the right and left pulmonary arteries to grow. This procedure is indicated when newborns have TOF, PA, severe cyanosis while younger than 6 months, unmanageable "tet" spells, or hypoplastic pulmonary artery where corrective surgery is difficult (Park & Salamat, 2021). There are some neonatal centers that will perform the surgery before 6 months of age (Goff, 2020). The corrective procedure is performed after 6 months of age. It can be delayed until ages 2 to 4 years in asymptomatic children or those who have received the palliative procedure. This procedure requires cardiopulmonary bypass and consists of a patch closure of the VSD, excision of the PS, and widening of the right ventricular outflow tract (Goff, 2020). The postoperative mortality rate is about 1.1% if the TOF is uncomplicated with the first 2 years in uncomplicated TOF and higher in more severe cases (Goff, 2020).

REFERENCES

Dipchand, A., Giuffre, M., & Freedom, R. (1999). Tetralogy of Fallot with non-confluent pulmonary arteries and aortopulmonary septal defect. *Cardiology in the Young, 9*(1), 75–77. https://doi.org/10.1017/S1047951100007549

Goff, D. A. (2020). Cardiovascular system. In C. Kenner, L. B. Altimier, & M. V. Boykova (Eds.), *Comprehensive neonatal nursing care* (6th ed., pp. 147–178). Springer Publishing Company.

Park, M. K., & Salamat, M. (2021). *Park's pediatric cardiology for practitioner* (7th ed.). Mosby.

COARCTATION OF THE AORTA

Incidence

◼ It accounts for 8% of all CHDs.

◼ It is found in 30% of newborns with Turner syndrome (Park & Salamat, 2021).

◼ Male-to-female ratio is 2:1.

Physiology

Coarctation of the aorta (COA) is the narrowing or constriction of the aortic arch. It is more commonly seen below the left subclavian artery. COA can occur as a single lesion related to improper development of the aorta or because of the constriction of the DA. The severity depends on the degree of constriction and location. Preductal COA (proximal to the DA) accounts for 40% of cases. Other defects associated with preductal COA are VSD, transposition of the great arteries (TGA), and PDA. Collateral circulation is more effective with postductal COA versus preductal COA. There are normally no other defects with postductal COA and they are usually asymptomatic. In newborns with COA, there is a greater than 50% chance that they will have a bicuspid valve (Park, 2014). COA is shown in Figure 2.7.

Hemodynamics

COA causes an obstruction to blood flow, which causes varying pressure across the aortic arch. An obstruction proximal to the constriction of the aorta results in elevated pressure and causes increased left ventricular pressure. This increased

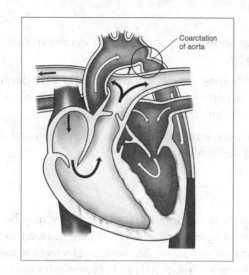

Coarctation
of aorta

FIGURE 2.7 COA is a narrowing or constriction of the aorta near the DA.
COA, coarctation of the aorta; DA, ductus arteriosus.
Source: Adapted and modified from Ross Laboratories (1985).

pressure results in left ventricular hypertrophy and dilation. The compensatory mechanism is collateral circulation (develops proximal to distal arteries to bypass the constriction). This increases blood flow to the lower extremities and abdomen, which produces a lower pulse (Park & Salamat, 2021).

Clinical Manifestations/Diagnosis

The severity depends on the degree of constriction and location as well as the time of appearance of symptoms and the presence of associated cardiac defects. Some symptoms of COA include signs of CHF, as well as weak, absent, or delayed lower extremity pulses. If CHF is present, then all pulses may be weak. With severe COA, auscultation will reveal a loud and single S2, an ejection click may be audible at the apex if a bicuspid aortic valve (AV) or systemic hypertension is present, and a grade 2/6 to 3/6 SEM is heard at the upper right and middle or LLSB and left interscapular area in newborns. In newborns, greater than 50% will have no murmurs in COA (Park & Salamat, 2021).

Diagnosis is based on history, physical findings, radiograph, ECG, and echocardiograph.

Radiograph

■ Asymptomatic newborns—may show a normal or slightly enlarged heart and may see dilation of the ascending aorta. On a barium swallow study, an "E" sign may appear. The "E" sign is due to the large proximal aortic segment or prominent subclavian artery above the poststenotic dilation of the descending aorta below the constricted segment (Park & Salamat, 2021).

■ Symptomatic newborns—reveals cardiomegaly and increased pulmonary venous congestion.

Echocardiogram

■ Asymptomatic newborns—may show left axis deviation of the QRS and left ventricular hypertrophy.

■ Symptomatic newborns—reveals normal or right axis deviation of the QRS, right ventricular hypertrophy, or right bundle branch block in newborns. In older children, a left ventricular hypertrophy is present.

A two-dimensional echocardiogram reveals the location and degree of constriction and other associated cardiac defects.

Management

The definitive treatment is surgical correction. Surgery may be delayed until the patient is 3 to 5 years of age if medically controlled; however, severe symptomatic newborns require immediate surgery. Medical management is used to provide adequate oxygenation, prevent or treat CHF, and prevent subacute infective endocarditis (SAIE). Prostaglandin (PGE) may be used if the constricted segment is at the DA to maintain ductal patency (Park & Salamat, 2021).

Surgical intervention involves excision of the constricted segment with end-to-end anastomosis, patch graft, bypass tube graft, or Dacron graft (Park & Salamat, 2021). Another alternative may be a subclavian flap aortoplasty. If CHF is present, then surgery is indicated even without circulatory shock. The mortality rate for surgical correction is less than 5% (Goff, 2020). Almost 20% of postoperative complications include renal failure and recoarctation.

REFERENCES

Goff, D. A. (2020). Cardiovascular system. In C. Kenner, L. B. Altimier, & M. V. Boykova (Eds.), *Comprehensive neonatal nursing care* (6th ed., pp. 147–178). Springer Publishing Company.

Park, M. K. (2014). *Pediatric cardiology for practitioners.* Mosby.

Park, M. K., & Salamat, M. (2021). *Park's pediatric cardiology for practitioner* (7th ed.). Mosby.

3

Neurologic System

GEORGIA R. DITZENBERGER, SUSAN TUCKER BLACKBURN,
BETH BROWN, AND LESLIE B. ALTIMIER

The neurologic system is one of the most complex systems in the body and critical to the function and integration of other body systems. Alterations in neurologic function can arise from alterations in developmental processes or from insults prior to, during, or after birth with immediate and long-term consequences for the infant (Ditzenberger & Blackburn, 2020). Neurologic development is influenced by many factors and substances including neuroendocrine, neuroimmune, genetic, transcriptional, and signaling factors; neurotropic proteins; vitamins; and the microbiome (Blackburn, 2018).

Neurologic development begins in the third week of gestation with the formation of the neural plate, neural folds, and neural tube. Once the tube is formed and becomes a closed system, different regions of the brain begin to develop. At 4 weeks' gestation, the brain differentiates into the forebrain, midbrain, and hindbrain. The forebrain translates input from the senses and is responsible for memory formation, thinking, reasoning, and problem solving. The midbrain functions as a relay station, coordinating messages to their final destination. Regulating the heart, breathing, and muscle movements are the functions of the hindbrain. At 7 weeks' gestation, the brain has the first detectable brain waves. From 9 to 11 weeks' gestation, the basic brain structure develops. As these different regions of the brain begin to form, the development of the central nervous system (CNS) is characterized by the following distinct overlapping processes: neurulation (primary and secondary), prosencephalic development (ventral induction), neuronal and glial cell proliferation, neuronal and glial cell migration, organization, and myelination. These processes, especially organization and myelination, continue past birth. The first section of this chapter reviews CNS development.

CENTRAL NERVOUS SYSTEM DEVELOPMENT

GEORGIA R. DITZENBERGER AND SUSAN TUCKER BLACKBURN

Development of the central nervous system (CNS) is divided into six overlapping stages. Development progresses at different rates in various sections of the CNS.

Many disorders of the neurologic system are related to defects in the development of the CNS. The stages of CNS development are as follows:

■ Neurulation is the process by which the early brain and spinal cord are formed via inductive events within the dorsal area of the embryo. The inductive events are separated into two stages:

● Primary neurulation (formation of the brain and spinal cord excluding the caudal segments of the lumbar region) occurs during the first 3 to 4 weeks of gestation. The brain and spinal cord develop from the neural plate and neural folds, which fuse to eventually form the forebrain, midbrain, hindbrain, and spinal cord. Closure of the neural tube begins in the area of the future medulla and takes place between 22 and 28 days' gestation. Failure of part of the neural tube to close leads to neural tube defects (NTDs).

● Secondary neurulation (caudal neural tube formation) occurs from 4 to 7 weeks. The caudal neural tube arises from a caudal cell mass at the end of the neural tube that fuses with the neural tube; much of this mass later regresses.

● During this time other cells form the neural crest, which later gives rise to ganglia, peripheral nerves, glial cells, the autonomic nervous system, parts of the meninges, and other supportive structures (Ditzenberger & Blackburn, 2020; du Plessis & Volpe, 2018a; Moore et al., 2020).

■ Prosencephalic development, or ventral induction, involves early development of the brain and ventricular system during the second to third month of gestation. The brain develops from the cranial end of the neural tube beginning at the end of the fourth week. Since development of the face is associated with prosencephalic development, alterations in brain development often result in facial malformations (Ditzenberger & Blackburn, 2020; du Plessis & Volpe, 2018b; Fleiss et al., 2018).

■ Neuronal and glial cell proliferation involves development and proliferation of neurons and glial cells in the subependymal germinal matrix. The peak period of neuronal proliferation is from 2 to 4 months' gestation. Proliferation of other glia and derivatives (including astrocytes and oligodendrocytes) occurs intensively at 5 to 8 months' gestation. Damage to the premyelinating oligdendrocytes is characteristic of periventricular leukomalacia (PVL) in preterm infants. During the most intense period of proliferation, before 32 to 34 weeks' gestation, the periventricular area receives a large proportion of the cerebral blood flow. This area is vulnerable to germinal matrix–intraventricular hemorrhage (GM-IVH) in preterm infants. The germinal matrix involutes by 34 to 36 weeks' gestation (Blackburn, 2018; Ditzenberger & Blackburn, 2020; Poduri & Volpe, 2018b).

■ Neuronal and glial cell migration is characterized by the movement of millions of cells from their origin in the germinal matrix of the periventricular region to their eventual loci in the cerebral cortex. Neuronal migration peaks at 3 to

5 months in the cerebrum and is critical to the formation of the cortex, gyri, and deep nuclear structures; glial migration occurs later. Endogenous alterations or exogenous insults before or after birth can alter migration. The preterm infant may be especially vulnerable to gyral alterations. Rapid development of the gyri begins at 26 to 28 weeks' gestation and continues through the third trimester into the postbirth period. Gyral development markedly increases cerebral surface area (Ditzenberger & Blackburn, 2020; Poduri & Volpe, 2018a).

■ Organization allows the nervous system to act as an integrated whole. Organizational processes include:

● Attainment of the proper alignment, orientation, and layering of cortical neurons. Establishment of subplate neurons is critical for neocortex development and is particularly vulnerable from 24 to 32 weeks' gestation.

● Arborization or differentiation and branching of axons and dendrites.

● Differentiation of the glial cells including astrocytes (critical for brain development, blood–brain barrier function, and CNS organization), oligodendrocytes (needed for CNS development and myelination), and microglia (brain macrophages, which also have role in brain development).

● Development of synaptic connections ("wiring" of the brain).

● Balancing of excitatory and inhibitory synapses.

● Cell death and selective elimination of excess neuronal processes adjust the size of neuron groups to anticipated use; part of brain plasticity.

The peak period for organization is from the fifth month of gestation to a few years after birth. However, organizational processes continue throughout childhood and adolescence. Some processes, such as synaptogenesis, continue throughout life. A marked increase in cerebral cortical volume and gyri occurs during this stage, especially from around 28 to 40 weeks' gestation with a four-fold increase in cortical gray matter volume. Organization of the brain is susceptible to insults from errors of metabolism, abnormal chromosomes, and perinatal events and is particularly vulnerable in the preterm infant being cared for in an ICU during this period (Blackburn, 2018; Ditzenberger & Blackburn, 2020; Fleiss et al., 2018; Kinney & Volpe, 2018b).

■ Myelination involves development of myelin sheaths around nerve fibers in the nervous system. Myelination of fiber tracts tends to occur before maturation of functional ability. Myelination begins during gestation and is prominent from 8 months' gestation to 2 years postbirth but continues to adulthood. Myelination is susceptible to damage from diverse exogenous influences, particularly malnutrition, which can lead to a range of neurologic deficits in which hypoplasia of the cerebral white matter occurs (Ditzenberger & Blackburn, 2020; Kinney & Volpe, 2018a; Moore et al., 2020).

REFERENCES

Blackburn, S. T. (2018). *Maternal, fetal and neonatal physiology: A clinical perspective* (5th ed.). Elsevier.

Ditzenberger, G. R., & Blackburn, S. T. (2020). Neurologic system. In C. Kenner, L. B. Altimer, & M. V. Boykova (Eds.), *Comprehensive neonatal nursing care* (6th ed., pp. 373–416). Springer Publishing Company.

du Plessis, A. J., & Volpe, J. J. (2018a). Neural tube development. In J. J. Volpe, T. E. Inder, B. T. Darras, L. S. De Vries, A. J. du Plessis, J. Neil, & J. M. Perlman (Eds.), *Volpe's neurology of the newborn* (6th ed., pp. 3–33). Elsevier.

du Plessis, A. J., & Volpe, J. J. (2018b). Prosencephalic development. In J. J. Volpe, T. E. Inder, B. T. Darras, L. S. De Vries, A. J. du Plessis, J. Neil, & J. M. Perlman (Eds.), *Volpe's neurology of the newborn* (6th ed., pp. 34–57). Elsevier.

Fleiss, B., Stolp, H., Metzger, V., & Gressens, P. (2018). Central nervous system development. In C. A. Gleason & S. E. Juul (Eds.), *Avery's diseases of the newborn* (10th ed., pp. 852–856). Elsevier.

Kinney, H. C., & Volpe, J. J. (2018a). Myelination events. In J. J. Volpe, T. E. Inder, B. T. Darras, L. S. De Vries, A. J. du Plessis, J. Neil, & J. M. Perlman (Eds.), *Volpe's neurology of the newborn* (6th ed., pp. 176–190). Elsevier.

Kinney, H. C., & Volpe, J. J. (2018b). Organizational events. In J. J. Volpe, T. E. Inder, B. T. Darras, L. S. De Vries, A. J. du Plessis, J. Neil, & J. M. Perlman (Eds.), *Volpe's neurology of the newborn* (6th ed., pp. 145–175). Elsevier.

Moore, K. L, Persaud, T. V. N., & Torchia, M. G. (2020). *The developing human: Clinically oriented embryology* (11th ed.). Elsevier.

Poduri, A., & Volpe, J. J. (2018a). Neuronal migration. In J. J. Volpe, T. E. Inder, B. T. Darras, L. S. De Vries, A. J. du Plessis, J. Neil, & J. M. Perlman (Eds.), *Volpe's neurology of the newborn* (6th ed., pp. 120–144). Elsevier.

Poduri, A., & Volpe, J. J. (2018b). Neuronal proliferation. In J. J. Volpe, T. E. Inder, B. T. Darras, L. S. De Vries, A. J. du Plessis, J. Neil, & J. M. Perlman (Eds.), *Volpe's neurology of the newborn* (6th ed., pp. 100–119). Elsevier.

ASSESSMENT OF NEUROLOGIC FUNCTION

GEORGIA R. DITZENBERGER AND SUSAN TUCKER BLACKBURN

Assessment of neurologic function is an initial step in evaluating an infant's response to the transition to extrauterine life and the impact of perinatal events and pathophysiologic problems on the central and peripheral nervous systems. Assessment of neurologic function and identification of dysfunction encompass several components: history, physical examination, neurologic examination, laboratory tests, and other diagnostic techniques.

HISTORY

■ Family history: neural tube defects (NTDs), chromosomal or genetic abnormalities, or other malformations

■ Maternal history: substance abuse, chronic health problems, age, nutritional status, exposure to teratogens

■ Obstetrical history: prematurity, postmaturity, placental problems (e.g., abruptio placentae and placenta previa), use of analgesia or anesthesia, maternal problems (e.g., infection, hypertension, and substance abuse), large-for-gestational-age infant, prolonged labor, precipitate labor, forceps delivery, abnormal presentation, intrauterine growth restriction, polyhydramnios, fetal distress, hypoxia, ischemia, low Apgar scores

■ Postnatal history: status at birth, required resuscitation, hypoxic episodes, shock, hypoperfusion ± subsequent reperfusion, hemorrhage, infection, metabolic or electrolyte aberrations

PHYSICAL EXAMINATION

■ Vital signs: temperature, heart rate, respiratory pattern, blood pressure, color
■ Signs of infection, birth trauma: ecchymosis, petechiae, edema, lacerations, fractures
■ Signs of vascular alterations
■ Seizures; alterations in activity, tone, and state
■ Infant's cry: robustness, presence in response to aversive stimuli, and pitch
■ Head size, shape, growth
  ● Occipital–frontal (head) circumference (OFC; HC): at birth, daily, or weekly per underlying condition
    • Term infants: average 32.6 to 37.2 cm at birth
    • Infants 24 to 40 weeks' gestation, average growth: 0.1 to 0.6 cm/wk
  ● Sutures: proximity, widened, overlapping, asymmetrical
    • Normal: up to 4- to 5-mm separation of all sutures except squamosal (temporoparietal)
    • Squamosal suture: no more than 2 to 3 mm
    • Overriding bone plates, molding; resolve after first few days postbirth
    • Abnormal: persistent suture separation, increased separation
    • Increased/increasing separation: increased intracranial pressure (ICP)
    • Craniosynostosis: premature closure of one or more sutures
  ● Fontanelles
    • Anterior: diamond shaped, 3 to 4 cm long by 1 to 3 cm wide in term infants
      – Closes at 8 to 16 months of age
      – May bulge slightly when the infant cries
      – May be slightly depressed in upright position
    • Posterior: usually closed but, if open, triangular shaped, 1 to 3 cm wide
      – Closes sometime between 8 months' gestation to 2 months after birth

- "Third fontanelle": parietal bone defect; rare
  - Can be palpated in normal infants
  - Often present with Down syndrome (trisomy 21) or hypothyroidism
- Sunken, depressed: dehydration
- Bulging: increased ICP
● Presence/absence of major and/or minor anomalies
  - Low-set or abnormally shaped ears, micrognathia, hypertelorism
  - Hydrocephalus
● Vertebral column: NTDs; hair tufts, dimples, fistulae
● Cranial bones: fractures, extradural hemorrhage, edema, and areas of uneven ossification

NEUROLOGIC EXAMINATION

■ Goal: evaluate for presence, determining the extent of neurologic dysfunction; monitor recovery; prognostic indicator; perform serial evaluations if concerns arise during examination or if clinical indications arise for issues that may affect neurologic status

■ Consider when interpreting findings: gestational age, health status, infant state, medications, and feeding timing (LaBronte, 2019)

■ Optimum infant state during exam: quiet and alert

■ Level of consciousness: hyperalert, lethargy, and stupor or coma

  ● Hyperalert: increased sensitivity to sensory stimulation, wide-open eyes, diminished blink response, diminished ability to fixate and follow

  ● Lethargy: delayed response to tactile or noxious stimuli

  ● Stupor (obtunded): limited response to tactile or noxious stimuli

  ● Coma: no response to tactile or noxious stimuli

■ Posture, tone, and activity

  ● Normal posture, tone, and activity requires integrated functioning of the entire nervous system.

  ● Disturbances in either the central or peripheral nervous system manifest in alterations in neonatal position, tone, and activity.

  ● Assess resting position.

  ● Quality symmetry of activity with spontaneous and elicited movement

  ● Alterations in symmetry of trunk, face, and extremities at rest or with spontaneous movement: congenital anomalies, birth injury, or neurologic insult

  ● Abnormal findings: tight fisting, persistent cortical thumb; opisthotonos; decerebrate or decorticate posturing

- Abnormal movements: jitteriness, tremors
  - May be normal; occurs infrequently in newborns
  - Must be differentiated from seizures
  - Tremors: vary with the underlying disorder
    - Metabolic abnormalities, asphyxia, drug or nicotine (occurs with mother with a history of tobacco use) withdrawal: low-amplitude, high-frequency movements
    - Central nervous system (CNS) complications: high-amplitude, low-frequency movements
  - Jitteriness: common finding due to lack of myelinization of pyramidal tracts
    - Stimulus sensitive; not marked by gaze or eye deviations
    - Predominant movement in jitteriness is tremulousness
    - Stops with passive flexion
    - Can be initiated with spontaneous or elicited movement
- Tone: resting, passive, active; hypotonia, hypertonia
  - Resting: observe supine infant at rest
  - Passive: evaluate extensibility through righting reactions of legs and trunk and examination of neck flexors and extensors
  - Active: alter infant's posture to obtain directed motor responses
  - Hypotonia with muscle weakness: peripheral nerve injuries, neuromuscular disorders, alterations at the neuromuscular junction, and spinal cord injuries
  - Hypotonia without muscle weakness: CNS disturbances secondary to asphyxia, intracranial hemorrhage, chromosomal disorders or other genetic defects, or metabolic disturbances
  - Marked extensor hypertonia, opisthotonus: severe hypoxic–ischemic injury, bacterial meningitis, or massive IVH
- Reflexes
  - Primary reflexes: affected by gestational age, present to some degree by 28 to 32 weeks' gestation
    - Sucking, grasping, crossed extension, automatic walking (stepping), Moro reflex, startle reflex
      - Present, symmetric, and reproducible
      - Gradually disappear during infancy
    - Tendon reflexes: biceps, knee, and ankle jerk
      - Present after about 33 weeks' gestation
      - Not very helpful beyond confirming symmetry

■ Selected cranial nerves

- Fixation and following, pupillary responses, doll's eye response, hearing, vestibular response, suck/swallow

LABORATORY TESTS, OTHER DIAGNOSTIC TECHNIQUES

■ Laboratory tests:

- Cerebrospinal fluid (CSF): hemorrhage (increased red blood cells, increased protein, decreased glucose, xanthochromia); rule out infection (culture, turbidity of the fluid, increased or decreased white cells, protein, and/or glucose)

- Blood: complete blood count with differential, serum glucose, calcium levels, electrolyte levels, blood gases, acid–base status

- Sepsis workup; screening for toxoplasmosis, rubella, cytomegalovirus, herpes simplex, and syphilis (suspect infection)

- Genetic workup and other metabolic studies (suspect inborn errors of metabolism [IEM], inherited conditions)

■ Other diagnostic techniques:

- EEG; ≥24 hours with video preferred

- Bedside amplitude-integrated EEG (aEEG); particularly important for continuous monitoring during therapeutic hypothermia treatment

- Head ultrasonography (HUS), CT, and MRI

- Doppler sonography (part of complete HUS)

- Brainstem auditory evoked responses, visual evoked responses, somatosensory evoked responses

GENERALIZED NURSING CARE

GEORGIA R. DITZENBERGER AND SUSAN TUCKER BLACKBURN

■ Monitor infant's state, activity level, responsiveness, eye movements, head circumference, and vital signs; seizure activity; signs of increased intracranial pressure (ICP).

■ Monitor fluid and electrolyte status.

■ Maintain adequate ventilation and perfusion.

■ Position in alignment and change position regularly, particularly for newborns with minimal spontaneous movement.

■ Promote skin integrity; monitor for pressure sores, skin breakdown.

■ Maintain head in midline, slightly elevated to reduce ICP.

■ Massage skin gently to stimulate circulation.

■ Maintain an appropriate thermal environment.

■ Reduce environmental stressors: minimal handling, decreased noise, light.

■ Use sterile technique for dressing changes, wound care.

■ Monitor for signs of localized infection or neonatal sepsis.

■ Provide parent/family support including condition-specific information and teaching; discharge preparation (Amiel-Tison & Gosselin, 2009; Bennett & Meier, 2019; Ditzenberger, 2020; Ditzenberger & Blackburn, 2020; Fenichel, 2007; Heaberlin, 2019; Honeyfield, 2019; Romeo et al., 2017; Rousseau et al., 2017; Simbruner et al., 2010; Smith, 2012; Trollmann et al., 2010).

REFERENCES

Amiel-Tison, C., & Gosselin, J. (2009). Clinical assessment of the infant nervous system. In M. I. Leven & F. A. Chervenak (Eds.), *Fetal and neonatal neurology and neurosurgery* (4th ed., pp. 128–154). Churchill Livingstone/Elsevier.

Bennett, M., & Meier, S. R. (2019). Assessment of the dysmorphic infant. In E. P. Tappero & M. E. Honeyfield (Eds.), *Physical assessment of the newborn: A comprehensive approach to the art of physical examination* (6th ed., Chapter 13, Kindle Version). NICU Ink.

Ditzenberger, G. R. (2020). Nutritional management. In M. T. Verklan, M. Walden, & S. Forest (Eds.), *Core curriculum for neonatal intensive care nursing* (5th ed., pp. 152–171). Saunders/Elsevier.

Ditzenberger, G. R., & Blackburn, S. T. (2020). Neurologic system. In C. Kenner, L. B. Altimier, & M. V. Boykova (Eds.), *Comprehensive neonatal nursing care* (6th ed., pp. 373–416). Springer Publishing Company.

Fenichel, G. M. (2007). *Neonatal neurology* (4th ed.). Churchill/Livingstone/Elsevier.

Heaberlin, P. D. (2019). Neurologic assessment. In E. P. Tappero & M. E. Honeyfield (Eds.), *Physical assessment of the newborn: A comprehensive approach to the art of physical examination* (6th ed., Chapter 11, Kindle Version). NICU Ink.

Honeyfield, M. E. (2019). Principles of physical assessment. In E. P. Tappero & M. E. Honeyfield (Eds.), *Physical assessment of the newborn: A comprehensive approach to the art of physical examination* (6th ed., Chapter 1, Kindle Version). NICU Ink.

LaBronte, K. H. (2019). Recording and evaluating the neonatal history. In E. P. Tappero & M. E. Honeyfield (Eds.), *Physical assessment of the newborn: A comprehensive approach to the art of physical examination* (6th ed., Chapter 2, Kindle Version). NICU Ink.

Romeo, D. M., Bompard, S., Cocca, C., Serrao, F., DeCarolis, M. P., Zuppa, A. A., Ricci, D., Gallini, F., Madaloni, C., Romagnoli., C., & Mercuri, E. (2017). Neonatal neurological examination during the first 6 h after birth. *Early Human Development, 108*, 41–44. https://doi.org/10.1016/j.earlhumdev.2017.03.013

Rousseau, P., Maton, F., Lecuyer, R., & Lahaye, W. (2017). The moro reaction: More than a reflex, a ritualized behavior of nonverbal communication. *Infant Behavior and Development, 46*, 169–177. https://doi.org/10.1016/j.infbeh.2017.01.004

Simbruner, G., Mittal, R. A., Rohlmann, F., Muche, R., & neo.nEURO.network Trial Participants. (2010). Systemic hypothermia after neonatal encephalopathy: Outcomes of neo.nEURO .network RCT. *Pediatrics, 126*(4), e771–e778. https://doi.org/10.1542/peds.2009-2441

Smith, J. B. (2012). Initial evaluation: History and physical examination of the newborn. In C. A. Gleason & S. Devaskar (Eds.), *Avery's diseases of the newborn* (9th ed., pp. 277–299). Elsevier.

Trollmann, R., Nüsken, E., & Wenzel, D. (2010). Neonatal somatosensory evoked potentials: Maturational aspects and prognostic value. *Pediatric Neurology, 42*(6), 427–433. https://doi.org/10.1016/j.pediatrneurol.2009.12.007

CONGENITAL DISORDERS OF THE CENTRAL NERVOUS SYSTEM

Neural Tube Defects/Disorders of Primary Neurulation

Congenital spinal anomalies that occur during primary neurulation result from alternations in neural tube closure. The defects include abnormal/absent closure that may include vertebral bodies and meningeal, vascular, and dermal structures. Eighty percent of these defects occur in the cranial or caudal end of the neural tube (Blackburn, 2018; Ditzenberger & Blackburn, 2020; du Plessis & Volpe, 2018a; Moore et al., 2020).

Incidence

■ Occurs in 0.5 to 5 per 1,000 live births (Back & Plawner, 2012; Kanekar et al., 2011)

■ Varies with ethnicity, diet, geographical area, socioeconomic status

■ Folic acid supplementation at conception reduces the rate of neural tube defects (NTDs; American Academy of Pediatrics Committee on Genetics, 1999; reaffirmed 2012)

Physiology/Pathophysiology

NTDs include anencephaly, encephalocele, spina bifida occulta, and spina bifida cystica (meningocele, myelomeningocele, and myeloschisis). NTDs are usually accompanied by alterations in vertebral, meningeal, vascular, and dermal structures. NTDs arise from genetic, nutritional, and/or environmental influences. NTDs can be diagnosed prior to birth using maternal serum alpha-fetoprotein (AFP, a fetal glycoprotein) screening at 15 to 20 weeks, ultrasound examination, and/or measurement of the AFP level of the amniotic fluid (Blackburn, 2018; Copp et al., 2015; Ditzenberger & Blackburn, 2020; du Plessis & Volpe, 2018a, 2018b; Stoll et al., 2011).

REFERENCES

American Academy of Pediatrics Committee on Genetics. (1999). Folic acid for the prevention of neural tube defects. *Pediatrics, 104*(2), 325–327. https://doi.org/10.1542/peds.104.2.325

Back, S., & Plawner, L. L. (2012). Congenital malformations of the central nervous system. In H. W. Taeusch, R. A. Ballard, & C. A. Gleason (Eds.), *Avery's diseases of the newborn* (9th ed., pp. 844–867). Elsevier/Saunders.

Blackburn, S. T. (2018). *Maternal, fetal and neonatal physiology: A clinical perspective* (5th ed.). Elsevier.

Copp, A. J., Adzick, N. S., Chitty, L. S., Fletcher, J. M., Holmbeck, G. N., & Shaw, G. M. (2015). Spina bifida. *Nature Reviews Disease Primers, 1*, 15007. https://doi.org/10.1038/nrdp.2015.7

Ditzenberger, G. R., & Blackburn, S. T. (2020). Neurological system. In C. Kenner, L. B. Altimier, & M. V. Boykova (Eds.), *Comprehensive neonatal nursing care* (6th ed.). Springer Publishing Company.

du Plessis, A. J., & Volpe, J. J. (2018a). Neural tube development. In J. J. Volpe, T. E. Inder, B. T. Darras, L. S. deVries, A. J. du Plessis, & J. M. Perlman (Eds.), *Volpe's neurology of the newborn* (6th ed., pp. 3–33). Elsevier.

du Plessis, A. J., & Volpe, J. J. (2018b). Prosencephalic development. In J. J. Volpe, T. E. Inder, B. T. Darras, L. S. De Vries, A. J. du Plessis, J. Neil, & J. M. Perlman (Eds.), *Volpe's neurology of the newborn* (6th ed., pp. 34–57). Elsevier.

Kanekar, S., Shively, A., & Kaneda, H. (2011). Malformations of ventral induction. *Seminars in Ultrasound, CT, and MRI, 32*(3), 200–210. https://doi.org/10.1053/j.sult.2011.02.012

Moore, K. L., Persaud, T. V. N., & Torchia, M. G. (2020). *The developing human: Clinically oriented embryology* (11th ed.). Elsevier.

Stoll, C., Dott, B., Alembik, Y., & Roth, M.-P. (2011). Associated malformations among infants with neural tube defects. *American Journal of Medical Genetics Part A, 155A*(3), 565–568. https://doi.org/10.1002/ajmg.a.33886

DISORDERS OF PRIMARY NEURULATION

BETH BROWN AND LESLIE B. ALTIMIER

CRANIORACHISCHISIS TOTALIS

Risk Factors

■ Associations between selective serotonin reuptake inhibitors (SSRIs; venlafaxine) and non-congenital heart disease (CHD) birth defects

Incidence

■ Unknown; most result in spontaneous abortion in early pregnancy

■ Occurs more in females than males

■ Solitary midline closure defects are more prevalent in babies with trisomy 18 (du Plessis & Volpe, 2018; Tobin et al., 2019)

Pathophysiology

■ Total failure of primary neurulation very early; results in no closure and exposure of the entire neural plate, absent brain and skull, open vertebra column

Prognosis

■ Death, either spontaneous abortion, stillbirth, or soon after delivery (Alghamdi et al., 2017; Anderson et al., 2020; Dong et al., 2020; du Plessis & Volpe, 2018; Gayathri et al., 2016; Guerrero et al., 2020; Juriloff et al., 2018; Orphanet, 2010; Schoenwolf et al., 2015)

REFERENCES

Alghamdi, M. A., Ziermann, J. M., Gregg, L., & Diogo, R. (2017). A detailed musculoskeletal study of a fetus with anencephaly and spina bifida (craniorachischisis), and comparison with other cases of human congenital malformations. *Journal of Anatomy, 230*(6), 842–858. https://doi.org/10.1111/joa.12601

Anderson, K. N., Lind, J. N., Simeone, R. M., Bobo, W. V., Mitchell, A. A., Riehle-Colarusso, T., Polen, K. N., & Reefhuis, J. (2020). Maternal use of specific antidepressant medications during early pregnancy and the risk of selected birth defects. *JAMA Psychiatry, 77*(12), 1246–1255. https://doi.org/10.1001/jamapsychiatry.2020.2453

Dong, N., Gu, H., Liu, D., Wei, X., Ma, W., Ma, L., Liu, Y., Wang, Y., Jia, S., Huang, J., Wang, C., He, X., Huang, T., He, Y., Zhang, Q., An, D., Bai, Y., & Yuan, Z. (2020). Complement factors and alpha-fetoprotein as biomarkers for noninvasive prenatal diagnosis of neural tube defects. *Annals of the New York Academy of Sciences, 1478*(1), 75–91. https://doi.org/10.1111/nyas.14443

du Plessis, A. J. & Volpe, J. J. (2018). Neural tube development. In J. J. Volpe, T. E. Inder, B. T. Darras, L. S. deVries, A. J. du Plessis, & J. M. Perlman (Eds.), *Volpe's neurology of the newborn* (6th ed., pp. 3–33). Elsevier.

Gayathri, P., Saritha, S., Nagajyothi1, D., Ramani, T. V., & Himabindu, N. (2016). A fetal study of craniorachischisis, with emphasis on prenatal diagnosis and prevention. *Journal of Medical Science and Clinical Research, 4*(4), 10140–10145. https://doi.org/10.18535/jmscr/v4i4.27

Guerrero, J., Heller, D. S., & de Leon, A. B. (2020). Craniorachischisis with exencephaly. *Fetal and Pediatric Pathology*, 1–4. https://doi.org/10.1080/15513815.2020.1716282

Juriloff, D. M., & Harris, M. J. (2018). Insights into the etiology of mammalian neural tube closure defects from developmental, genetic and evolutionary studies. *Journal of Developmental Biology, 6*(3), 22. https://doi.org/10.3390/jdb6030022

Orphanet. (2010). *Craniorachischisis.* https://www.orpha.net/consor/cgi-bin/Disease_Search .php?lng=EN&data_id=10817&disease=Craniorachischisis&search=Disease_Search _Simple

Schoenwolf, G. C., Bleyl, S. B., Brauer, P. R., & Francis-West, P. H. (2015). *Larsen's human embryology* (5th ed.). Elsevier Saunders.

Tobin, M., Gunaji, R., Walsh, J. C., & Grice, G. P. (2019). A review of genetic factors underlying craniorachischisis and omphalocele: Inspired by a unique trisomy 18 case. *American Journal of Medical Genetics Part A, 179*(8), 1642–1651. https://doi.org/10.1002/ajmg.a.61255

ANENCEPHALY

Risk Factors

■ Genetic predisposition accounts for most of the risk of neural tube defects (NTDs), and genes that regulate folate one-carbon metabolism and planar cell polarity have been strongly implicated.

■ Environmental factors also appear to be involved in the development of anencephaly; many of these infants have other anomalies (Copp et al., 2013; du Plessis & Volpe, 2018; Gole et al., 2014).

■ Increase risk with low socioeconomic status and history of affected siblings.

■ More common in White patients

■ More common in females

Incidence

■ Occurs in 0.28 out of 1,000 live births in the United States

■ Prior to folic acid fortification: 2.5 per 1,000 live births worldwide

■ After universal folic acid fortification: 0.5 per 1,000 live births worldwide

■ Seventy-five percent are stillborn (Cook et al., 2008; Danzer et al., 2017; du Plessis & Volpe, 2018; Gole et al., 2014; Gressens & Huppi, 2015; Huang & Doherty, 2018; Kancherla & Black, 2018; Kancherla et al., 2020; Pfeiffer et al., 2019; Yuskaitis & Pomeroy, 2017)

Pathophysiology

■ Anencephaly occurs when the neural tube fails to close anteriorly during primary neurulation. It most commonly involves the forebrain and variable amounts of the upper brainstem. Because the anterior neural tube forms the forebrain, failure of fusion causes minimal development of brain tissue (cerebrum, cerebellum, brainstem, and spinal cord). The brain tissue that does develop is poorly differentiated and becomes necrotic with exposure to amniotic fluid. In this defect, much of the posterior skull is missing.

■ Anencephaly begins within the first 24 to 26 days of gestation (du Plessis & Volpe, 2018; Huang & Doherty, 2018; Kancherla et al., 2020; Pfeiffer et al., 2019).

Clinical Manifestations

■ Exposed neural tissue

Diagnosis

■ Amniotic fluid reveals high levels of maternal serum alpha-fetoprotein (MSAFP) in the first trimester.

■ The primary screening test for the detection of fetal structural abnormalities including open/closed NTDs (anencephaly, encephalocele, spina bifida) is a second-trimester anatomical ultrasound with detailed fetal intracranial and spinal imaging and assessment. Prenatal detection of anencephaly by ultrasound is possible in almost 100% of cases.

■ It is apparent upon visual inspection after birth (American College of Obstetricians and Gynecologists [ACOG], 2017; Cameron & Moran, 2009; Cavalheiro et al., 2017; Johnson et al., 1997).

Treatment/Management

■ Prevention: Folic acid was proven in 1991 to prevent most cases of spina bifida and anencephaly.

- ● In 1998, the United States mandated fortification of enriched cereal grain products (Williams et al., 2015).

- ● In 2008, less than 10% of folic acid–preventable spina bifida and anencephaly (FAPSBA) was prevented through folic acid fortification programs. The proportion of FAPSBA prevented globally with various types of folic acid fortification as of 2012 is estimated to be 25% (Youngblood et al., 2013).

■ Management of infants with anencephaly is supportive, involving provision of warmth and comfort until the infant dies.

■ Families require emotional support and assistance in coping with their grief over the birth of an infant with a defect and the death of their infant (Blackburn, 2018).

Prognosis

■ Seventy-five percent of anencephalic infants are stillborn.

■ Live-borns die in the first days or month of life, generally by the end of the 1st week (Ditzenberger & Blackburn, 2020; du Plessis & Volpe, 2018; Huang & Doherty, 2018; Kancherla et al., 2020; Pfeiffer et al., 2019).

REFERENCES

American College of Obstetricians and Gynecologists, Committee on Practice Bulletins-Obstetrics. (2017). Practice bulletin no.187: Neural tube defects. *Obstetrics and Gynecology, 130*(6), e279–e290. https://doi.org/10.1097/AOG.0000000000002412

Blackburn, S. T. (2018). *Maternal, fetal and neonatal physiology: A clinical perspective* (5th ed.). Elsevier.

Cameron, M., & Moran, P. (2009). Prenatal screening and diagnosis of neural tube defects. *Prenatal Diagnosis, 29*(4), 402–411. https://doi.org/10.1002/pd.2250

Cavalheiro, S., da Costa, M. D. S., Moron, A. F., & Leonard J. (2017). Comparison of prenatal and postnatal management of patients with myelomeningocele. *Neurosurgical Clinics of North America, 28*, 439–448. https://doi.org/10.1016/j.nec.2017.02.005

Cook, R. J., Erdman, J. N., Hevia, M., & Dickens, B. M. (2008). Prenatal management of anencephaly. *International Journal of Gynaecology & Obstetrics, 102*(3), 304–308. https://doi.org/10.1016/j.ijgo.2008.05.002

Copp, A. J., Stanier, P., & Greene, N. E. (2013). Neural tube defects: Recent advances, unsolved questions, and controversies. *Lancet Neurology, 12*(8), 799–810. https://doi.org/10.1016/S1474-4422(13)70110-8

Danzer, E., Rintoul, N. E., & Adzick, N. S. (2017). Pathophysiology of neural tube defect. In R. A. Polin, S. H. Abram, D. H. Rowitch, W. E. Benita, & W. W. Fox (Eds.), *Fetal and neonatal physiology* (5th ed., pp. 1724–1732). Elsevier Saunders.

Ditzenberger, G. R., & Blackburn, S. T. (2020). Neurologic system. In C. Kenner, L. B. Altimer, & M. V. Boykova (Eds.), *Comprehensive neonatal nursing care* (6th ed., pp. 373–416). Springer Publishing Company.

du Plessis, A. J., & Volpe, J. J. (2018). Neural tube development. In J. J. Volpe, T. E. Inder, B. T. Darras, L. S. deVries, A. J. du Plessis, & J. M. Perlman (Eds.), *Volpe's neurology of the newborn* (6th ed., pp. 3–33). Elsevier.

Gole, R. A., Meshram, P. M., & Hattangdi, S. S. (2014). Anencephaly and its associated malformations. *Journal of Clinical and Diagnostic Research, 8*(9), AC07–AC9. https://doi .org/10.7860/JCDR/2014/10402.4885

Gressens, P., & Huppi, P. S. (2015). The central nervous system, part 1: Normal and abnormal brain development. In R. J. Martin, A. A. Fanaroff, & M. C. Walsh (Eds.), *Neonatal and perinatal medicine: Diseases of the fetus and infant* (10th ed.). Mosby/Elsevier.

Huang, S. B., & Doherty, D. (2018). Congenital malformations of the central nervous system. In C. A. Gleason & S. E. Juul (Eds.), *Avery's diseases of the newborn* (10th ed., pp. 857–878). Elsevier.

Johnson, D. D., Pretorius, D. H., Riccabona, M., Budorick, N. E., & Nelson, T. R. (1997). Three-dimensional ultrasound of the fetal spine. *Obstetrics & Gynecology, 89*, 434–438. https://doi.org/10.1007/s00247-015-3441-6

Kancherla, V., & Black, R. E. (2018). Historical perspective on folic acid and challenges in estimating global prevalence of neural tube defects. *Annals of the New York Academy of Sciences, 1414*, 20–30. https://doi.org/10.1111/nyas.13601

Kancherla, V., Wagh, K., Pachón, H., & Oakley, G. P., Jr. (2020). A 2019 global update on folic acid-preventable spina bifida and anencephaly. *Birth Defects Research, 113*, 77–98. https://doi.org/10.1002/bdr2.1835

Pfeiffer, C. M., Sternberg, M. R., Zhang, M., Fazili, Z., Storandt, R. J., Crider, K. S., Yamini, S., Gahche, J. J., Juan, W., Wang, C.-Y., Potischman, N., Williams, J., & LaVoie, D. J. (2019). Folate status in the US population 20 y after the introduction of folic acid fortification. *American Journal of Clinical Nutrition, 110*(5), 1088–1097. https://doi.org/10.1093/ajcn/nqz184

Williams, J., Mai, C. T., Mulinare, J., Isenburg, J., Flood, T. J., Ethen, M., Frohnert, B., & Kirby, R. S. (2015). Updated estimates of neural tube defects prevented by mandatory folic acid fortification—United States, 1995–2011. *Morbidity and Mortality Weekly Report, 64*(1), 1–5. https://www.cdc.gov/mmwr/preview/mmwrhtml/mm6401a2.htm

Youngblood, M. E., Williamson, R., Bell, K. N., Johnson, Q., Kancherla, V., & Oakley, G. J. (2013). 2012 Update on global prevention of folic acid-preventable spina bifida and anencephaly. *Birth Defects Research Part A Clinical and Molecular Teratology, 97*(10), 658–663. https://doi.org/10.1002/bdra.23166

Yuskaitis, C. J., & Pomeroy, S. L. (2017). Development of the nervous system. In R. A. Polin, S. H. Abram, D. H. Rowitch, W. E. Benita, & W. W. Fox (Eds.), *Fetal and neonatal physiology* (5th ed., pp. 1294–1313). Elsevier.

ENCEPHALOCELE

Risk Factors

■ Environmental and genetic factors

Incidence

■ Occurs in between 0.8 to 5.6 per 10,000 live births

■ Occurs in association with chromosomal abnormalities, such as trisomy 13, 18, and 21; Meckel–Gruber syndrome; or Walker–Warburg syndrome

- Seventy percent occurs in males
- Most result in spontaneous abortion (du Plessis & Volpe, 2018; Markovic, 2020; Tse et al., 2020)

Anatomy and Physiology

- Encephalocele is a congenital anomaly in which intracranial structures (brain tissue, meninges, and cerebrospinal fluid [CSF]) protrude out of the cranium.

Pathophysiology

- Encephaloceles form within the first 24 to 26 days of gestation.
- Encephaloceles not only arise from the failure of closure of the anterior portion of the neural tube in restricted areas but are also possibly post-closure defects.
- Between 70% and 80% occur in the occipital region.
- Less commonly, it occurs in the frontal, temporal, or parietal regions.
- Hydrocephalus is a common complication, occurring at birth or developing after the repair of the encephalocele (Demir et al., 2014; Ditzenberger & Blackburn, 2020; du Plessis & Volpe, 2018; Gressens & Huppi, 2015; Huang & Doherty, 2018; Marinho et al., 2020; Tse et al., 2020).

Clinical Manifestations

- Protruding midline skin-covered sac is observed from the head or base of the neck.
- The protruding sac may vary greatly in size; the size of the defect does not always correlate with the presence of neural tissue and is connected to the central nervous system (CNS) by a narrow stalk.
- Majority of sacs occur in the occipital region (Ditzenberger & Blackburn, 2020; Gressens & Huppi, 2015).

Diagnosis

- Second-trimester intrauterine ultrasonography
- Cranial ultrasonography
- CT scan
- MRI (Ditzenberger & Blackburn, 2020; Marinho et al., 2020; Markovic et al., 2020)

Treatment/Management

- Maintain normal body temperature.

■ If the defect is covered by skin, surgery is delayed pending a full evaluation.

■ If the sac is leaking CSF at birth, immediate surgical repair is necessary.

■ Insert a ventriculoperitoneal (VP) shunt if a hydrocephalus is present.

■ Treat seizure activity.

■ Prevent infection.

■ Position infant to avoid pressure on the defect.

■ Postoperative management: assessment of ventilation and perfusion, comfort measures, monitoring of neurologic and motor function, promotion of normothermia, prevention of infection, positioning to prevent pressure on the operative site, and monitoring of the site for CSF leakage

■ Support family with initial and continuing support and counseling.

■ Discharge teaching includes skin care, positioning, exercises, handling and feeding techniques, and activities to promote growth and development.

Prognosis

■ Mortality rate and later outcome are significantly better for infants with anterior defects than for those with posterior defects.

■ Prognosis is poor if significant brain tissue is contained within the sac (Back & Plawner, 2012; Blackburn, 2018; Ditzenberger & Blackburn, 2020; Huang & Doherty, 2018; Markovic et al., 2020; Wang et al., 2014).

REFERENCES

Back, S., & Plawner, L. L. (2012). Congenital malformations of the central nervous system. In H. W. Taeusch, R. A. Ballard, & C. A. Gleason (Eds.), *Avery's diseases of the newborn* (9th ed., pp. 844–867). Elsevier/Saunders.

Blackburn, S. T. (2018). *Maternal, fetal and neonatal physiology: A clinical perspective* (5th ed.). Elsevier.

Demir, S., Demir, B., Demir, F., Bingöl, G., Kaya, E., Balsak, D., & Sakar, M. N. (2014). Encephalocele: A case report. *Perinatal Journal/Perinatoloji Dergisi, 22*, SE18. https://www.perinataljournal.com/Files/Archive/en-US/Articles/PJ-918d9e1b-4722-4b42-b57e-60169feddf36.pdf

Ditzenberger, G. R., & Blackburn, S. T. (2020). Neurological system. In C. Kenner, L. B. Altimier, & M. V. Boykova (Eds.), *Comprehensive neonatal nursing care* (6th ed., pp. 373–416). Springer Publishing Company.

du Plessis, A. J., & Volpe, J. J. (2018). Neural tube development. In J. J. Volpe, T. E. Inder, B. T. Darras, L. S. deVries, A. J. du Plessis, & J. M. Perlman (Eds.), *Volpe's neurology of the newborn* (6th ed., pp. 3–33). Elsevier.

Gressens, P., & Huppi, P. S. (2015). The central nervous system, part 1: Normal and abnormal brain development. In R. J. Martin, A. A. Fanaroff, & M. C. Walsh (Eds.), *Neonatal and perinatal medicine: Diseases of the fetus and infant* (10th ed.). Mosby/Elsevier.

Huang, S. B., & Doherty, D. (2018). Congenital malformations of the central nervous system. In C. A. Gleason & S. E. Juul (Eds.), *Avery's diseases of the newborn* (10th ed., pp. 857–878). Elsevier.

Marinho, M., Lourenço, C., Nogueira, R., & Valente, F. (2020). Prenatal diagnosis of frontal encephalocele. *Journal of Clinical Ultrasound: JCU, 48*(9), 557–559. https://doi.org/10.1002/jcu.22848

Markovic, I., Bosnjakovic, P., & Milenkovic, Z. (2020). Occipital encephalocele: Cause, incidence, neuroimaging and surgical management. *Current Pediatric Reviews, 16*(3), 200–205. https://doi.org/10.2174/1573396315666191018161535

Tse, G. T., Frydman, A. S., O'Shea, M. F., Fitt, G. J., Weintrob, D. L., Murphy, M. A., Fabinyi, G. C., Bulluss, K. J., Cook, M. J., & Berkovic, S. F. (2020). Anterior temporal encephaloceles: Elusive, important, and rewarding to treat. *Epilepsia, 61*(12), 2675–2684. https://doi.org/10.1111/epi.16729

Wang, J., Amin, A., Jallo, G., & Ahn, E. (2014). Ventricular reservoir versus ventriculosubgaleal shunt for posthemorrhagic hydrocephalus in preterm infants: Infection risks and ventriculoperitoneal shunt rate. *Journal of Neurosurgery: Pediatrics, 14*(5), 447–454. https://doi.org/10.3171/2014.7.PEDS13552

SPINA BIFIDA

Risk Factors

■ Family history exists of a previous pregnancy resulting in an NTD

■ Women with insulin-dependent diabetes

■ Maternal obesity may be a risk factor as a result of hyperinsulinemia

■ Maternal folic acid deficiency before conception and in early pregnancy

■ Maternal malabsorption may result in nutritional deficiencies

■ Lower socioeconomic groups (Cao et al., 2020; Centers for Disease Control and Prevention [CDC], 2020; Ditzenberger & Blackburn, 2020; DeMarco et al., 2011; Kancherla et al., 2020; Pfeiffer et al., 2019)

Incidence

■ Spina bifida occulta is estimated to occur in 3% to 20% of the normal population.

■ Spina bifida cystica occurs in approximately one in 1,000 live births.

■ Myelomeningocele (MMC) occurs in approximately 0.3 to 0.72 per 1,000 births.

■ Higher incidence in White than Black ethnicity

■ Higher incidence in women less than 20 years of age and greater than 35 years of age (Cavalheiro et al., 2017; CDC, 2020; S. Liu et al., 2019; Moore et al., 2020)

Anatomy and Physiology

Spina bifida is a defect in caudal neurulation associated with malformations of the spinal cord and vertebrae. The two major forms are spina bifida cystica (failure of closure of the caudal portion of the neural tube during primary neurulation) and spina bifida occulta (alterations in secondary neurulation).

■ Spina bifida occulta: a vertebral defect at L5 or S1 arising from failure of the vertebral arch to grow and fuse between 5 weeks' gestation and the early fetal period. The dermal layer is intact over the vertebral defect; occasionally, the defect is indicated by a dimple, lipoma, or tuft of hair. Many are unrecognized due to minimal/no physical problems arising from the presence of this defect.

■ Spina bifida cystica: a cystic sac containing meninges or spinal cord elements, or both, along with vertebral defects. The level of the impairment of the spinal cord determines the severity of the neurologic deficit with impairment of nerve tissues below the sac. If the sac is covered with meninges, there is a risk of rupture and leakage of CSF during delivery with the risk of infection and dehydration.

● Occurs anywhere along the spinal column; seen most often in lumbar or lumbosacral area

● Three main forms: meningocele, MMC (most common), and myeloschisis

• Meningocele: sac containing meninges and CSF; spinal cord and nerve roots in normal position.

— Not typically associated with neurologic deficits

• Meningomyelocele (or MMC): In this type, CNS cord tissue extends into the meningocele sac. This is the most significant and common type, accounting for 94% of cases.

— Approximately 75% of MMC have a lumbar localization (thoracolumbar, lumbar, or lumbosacral).

— Hydrocephalus is present in 70% of cases, especially when the lumbar region is involved.

— Chiari II malformation is almost always present in lumbar MMC.

• Myeloschisis (limited dorsal myeloschisis): severe defect; no cystic covering; spinal cord open and exposed.

— Poor prognosis; significant neurologic deficits; many die of sepsis in neonatal period.

— If limited dorsal myeloschisis, may have a more favorable functional prognosis (Blackburn, 2018; Cavalheiro et al., 2017; Ditzenberger & Blackburn, 2020; du Plessis & Volpe, 2018; Eibach et al., 2017; Gressens & Huppi, 2015; Gressens et al., 2020; Hills & Tomei, 2020; Moore et al., 2020; Russell et al., 2012; Sandler, 2010).

Assessment/Clinical Manifestations

■ Lesions that are usually apparent at birth

■ Often altered lower extremity tone and activity; may assume a froglike posture

■ If bowel and bladder involved, dribbling of urine and feces

■ Frequently associated with Arnold-Chiari malformation type II (alterations of lower portion of brain) with noncommunicating hydrocephalus

■ Monitor for associated anomalies including renal dysfunction, as well as cardiac, intestinal, orthopedic, and other neurologic anomalies

Diagnosis

■ Prenatal ultrasound

■ MSAFP

■ Amniocentesis

■ Prenatal MRI

■ Ultrasonography, CT, or MRI can be used to determine the size of the ventricular system, to rule out Chiari type II malformation, and to monitor ventricular status and the development of hydrocephalus (Blackburn, 2018; Ditzenberger & Blackburn, 2020; du Plessis & Volpe, 2018; Gressens & Huppi, 2015; Moore et al., 2020; Sandler, 2010)

Treatment/Management

■ Immediate management for spina bifida includes:

- ● Stabilize in delivery room: prevent trauma to or infection of sac and contents
- ● Provide warmth and hydration and monitor fluid and electrolyte status
- ● Latex-free environment

■ Immediate closure of meningomyelocele for most infants; reduces infection risk, improves prognosis by reducing further deterioration of the spinal cord and nerve tracts; facilitates caregiving

■ Multidisciplinary follow-up: neurologic, urologic, orthopedic, psychologic

■ In utero repair of MMC, performed before 26 weeks' gestation, has been reported with mixed results to reduce the need for postnatal shunting, improve motor outcomes, and reduce postnatal complications, such as hindbrain herniation, hydrocephalus, and urologic dysfunction (Adzick et al., 2011; Danzer et al., 2012; Ditzenberger & Blackburn, 2020; Hockley & Salanki, 2009; Kelly & Sussman, 2017; NIOSH, 2020; Piatt, 2010)

Specific Nursing Care (In Addition to Generalized Nursing Care)

■ Monitor signs of infection, including signs of sepsis or meningitis and localized infection, including redness or discharge from the sac.

■ Provide comfort measures, including gentle handling, pacifiers, sucrose, and medications as ordered.

■ Position prone or on the side to reduce tension on the sac.

■ Change position from prone to side-lying or side to side.

■ Provide range-of-motion exercises; this prevents skin breakdown and contractures.

■ Keep lumbar/sacral defects free of fecal or urine contamination.

- Observe the timing and characteristics of urination and stool excretion: help determine degree of deficit.

■ Provide meticulous skin care.

■ Provide family teaching regarding skin care, positioning, exercises, handling, and feeding techniques, as well as provision of activities to promote development.

■ Coordinate multidisciplinary follow-up and care to deal with neurologic, urologic, orthopedic, and psychologic problems.

■ Provide "Guidelines for the Care of People With Spina Bifida" to families of infants with spina bifida (Dicianno et al., 2020; Kritikos et al., 2020)

■ Provide "Spina Bifida Mental Health Guidelines" to families of infants with spina bifida (Dicianno et al., 2020; Ditzenberger & Blackburn, 2020; Hills & Tomei, 2020; Kritikos et al., 2020; Lo et al., 2020)

Prognosis

■ Varies with the level and severity of the defect.

■ Prognosis of infants with meningomyelocele has improved with the current early and aggressive treatment of infants without major cerebral lesions, hemorrhage, infection, high spinal cord lesions, or advanced hydrocephalus.

■ After fetal surgeries, 79% of infants at 10 years of age were community ambulators, 14% wheelchair dependent, and 26% had normal bladder function (Danzer et al., 2016).

■ At risk for mental health concerns (Kritikos et al., 2020)

■ Head circumference ≥38 cm at birth is a significant risk factor for shunt revision (Protzenko et al., 2019).

■ Main causes of morbidity and mortality in patients with MMC are shunt failures and repeated UTIs (Danzer et al., 2016; Ditzenberger & Blackburn, 2020; du Plessis & Volpe, 2018; Kritikos et al., 2020; Protzenko et al., 2019; Thompson, 2009)

REFERENCES

Adzick, N. S., Thom, E. A., Spong, C. Y., Brock, J. W., Burrows, P. K., Johnson, M. P., & Farmer, D. L. (2011). A randomized trial of prenatal versus postnatal repair of myelomeningocele. *New England Journal of Medicine, 364*(11), 993–1004. https://doi.org/10.1056/NEJMoa1014379

Blackburn, S. T. (2018). *Maternal, fetal and neonatal physiology: A clinical perspective* (5th ed.). Elsevier.

Cao, S., Reece, E. A., Shen, W.-B., & Yang, P. (2020). Restoring BMP4 expression in vascular endothelial progenitors ameliorates maternal diabetes-induced apoptosis and neural tube defects. *Cell Death & Disease, 11*(10), 859. https://doi.org/10.1038/s41419-020-03078-5

Cavalheiro, S., da Costa, M. D. S., Moron, A. F., & Leonard, J. (2017). Comparison of prenatal and postnatal management of patients with myelomeningocele. *Neurosurgery Clinics of North America, 28*, 439–448. https://doi.org/10.1016/j.nec.2017.02.005

Centers for Disease Control and Prevention. (2020). *Facts about microcephaly.* https://www .cdc.gov/ncbddd/birthdefects/microcephaly.html

Danzer, E., Johnson, M. P., & Adzick, N. S. (2012). Fetal surgery for myelomeningocele: Progress and perspectives. *Developmental Medicine & Child Neurology, 54*(1), 8–14. https://doi.org/10.1111/j.1469-8749.2011.04049.x

Danzer, E., Thomas, N. H., Thomas, A., Friedman, K. B., Gerdes, M., Koh, J., Adzick, N. S., & Johnson, M. P. (2016). Long-term neurofunctional outcome, executive functioning, and behavioural adaptive skills following fetal myelomeningocele surgery. *American Journal of Obstetrics and Gynecology, 214*(2), 269.e1–269.e8. https://doi.org/10.1016/j.ajog.2015.09.094

De Marco, P., Merello, E., Calevo, M. G., Mascelli, S., Pastorino, D., Crocetti, L., De Biasio, P., Piatelli, G., Cama, A., & Capra, V. (2011). Maternal periconceptional factors affect the risk of spina bifida-affected pregnancies: An Italian case-control study. *Child's Nervous System ,* 27(7), 1073–1081. https://doi.org/10.1007/s00381-010-1372-y

Dicianno, B. E., Beierwaltes, P., Dosa, N., Raman, L., Chelliah, J., Struwe, S., Panlener, J., & Brei, T. J. (2020). Scientific methodology of the development of the Guidelines for the Care of People With Spina Bifida: An initiative of the Spina Bifida Association. *Disability and Health Journal, 13*(2), 100816. https://doi.org/10.1016/j.dhjo.2019.06.005

Ditzenberger, G. R., & Blackburn, S. T. (2020). Neurologic system. In C. Kenner, L. B. Altimer, & M. V. Boykova (Eds.), *Comprehensive neonatal nursing care* (6th ed., pp. 373–416). Springer Publishing Company.

du Plessis, A. J., & Volpe, J. J. (2018). Neural tube development. In J. J. Volpe, T. E. Inder, B. T. Darras, L. S. deVries, A. J. du Plessis, & J. M. Perlman (Eds.), *Volpe's neurology of the newborn* (6th ed., pp. 3–33). Elsevier.

Eibach, S., Moes, G., Zovickian, J., & Pang, D. (2017). Limited dorsal myeloschisis associated with dermoid elements. *Child's Nervous System, 33*(1), 55–67. https://doi.org/10.1007/s00381-016-3207-y

Gressens, P., & Huppi, P. S. (2015). The central nervous system, part 1: Normal and abnormal brain development. In R. J. Martin, A. A. Fanaroff, & M. C. Walsh (Eds.), *Neonatal and perinatal medicine: Diseases of the fetus and infant* (10th ed.). Mosby/Elsevier.

Gressens, P., Passemard, S., & Huppi, P. S. (2020). Normal and abnormal brain development. In R. J. Marttin, A. A. Fanaroff, & M. C. Walsh (Eds.), *Fanaroff and Martin's neonatal-perinatal medicine: Diseases of the fetus and infant* (11th ed., pp. 914–946). Elsevier.

Hills, B., & Tomei, K. (2020). Spinal dysraphisms. Normal and abnormal brain development. In R. J. Marttin, A. A. Fanaroff, & M. C. Walsh (Eds.), *Fanaroff and Martin's neonatal-perinatal medicine: Diseases of the fetus and infant* (11th ed., pp. 1073–1080). Elsevier.

Hockley, A. D., & Salanki, G. A. (2009). Surgical management of neural tube defects. In M. I. Levene & F. A. Chervenak (Eds.), *Fetal and neonatal neurology and neurosurgery* (4th ed., pp. 847–855). Churchill Livingstone/Elsevier.

Kancherla, V., Wagh, K., Pachón, H., & Oakley, G. P., Jr. (2020). A 2019 global update on folic acid-preventable spina bifida and anencephaly. *Birth Defects Research, 113*, 77. https://doi.org/10.1002/bdr2.1835

Kritikos, T. K., Smith, K., & Holmbeck, G. N. (2020). Mental health guidelines for the care of people with spina bifida. *Journal of Pediatric Rehabilitation Medicine, 13*(4), 525–534. https://doi.org/10.3233/PRM-200719

Liu, S., Evans, J., MacFarlane, A. J., Ananth, C. V., Little, J., Kramer, M. S., & Joseph, K. S. (2019). Association of maternal risk factors with the recent rise of neural tube defects in Canada. *Paediatric and Perinatal Epidemiology, 33*(2), 145–153. https://doi.org/10.1111/ppe.12543

Lo, W. B., Herbert, K., Rodrigues, D., & Afshari, F. T. (2020). The "transverse guard" wound dressing technique to reduce faecal contamination after spinal surgery in neonates and infants. *British Journal of Nursing*, 29(12), S12–S15. https://doi.org/10.12968/bjon.2020.29.12.S12

Moore, K. L., Persaud, T. V. N., & Torchia, M. G. (2020). *The developing human: Clinically oriented embryology* (11th ed.). Elsevier.

National Institute for Occupational Safety and Health. (2020). *Preventing allergic reactions to natural rubber latex in the workplace*. DHHS (NIOSH) Publication Number 97–135. https://www.cdc.gov/niosh/docs/97-135/

Piatt, J. H. (2010). Treatment of myelomeningocele: A review of outcomes and continuing neurosurgical considerations among adults. *Journal of Neurosurgery: Pediatrics*, 6(6), 515–525. https://doi.org/10.3171/2010.9.PEDS10266

Protzenko, T., Bellas, A., Pousa, M. S., Protzenko, M., Fontes, J. M., de Lima Silveira, A. M., Sá, C. A., Pereira, J. P., Salomão, R. M., Salomão, J. F. M., & Dos Santos Gomes, S. C. (2019). Reviewing the prognostic factors in myelomeningocele. *Neurosurgical Focus*, 47(4), E2. https://doi.org/10.3171/2019.7.FOCUS19462

Russell, N. E., Chalouhi, G. E., Desveaux, C., Benzina, N., Dirocco, F., Zerah, M., Millischer, A., Salomon, L. J., & Ville, Y. (2012). P19.16: Not all large neural tube defects have a poor prognosis: A case report of prenatally diagnosed limited dorsal myeloschisis. *Ultrasound in Obstetrics & Gynecology*, 40, 247–248. https://doi.org/10.1002/uog.12033

Sandler, A. D. (2010). Children with spina bifida: Key clinical issues. *Pediatric Clinics of North America*, 57(4), 879–892. https://doi.org/10.1016/j.pcl.2010.07.009

Thompson, D. N. P. (2009). Postnatal management and outcome for neural tube defects including spina bifida and encephalocoeles. *Prenatal Diagnosis*, 29(4), 412–419. https://doi.org/10.1002/pd.2199

DISORDERS OF PROENCEPHALIC DEVELOPMENT

BETH BROWN AND LESLIE B. ALTIMIER

Prosencephalic development, or ventral induction, involves early development of the brain and ventricular system, which occurs during the second to third month of gestation (peaking at 5–6 weeks). The brain develops from the cranial end of the neural tube, beginning at the end of the fourth week. During this period, the three primary brain bulges (or vesicles) and cavities are formed, after fusion of the neural folds in the cranial area. During prosencephalic development, the major event following neurulation results in the structures most recognizable as the essential form of the central nervous system (CNS). The primary brain bulges are the forebrain (prosencephalon), the midbrain (mesencephalon), and the hindbrain (rhombencephalon). The midbrain (mesencephalon) and the hindbrain (rhombencephalon) ultimately form the cerebral hemispheres and diencephalic structures (thalamus and hypothalamus; Ditzenberger & Blackburn, 2020; du Plessis & Volpe, 2018).

Malformations that occur during this period are thought to arise around the fifth to sixth weeks of gestation and occur during the period of prosencephalic formation development (aprosencephaly/atelencephaly), the period of prosencephalic cleavage (holoprosencephaly/holotelencephaly), or the period of midline prosencephalic development (agenesis of corpus callosum, agenesis of septum pel-lucidum, septo-optic dysplasia, or septo-optic-hypothalamic dysplasia). Infants with these anomalies have a poor prognosis, and many are lost in early pregnancy or are stillborn. Malformations of the forebrain include holoprosencephaly and holotelencephaly (Addissie et al., 2020; Petrikovsky et al., 2018).

Holoprosencephaly, holotelencephaly, congenital hydrocephaly, microcephaly, and facial anomalies may all be seen with disorders of proencephalic development (Back & Plawner, 2012; Ditzenberger & Blackburn, 2020; J. J. Volpe, 2008; P. Volpe et al., 2009).

HOLOPROSENCEPHALY

Risk Factors

■ Maternal diabetes mellitus

■ Trisomy 13 and 18

■ Twinning possibly due to cleavage disorders of the midline field

■ Alcohol consumption

■ Synthetic cannabinoids

■ Exposure to retinoic acid (Billington et al., 2015; Gabbay-Benziv et al., 2015; Gilbert et al., 2016; Hong & Krauss, 2017; Weber & Sebire, 2010)

Incidence

■ Holoprosencephaly is the most common human brain malformation.

■ Prevalence of one in 250 in the developing embryo

■ Occurs in one per 10,000 to 20,000 live births (Cohen, 1989; Summers et al., 2018; Yi et al., 2019)

Anatomy and Physiology

■ Abnormality in cleavage of the hemispheres that arises from genetic or possibly environmental alterations

■ Defect involves a variable degree of incomplete cleavage of the proencephalon along one or more of its three major planes (horizontal, transverse, and/or sagittal).

■ The spectrum includes alobar, semilobar, and lobar types, all of which have the unifying diagnostic feature of a single ventricular cerebral mass enclosed by a membrane; aplasia of the optic tract with absence of the olfactory tracts and bulbs; and agenesis of the corpus callosum (Addissie et al., 2020; Huang & Doherty, 2018; Moore et al., 2020).

Pathophysiology

■ Cyclopia (a single central eye) with a nose-like structure (proboscis) above the eye

■ Cebocephaly (a flattened single nostril situated centrally between the eyes)

■ Median cleft lip

■ Mildly affected infants may display a single central incisor or hypotelorism (Huang & Doherty, 2018; Kanekar et al., 2011)

Clinical Manifestations

■ Neurologic impairment (degree relates to severity of the cerebral malformation)

■ Apneic episodes in association with intractable seizures

■ Temperature instability and hypothermia

■ Hypernatremia or hyponatremia (diabetes insipidus, inappropriate secretion of antidiuretic hormone, or both)

■ Failure to thrive (impaired suck and swallow)

■ Abnormalities of other systems (cardiac, genitourinary, gastrointestinal)

■ Microcephaly is the norm.

■ Persistent primitive reflexes

■ Lack of social smile

Diagnosis

■ CT scan

■ MRI

Treatment/Management

■ Supportive and comfort measures

Prognosis

■ Survival correlates with the severity of the brain malformations.

■ Severely affected infants often are stillborn or rarely survive beyond the first year of life.

HOLOTELENCEPHALY

Parts of the brain that develop from the telencephalon form a single spheroid structure; the diencephalon and its derivatives are less affected.

Congenital hydrocephalus and agenesis of the corpus callosum can also occur.

Development of the face is associated with prosencephalic development of the CNS; consequently, alterations in brain development often result in facial malformations (Huang & Doherty, 2018; Kanekar et al., 2011).

Pathophysiology

■ Cyclopia (a single central eye) with a nose-like structure (proboscis) above the eye
■ Cebocephaly (a flattened single nostril situated centrally between the eyes)
■ Median cleft lip
■ Mildly affected infants may display a single central incisor or hypotelorism
■ Cyclopia (a single central eye) with a nose-like structure (proboscis) above the eye
■ Cebocephaly (a flattened single nostril situated centrally between the eyes)
■ Median cleft lip
■ Mildly affected infants may display a single central incisor or hypotelorism

Clinical Manifestations

■ Neurologic impairment (degree relates to severity of the cerebral malformation)
■ Apneic episodes in association with intractable seizures
■ Temperature instability and hypothermia
■ Hypernatremia or hyponatremia (diabetes insipidus, inappropriate secretion of antidiuretic hormone, or both)
■ Failure to thrive (impaired suck and swallow)
■ Abnormalities of other systems (cardiac, genitourinary, gastrointestinal)
■ Microcephaly is the norm
■ Persistent primitive reflexes
■ Lack of social smile

Diagnosis

■ CT scan
■ MRI

Treatment

■ Supportive and comfort measures

Prognosis

■ Survival correlates with the severity of the brain malformations.
■ Severely affected infants often are still born or rarely survive beyond the first year of life. (Gressens et al., 2020).

CONGENITAL HYDROCEPHALUS

At about 6 weeks' gestation, three critical events occur that are related to the formation and circulation of the cerebrospinal fluid (CSF): (a) development of secretory epithelium in the choroid plexus, (b) perforation of the roof of the fourth ventricle, and (c) formation of the subarachnoid space. Alterations in the second and third events give rise to a communicating form of hydrocephalus (Ditzenberger & Blackburn, 2020; du Plessis et al., 2018; Huang & Doherty, 2018; Kanekar et al., 2011).

Risk Factors

■ First-born newborns

■ Mothers utilizing antidepressants during the first trimester

■ Male gender, multiples, and maternal diabetes (Cao et al., 2020; Ditzenberger & Blackburn, 2020)

Incidence

■ Incidence depends on etiology of the hydrocephalus.

Anatomy and Physiology

■ Hydrocephalus, which is usually associated with neural tube defects (NTDs), develops as a result of outflow tract obstruction of the CSF from the ventricular system because of downward displacement of the brain.

■ Excess CSF in the ventricles of the brain occurs due to a decrease in reabsorption or overproduction.

■ Associated with ventriculomegaly (Ditzenberger & Blackburn, 2020; du Plessis et al., 2018; Huang & Doherty, 2018; Kanekar et al., 2011).

Pathophysiology

■ Excessive CSF production

■ Inadequate CSF absorption secondary to abnormal circulation

■ Excess ventricular CSF secondary

Clinical Manifestations

■ Large head

■ Widened sutures

■ Full (bulging) and tense fontanelles

■ Increased or increasing frontal-occipital circumference (FOC)

■ Setting-sun eyes

■ Vomiting, lethargy, irritability

■ Visible scalp veins

Diagnosis

■ Increase in FOC measurements

■ CT scan

■ Cranial ultrasonography

■ MRI

Treatment/Management

■ Maintain lumbar or ventricular pressure at approximately 5 cm H_2O while evaluating for shunt placement

■ Ventriculoperitoneal (VP) shunt

Prognosis

■ Poor outcomes are likely when cerebral decompression does not occur after VP shunt placement.

■ Motor and cognitive deficits are likely.

REFERENCES

Addissie, Y. A., Troia, A., Wong, Z. C., Everson, J. L., Kozel, B. A., Muenke, M., Lipinski, R. J., Malecki, K. M. C., & Kruszka, P. (2020). Identifying environmental risk factors and gene-environment interactions in holoprosencephaly. *Birth Defects Research, 113*, 63–76. https://doi.org/10.1002/bdr2.1834

Back, S., & Plawner, L. L. (2012). Congenital malformations of the central nervous system. In H. W. Taeusch, R. A. Ballard, & C. A. Gleason (Eds.), *Avery's diseases of the newborn* (9th ed., pp. 844–867). Elsevier.

Cao, S., Reece, E. A., Shen, W.-B., & Yang, P. (2020). Restoring BMP4 expression in vascular endothelial progenitors ameliorates maternal diabetes-induced apoptosis and neural tube defects. *Cell Death & Disease, 11*(10), 859. https://doi.org/10.1038/s41419-020-03078-5

Cohen, M. M., Jr. (1989). Perspectives on holoprosencephaly: Part I. Epidemiology, genetics, and syndromology. *Teratology, 40*, 211–235. https://doi.org/10.1002/tera.1420400304

Ditzenberger, G. R., & Blackburn, S. T. (2020). Neurological system. In C. Kenner, L. B. Altimier, & M. V. Boykova (Eds.), *Comprehensive neonatal nursing care* (6th ed., pp. 373–416). Springer Publishing Company.

du Plessis, A. J., & Volpe, J. J. (2018). Prosencephalic development. In J. J. Volpe, T. E. Inder, B. T. Darras, L. S. deVries, A. J. du Plessis, & J. M. Perlman (Eds.), *Volpe's neurology of the newborn* (6th ed., pp. 34–57). Elsevier.

Gressens, P., Passemard, S., & Huppi, P. S. (2020). Normal and abnormal brain development. In R. J. Marttin, A. A. Fanaroff, & M. C. Walsh (Eds.), *Fanaroff and Martin's neonatal-perinatal medicine: Diseases of the fetus and infant* (11th ed., pp. 914–946). Elsevier.

Huang, S. B., & Doherty, D. (2018). Congenital malformations of the central nervous system. In C. A. Gleason & S. E. Juul (Eds.), *Avery's diseases of the newborn* (10th ed., pp. 857–878). Elsevier.

Kanekar, S., Kaneda, H., & Shively, A. (2011). Malformations of dorsal induction. *Seminars in Ultrasound, CT, and MRI, 32*, 189–199. https://doi.org/10.1053/j.sult.2011.02.009

Moore, K. L., Persaud, T. V. N., & Torchia, M. G. (2020). *The developing human: Clinically oriented embryology* (11th ed.). Elsevier.

Petrikovsky, B. M., Cohen, H. L., & Cohen, D. (2018). Update on holoprosencephaly. *Neonatal Intensive Care, 31*(3), 24–26. https://www.nicmag.ca/pdf/NIC.31-3.Summer.2018.R13.pdf

Summers, A. D., Reefhuis, J., Taliano, J., & Rasmussen, S. A. (2018). Nongenetic risk factors for holoprosencephaly: An updated review of the epidemiologic literature. *American Journal of Medical Genetics Part C, Seminars in Medical Genetics, 178*(2), 151–164. https://doi .org/10.1002/ajmg.c.31614

Volpe, J. J. (2008). *Neurology of the newborn* (5th ed.). Saunders/Elsevier.

Volpe, P., Campobasso, G., De Robertis, V., & Rembouskos, G. (2009). Disorders of prosencephalic development. *Prenatal Diagnosis, 29*(4), 340–354. https://doi.org/10.1002/pd.2208

DISORDERS OF NEURONAL PROLIFERATION

BETH BROWN AND LESLIE B. ALTIMIER

Alterations in neuronal proliferation can lead to increases or decreases in the number and size of cells in the brain and associated structures. The actual number of neurons is determined early in gestation, because mature neurons cannot divide. Insults may alter the neuronal-glial stem cells, which reduce the number of neuronal or glial cells, or may alter cell growth, which result in smaller cells. The resulting disorders include micrencephaly, macrencephaly, and neurofibromatosis (Abuelo, 2007; Ditzenberger & Blackburn, 2020; Huang & Doherty, 2018; Olney, 2007; Poduri & Volpe, 2018).

MICRENCEPHALY

Risk Factors

■ Maternal:

- Viral infections (TORCH spectrum, rubella, cytomegalovirus, HIV, Zika)
- Exposure to radiation
- Metabolic conditions
  - Diabetes mellitus
  - Hyperphenylalaninemia in nonphenyl ketonuric infants
- Use of prescription and/or street drugs (alcohol, cocaine, etc.), especially in first trimester
- Genetic (autosomal recessive, autosomal dominant, X-linked, or translocation)
- Malnutrition is the most common etiology worldwide.

■ Fetal:

- Prenatal/perinatal insult: inflammation; hypoxia; birth trauma

■ Neonatal:

- Very-low-birthweight infant
- Hypoxic–ischemic encephalopathy (HIE)
- Nutrition: most common worldwide cause (Messinger et al., 2020; Rubin et al., 2016)

Incidence

■ Primary microcephalies are rare: less than one per 10,000 live births (Gressens et al., 2020).

Anatomy and Physiology

Micrencephaly is a disorder in which the primary defect is a marked reduction in the size of the brain or of the cerebral hemispheres. Microcephaly denotes a small cranial vault (defined as a frontal-occipital circumference [FOC] ≥2 standard deviations below the normative curves for age) that is associated with either micrencephaly or acquired brain atrophy. Micrencephaly arises from a decrease in size or number of neuronal-glial stem cell units. Small brain implies neurologic impairment.

Primary micrencephaly is impaired neuronal proliferation resulting in too few neurons. Secondary micrencephaly is due to destructive disease such as hypoxic ischemic, infectious, metabolic, or other destructive events that usually occur following completion of cerebral neuronal proliferation events near the end of the fourth month of gestation (Abuelo, 2007; Back & Plawner, 2012; Blackburn, 2018; Ditzenberger & Blackburn, 2020; Huang & Doherty, 2018; Inder & Volpe, 2018; Olney, 2007; Perlman & Volpe, 2018; Poduri & Volpe, 2018; Verklan & Walden, 2010; Volpe, 2008).

Pathophysiology

■ Neuronal proliferation defect

■ Occurs between 3 and 4 months' gestation

■ Destructive micrencephaly occurs when the normal brain suffers prenatal/perinatal insult.

Clinical Manifestations

■ Small head, backward sloping of the forehead, small cranial volume

■ Do not have marked neurologic deficits or seizures during neonatal period

■ Mental delays manifest later in infants

Diagnosis

■ Complete physical assessment with thorough neurologic assessment

■ Maternal history

■ CT scan or MRI

Treatment/Management

■ Record accurate measurement of FOC, length, and weight weekly (note percentiles)

■ Genetic counseling

■ Infectious disease consult

■ Supportive and comfort measures

Prognosis

■ Dependent on severity

■ Frequently associated with developmental delays

■ Intellectual disability (decreased ability to learn and function in daily life)

■ Problems with movement and balance

■ Feeding problems, such as difficulty swallowing

■ Hearing loss

■ Vision problems (Centers for Disease Control and Prevention [CDC], 2020)

MACRENCEPHALY

Excessive proliferation (macrencephaly) may have a familial base, occur with growth disturbances and chromosomal disorders, or have unknown causes. Macrencephaly results in a large brain size because of excessive proliferation of neuronal elements, nonneuronal elements, or a combination of both. It can affect one (hemimegalencephaly) or both hemispheres (symmetric megalencephaly). Like microcephaly, macrocephaly is a feature of a heterogeneous group of disorders in which the brain is generally well formed but unusually large (Blackburn, 2018; Ditzenberger & Blackburn, 2020; Huang & Doherty, 2018; Kanekar et al., 2011; Poduri & Volpe, 2018).

Risk Factors

■ Maternal:

● Genetic disorders

* Beckwith–Wiedemann syndrome

* Sturge–Weber syndrome

* Weaver syndrome

* Achondroplasia

● Chromosomal disorders

* Klinefelter and fragile X syndromes

* Partial trisomy of chromosome 7

● Multiple hemangiomas

● Neurocutaneous disorders

* Neurofibromatosis (autosomal-dominant genetic disorder involving excessive proliferation of nonneuronal elements in the central nervous system [CNS] and mesodermal structures of the body with cutaneous stigmata)

* Lipomas, hemangiomas, lymphangiomas, pseudopapilledema (Bannayan–Riley–Ruvalcaba)

* Asymmetric hypertrophy, hemangioma, varicosities (Klippel–Trénaunay–Weber)

- Asymmetric hypertrophy, telangiectatic lesions, flame nevus of the face
- Neurofibromatosis, "tuberous sclerosis," Sturge–Weber syndrome
- Epidermal nevus syndrome (Back & Plawner, 2012; Blackburn, 2018; Ditzenberger & Blackburn, 2020; Isaacs, 2010; Jett & Friedman, 2010; Kanekar et al., 2011; Poduri & Volpe, 2018; Volpe, 2008)
- Clinical manifestations include:
  - Altered skin pigmentation (café-au-lait macules)
  - Lisch nodules of the iris
  - Bupthalmos (enlarged eyeball)
  - Skin nodules
  - Multiple benign neurofibromas
  - Associated with learning disabilities
  - Skeletal abnormalities
  - Vascular disease
  - CNS tumors
  - Malignant peripheral nerve sheath tumors

Anatomy and Physiology

■ Macrencephaly refers to a diverse group of conditions characterized by a large brain size, believed to arise from excessive proliferation of neuronal elements, nonneuronal elements, or a combination of both. Macrencephaly manifests most commonly as an isolated finding in familial (autosomal dominant or autosomal recessive) and sporadic causes.

Pathophysiology

■ Neuronal proliferation defect
■ Occurs between 3 and 4 months' gestation

Clinical Manifestations

■ Large brain size—at birth, head circumference in 50% of cases is greater than 90th percentile.
■ Autosomal-dominant macrencephaly (macrocephaly in either parent) is generally associated with favorable outcome.
■ Autosomal-recessive inheritance is commonly associated with mental retardation and epilepsy.
■ Extracerebral fluid collections enlarge the subarachnoid spaces (rarely requires shunt; Alvarez et al., 1986).

Diagnosis

■ Complete physical assessment with thorough neurologic assessment

■ Parental history (macrocephaly in either parent)

■ CT scan or MRI

Treatment/Management

■ Record accurate measurement of FOC, length, and weight weekly (note percentiles)

■ Genetic counseling

■ Supportive and comfort measures

Prognosis

■ Dependent on severity

■ Frequently associated with developmental delays

NEUROFIBROMATOSIS

Anatomy and Physiology

Neurofibromatosis is an autosomal-dominant genetic disorder involving excessive proliferation of nonneuronal elements in the CNS and mesodermal structures of the body, with cutaneous stigmata.

Pathophysiology

■ Neuronal proliferation defect.

■ Occurs during gestation months 3 and 4; however, this time period may be prolonged in disorders of excessive proliferation.

■ Alternatively, abnormal proliferation may occur at the appropriate time during development but at an excessive rate.

Clinical Manifestations

■ Varies from no apparent neurologic deficit (autosomal dominant, isolated macrocephaly) to severe seizures (epilepsy) and intellectual disability (autosomal recessive, isolated macrocephaly, or unilateral macrocephaly)

■ Large brain size: at birth, head circumference >90th percentile in 50% of cases

■ Altered skin pigmentation (café-au-lait macules)

■ Forty percent of infants have more than five café-au-lait macules larger than 5 mm in diameter at birth.

■ Lisch nodules of the iris

- Bupthalmos (enlarged eyeball)
- Skin nodules
- Multiple benign neurofibromas
- Associated with learning disabilities
- Skeletal abnormalities
- Vascular disease
- CNS tumors
- Malignant peripheral nerve sheath tumors
- Other types of this disorder may have extraneural features (associated growth disorders and certain neurocutaneous syndromes; Aagaard et al., 2020; Blackburn, 2018; Jett & Friedman, 2010; Lalor et al., 2020; Poduri & Volpe, 2018)

Diagnosis

- Complete physical assessment with thorough neurologic assessment
- Parental history (macrocephaly in either parent)
- CT scan or MRI

Treatment/Management

- Record accurate measurement of FOC, length, and weight weekly (note percentiles)
- Genetic counseling
- Supportive and comfort measures

Prognosis

- Dependent on severity
- Frequently associated with developmental delays (Blackburn, 2018; Huang & Doherty, 2018; Kanekar et al., 2011; Poduri & Volpe, 2018)

REFERENCES

Aagaard, K., Matthiesen, N. B., Bach, C. C., Larsen, R. T., & Henriksen, T. B. (2020). Head circumference at birth and intellectual disability: A nationwide cohort study. *Pediatric Research, 87*(3), 595–601. https://doi.org/10.1038/s41390-019-0593-3

Abuelo, D. (2007). Microcephaly syndromes. *Seminars in Pediatric Neurology, 14*, 118–127. https://doi.org/10.1016/j.spen.2007.07.003

Alvarez, L. A., Maytal, J., & Shinnar, S. (1986). Idiopathic external hydrocephalus: Natural history and relationship to benign familial macrocephaly. *Pediatrics, 77*(6), 901–907. https://pediatrics.aappublications.org/content/77/6/901

Back, S., & Plawner, L. L. (2012). Congenital malformations of the central nervous system. In H. W. Taeusch, R. A. Ballard, & C. A. Gleason (Eds.), *Avery's diseases of the newborn* (9th ed., pp. 844–867). Elsevier/Saunders.

Blackburn, S. T. (2018). *Maternal, fetal and neonatal physiology: A clinical perspective* (5th ed.). Saunders/Elsevier Science.

Centers for Disease Control and Prevention. (2020). *Microcephaly.* https://www.cdc.gov/ncbddd/birthdefects/microcephaly.html

Ditzenberger, G. R., & Blackburn, S. T. (2020). Neurologic system. In C. Kenner, L. B. Altimier, & M. B. Boykova (Eds.), *Comprehensive neonatal nursing care* (6th ed., pp. 373–416). Springer Publishing Company.

Gressens, P., Passemard, S., & Huppi, P. S. (2020). Normal and abnormal brain development. In R. J. Marttin, A. A. Fanaroff, & M. C. Walsh (Eds.), *Fanaroff and Martin's neonatal-perinatal medicine: Diseases of the fetus and infant* (11th ed., pp. 914–94). Elsevier.

Huang, S. B., & Doherty, D. (2018). Congenital malformations of the central nervous system. In C. A. Gleason & S. E. Juul (Eds.), *Avery's diseases of the newborn* (10th ed., pp. 857–878). Elsevier.

Inder, T. E., & Volpe, J. J. (2018). Hypoxic-ischemic injury in the term infant: Clinical-neurological features, diagnosis, imaging, prognosis, therapy. In J. J. Volpe, T. E. Inder, B. T. Darras, L. S. deVries, A. J. du Plessis, & J. M. Perlman (Eds), *Volpe's neurology of the newborn* (6th ed., pp. 510–563). Elsevier.

Isaacs, H. (2010). Perinatal neurofibromatosis: Two case reports and review of the literature. *American Journal of Perinatology, 27,* 285–292. https://doi.org/10.1055/s-0029-1241737

Jett, K., & Friedman, J. M. (2010). Clinical and genetic aspects of neurofibromatosis. *Genetics in Medicine, 362,* 2185–2193. https://doi.org/10.1097/GIM.0b013e3181bf15e3

Kanekar, S., Kaneda, H., & Shively, A. (2011). Malformations of dorsal induction. *Seminars in Ultrasound, CT, and MRI, 32*(3), 189–199. https://doi.org/10.1053/j.sult.2011.02.009

Lalor, L., Davies, O. M. T., Basel, D., & Siegel, D. H. (2020). Café au lait spots: When and how to pursue their genetic origins. *Clinics in Dermatology, 38*(4), 421–431. https://doi.org/10.1016/j.clindermatol.2020.03.005

Messinger, C. J., Lipsitch, M., Bateman, B. T., He, M., Huybrechts, K. F., MacDonald, S., Mogun, H., Mott, K., & Hernández-Díaz, S. (2020). Association between congenital cytomegalovirus and the prevalence at birth of microcephaly in the United States. *JAMA Pediatrics, 174,* 1159–1167. https://doi.org/10.1001/jamapediatrics.2020.3009

Olney, A. H. (2007). Macrocephaly syndromes. *Seminars in Pediatric Neurology, 14*(3), 128–135. https://doi.org/10.1016/j.spen.2007.07.004

Perlman, J. M., & Volpe, J. J. (2018) Amino acids. In J. J. Volpe, T. E. Inder, B. T. Darras, L. S. deVries, A. J. du Plessis, & J. M. Perlman (Eds.), *Volpe's neurology of the newborn* (6th ed., pp. 763–792). Elsevier.

Poduri, A., & Volpe, J. J. (2018). Neuronal proliferation. In J. J. Volpe, T. E. Inder, B. T. Darras, L. S. deVries, A. J. du Plessis, & J. M. Perlman (Eds.), *Volpe's neurology of the newborn* (6th ed., pp. 100–119). Elsevier.

Rubin, E. J., Greene, M. F., & Baden, L. R. (2016). Zika virus and microcephaly. *New England Journal of Medicine, 374*(10), 984–985. https://doi.org/10.1056/NEJMe1601862

Verklan, M. T., & Walden, M. (2010). *Core curriculum for neonatal intensive care nursing* (4th ed.). Saunders, Elsevier.

Volpe, J. J. (2008). *Neurology of the newborn* (5th ed.). Saunders/Elsevier.

NEURONAL MIGRATION DISORDERS

BETH BROWN AND LESLIE B. ALTIMIER

■ Disorders of migration alter gyral development and lead to hypoplasia or agenesis of the corpus callosum. Gyral development is most dominant during the last 3 months of gestation with the most rapid increase between 26 and 28 weeks and enlarges from 15 to 34 weeks. Gyral development overlaps the end of the peak period for the neuronal migration stage, which occurs primarily from 12 to 20 weeks' gestation and most rapidly between 26 and 28 weeks of gestation in the cerebrum, and 16 to 20 weeks' gestation to 10 months postnatally in the cerebellum.

■ There are three distinctive layers of the brain that develop as the brain matures: the brainstem, limbic system, and cerebral cortex. The brainstem (medulla, cerebellum, pons) is first fashioned around the 33rd day of gestation and is nearly complete around the seventh month of gestation. The brainstem receives sensory messages and relays the information to the cerebral cortex. It processes vestibular sensations necessary for hearing, balance, vision, and focusing attention. It also regulates autonomic functions of internal organs, such as breathing, heartbeat, and digestion.

■ The limbic system (basal ganglia, hippocampus, amygdala, and hypothalamus) is located in the center of the brain.

■ The cognitive brain (cerebrum) is known as the cerebral cortex and performs the most complex organizing of sensory input. The cerebral cortex is highly specialized and contains specific areas for dealing with voluntary functions in the body. Although the neurologic system is one of the earliest systems to develop in the embryo, it is not fully matured until adulthood (Altimier & White, 2020; Blackburn, 2018; Ditzenberger & Blackburn, 2020; McQuillen & Ferriero, 2005; Oegema et al., 2020; Yuskaitis & Pomeroy, 2017).

Risk Factors

■ Maternal infections (cytomegalovirus infection or toxoplasmosis)

■ Maternal metabolic disorders (e.g., diabetes mellitus, phenylketonuria, hypothyroidism)

■ Trauma

■ Substance abuse (exposure to ethanol/cocaine)

■ Exposure to ionizing radiation (Gressens et al., 2020)

Incidence

■ More than 500 different diseases with neuronal migration disorder (NMD) are currently known (Schiller et al., 2020).

■ These are rare diseases with an estimated incidence of 1:100.000 to 1:250.000 newborns (Schiller et al., 2020).

Anatomy and Physiology

■ Neuronal migration forms the deepest layers of the cortex, progressing from the inside out (Gressens et al., 2020).

■ The period of early migration overlaps with the proliferative period, and the period of late migration overlaps with later cortical organization.

■ Neuronal migration is a series of events whereby millions of neurons move from their sites of origin in the ventricular and subventricular zones to the loci within the central nervous system (CNS), where they will reside for life. Timing and direction of these migrations must be highly ordered, and if not, disorders of neuronal migration can occur (Poduri & Volpe, 2018).

■ The peak period for the neuronal migration stage is 3 to 5 months gestation (most rapidly between 26 and 28 weeks of gestation) in the cerebrum and 4 months gestation to 10 months postnatally in the cerebellum (Yuskaitis & Pomeroy, 2017).

■ Timing and direction of these migrations must be highly ordered, and if not, disorders of neuronal migration can occur (Poduri & Volpe, 2018).

Pathophysiology

■ Disorders of neuronal migration usually cause overt disturbances of neuronal function.

■ Clinical deficits often appear within the first days of life.

■ Hallmark of migration disorders is the alteration of gyral development.

■ Common feature: hypoplasia or agenesis of the corpus callosum

■ Extremely premature newborns may be especially vulnerable to gyral alterations, as the formation of secondary and tertiary gyri occurs most rapidly at 26 and 28 weeks and enlarges from 15 to 34 weeks.

■ Many are genetic.

■ They include a wide spectrum of disorders with various phenotypical manifestations; classified based on visible morphologic anomalies of the cortex

● Lissencephaly spectrum (agyria, pachygyria, cobblestone)

• Agyria (no gyri), pachygyria (few gyri): thickened cortex with fewer than six layers and an absent or reduced formation of gyri and sulci

• Classical lissencephaly (type I lissencephaly)

• Cobblestone lissencephaly (type II lissencephaly)

● Polymicrogyria: Hypoplasia or agenesis of the corpus callosum; characterized by excessive number of small gyri and a disturbed cortical layering

● Schizencephaly: Extremely rare cortical malformation; cleft lined with dysplastic gray matter extending from the ependyma to the pia mater; sometimes only clefts filled with cerebrospinal fluid (CSF) are considered as schizencephaly

● Neuronal heterotopia: Gray matter heterotopias; band or nodules of neurons within the normally underlying white matter (Altimier & White, 2020; Blackburn, 2018; Braga et al., 2018; Gressens et al., 2020; Lasser et al., 2018; McQuillen & Ferriero, 2005; Moffat et al., 2015; Oegema et al., 2020; Parrini et al., 2016; Poduri & Volpe, 2018; Severino et al., 2020; Yuskaitis & Pomeroy, 2017)

■ Errors or exogenous insults before/after birth can alter migration of neurons and glial cells, resulting in:

● Hypoplasia or agenesis of the corpus callosum

● Agenesis/dysgenesis of a part of the cerebral wall (schizencephaly)

■ Inborn errors of metabolism (IEM) or errors of metabolism (EM): Accumulation of toxic intermediates, reduced ability to synthesize metabolites, or the defects in energy supply can severely interfere with the complex and finely tuned process of early brain development (Fleiss et al., 2018; Hutton et al., 2014; Juul et al., 2018; Poduri & Volpe, 2018; Schiller et al., 2020)

Clinical Manifestations

■ Severe psychomotor developmental delay

■ Severe intellectual disability

■ Intractable epilepsy or seizures

■ Dysmorphisms

■ Multiple developmental disorders (dyslexia, schizophrenia, autism spectrum disorders)

Diagnosis

■ Prenatal ultrasound

■ Fetal MRI

■ Early neonatal MRI

■ Magnetoencephalography

■ Magnetic resonance spectroscopy (MRS)

■ PET

■ PET fused with MRI (can provide data related to metabolic activity unique to neurometabolic diseases [NMDs])

■ Computational analysis (can detect subtle pathology in apparently unremarkable MR images)

■ Electroencephalography recordings with pattern recognition aids in diagnosis of lissencephaly

■ Genetic testing

■ Laboratory testing for infections

Treatment/Management

■ Record accurate measurement of occipital frontal circumference (OFC)

■ Genetic counseling

■ Supportive and comfort measures

Prognosis

■ Dependent on severity of NMD

● NMD with visible lesions on MR have better surgical outcomes.

■ Frequently associated with developmental delays (Boia et al., 2016; Dudink et al., 2015; Irwin et al., 2016; Jauhari et al., 2020; Kini et al., 2016; Pan et al., 2019; Roberts, 2018; Schiller et al., 2020; Shin et al., 2015)

REFERENCES

Altimier, L., & White, R. (2020). The neonatal intensive care unit (NICU) environment. In C. Kenner, L. B. Altimier, & M. V. Boykova (Eds.), *Comprehensive neonatal nursing care* (6th ed., pp. 713–726). Springer Publishing Company.

Blackburn, S. T. (2018). *Maternal, fetal and neonatal physiology: A clinical perspective* (5th ed.). Elsevier.

Boia, M., Cioboata, D., Doandes, F., Dobre, M.-C., Bilav, O., D. VL, & Manea, A. (2016). Clinical-imaging correlation and early diagnosis in brain malformations. *Jurnaul Pediatrului*, *19*(73/74), 19–25. http://www.jurnalulpediatrului.ro/archive/73-74/73-74-05.pdf

Braga, V. L., da Costa, M. D. S., Riera, R., Dos Santos Rocha, L. P., de Oliveira Santos, B. F., Matsumura Hondo, T. T., de Oliveira Chagas, M., & Cavalheiro, S. (2018). Schizencephaly: A review of 734 patients. *Pediatric Neurology*, *87*, 23–29. https://doi.org/10.1016/j.pediatrneurol.2018.08.001

Ditzenberger, G. R., & Blackburn, S. T. (2020). Neurological system. In C. Kenner, L. B. Altimier, & M. V. Boykova (Eds.), *Comprehensive neonatal nursing care* (6th ed., pp. 373–416). Springer Publishing Company.

Dudink, J., Pieterman, K., Leemans, A., Kleinnijenhuis, M., van Cappellen van Walsum, A. M., & Hoebeek, F. E. (2015). Recent advancements in diffusion MRI for investigating cortical development after preterm birth—Potential and pitfalls. *Frontiers in Human Neuroscience*, *8*, 1066. https://doi.org/10.3389/fnhum.2014.01066

Fleiss, B., Stolp, H., Metzger, V., & Gressens, P. (2018). Central nervous system development. In C. A. Gleason & S. E. Juul (Eds.), *Avery's diseases of the newborn* (10th ed., pp. 852–856). Elsevier.

Gressens, P., Passemard, S., & Huppi, P. S. (2020). Normal and abnormal brain development. In R. J. Marttin, A. A. Fanaroff, & M. C. Walsh (Eds.), *Fanaroff and Martin's neonatal-perinatal medicine: Diseases of the fetus and infant* (11th ed., pp. 914–946). Elsevier.

Hutton, L. C., Yan, E., Yawno, T., Castillo-Melendez, M., Hirst, J. J., & Walker, D. W. (2014). Injury of the developing cerebellum: A brief review of the effects of endotoxin and asphyxial challenges in the late gestation sheep fetus. *The Cerebellum*, *13*(6), 777–786. https://doi.org/10.1007/s12311-014-0602-3

Irwin, K., Henry, A., Gopikrishna, S., Taylor, J., & Welsh, A. W. (2016). Utility of fetal MRI for workup of fetal central nervous system anomalies in an Australian maternal-fetal medicine cohort. *Australian & New Zealand Journal of Obstetrics & Gynaecology*, *56*(3), 267–273. https://doi.org/10.1111/ajo.12440

Jauhari, P., Farmania, R., Chakrabarty, B., Kumar, A., & Gulati, S. (2020). Electrographic pattern recognition: A simple tool to predict clinical outcome in children with lissencephaly. *Seizure*, *83*, 175–180. https://doi.org/10.1016/j.seizure.2020.10.020

Juul, S. E., Fleiss, B., McAdams, R. M., & Gressens, P. (2018). Neuroprotection strategies for the newborn. In C. A. Gleason & S. E. Juul (Eds.), *Avery's diseases of the newborn* (10th ed., pp. 910–921). Elsevier.

Kini, L. G., Gee, J. C., & Litt, B. (2016). Computational analysis in epilepsy neuroimaging: A survey of features and methods. *NeuroImage Clinical*, *11*, 515–529. https://doi.org/10.1016/j.nicl.2016.02.013

Lasser, M., Tiber, J., & Lowery, L. A. (2018). The role of the microtubule cytoskeleton in neurodevelopmental disorders. *Frontiers in Cellular Neuroscience*, *12*, 165. https://doi.org/10.3389/fncel.2018.00165

McQuillen, P. S., & Ferriero, D. M. (2005). Perinatal subplate neuron injury: Implications for cortical development and plasticity. *Brain Pathology, 15*(3), 250–260. https://doi.org/10.1111/j.1750-3639.2005.tb00528.x

Moffat, J. J., Ka, M., Jung, E.-M., & Kim, W.-Y. (2015). Genes and brain malformations associated with abnormal neuron positioning. *Molecular Brain, 8,* 72. https://doi.org/10.1186/s13041-015-0164-4

Oegema, R., Barakat, T. S., Wilke, M., Stouffs, K., Amrom, D., Aronica, E., Bahi-Buisson, N., Conti, V., Fry, A. E., Geis, T., Andres, D. G., Parrini, E., Pogledic, I., Said, E., Soler, D., Valor, L. M., Zaki, M. S., Mirzaa, G., Dobyns, W. B., ... Di Donato, N. (2020). International consensus recommendations on the diagnostic work-up for malformations of cortical development. *Nature Reviews Neurology, 16*(11), 618–635. https://doi.org/10.1038/s41582-020-0395-6

Pan, Y.-H., Wu, N., & Yuan, X.-B. (2019). Toward a better understanding of neuronal migration deficits in autism spectrum disorders. *Frontiers in Cell and Developmental Biology, 7,* 205. https://doi.org/10.3389/fcell.2019.00205

Parrini, E., Conti, V., Dobyns, W. B., & Guerrini, R. (2016). Genetic basis of brain malformations. *Molecular Syndromology, 7*(4), 220–233. https://doi.org/10.1159/000448639

Poduri, A., & Volpe, J. J. (2018). Neuronal migration. In J. J. Volpe, T. E. Inder, B. T. Darras, L. S. deVries, A. J. du Plessis, & J. M. Perlman (Eds.), *Volpe's neurology of the newborn* (6th ed., pp. 120–144). Elsevier.

Roberts, B. (2018). Neuronal migration disorders. *Radiologic Technology, 89*(3), 279–295. http://www.radiologictechnology.org/content/89/3/279.abstract

Schiller, S., Rosewich, H., Grünewald, S., & Gärtner, J. (2020). Inborn errors of metabolism leading to neuronal migration defects. *Journal of Inherited Metabolic Disease, 43*(1), 145–155. https://doi.org/10.1002/jimd.12194

Severino, M., Geraldo, A. F., Utz, N., Tortora, D., Pogledic, I., Klonowski, W., Triulzi, F., Arrigoni, F., Mankad, K., Leventer, R. J., Mancini, G. M. S., Barkovich, J. A., Lequin, M. H., & Rossi, A. (2020). Definitions and classification of malformations of cortical development: Practical guidelines. *Brain, 143*(10), 2874–2894. https://doi.org/10.1093/brain/awaa174

Shin, H. W., Jewells, V., Sheikh, A., Zhang, J., Zhu, H., An, H., Gao, W., Shen, D., Hadar, E., & Lin, W. (2015). Initial experience in hybrid PET-MRI for evaluation of refractory focal onset epilepsy. *Seizure, 31,* 1–4. https://doi.org/10.1016/j.seizure.2015.06.010

Yuskaitis, C. J., & Pomeroy, S. L. (2017). Development of the nervous system. In R. A. Polin, S. H. Abram, D. H. Rowitch, W. E. Benita, & W. W. Fox (Eds.), *Fetal and neonatal physiology* (5th ed., pp. 1294–1313). Elsevier.

NEONATAL SEIZURES

GEORGIA R. DITZENBERGER AND SUSAN TUCKER BLACKBURN

The neonatal period is the most frequent time of life to have epileptic seizures. However, neonates can also exhibit unusual movements that are not epileptic seizures. Differentiating between epileptic and nonepileptic movements can be difficult. Most neonatal epileptic seizures are provoked by an underlying condition, such as hypoxic brain injury, hemorrhage, hypoglycemia, head trauma, electrolyte imbalance, or cerebral infections (Glass, 2014). These are called acute symptomatic seizures and are not epilepsy. Epileptic seizures are a group of conditions in which the seizures are unprovoked or symptomatic of an underlying condition. Because neonates exhibit a wide range of paroxysmal movements, which may or may not be epileptic seizures, a thorough neurophysiologic assessment should be performed before treatment is instigated (Hart et al., 2015).

Risk Factors

■ Hypoxic brain injury
■ Brain hemorrhage
■ Hypoglycemia
■ Head trauma
■ Electrolyte imbalance
■ Cerebral infections

Incidence

■ Occurs in 1.8 to 5 per 1,000 live term births
■ Occurs in 30 to 130 per 1,000 live preterm births

Anatomy and Physiology/Pathophysiology

■ Result of excessive, synchronous electrical discharge, or depolarization in the brain; produces stereotypic, repetitive behaviors
   ● Nerve depolarization–repolarization caused by movement of sodium and potassium across the cell membrane.
■ Specific mechanism causing neonatal seizures unknown; might be the result of one or more:
   ● Disturbances in energy production and the Na^+ to K^+ pump
   ● Altered neuronal membrane permeability to sodium
   ● Imbalances in excitatory and inhibitory neurotransmitters
■ Biochemical effects
   ● Increased energy expenditure
   ● Increased blood pressure
   ● Increased cerebral blood flow
   ● Marked decrease in brain glucose concentrations
■ Seizure activity in neonates: arise from temporal lobe, subcortical, limbic area
   ● Limbic area involved in sucking, drooling, chewing, swallowing, oculomotor deviations, and apneic episodes; subtle seizures in infant seizures
■ Seizure activity may be acute, recurrent, or chronic
   ● Usually acute: One-third occur on the first day of life, another one-third on the second day of life, then disappear within the first few weeks after birth.

■ Perinatal hypoxia–ischemia accounts for 50% to 60% of all neonatal seizures.

■ It is a signal of underlying disease processes resulting in acute disturbance in the brain.

● Primary central nervous system (CNS) disorders, hypoxic–ischemic events, stroke, hypoglycemia, hypocalcemia, intracranial hemorrhage, infection (meningitis, congenital viral infections, viral encephalopathy), congenital anomalies, other metabolic disturbances (alkalosis, hypomagnesemia, hypernatremia, hyponatremia)

● Less common: drug withdrawal (opiates or barbiturates), inborn errors of metabolism (IEM), kernicterus, hyperviscosity, local anesthetic intoxication

■ If left untreated, it can lead to permanent CNS damage or other issues.

■ Types: subtle, tonic, clonic (multifocal or migratory, and focal), and myoclonic

● Subtle: most common

• Horizontal deviations of the eyes with or without nystagmoid jerking; repetitive blinking or eyelid fluttering; drooling, sucking, or tongue thrusting; swimming or rowing movements of arms; and bicycling movements of legs

• Apnea, increased blood pressure

● Generalized tonic: more common in preterm infants

• Extremity extension; sometimes limited to one extremity

• Eye deviations, apnea, occasional clonic movements, and decerebrate-type postures

● Clonic, multifocal, or focal: more frequent in term infants; occasionally observed in older preterm infants

• Rhythmic, jerky clonic movements of one or more limbs; migrate to other parts of the body randomly

• Can be confused with jitteriness

• Associated with focal traumatic CNS injuries: cerebral contusions and infarcts; severe metabolic disturbance or asphyxia

● Myoclonic: uncommon in term infants, rare in preterm infants

• Single or multiple sudden jerks with flexion of the upper (most common) or lower extremities; occasionally observed on the trunk and neck

• Associated with IEM and other metabolic problems

Assessment

■ Determine cause: perinatal and neonatal history, a physical examination, laboratory evaluation, other diagnostic studies

■ Physical examination: general health and neurologic status

Clinical Manifestations/Diagnosis

▪ Difficult to recognize in neonates: often subtle; can be associated with other disorders or masked by seemingly normal newborn behaviors (grimacing, startle, sucking, and twitching); can occur with minimal or no outward sign

▪ Abnormal movements or altered tone of trunk or extremities

▪ Abnormal, repetitive facial, oral, tongue, or ocular movements: blinking, lip-smacking, or chewing motions

▪ Increased blood pressure; apneic events

▪ Laboratory studies: electrolyte levels; glucose, calcium, magnesium, and blood urea nitrogen levels; hematocrit value; blood gases; and pH; blood culture and lumbar puncture; screening for congenital viral infections; amino acid screening (for IEM)

▪ Diagnostic studies: CT, ultrasonography, MRI, skull radiography, EEG, and continuous video-EEG (gold standard); aEEG may miss seizures arising from areas of the brain not monitored by one to three probe placement

Treatment/Management

▪ Treatment of the underlying cause of the seizure is a priority for preventing more seizures and neurologic damage.

▪ Continual monitoring: blood gases, acid–base status, serum glucose, and fluid and electrolyte status

▪ Intravenous glucose administration; seizure activity depletes brain glucose and energy supplies

▪ Fluid and electrolyte management should be appropriate to the underlying cause of the seizures.

▪ Anticonvulsant drugs

  ● Phenobarbital, phenytoin, and fosphenytoin doses are given incrementally to reach therapeutic blood levels.

    * Phenobarbital is currently the most recommended and most commonly used first anticonvulsant drug; has potential for adverse neurodevelopmental effects.

    * Phenytoin and fosphenytoin are used as secondary agents.

    * Levetiracetam has been increasingly used in recent years; few clinical trials are available to demonstrate efficacy or safety.

  ● Blood levels are monitored carefully to maintain therapeutic effect and prevent toxicity.

▪ Refractory seizure may require alternative agents: clonazepam, lidocaine (used more in European countries and not in the United States), carbamazepine, diazepam, valproate, primidone

Specific Nursing Care (in Addition to Generalized Nursing Care)

■ Document seizure activity

- ● Time the seizure begins and ends
- ● Body parts involved (e.g., extremities, eyes, head)
- ● Description of movement, eye deviations, pupillary reactions
- ● Respiratory status, color, state, level of consciousness, postictal status

■ Protect from injury during the seizure: do not force anything into the infant's mouth or try to restrain the infant's extremities

■ Maintain infant's head to the side during seizure, if possible

■ Parent teaching: help family understand cause, significance of seizures, diagnostic tests, recognition of seizure activity, care during and after a seizure, anticonvulsants (dosage and side effects) if continued after discharge

Prognosis

■ Mortality: less than 15%

■ Morbidity: two-thirds of infants with seizures: adverse neurologic sequelae, epilepsy (20%–25%), motor deficits, mental retardation, learning disabilities, or poor social adjustment in teen years

■ Preterm infants tend to recover more rapidly from a seizure than do term infants; however, mortality and later morbidity are higher in preterm infants.

■ Prognosis is influenced by time of onset, cause, EEG results, treatment response, and frequency, duration.

- ● Good prognosis: onset after 4 days of life; benign seizures in otherwise healthy infants during first week of life; associated with late hypocalcemia, hyponatremia, uncomplicated subarachnoid hemorrhage (SAH)
- ● Clonic seizures have a better prognosis than other types of seizures.
- ● Poor prognosis: onset less than 48 hours after birth
- ● Poorest prognosis: seizures associated with severe hypoxic–ischemic injury, grade III or grade IV IVH, herpes infection, some bacterial meningitis, CNS malformations
- ● Infants with seizures secondary to late hypocalcemia, hyponatremia, and uncomplicated SAH seem to have the best prognosis.
- ● EEG results appear to be better prognostic signs in term than in preterm infants (Abend et al., 2018; Bassan et al., 2008; Blackburn, 2009; Bonifacio et al., 2011; Ditzenberger & Blackburn, 2020; Fenichel, 2007; Glass & Wirrell, 2009; Hellstrom-Westas & de Vries, 2007; Hill et al., 2017; Jensen, 2009; Rao et al., 2018; Rennie & Boylan, 2009; Scher, 2012a, 2012b; Shah et al., 2012; Soul, 2018; Tao & Mathur, 2010; Toet & deVries, 2012; Toet & Lemmers, 2009; Volpe, 2008)

REFERENCES

Abend, N. S., Jensen, F. E., Inder, T. E., & Volpe, J. J. (2018). Neonatal seizures. In J. J. Volpe, T. E. Inder, B. T. Darras, L. S. de Vries, A. J. du Plessis, J. Neil, & J. M. Perlman (Eds.), *Volpe's neurology of the newborn* (6th ed., pp. 275–372). Elsevier.

Bassan, H., Bental, Y., Shany, E., Berger, I., Froom, P., Levi, L., & Shiff, Y. (2008). Neonatal seizures: Dilemmas in workup and management. *Pediatric Neurology, 38*(6), 415–421. https://doi.org/10.1016/j.pediatrneurol.2008.03.003

Blackburn, S. T. (2009). Central nervous system vulnerabilities in preterm infants, part II. *Journal of Perinatal & Neonatal Nursing, 23*(2), 108–110. https://doi.org/10.1097/JPN.0b013e3181a3924b

Bonifacio, S. L., Glass, H. C., Peloquin, S., & Ferriero, D. M. (2011). A new neurological focus in neonatal intensive care. *Nature Review Neurology, 7*(9), 485–494. https://doi.org/10.1038/nrneurol.2011.119

Ditzenberger, G. R., & Blackburn, S. T. (2020). Neurologic system. In C. Kenner, L. B. Altimier, & M. V. Boykova (Eds.), *Comprehensive neonatal nursing care* (6th ed., pp. 373–416). Springer Publishing Company.

Fenichel, G. M. (2007). *Neonatal neurology* (4th ed.). Churchill/ Livingstone/Elsevier.

Glass, H. C. (2014). Neonatal seizures: Advances in mechanisms and management. *Clinics in Perinatology, 41*, 177–190. https://doi.org/10.1016/j.clp.2013.10.004

Glass, H. C., & Wirrell, E. (2009). Controversies in neonatal seizure management. *Journal of Child Neurology, 24*, 591–599. https://doi.org/10.1177/0883073808327832

Hart, A. R., Pilling, E. L., Alix, J. J., & Alix, J. P. (2015). Neonatal seizures-part 1: Not everything that jerks, stiffens and shakes is a fit. *Archives of Disease in Childhood—Education & Practice Edition, 100*(4), 170–175. https://doi.org/10.1136/archdischild-2014-306385

Hellstrom-Westas, L., & de Vries, L. S. (2007). EEG and evoked potentials in the neonatal period. In M. I. Levene & F. A. Chervenak (Eds.), *Fetal and neonatal neurology and neurosurgery* (4th ed., pp. 192–221). Churchill Livingstone/Elsevier.

Hill, E., Glass, H. C., Kelley, K., Barnes, M., Rau, S., Franck, L., & Shellhaas, R. A. (2017). Sezures and antiseizure medications are important to parents of newborns with seizures. *Pediatric Neurology, 67*, 40–44. https://doi.org/10.1016/j.pediatrneurol.2016.10.003

Jensen, F. E. (2009). Neonatal seizures: An update on mechanisms and management. *Clinics in Perinatology, 36*(4), 1–20. https://doi.org/10.1016/j.clp.2009.08.001

Rao, L. M., Hussain, S. A., Zaki, T., Cho, A., Chanlaw, T., Garg, M., & Sankar, R. (2018). A comparison of levetiracetam and phenobarbital for the treatment of neonatal seizures associated with hypoxic-ischemic encephalopathy. *Epilepsy & Behavior, 88*, 212–218. https://doi.org/10.1016/j.yebeh.2018.09.015

Rennie, J. M., & Boylan, G. B. (2009). Seizure disorders of the neonate. In M. I. Levene & F. A. Chervenak (Eds.), *Fetal and neonatal neurology and neurosurgery* (4th ed., pp. 698–710). Churchill Livingstone/Elsevier.

Scher, M. S. (2012a). Diagnosis and treatment of neonatal seizures. In J. M. Perlman (Ed.), *Neurology* (2nd ed., pp. 109–141). Saunders/Elsevier.

Scher, M. S. (2012b). Neonatal seizures. In C. A. Gleason & S. Devaskar (Eds.), *Avery's diseases of the newborn* (9th ed., pp. 901–919). Saunders/Elsevier.

Shah, D. K., Boylan, G. B., & Rennie, J. M. (2012). Monitoring of seizures in the newborn. *Archives of Disease in Childhood—Fetal and Neonatal Edition, 97*(1), F65–F69. https://doi.org/10.1136/adc.2009.169508

Soul, J. (2018). Acute symptomatic seizures in term neonates: Etiologies and treatments. *Seminars in Fetal & Neonatal Medicine, 23*, 183–190. https://doi.org/10.1016/j.siny.2018.02.002

Tao, J. D., & Mathur, A. M. (2010). Using amplitude-integrated EEG in neonatal intensive care. *Journal of Perinatology, 30*(S1), S73–S81. https://doi.org/10.1038/jp.2010.93

Toet, M. C., & deVries, L. S. (2012). Amplitude-integrated EEG and its potential role in augmenting management within the NICU. In J. M. Perlman (Ed.), *Neurology* (2nd ed., pp. 263–284). Saunders/Elsevier.
Toet, M. C., & Lemmers, P. M. A. (2009). Brain monitoring in neonates. *Early Human Development, 85*(2), 77–84. https://doi.org/10.1016/j.earlhumdev.2008.11.007
Volpe, J. J. (2008). *Neurology of the newborn* (5th ed.). Saunders/Elsevier.

BRAIN INJURY IN PRETERM INFANTS

GEORGIA R. DITZENBERGER AND SUSAN TUCKER BLACKBURN

Preterm infants are vulnerable to alterations in brain maturation and injury from pathophysiologic events because after birth, when they are cared for in the NICU, it is "at a time of peak brain growth, synaptogenesis, developmental regulation of specific receptor populations, and central nervous system (CNS) organization and differentiation" (Symes, 2016, p. 1157). Severe neurobehavioral sequelae (including impairment and cerebral palsy) have been described in 5% to 15% of very preterm infants. Milder cognitive defects, learning disabilities, and behavioral sequelae are seen in up to 25% to 50% of very preterm infants (Schneider & Miller, 2019). The pathophysiologic events leading to brain injury are hypoxemia ischemia and inflammation infection (Back & Miller, 2018; Kinney & Volpe, 2018). Multiple brain lesions are seen in preterm infants. The most common are the result of germinal matrix hemorrhage–intraventricular hemorrhage (GMH-IVH), including periventricular hemorrhagic infarction (PVHI); white matter injury (WMI); periventricular leukomalacia (PVL); and cerebellar injury. These disorders are the leading causes of neurologic disability in preterm infants with motor, cognitive, learning, and neurobehavioral sequelae.

GERMINAL MATRIX–INTRAVENTRICULAR HEMORRHAGE

Risk Factors

■ Resuscitation

■ Low gestational age (prematurity)

■ Hypotension

■ Multiple birth

■ Low birth weight (Lim & Hagen, 2019)

Incidence

■ Most common type of intracranial hemorrhage seen in the neonatal period

■ Seen almost exclusively in preterm infants, particularly those less than 1,500 g

■ Incidence of GMH-IVH in premature infants weighing less than 1,500 g is 15% to 25%; and higher in infants weighing less than 750 g (Back & Miller, 2018; Inder et al., 2018).

■ Incidence has declined in general but not for more severe hemorrhages and post-hemorrhagic ventricular dilatation (PHVD), which is seen in 30% to 50% of infants with large hemorrhages (Back & Miller, 2018; Ditzenberger & Blackburn, 2020; Inder et al., 2018; Leijser & de Vries, 2019).

Anatomy and Physiology

In preterm infants, GMH-IVH generally arises from the periventricular subependymal germinal matrix (site where neurons and glial cells originate before migrating to the cerebral cortex) at the head of the caudate nucleus near the foramen of Monro. GMH-IVH is rare after 35 to 36 weeks' gestation due to involution of the germinal matrix and changes in cerebral blood flow patterns. If GMH-IVH occurs later, bleeding usually arises from the choroid plexus (Back & Miller, 2018; Ditzenberger & Blackburn, 2020; Inder et al., 2018).

Pathophysiology

The major risk factors for GMH-IVH in the neonate are prematurity and hypoxic events interrelated with the anatomic and physiologic processes that make the periventricular germinal matrix site particularly vulnerable. Any perinatal or neonatal event that results in hypoxia or alters cerebral blood flow or intravascular pressure increases the risk of GMH-IVH. Several classification systems are available based on location and severity of the hemorrhage. Using Volpe's system (Back & Miller, 2018; Inder et al., 2018), GMH-IVH can be classified as:

■ Grade I or slight hemorrhage: isolated GMH

■ Grade II or small hemorrhage: small GMH-IVH (extends into the ventricle) with normal ventricular size

■ Grade III or moderate hemorrhage: moderate GMH-IVH with ventricular dilation and hemorrhage filling greater than 75% of the ventricle

■ PVHI, also referred to as Grade IV hemorrhage: severe hemorrhage involving both intraventricular and brain parenchyma hemorrhage with acute ventricular dilatation. PVHI accounts for 3% to 15% of all GMH-IVH (Leijser & de Vries, 2019)

The pathophysiology of GMH-IVH involves a complex interaction of intravascular, vascular, and extravascular factors. In many preterm infants, the hemorrhage begins as a microvascular event in the germinal matrix and may be confined to the subependymal area. The original hemorrhage may also rupture into the lateral ventricles and then into the third and fourth ventricles. The blood eventually collects in the subarachnoid space of the posterior fossa, often extending into the basal cistern. Progressive ventricular dilation may occur as the result of obstruction of cerebrospinal fluid (CSF) flow by obliterative arachnoiditis or as the result of blood clots at the aqueduct of Sylvius or the foramen of Monro. With severe hemorrhages, blood may also be found in the periventricular white matter (PVHI). This usually arises from an associated insult in the white matter and increases the risk of adverse neuromotor outcome.

Neuropathologic consequences of GMH-IVH include (a) destruction of the germinal matrix and its glial precursor cells; (b) infarction and necrosis of periventricular WMI; (c) alterations in central brain development, myelination, and axonal maturation; (d) PHVD; and (e) cerebellar changes. PVHI and intraparenchymal echodensities may develop in the white matter. The appearance of these parenchymal lesions is associated with increased mortality and neurodevelopmental sequelae. Infants with GMH-IVH may also have WMI or PVL. PVL may be a consequence of hypoxic–ischemic injury and not directly the result of the GMH-IVH. In up to 65% of infants with PHVD, the ventricular dilation progresses slowly then arrests, sometimes with reduction in the extent of the dilation. In 35% of infants with PHVD, a rapid increase in ventricular size occurs over days or weeks (Back & Miller, 2018; Ditzenberger & Blackburn, 2020; Inder et al., 2018; Leijser & de Vries, 2019).

Assessment

Risk Factors for Germinal Matrix Hemorrhage–Intraventricular Hemorrhage

■ Perinatal events associated with fetal and neonatal hypoxia, such as maternal bleeding, fetal distress, perinatal hypoxia ischemia, prolonged labor, maternal infection, preterm labor, and abnormal presentation

■ Neonatal hypoxic events, such as respiratory distress, apnea, and hypotension, which further increase the risk of GMH-IVH

■ Events leading to impairment of venous return or increased venous pressure, such as assisted ventilation, high-positive inspiratory pressure, prolonged duration of inspiration, continuous positive airway pressure, and air leak

■ Other factors that increase venous pressure, such as compression of the infant's skull during vaginal delivery, application of forceps, and use of constricting headbands (tight bilirubin band masks)

■ Rapid administration of hypertonic solutions or arterial blood withdrawal, rapid volume expansion, hypernatremia, hypercarbia, caregiving interventions, and environmental stress can increase cerebral blood flow and pressure.

■ Repeated or prolonged seizures raise the blood pressure and can also lead to hypoxia (Bissinger et al., 2019; Ditzenberger & Blackburn, 2020; Inder et al., 2018; Leijser & de Vries, 2019; Sandoval et al., 2019).

Clinical Manifestations

■ Over 90% bleed within the first 72 hours after birth; 50% of the bleeding occurs in the first 24 hours.

■ Late hemorrhages are seen after a few days or weeks in about 10% of infants, primarily preterm infants with severe, prolonged respiratory problems; new hemorrhage or an extension of a previous one may develop.

■ Signs are often subtle and nonspecific although a few may present with catastrophic deterioration if the hemorrhage is rapid and severe.

- Full anterior fontanelle; changes in activity level; decreased/increased tone
- Impaired visual tracking; altered lower extremity tone, hypotonia of the neck, brisk tendon reflexes
- Catastrophic deterioration usually involves major hemorrhages that evolve rapidly over several minutes or hours.
  - Present with stupor progressing to coma, respiratory distress progressing to apnea, generalized tonic seizures, decerebrate posturing, and fixation of pupils to light and flaccid quadriparesis
  - Associated with a declining hematocrit value, bulging fontanelle, hypotension, bradycardia, temperature alterations, hypoglycemia, syndrome of inappropriate antidiuretic hormone

Diagnosis

- Cranial ultrasonography to determine the presence, severity, and progression of the hemorrhage; monitor later complications (PVL, PHVD, and posthemorrhagic hydrocephalus). MRI is useful to identify concomitant WMI and cerebellar hemorrhage.
- Laboratory findings: declining hematocrit; failure of the hematocrit to increase after transfusion; and spinal fluid findings: increased red blood cell levels, increased protein levels, decreased glucose levels, and xanthochromia (Back & Miller, 2018; Ditzenberger & Blackburn, 2020; Dorner et al., 2018; Inder et al., 2018; Leijser & de Vries, 2019)

Treatment/Management

- Acute treatment of infants with or at risk for GMH-IVH
  - Prompt cardiopulmonary resuscitation by a trained NICU team and interventions to prevent or reduce hypoxic or ischemic events.
  - Provide physiologic support to maintain arterial perfusion and oxygenation; avoid hypotension, hypertension, acidosis, hypercarbia, and hypocarbia.
  - Minimize physical manipulations, handling, and environmental stressors to reduce the risk of hypoxia and of fluctuations in arterial blood pressure and cerebral blood flow.
  - Position head in the midline or to the side, without flexing the neck. The head of the bed can be elevated slightly; avoid the Trendelenburg position.
  - Provide fluid, as well as nutritional and metabolic support; maintain normothermia, normoglycemia, oxygenation, and perfusion.
  - Monitor vital signs, blood pressure, tone, activity, and level of consciousness.
- Routine ultrasonographic screening of infants at risk for GMH-IVH to identify infants with silent bleeding or bleeding with nonspecific symptoms
- Prevention or risk reduction in the perinatal period, with the prevention of preterm birth, perinatal hypoxic–ischemic injury, and birth trauma

- Antenatal glucocorticoid steroids associated with decreased incidence of GMH-IVH
■ Postbirth prevention and risk-reduction activities beginning immediately at birth
■ Prevent rapid changes in cerebral blood flow, fluctuations in systemic blood pressure, and hyperosmolarity; prevent or minimize fluctuations in intracranial pressure (ICP).
■ Management of PHVD:
  - Initial treatment is observation since ventricular growth often arrests spontaneously without therapy.
  - Progressive ventricular dilation with increasing ICP is managed with a ventricularperitoneal (VP) shunt or, if the infant cannot tolerate surgery, with temporary ventricular drainage via a reservoir or serial lumbar puncture (Bissinger et al., 2019; Blackburn, 2018; Chiriboga et al., 2018; de Bijl-Marcus et al., 2020; Ditzenberger & Blackburn, 2020; Inder et al., 2018; Klebel et al., 2020; Leijser & de Vries, 2019; Lim & Hagen, 2019; Sandoval et al., 2019).

Specific Nursing Care (In Addition to Generalized Nursing Care)

■ Avoid or minimize activities and environmental stressors that can increase ICP or cause wide swings in arterial or venous pressure, especially during the first 72 hours after birth.
■ Provide interventions, such as containment or swaddling, during aversive procedures such as endotracheal suctioning to promote greater physiologic stability and a more rapid return to baseline.
■ Assess and monitor pain and stress implementing pharmacologic and nonpharmacologic therapies if needed.
■ Monitor for signs of progressive PHVD.
■ Assess head size: head size can increase without increases in ICP (normopressive hydrocephalus).
■ Assess fontanelles (tense fontanelle may only be noted when the infant is placed in an upright position).
■ Observe for signs of increased ICP (bulging anterior fontanelle, setting-sun sign, dilated scalp veins, and widely separated sutures).
■ Administer hypertonic solutions and volume expanders slowly, with careful monitoring of vital signs and color; avoid rapid IV flushes and rapid arterial blood withdrawal.
■ Position head in the midline and raise head of bed slightly to reduce ICP.
■ Avoid turning head sharply; turn body as a unit.
■ Keep head of bed flat, avoid raising the feet above the head, such as with a diaper change.
■ Minimize handling and stimuli.

■ Since GMH-IVH usually occurs in the first few days after birth in infants less than 1,500 g, GMH-IVH prevention bundles have been implemented for the first 72 hours. These bundles minimize activities that increase ICP or lead to alterations in venous and arterial pressure or hypoxemia and promote neutral head positioning (Bissinger et al., 2019; Chiriboga et al., 2018; de Bijl-Marcus et al., 2020; Ditzenberger & Blackburn, 2020). Few randomized controlled trials of the effects of neutral head positioning on the incidence of IVH have been conducted and data are inconclusive (Romantsik et al., 2020).

■ Family support and teaching include how to interact with and care for the infant at risk for GMH-IVH in a developmentally appropriate manner, promoting opportunities for interaction while minimizing stressful events (Bissinger et al., 2019; Blackburn, 2018; Chiriboga et al., 2018; de Bijl-Marcus et al., 2020; Ditzenberger & Blackburn, 2020; Romantsik et al., 2020).

Care of an Infant With a Ventriculoperitoneal Shunt

■ Position after surgery on the side opposite the shunt, with the head of the bed flat or slightly elevated to prevent rapid loss of cerebrospinal fluid (CSF) and decompression.

■ Position can be rotated to supine every few hours to prevent skin breakdown.

■ Keep the skin around the shunt clean and dry.

■ Observe for signs of localized or systemic infection.

  ● Shunt infection may appear as localized redness or drainage around the incision, temperature instability, altered activity, or poor feeding.

■ Observe for shunt obstruction (accumulation of CSF, enlargement of the head, and signs of increased ICP).

■ Monitor fluid status and intake and output; observe for signs of dehydration from too rapid loss of CSF (sunken fontanelle, agitation or restlessness, increased urine output, and electrolyte abnormalities).

■ Provide parent teaching: care of the infant and shunt, including positioning and skin care, signs of shunt malfunction, increased ICP, infection, and dehydration (Ditzenberger & Blackburn, 2020; Joseph et al., 2017).

Prognosis

■ Severity and extent of hemorrhage and the presence of associated problems influence mortality and morbidity.

■ The milder or smaller the hemorrhage, the lower the mortality and the incidence of major neurologic sequelae and PHVD.

■ Incidence of neurologic sequelae ranges from 15% to 20% in infants with moderate hemorrhage up to 50% in infants with grade III hemorrhage and up to 75% in infants with PVHI.

■ Sequelae include cerebral palsy, developmental delay, sensory and attention problems, learning disorders, and hydrocephalus (Ditzenberger & Blackburn, 2020; Gotardo et al., 2019; Inder et al., 2018; Reubsaet et al., 2017).

WHITE MATTER INJURY IN PRETERM INFANTS

Risk Factors

■ Antenatal infection/chorioamnionitis

■ Hypoxia-ischemia

■ Various postnatal events such as oxidative stress, sepsis, mechanical ventilation, hemodynamic variances (Ditzenberger & Blackburn, 2020)

Incidence

■ WMI and its associated neuronal and axonal alterations (referred to as the encephalopathy of prematurity) is the most common severe neurologic insult seen in preterm infants. Encephalopathy of prematurity is characterized by "multifaceted gray and white matter lesions in the preterm brain that reflect acquired and developmental factors in combination" (Kinney & Volpe, 2018, p. 389).

■ Focal cystic necrotic lesions are seen in fewer than 5% of infants born at 24 to 32 weeks; the more common noncystic and diffuse lesions associated with disturbances in myelination are seen in up to 25% to 50%.

■ Time of onset is variable. Onset of injury is most likely perinatal, especially in the early postbirth period. Late onset after severe illness is sometimes seen.

■ Greatest risk of WMI is in infants born at 23 to 32 weeks' gestation (Back & Miller, 2018; Kinney & Volpe, 2018; Neil & Volpe, 2018; Schneider & Miller, 2019).

Physiology/Pathophysiology

WMI involves both cystic and noncystic focal necrotic lesions as well as diffuse WMI with damage to the premyelinating oligodendrocytes, astrogliosis, and microglial infiltration. This injury is referred to as PVL. PVL is a symmetric, nonhemorrhagic, usually bilateral lesion caused by ischemia from alterations in arterial circulation. Leukomalacia refers to change in the brain's white matter reflective of softening. WMI often is associated with GMH-IVH, but it is a separate lesion that may also occur in the absence of GMH-IVH (Back & Volpe, 2018; Ditzenberger & Blackburn, 2020; Neil & Volpe, 2018; Schneider & Miller, 2019).

PVL begins with ischemic necrosis of the white matter dorsal and lateral to the external angles of the lateral ventricles. Pathologic changes begin with patchy areas of focal ischemic coagulation that may occur as early as 5 to 8 hours after the initial hypoxic–ischemic insult. This is followed within a few days by proliferation of macrophages and astrocytes, along with endothelial and glial infiltration. Later changes include thinning of the white matter and liquefaction in the central portion of the necrotic area, as well as cavitation, cystic changes, and decreased myelinization. Cerebral atrophy leads to expansion of the lateral ventricles and hydrocephalus.

The pathogenesis of WMI involves an interaction between three maturation-dependent factors: (a) immature vascular supply to the WM (reducing oxygen delivery to areas of the brain that are vulnerable to ischemic injury); (b) impairments in cerebral autoregulation; and (c) vulnerability of premyelinating oligodendrites to damage from oxidative stress, glutamate (excitotoxicity), adenosine, and cytokines. Damage to the premyelinating oligodendrocytes leads to further release of cytokines (indicating an inflammatory process), glutamate, and free radicals. Oligodendrocyte development and survival are impaired, leading to hypomyelinization with subsequent motor, cognitive, behavioral, and neurodevelopmental problems. Axonal damage and disruption also occur. Perinatal infection and an immune-mediated inflammatory response with release of proinflammatory cytokines are thought to play a prominent role in the pathogenesis of PVL (Back & Volpe, 2018; Blackburn, 2018; Ditzenberger & Blackburn, 2020; Kinney & Volpe, 2018; Neil & Volpe, 2018; Schneider & Miller, 2019).

Clinical Manifestations

■ Often no clinical findings specific to PVL are seen during the first weeks of life unless the damage is severe.

Diagnosis

■ Cranial ultrasonography can identify infants at risk for, or who have early signs of, PVL.

■ MRI can identify changes early and is especially useful with diffuse WMI (Ditzenberger & Blackburn, 2020; Neill & Volpe, 2018).

Treatment/Management

■ Initial treatment focuses on treating the primary insult and its attendant complications and preventing further hypoxic–ischemic damage, including preventing or minimizing hypotension, hypoxia, acidosis, and severe apneic and bradycardic episodes.

● Prompt cardiopulmonary resuscitation by a trained NICU team and interventions to prevent or reduce hypoxic or ischemic events.

● Provide physiologic support to maintain arterial perfusion and oxygenation; avoid hypotension, hypertension, acidosis, hypercarbia, and hypocarbia.

● Identify signs of hypoxia and ischemia and institute interventions to prevent further ischemic damage.

● Provide fluid, nutritional, and metabolic support; maintain normothermia, normoglycemia, oxygenation, and perfusion.

● Monitor vital signs, blood pressure, tone, activity, and level of consciousness.

■ Prevention or risk reduction in the perinatal period, with the prevention of preterm birth, perinatal hypoxic–ischemic injury, and birth trauma. Antenatal magnesium sulfate reduces the risk of cerebral palsy (Shepherd et al., 2017).

■ Head ultrasound and MRI are used serially to diagnose PVL and to follow its progression in infants at risk (Back & Volpe, 2018; Ditzenberger & Blackburn, 2020; Neil & Volpe, 2018; Schneider & Miller, 2019).

Specific Nursing Care (In Addition to Generalized Nursing Care)

■ Identify signs of hypoxia and ischemia and institute physiologic and neuroprotective interventions to prevent further ischemic damage (see the section on GMH-IVH).

■ Minimize physical manipulations, handling, and environmental stressors to reduce the risk of hypoxia and of fluctuations in arterial blood pressure and cerebral blood flow.

■ Parent teaching on promoting an understanding of the infant's health status and care, providing anticipatory guidance, and discussing how to interact with and care for their infant in a developmentally appropriate manner (Bissinger et al., 2019; Ditzenberger & Blackburn, 2020; Neil & Volpe, 2018; Schneider & Miller, 2019).

Prognosis

■ Infants are at higher risk for later problems that affect motor, cognitive, and visual function.

■ The most prominent neuromotor sequelae in survivors is spastic diplegia, although the incidence of spastic diplegia has decreased in recent years.

■ Infants with diffuse WMI are more likely to develop visual, cognitive, and neurobehavioral impairments, such as autism spectrum disorders (Ditzenberger & Blackburn, 2020; Gotardo et al., 2019; Neil & Volpe, 2018; Schneider & Miller, 2019).

CEREBELLAR INJURY IN PRETERM INFANTS

Incidence and Risk Factors

■ The cerebellum is one of the later structures to mature, with critical developmental events occurring at the end of the second and in the third trimester. There is a rapid cerebellar growth spurt from 24 to 40 weeks with a five-fold increase in cerebellar volume and 30-fold increase in surface area. The cerebellum is vulnerable to alterations during this period as neuronal proliferation, migration, and arborization are prominent (Gano & Barkovich, 2019; Tam, 2018; Yuskaitis & Pomeroy, 2017).

■ The cerebellum is important in regulation of cognition, motor function, emotion, and social behavior and acts as a neural distribution node with interconnections with the thalamus and cortex (Ditzenberger & Blackburn, 2020).

Preterm infants are at risk for cerebellar injury. The greatest risk of cerebellar injury is in infants less than 28 weeks' gestation, with an increased incidence with decreasing gestation. These injuries may alter motor and language development and cognitive, socio-emotional, and behavioral function.

■ Risk factors for cerebellar injury are similar to those for GMH-IVH and WMI (see the sections on GMH-IVH and WMI; Gano & Barkovich, 2019; Limperopoulos et al., 2018; Tam, 2018; Yuskaitis & Pomeroy, 2017).

Pathophysiology

■ Two forms of cerebellar injury are seen in preterm infants: primary and secondary. Primary injury is usually due to cerebellar hemorrhage or infarction. Secondary injury (cerebellar hypoplasia) involves alterations in cerebellar growth and development. Associated factors include PVL, GMC-IVH, postnatal glucocorticoids, exposure to pain and stress, postnatal opioids, nutritional and growth alterations, and cardiorespiratory instability (Gano & Barkovich, 2019; Limperopoulos et al., 2018; Tam, 2018; Yuskaitis & Pomeroy, 2017).

Clinical Manifestations

■ Assessment is similar to GMH-IVH and WMI (see the sections on GMH-IVH and WMI).

■ Clinical manifestations of cerebral hypoplasia may be subtle or nonspecific unless a severe cerebellar hemorrhage develops in this case tissue and is connected to the CNS by a narrow stalk.

■ Infants with significant cerebellar hemorrhage may be critically ill from birth. Other infants are less ill initially, and symptoms develop up to 2 to 3 weeks of age.

■ Clinical manifestations include apnea, bradycardia, hoarse or high-pitched cry, eye deviations, opisthotonos, seizures, vomiting, hypotonia, and altered Moro reflex (Ditzenberger & Blackburn, 2020; Inder et al., 2018).

Diagnosis

■ MRI and cranial ultrasound via posterior fontanelle may be used. MRI is preferred as a smaller hemorrhage may be unseen on cranial ultrasound. Using MRI, smaller hemorrhages have been reported in 10% to 30% of preterm infants (Tam, 2018).

Treatment/Management

■ Management involves primarily supportive care and is similar to that for GMH-IVH (see the section on GMH-IVH).

■ Parent teaching on promoting an understanding of the infant's health status and care, providing anticipatory guidance, and discussing how to interact with and care for their infant in a developmentally appropriate manner

Prognosis

▪ Higher mortality rates are seen in infants with severe cerebellar hemorrhage. Survivors of severe cerebellar hemorrhage are at risk for microcephaly, developmental delay, and hypotonia. Better outcomes are seen in infants with smaller hemorrhages with an increased risk of mild-to-moderate motor impairments (Tam, 2018).

▪ Infants with cerebellar hypoplasia are at increased risk for altered cognitive and motor outcomes (Gano & Barkovich, 2019; Limperopoulos et al., 2018; Tam, 2018; Yuskaitis & Pomeroy, 2017).

REFERENCES

Back, S. A., & Miller, S. P. (2018). Brain injury in the preterm infant. In C. A. Gleason & S. E. Juul (Eds.), *Avery's diseases of the newborn* (10th ed., pp. 879–896). Elsevier.

Back, S. A., & Volpe, J. J. (2018). Encephalopathy of prematurity: Pathophysiology. In J. J. Volpe, T. E. Inder, B. T. Darras, L. S. deVries, A. J. du Plessis, & J. M. Perlman (Eds.), *Volpe's neurology of the newborn* (6th ed., pp. 405–424). Elsevier.

Bissinger, R. L., Annibale, D. J., & Fanning, B. (2019). *Golden hours: Care of the very low birth weight infant* (2nd ed.). The National Certification Corporation.

Blackburn, S. T. (2018). *Maternal, fetal and neonatal physiology: A clinical perspective* (5th ed.). Elsevier.

Chiriboga, N., Cortez, J., Pena-Ariet, A., Makker, K., Smotherman, C., Gautam, S., Trikardos, A. B., Knight, H., Yeoman, M., Burnett, E., Beier, A., Cohen, I., & Hudak, M. L. (2018). Successful implementation of an intracranial hemorrhage (ICH) bundle in reducing severe ICH: A quality improvement project. *Journal of Perinatology, 39,* 143–151. https://doi.org/10.1038/s41372-018-0257-x

de Bijl-Marcus, K., Brouwer, A. J., de Vries, L. S., Groenendaal, F., & van Wezel-Meijler, G. (2020). Neonatal care bundles are associated with a reduction in the incidence of intraventricular haemorrhage in preterm infants: A multicentre cohort study. *Archives of Disease in Childhood - Fetal and Neonatal Edition, 105,* F419–F424. https://doi.org/10.1136/archdischild-2018-316692

Ditzenberger, G. R., & Blackburn, S. T. (2020). Neurologic system. In C. Kenner, L. B. Altimer, & M. V. Boykova (Eds.), *Comprehensive neonatal nursing care* (6th ed., pp. 373–416). Springer Publishing Company.

Dorner, R. A., Burton, V. J., Allen, M. C., Robinson, S., & Soares, B. P. (2018). Preterm neuroimaging and neurodevelopmental outcome: A focus on intraventricular hemorrhage, post-hemorrhagic hydrocephalus, and associated brain injury. *Journal of Perinatology, 38,* 1431–1443. https://doi.org/10.1038/s41372-018-0209-5

Gano, D., & Barkovich, J. (2019). Cerebellar hypoplasia of prematurity: Causes and consequences. In L. S. de Vries & H. C. Glass (Eds.), *Handbook of clinical neurology* (Vol. 162, pp. 201–206). Elsevier.

Gotardo, J. W., Volkmer, N. V., Stangler, G. P., Dornelles, A. D., Bohrer, B. B., & Carvalho, C. G. (2019). Impact of peri-intraventricular haemorrhage and periventricular leukomalacia in the neurodevelopment of preterms: A systematic review and meta-analysis. *PLoS One, 14*(10), e02234275. https://doi.org/10.1371/journal.pone.0223427

Inder, T. E., Perlman, J. M., & Volpe, J. J. (2018). Preterm intraventricular hemorrhage/posthemorrhagic hydrocephalus. In J. J. Volpe, T. E. Inder, B. T. Darras, L. S. deVries, A. J. du Plessis, & J. M. Perlman (Eds.), *Volpe's neurology of the newborn* (6th ed., pp. 637–698). Elsevier.

Joseph, R. A., Killian, M. R., & Brady, E. E. (2017). Nursing care of infants with a ventriculoperitoneal shunt. *Advances in Neonatal Care, 17,* 430–439. https://doi.org/10.1097/ANC.0000000000000439

Kinney, H. C., & Volpe, J. J. (2018). Encephalopathy of prematurity: Neuropathology. In J. J. Volpe, T. E. Inder, B. T. Darras, L. S. deVries, A. J. du Plessis, & J. M. Perlman (Eds.), *Volpe's neurology of the newborn* (6th ed., pp. 389–404). Elsevier.

Klebel, D., McBride, D., Krafft, P. R., Flores, J. J., Tang, J., & Zhang, J. H. (2020). Posthemorrhagic hydrocephalus development after germinal matrix hemorrhage: Established mechanisms and proposed pathways. *Neuroscience Research, 98,* 105–120. https://doi.org/10.1002/jnr.24394

Leijser, L. M., & de Vries, L. S. (2019). Preterm brain injury: Germinal matrix–intraventricular hemorrhage and post-hemorrhagic ventricular dilatation. In L. S. de Vries & H. C. Glass (Eds.), *Handbook of clinical neurology* (Vol. 162, pp. 173–199). Elsevier.

Lim, J., & Hagen, E. (2019). Reducing germinal matrix-intraventricular hemorrhage: Perinatal and delivery room factors. *NeoReviews, 20,* e452. https://doi.org/10.1542/neo.20-8-e452

Limperopoulos, C., du Plessis, A. J., & Volpe, J. J. (2018). Cerebellar hemorrhage. In J. J. Volpe, T. E. Inder, B. T. Darras, L. S. deVries, A. J. du Plessis, & J. M. Perlman (Eds.), *Volpe's neurology of the newborn* (6th ed., pp. 623–636). Elsevier.

Neil, J. J., & Volpe, J. J. (2018). Encephalopathy of prematurity: Clinical-neurological features, diagnosis, imaging, prognosis, therapy. In J. J. Volpe, T. E. Inder, B. T. Darras, L. S. deVries, A. J. du Plessis, & J. M. Perlman (Eds.), *Volpe's neurology of the newborn* (6th ed., pp. 425–457). Elsevier.

Reubsaet, P., Brouwer, A. J., van Haastert, I. C., Brouwer, M. J., Koopman, C., Groenendaal, F., & de Vries, L. S. (2017). The impact of low-grade germinal matrix-intraventricular hemorrhage on neurodevelopmental outcome of very preterm infants. *Neonatology, 112,* 203–210. https://doi.org/10.1159/000472246

Romantsik, O., Calevo, M. G., & Bruschettini, M. (2020). Head midline position for preventing the occurrence or extension of germinal matrix-intraventricular haemorrhage in preterm infants. *Cochrane Database of Systematic Reviews, 7*(7), CD012362. https://doi.org/10.1002/14651858.CD012362.pub3

Sandoval, V. P., Rosales, P. H., Hernández, D. G. Q., Naranjo, E. A. C., & Navarro, V. C. (2019). Intraventricular hemorrhage and posthemorrhagic hydrocephalus in preterm infants: Diagnosis, classification, and treatment options. *Child's Nervous System, 35,* 917–927. https://doi.org/10.1007/s00381-019-04127-x

Schneider, J., & Miller, S. P. (2019). Preterm brain injury: White matter. In L. S. de Vries & H. C. Glass (Eds.), *Handbook of clinical neurology* (Vol. 162, pp. 155–178). Elsevier.

Shepherd, E., Salam, R. A., Middleton, P., Makrides, S., McIntyre, S., Badawi, N., & Crowther, C. A. (2017). Antenatal and intrapartum interventions for preventing cerebral palsy: An overview of Cochrane systematic reviews. *Cochrane Database of Systematic Reviews, 8*(8), CD012077. https://doi.org/10.1002/14651858.CD012077.pub2

Symes, A. (2016). Developmental outcomes. In M. G. MacDonald & M. M. Seshia (Eds.), *Avery's neonatology: Pathophysiology & management of the newborn* (7th ed., pp. 1157–1168). Wolters Kluwer.

Tam, E. Y. W. (2018). Cerebellar injury in preterm infants. In M. Manto & T. A. G. M. Huisman (Eds.), *Handbook of clinical neurology* (Vol. 155, pp. 49–59). Elsevier.

Yuskaitis, C. J., & Pomeroy, S. L. (2017). Development of the nervous system. In R. A. Polin, S. H. Abram, D. H. Rowitch, W. E. Benita, & W. W. Fox (Eds.), *Fetal and neonatal physiology* (5th ed., pp. 1294–1313). Elsevier.

BRAIN INJURY IN TERM INFANTS

GEORGIA R. DITZENBERGER AND SUSAN TUCKER BLACKBURN

HYPOXIC–ISCHEMIC ENCEPHALOPATHY

Hypoxic–ischemic encephalopathy (HIE) is an injury to the brain caused by oxygen deficit resulting from either systemic hypoxemia (decreased oxygen in the blood supply), or ischemia (diminished cerebral blood perfusion), or a combination of the two conditions. The hypoxemia and ischemia may occur simultaneously or sequentially, and it appears from recent evidence that ischemia is the more important of the two oxygen deprivation states in causing the brain injury. In addition, the subsequent reperfusion of the affected brain area has been shown to be the time at which the majority of the injury to the brain occurs. Glucose deprivation also plays a part in the severity of the brain injury (Ditzenberger & Blackburn, 2020; Sorem et al., 2009; Volpe, 2008; Volpe et al., 2018).

HIE may occur secondary to prenatal, intrapartum, or postnatal insults in both preterm and term infants. The site of injury varies with maturational changes in the vascular anatomy and metabolic activity of the brain (Bonifacio et al., 2012; deVries & Jongmans, 2010; Dickey et al., 2011; Ditzenberger & Blackburn, 2020; Douglas-Escobar & Weiss, 2015; Simbruner et al., 2010; Volpe et al., 2018; Wachtel & Hendricks-Muñoz, 2011).

Risk Factors

■ Systemic hypoxemia

■ Cerebral ischemia

■ Oxygen deprivation

■ Prenatal, intrapartum, or postnatal hypoxic insults

Incidence

■ Between four to eight per 1,000 live births

■ Mortality and morbidity: one per 1,000

Physiology/Pathophysiology

■ Five types of lesions

● Selective neuronal necrosis

● Status marmoratus of the neurons of the basal ganglia and thalamus, with loss of neurons in these areas

● Parasagittal cerebral injury

● Periventricular leukomalacia (PVL; primarily in preterm infants)

● Focal or multifocal ischemic brain necrosis (Ditzenberger & Blackburn, 2020; Volpe, 2008)

■ Primary hypoxic injury: neuronal necrosis in cerebrum and cerebellum, with damage to the gray matter at the depths of the sulci

■ Primary ischemic injury: posterior portion of the parasagittal region secondary to watershed or border zone infarcts

■ After a hypoxic–ischemic insult, the entire cortex initially may be edematous, and further ischemic damage may occur as a result of compression of the cortex against the skull (Dickey et al., 2011; Ditzenberger & Blackburn, 2020; Johnston et al., 2011; Sorem et al., 2009; Stola & Perlman, 2008; Volpe, 2008; Volpe et al., 2018)

Clinical Manifestations

■ Characteristic pattern of neurologic findings over the first 72 hours of life: seizures, altered level of consciousness, altered tone, altered activity, irregular respirations, apnea, poor or absent Moro reflex, abnormal cry, poor suck, and altered pupillary responses, and eye movements

■ Clinical signs categorizing the severity of HIE classified in three stages (Sarnat & Sarnat, 1976):

● Stage 1 (mild): mild depression or hyperalertness, irritability, and sympathetic nervous system excitation (tachycardia, dilated pupils)

• Good Moro reflex and deep tendon reflexes; they typically are symptomatic for less than 24 hours.

● Stage 2 (moderate): lethargy interspersed with brief arousal, decreased tone, altered primary reflexes, and increased parasympathetic tone (bradycardia, decreased pupil size, and blood pressure) and may develop seizures

● Stage 3 (severe): varying levels of consciousness initially; then become stuporous or comatose

• Depressed deep tendon and Moro reflexes, hypotonia, and most develop seizures

■ Seizures occur in up to 60% infants with HIE.

● Onset at 12 to 14 hours of age

● Most often seen are multifocal clonic seizures in term infants.

● Occasionally, myoclonic, clonic, and subtle seizures

Diagnosis

■ Extensive workup to define the type, extent, and location of the injury may include cranial ultrasonography, brainstem auditory evoked potentials, MRI, EEG, and measurements of cerebral blood flow, intracranial pressure (ICP), and the creatinine kinase level.

■ Labs: glucose, calcium, magnesium, serum and urinary electrolyte levels, and osmolality; blood urea nitrogen, serum creatinine levels; fluid and electrolyte balance

■ At risk for hypocalcemia and hypoglycemia (Ditzenberger & Blackburn, 2020; Johnston et al., 2011; Volpe, 2008; Volpe et al., 2018)

Treatment/Management

Infants with HIE have multiorgan and multisystem problems that arise from the original hypoxic–ischemic insult (Sarkar et al., 2009; Tagin et al., 2012; Zanelli et al., 2011). As a result, management of these infants is complex and requires a coordinated team effort, preferably within a NICU/tertiary care center; transport to NICU/tertiary care center is strongly recommended within the first 6 hours of life.

■ Acute management
  ● Delivery room resuscitation and stabilization; consider mild passive cooling with decreased/no radiant heat provided during resuscitation for term, near-term newborns requiring significant resuscitation efforts
  ● Management of the primary problem and related alterations in the cardiovascular, pulmonary, gastrointestinal, and renal systems
  ● Prompt identification and treatment of seizures to prevent further alterations in ICP and cerebral blood flow
  ● Focuses on eliminating the cause of the original hypoxia, alleviation of tissue hypoxia, and promotion of adequate cerebral perfusion and brain oxygenation with maintenance of an adequate glucose supply (Ditzenberger & Blackburn, 2020; Stola & Perlman, 2008; Volpe, 2008; Wachtel & Hendricks-Muñoz, 2011; Wassink et al., 2019)
■ Passive cooling prior to controlled therapeutic hypothermia
  ● Recommendations for passive cooling are focused on use prior to/during transfer to NICU/tertiary care center, not for actual 72-hour active hypothermia therapy course.
  ● Primary intent for passive cooling is to initiate cooling within 1 to 3 hours of life to support ongoing controlled active hypothermia therapy within the NICU/tertiary care center.
  ● Important to consider initiation of passive cooling with NICU/tertiary care center guidance as soon as possible whenever HIE is suspected.
    • NICU/tertiary care center is required for continuous monitoring and intervention during critical period of acute adverse multiorgan effect resulting from initial insult of HIE and the need for controlled continuous therapeutic hypothermia to optimize newborn outcome.
  ● Current recommendations for passive cooling include the following:
    • Continuous monitoring of vital signs and rectal temperature
      − If cardio-respiratory monitoring and/or rectal temperature is not available, assess and record vital signs and rectal temperature every 15 minutes.
    • Rectal temperature during passive cooling is most accurate and strongly preferred.

- Skin and axillary temperatures are affected by surface, environmental temperatures.

- Rectal temperature (as does mid-esophageal temperature used during controlled active hypothermia) more accurately reflects core temperature, which in turn closely reflects brain temperature.

   ○ Current recommendations for goal rectal temperature during passive cooling is 33 °C to 35 °C.

■ Methods to achieve passive cooling prior to/during transport to NICU/tertiary care center:

● Turn off radiant heat source on radiant warmer; turn off incubator if in use and open all portholes

● Avoid using ice/cold packs—strongly recommended

   • Increases risk of overcooling, rapid temperature fluctuations

   • Causes increased risk of skin breakdown, fat necrosis at site of application

   • If necessary, room temperature water packs may be used; remove once rectal temperature is ~34.5 °C to 35 °C.

● Passive cooling increases risks of overcooling the newborn, causing increased risk of detrimental effects to newborn outcome.

● Passive cooling increases risk of temperature fluctuations, also causing increased risk of detrimental effects to newborn outcome.

● Guidelines and ongoing education for passive cooling for use in referral hospitals awaiting the transport team and during the transport arestrongly recommended (Arriagada et al., 2019; Chiang et al., 2017; Goel et al., 2016; Kendall et al., 2010; Lemyre et al., 2017; Monmany et al., 2019; Natarajan et al., 2018; Wassink et al., 2019)

■ NICU treatment

● Establish ventilation and adequate perfusion.

● Prevent/minimize hypotension, hypoxia, and acidosis; rapid alterations in cerebral blood flow and systemic blood pressure; and severe apneic and bradycardic episodes.

● Avoid hyperoxia: can result in cerebral vasoconstriction and diminished perfusion.

● Monitor and document neurologic status.

● Must be differentiated from other neurologic dysfunctions caused by trauma, infection, or central nervous system (CNS) anomalies (Ditzenberger & Blackburn, 2020; Gunny & Lin, 2012; Stola & Perlman, 2008; Tao & Mathur, 2010; Toet & deVries, 2012; Toet & Lemmers, 2009; Wachtel & Hendricks-Munoz, 2011; Walsh et al., 2011).

● Fluid management is critical not only for treating the cerebral edema but also for managing the alterations in renal function.

● Induced mild hypothermia has been shown to provide neuroprotection and reduce the extent of tissue injury and is increasingly the treatment of choice for infants ≥36 weeks' gestation with moderate-to-severe HIE (refer to whole body cooling protocol).

• For use only in NICU/high-acuity nurseries:

— Infants undergoing a cooling regimen, either selective head cooling or whole-body cooling, require optimal care and attention at the bedside; this intervention is only being done in tertiary NICU settings.

– Active therapeutic hypothermia with specialized equipment increasingly recommended for use during neonatal transport by experienced teams.

● Care should be taken that the infants not become hyperthermic with core temperatures greater than 37°C (Barks, 2008; Ditzenberger & Blackburn, 2020; Glass, 2010; Goel et al., 2016; Hoehn et al., 2008; Monmany et al., 2019; Pfister & Soll, 2010; Reynolds & Talmage, 2011; Selway, 2010; Zanelli et al., 2011).

● Therapeutic window: must begin within 6 hours of birth for neuroprotective interventions; early hypothermia studies indicate that cooling may be less effective if started after onset of seizures or in infants with most severe EEG changes before therapy.

● Studies indicate the earlier cooling begins, the better the outcome; indication for support of passive cooling after birth, while awaiting transport, and during transport to NICU/tertiary care center.

■ The cooling regimen continues for 72 hours.

■ Infants are assessed by a neonatologist team and/or pediatric neurologist to determine whether hypothermia criteria are met before the cooling regimen is initiated.

If newborn in referring hospital, contact with NICU/neonatologist as soon as possible is strongly recommended for guidance in initiating/maintaining passive cooling safely during wait for transport

■ Current criteria used to determine if a newborn is a candidate for hypothermia are:

● Term infants ≥36 weeks' gestation without major congenital anomalies, intrauterine growth restriction (IUGR; ≤1,800 g), or known chromosomal anomaly

● Admitted to NICU at ≤6 hours of age

● Assessed to be in Stage 2 moderate HIE, or Stage 3, severe HIE (Arriagada et al., 2019; Bonifacio et al., 2011, 2012; Chiang et al., 2017; Ditzenberger & Blackburn, 2020; Gancia & Pomero, 2011; Gluckman et al., 2005; Gunn et al., 2008; Hoehn et al., 2008; Kendall et al., 2010; Laptook, 2012; Lemyre et al., 2017; Natarajan et al., 2018; Stola & Perlman, 2008; Volpe, 2008; Volpe et al., 2018; Wassink et al., 2019)

Specific Nursing Care (In Addition to Generalized Nursing Care)

■ During acute phase and cooling phase:

● Fluctuations in systemic blood pressure with increased ICP and altered cerebral hemodynamics can occur as a result of caregiving or environmental stress, potentially worsening HIE complications.

● Developmentally supportive care of these infants to reduce stress is essential.

● Maintain minimal handling, as well as decreased auditory, visual, and sensory input.

● Positioning and skin care are important, especially for hypoactive, obtunded, or comatose infants.

● Monitor vital signs, neurologic status, and seizures.

■ During recovery following rewarming period through discharge and home

● Gradually introduce sensory experiences as tolerated.

• Will be easily overwhelmed; monitor response closely

● Continue monitoring physiologic and neurologic status.

● Observe for changes in level of consciousness, tone, and activity and seizures.

■ Parental support

● Teach reasons for lack of infant responsiveness if the infant is sedated, hypoactive, stuporous, or comatose.

● Prepare for possibility of death; consider the implications for later neurologic deficits.

● Focus on promoting an understanding of the infant's health status and care and providing anticipatory guidance regarding changes in the infant's state, as well as the outcome.

● Demonstrate how to interact with and care for their infant in a developmentally appropriate manner, with the goal of promoting opportunities for interaction while minimizing stressful events (Ditzenberger & Blackburn, 2020; Gudsnuk & Champagne, 2011; Hill et al., 2017; Long & Brandon, 2007; Selway, 2010; Sullivan et al., 2011).

Prognosis

■ Varies with the extent and severity of the insult and the resulting brain injury.

● Ranges from perinatal death to severe neurologic impairment to minimal or no sequelae.

● Specific sequelae are not apparent for several months or longer.

● Some infants make a significant recovery, although the rate and degree of recovery vary.

- MRI or CT can be used to assess the location, degree, and extent of the injury.

- Sequelae of HIE in term infants are related to the site of injury (e.g., the cortex) and include mental retardation, microcephaly, cortical blindness, hearing deficits, and epilepsy.

- Generally, infants with mild HIE do well.

- Those with moderate HIE or severe HIE have a higher mortality rate and later cognitive and motor problems (deVries & Jongmans, 2010; Ditzenberger & Blackburn, 2020; Epelman et al., 2012; Gunn et al., 2008; Gunny & Lin, 2012; Lodygensky et al., 2012; Lori et al., 2011; Volpe et al., 2018).

REFERENCES

Arriagada, S., Huang, H., Fletcher, K., & Giannone, P. (2019). Prevention of excessive hypothermia in infants with hypoxic ischemic encephalopathy prior to admission to a quaternary care center: A neonatal outreach educational project. *Journal of Perinatology, 39*, 1417–1427. https://doi.org/10.1038/s41372-019-0391-0

Barks, J. (2008). Technical aspects of starting a neonatal cooling program. *Clinics in Perinatology, 35*(4), 765–776. https://doi.org/10.1016/j.clp.2008.07.009

Bonifacio, S. L., Glass, H. C., Peloquin, S., & Ferriero, D. M. (2011). A new neurological focus in neonatal intensive care. *Nature Review Neurology, 7*(9), 485–494. https://doi.org/10.1038/nrneurol.2011.119

Bonifacio, S. L., Gonzalez, F., & Ferriero, D. M. (2012). Central nervous system injury and neuroprotection. In C. A. Gleason & S. Devaskar (Eds.), *Avery's diseases of the newborn* (9th ed., pp. 869–891). Saunders/Elsevier.

Chiang, M., Jong, Y., & Lin, C. (2017). Therapeutic hypothermia for neonates with hypoxic ischemic encephalopathy. *Pediatrics and Neonatology, 58*, 475–483. https://doi.org/10.1016/j.pedneo.2016.11.001

deVries, L. S., & Jongmans, M. J. (2010). Long-term outcome after neonatal hypoxic-ischaemic encephalopathy. *Archives of Disease in Childhood—Fetal and Neonatal Edition, 95*(3), F220–F224. https://doi.org/10.1136/adc.2008.148205

Dickey, E. J., Long, S. N., & Hunt, R. W. (2011). Hypoxic ischemic encephalopathy—What can we learn from humans? *Journal of Veterinary Internal Medicine, 25*(6), 1231–1240. https://doi.org/10.1111/j.1939-1676.2011.00818.x

Ditzenberger, G. R., & Blackburn, S. T. (2020). Neurologic system. In C. Kenner, L. B. Altimier, & M. V. Boykova (Eds.), *Comprehensive neonatal nursing care* (6th ed., pp. 373–416). Springer Publishing Company.

Douglas-Escobar, M., & Weiss, M. D. (2015). Hypoxic-ischemic encephalopathy: A review for the clinician. *JAMA Pediatrics, 169*(4), 397–403. https://doi.org/10.1001/jamapediatrics.2014.3269

Epelman, M., Daneman, A., Chauvin, N., & Hirsch, W. (2012). Head ultrasound and MR imaging in the evaluation of neonatal encephalopathy: Competitive or complementary imaging studies? *Magnetic Resonance Imaging Clinics of North America, 20*(1), 93–115. https://doi.org/10.1016/j.mric.2011.08.012

Gancia, P., & Pomero, G. (2011). Brain cooling and eligible newborns: Should we extend the indications? *Journal of Maternal-Fetal and Neonatal Medicine, 24*(S1), 53–55. https://doi.org/10.3109/14767058.2011.607617

Glass, H. C. (2010). Neurocritical care for neonates. *Neurocritical Care, 12*(3), 421–429. https://doi.org/10.1007/s12028-009-9324-7

Goel, N., Mohinuddin, S., Ratnavel, N., Kempley, S., & Sinha A. (2016). Comparison of passive and servo-controlled active cooling for infants with hypoxic-ischemic encephalopathy during neonatal transfers. *American Journal of Perinatology, 34,* 19–25. https://doi.org/10.1055/s-0036-1584151

Gudsnuk, K. M., & Champagne, F. A. (2011). Epigenetic effects of early developmental experiences. *Clinics in Perinatology, 38*(4), 703–718. https://doi.org/10.1016/j.clp.2011.08.005

Gunn, A. J. (2005). Selective head cooling with mild systemic hypothermia after neonatal encephalopathy: Multicentre randomised trial. *Lancet, 365*(9460), 663–670. https://doi.org/10.1016/S0140-6736(05)17946-X

Gunn, A. J., Wyatt, J. S., Whitelaw, A., Barks, J., Azzopardi, D., Ballard, R., Edwards, A. D., Ferriero, D. M., Gluckman, P. D., Polin, R. A., Robertson, C. M., Thoresen, M., & CoolCap Study Group. (2008). Therapeutic hypothermia changes the prognostic value of clinical evaluation of neonatal encephalopathy. *Journal of Pediatrics, 152*(1), 55–58.e51. https://doi.org/10.1016/j.jpeds.2007.06.003

Gunny, R. S., & Lin, D. (2012). Imaging of perinatal stroke. *Magnetic Resonance Imaging Clinics of North America, 20*(1), 1–33. https://doi.org/10.1016/j.mric.2011.10.001

Hill, E., Glass, H. C., Kelley, K., Barnes, M., Rau, S., Franck, L., & Shellhaas, R. A. (2017). Sezures and antiseizure medications are important to parents of newborns with seizures. *Pediatric Neurology, 67,* 40–44. https://doi.org/10.1016/j.pediatrneurol.2016.10.003

Hoehn, T., Hansmann, G., Bührer, C., Simbruner, G., Gunn, A. J., Yager, J., Levene, M., Hamrick, S. E. G., Shankaran, S., & Thoresen, M. (2008). Therapeutic hypothermia in neonates. Review of current clinical data, ILCOR recommendations and suggestions for implementation in neonatal intensive care units. *Resuscitation, 78*(1), 7–12. https://doi.org/10.1016/j.resuscitation.2008.04.027

Johnston, M. V., Fatemi, A., Wilson, M. A., & Northington, F. (2011). Treatment advances in neonatal neuroprotection and neurointensive care. *Lancet Neurology, 10*(4), 372–382. https://doi.org/10.1016/S1474-4422(11)70016-3

Kendall, G, Kapetanakis, A, Ratnavel, N, Azzopardi, D., Robertson, N., & on behalf of the Cooling on Retrieval Study Group. (2010). Passive cooling for initiation of therapeutic hypothermia in neonatal encephalopathy. *Archives in Diseases of Childhood Fetal Neonatal Edition, 95,* F408–F412. https://doi.org/10.1136/adc.2010.187211

Laptook, A. R. (2012). The use of hypothermia to provide neuroprotection for neonatal hypoxic-ischemic brain injury. In J. Perlman (Ed.), *Neurology* (2nd ed., pp. 63–76). Saunders/Elsevier.

Lemyre, B., Ly, L., Chau, V., Chacko, A., Barrowman, N., Whyte, H., & Miller, S. (2017). Initiation of passive cooling at referring centre is most predictive of achieving early therapeutic hypothermia in asphyxiated newborns. *Journal of Pediatrics & Child Health, 22,* 264–268. https://doi.org/10.1093/pch/pxx062

Lodygensky, G. A., Menache, C. C., & Huppi, P. S. (2012). Magnetic resonance imaging's role in the care of the infant at risk for brain injury. In J. M. Perlman (Ed.), *Neonatology* (2nd ed., pp. 285–324). Saunders/Elsevier.

Long, M., & Brandon, D. H. (2007). Induced hypothermia for neonates with hypoxic-ischemic encephalopathy. *Journal of Obstetric, Gynecologic, & Neonatal Nursing, 36*(3), 293–298. https://doi.org/10.1111/j.1552-6909.2007.00150.x

Lori, S., Bertini, G., Molesti, E., Gualandi, D., Gabbanini, S., Bastianelli, M. E., Pinto, F., & Dani, C. (2011). The prognostic role of evoked potentials in neonatal hypoxic-ischemic insult. *Journal of Maternal-Fetal and Neonatal Medicine, 24*(S1), 69–71. https://doi.org/10.3109/14767058.2011.607661

Monmany, N., Behrsin, J., & Leslie, A. (2019). Servo-controlled cooling during neonatal transport for babies with hypoxic-ischaemic encephalopathy is practical and beneficial: Experience from a large UK neonatal transport service. *Journal of Paediatrics and Child Health, 55,* 518–522. https://doi.org/10.1111/jpc.14232

Natarajan, G., Laptook, A., & Shankaran, S. (2018). Therapeutic hypothermia: How can we optimize this therapy to further improve outcomes? *Clinics in Perinatology, 45*, 241–255. https://doi.org/10.1016/j.clp.2018.01.010

Pfister, R., & Soll, R. (2010). Hypothermia for the treatment of infants with hypoxic–ischemic encephalopathy. *Journal of Perinatology, 30*, S82–S87. https://doi.org/10.1038/jp.2010.91

Reynolds, R., & Talmage, S. (2011). "Caution! Contents should be cold": Developing a whole-body hypothermia program. *Neonatal Network: Journal of Neonatal Nursing, 30*(4), 225–230. https://doi.org/10.1891/0730-0832.30.4.225

Sarkar, S., Barks, J., Bhagat, I., & Donn, S. (2009). Effects of therapeutic hypothermia on multiorgan dysfunction in asphyxiated newborns: Whole-body cooling versus selective head cooling. *Journal of Perinatology, 29*, 558–563. https://doi.org/10.1038/jp.2009.37

Sarnat, H., & Sarnat, M. (1976). Neonatal encephalopathy following fetal distress. A clinical and electroencephalographic study. *Archives of Neurology, 33*, 696–705. https://doi.org/10.1001/archneur.1976.00500100030012

Selway, L. D. (2010). State of the science: Hypoxic ischemic encephalopathy and hypothermic intervention for neonates. *Advances in Neonatal Care, 10*(2), 60–66. https://doi.org/10.1097/ANC.0b013e3181d54b30

Simbruner, G., Mittal, R. A., Rohlmann, F., Muche, R., & neo.nEURO.network Trial Participants. (2010). Systemic hypothermia after neonatal encephalopathy: Outcomes of neo.nEURO.network RCT. *Pediatrics, 126*(4), e771–e778. https://doi.org/10.1542/peds.2009-2441

Sorem, K., Smith, J. F., & Druzin, M. L. (2009). Antenatal prediction of asphyxia. In M. Levene & F. A. Chervenak (Eds.), *Fetal and neonatal neurology and neurosurgery.* Churchill Livingstone/Elsevier.

Stola, A., & Perlman, J. (2008). Post-resuscitation strategies to avoid ongoing injury following intrapartum hypoxia–ischemia. *Seminars in Fetal and Neonatal Medicine, 13*(6), 424–431. https://doi.org/10.1016/j.siny.2008.04.011

Sullivan, R., Perry, R., Sloan, A., Kleinhaus, K., & Burtchen, N. (2011). Infant bonding and attachment to the caregiver: Insights from basic and clinical science. *Clinics in Perinatology, 38*, 643–656. https://doi.org/10.1016/j.clp.2011.08.011

Tagin, M. A., Woolcott, C. G., Vincer, M. J., Whyte, R. K., & Stinson, D. A. (2012). Hypothermia for neonatal hypoxic ischemic encephalopathy: An updated systematic review and meta-analysis. *Archives of Pediatrics and Adolescent Medicine, 166*(6), 558–566. https://doi.org/10.1001/archpediatrics.2011.1772

Tao, J. D., & Mathur, A. M. (2010). Using amplitude-integrated EEG in neonatal intensive care. *Journal of Perinatology, 30*(S1), S73–S81. https://doi.org/10.1038/jp.2010.93

Toet, M. C., & deVries, L. S. (2012). Amplitude-integrated EEG and its potential role in augmenting management within the NICU. In J. M. Perlman (Ed.), *Neurology* (2nd ed., pp. 263–284). Saunders/Elsevier.

Toet, M. C., & Lemmers, P. M. A. (2009). Brain monitoring in neonates. *Early Human Development, 85*(2), 77–84. https://doi.org/10.1016/j.earlhumdev.2008.11.007

Volpe, J. J. (2008). *Neurology of the newborn* (5th ed.). Saunders/Elsevier.

Volpe, J. J., Inder, T. E., Darras, B. T., de Vries, L. S., du Plessis, A. J., Neil, J., & Perlman, J. M. (2018). *Volpe's neurology of the newborn* (6th ed.). Saunders/Elsevier.

Wachtel, E. V., & Hendricks-Muñoz, K. D. (2011). Current management of the infant who presents with neonatal encephalopathy. *Current Problems in Pediatric and Adolescent Health Care, 41*(5), 132–153. https://doi.org/10.1016/j.cppeds.2010.12.002

Walsh, B. H., Murray, D. M., & Boylan, G. B. (2011). The use of conventional EEG for the assessment of hypoxic ischaemic encephalopathy in the newborn: A review. *Clinical Neurophysiology, 122*(7), 1284–1294. https://doi.org/10.1016/j.clinph.2011.03.032

Wassink, G., Davidson, J., Dhillon, S., Zhou, K., Bennet, L., Thoresen, M., & Gunn, A. (2019). Therapeutic hypothermia in neonatal hypoxic-ischemic encephalopathy. *Current Neurology and Neuroscience Reports, 19*, 2–12. https://doi.org/10.1007/s11910-019-0916-0

Zanelli, S., Buck, M., & Fairchild, K. (2011). Physiologic and pharmacologic considerations for hypothermia therapy in neonates. *Journal of Perinatology, 31*(6), 377–386. https://doi .org/10.1038/jp.2010.146

BIRTH INJURIES

GEORGIA R. DITZENBERGER AND SUSAN TUCKER BLACKBURN

Traumatic injury to the central or peripheral nervous system can occur during the perinatal or postnatal period. Most of these injuries happen during the intrapartum period and may occur with perinatal hypoxic–ischemic events. Perinatal events most frequently associated with birth injury include midforceps delivery, shoulder dystocia, low-forceps delivery, birth weight exceeding 3,500 g, and second stage of labor lasting longer than 60 minutes. The incidence of injury has declined markedly in recent years as a result of improvement in obstetrical care and increased use of Cesarean sections for abnormal presentations. However, birth injuries can also arise from trauma during a Cesarean section or resuscitation. Injuries that occur before the intrapartum period usually are caused by compression or pressure injuries from an unusual fetal position. The risk of injury to the central or peripheral nervous system is greater with malpresentation (especially breech), prolonged or precipitate labor, prematurity, multiple gestation, shoulder dystocia, macrosomia, and instrumental delivery.

The most prevalent types of injury to the nervous system are extracranial hemorrhage, intracranial hemorrhage, skull fractures, spinal cord injury, and peripheral nerve injury (Bonifacio et al., 2012; Ditzenberger & Blackburn, 2020).

EXTRACRANIAL HEMORRHAGE

■ Caput succedaneum and cephalohematoma: most common types, most benign of birth injury
  ● Caput succedaneum: soft, pitting, superficial edema several millimeters thick; overlies presenting part in a vertex delivery; crosses suture lines
    • Edematous area above the periosteum
      − Edema consists of serum, blood, or both.
    • Infants with caput succedaneum may also have ecchymosis, petechiae, or purpura over the presenting part.
    • Occurs after a spontaneous vertex delivery or after use of a vacuum extractor.
    • Resolves within a few days after birth with no sequelae.
■ Cephalohematoma: firm, fluctuant mass; does not cross the suture lines
  ● Occurs in 1.5% to 2.5% of newborns; most often in males
  ● Subperiosteal bleeding, usually over the parietal bone but possibly over other cranial bones
    • Mass often enlarges slightly by 2 to 3 days of age.

- Occurs after the use of forceps; after a prolonged, difficult delivery; and in infants born to primiparas.
- Usually unilateral, can be bilateral
  - Approximately 5% of infants with unilateral and 18% with bilateral have a linear skull fracture underlying the mass.
- Generally asymptomatic
- Observe for symptoms of intracranial hemorrhage or skull fracture; hyperbilirubinemia
- Occasionally anemia develops with a large cephalohematoma.
- Resolve between 2 weeks and 6 months of age; most by 8 weeks.
  - Calcium deposits occasionally develop.
  - Swelling may remain for the first year (Bonifacio et al., 2012; Ditzenberger & Blackburn, 2020; Fenichel, 2007; Waller et al., 2012; Watchko, 2009)

■ Subgaleal hemorrhage
- Subgaleal or subaponeurotic hemorrhage is the most serious form of extracranial hemorrhage in newborns (Schierholz & Walker, 2014; Waller et al., 2012)
- Incidence: 1.5 to 30 per 10,000 births
  - Spontaneous vaginal deliveries: four per 10,000
  - Vacuum-assisted deliveries: 59 per 10,000
  - Increased with precipitous deliveries, macrosomia, and severe dystocia, and with failed vacuum deliveries requiring forceps

■ Mortality: 17% to 25% (Ditzenberger & Blackburn, 2020; Fenichel, 2007; Shah & Wusthoff, 2016; Volpe, 2008; Volpe et al., 2018)

Physiology/Pathophysiology

■ Traction or application of intense shearing forces to the scalp pull the aponeurosis from the vault and rupture large emissary veins. Blood collects in a large potential space between the galea aponeurotica and the periosteum of the skull through which the large emissary veins pass.

■ The area is called a potential space because it is not present until blood separates the galea aponeurotica from the periosteum of the skull. This space can quickly expand to accommodate 260 to 280 mL of blood.

■ Total newborn blood volume is 80 to 100 mL/kg. The amount of blood entering the subgalial space may be more than the entire blood volume of some newborns.

■ Subgaleal hemorrhage is a clinical emergency. These infants usually present at birth or within a few hours (Bonifacio et al., 2012; Ditzenberger & Blackburn, 2020; Fenichel, 2007; Schierholz & Walker, 2010, 2014; Shah & Wusthoff, 2016; Volpe, 2008; Volpe et al., 2018).

Assessment

■ Birth history

■ Observation during first hours of life; can develop over minutes following delivery; most rapid development over first 1 to 3 hours of life; few can develop slowly over 24 to 48 hours

Clinical Manifestations/Diagnosis

■ Firm, ballotable head mass crossing sutures and fontanelles

● Often extends from the orbital ridge, around the ears to the neck

■ Develops after birth and increases in size quickly within first 1 to 3 hours of life—most acute

■ Each centimeter of enlargement is estimated to be equivalent to 40 mL of blood loss

■ Mimics edema; shifts with head repositioning

■ Usually accompanied by pain on manipulation of the scalp or head

■ Symptoms: anemia, hypovolemia, pallor, hypotension, tachycardia, tachypnea, hypotonia, and other signs of shock

■ Laboratory results: rapidly falling hematocrit, platelets, clotting factors

Treatment/Management

■ Rapid recognition

■ Monitor cardiovascular (HR, BP), respiratory status

■ Check hematocrit/hemoglobin results at minimum every hour; d-dimers, fibrinogen levels every 2 to 4 hours during acute phase

■ Administer blood and volume expanders

■ Control bleeding with fresh frozen plasma and cryoprecipitate

■ Supportive care:

● Fluids, electrolytes, glucose

● Oxygen, ventilator support

■ Central lines (umbilical arterial and venous catheters) for immediate access, blood samples, cardiovascular support, blood products (Bonifacio et al., 2012; Ditzenberger & Blackburn, 2020; Fenichel, 2007; Schierholz & Walker, 2010, 2014; Shah & Wusthoff, 2016; Volpe, 2008; Volpe et al., 2018)

Prognosis

■ If infant survives initial acute hemorrhagic event and hypoxic–ischemic encephalopathy (HIE) does not develop, the condition usually resolves in 2 to 3 weeks.

■ Morbidity is related to neurologic deficits associated with HIE (Volpe, 2008; Volpe et al., 2018).

INTRACRANIAL HEMORRHAGE

Several clinically important types of intracranial bleeding can occur in the neonate, including intraventricular hemorrhage (IVH; described earlier), primary subarachnoid hemorrhage (SAH), subdural hemorrhage, and intracerebellar hemorrhage. These latter three types of hemorrhage arise from trauma or hypoxia during the perinatal period.

PRIMARY SUBARACHNOID HEMORRHAGE

Incidence

■ Rare; often is associated with severe asphyxial event and birth trauma
■ Most prevalent form of intracranial hemorrhage in neonates

Physiology/Pathophysiology

■ Hemorrhage into the subarachnoid space
  ● Newborns: venous blood; older children and adults: arterial blood
  ● Blood leaks from the leptomeningeal plexus, bridging veins, or ruptured vessels in the subarachnoid space.
  ● Associated with trauma or asphyxia (Ditzenberger & Blackburn, 2020; Hong & Lee, 2018; Levene & deVries, 2009; Shah & Wusthoff, 2016; Volpe, 2008; Volpe et al., 2018)

Assessment

■ Perinatal: birth trauma, prolonged labor, difficult delivery, fetal distress, perinatal hypoxic–ischemic events
■ Hemorrhage may be discovered accidentally with "bloody" lumbar puncture.

Clinical Manifestations/Diagnosis

■ Can be asymptomatic
■ May present at day 2 to 3 with isolated seizure for term; apnea for preterm
  ● Between seizures, infant appears and acts healthy.
■ Massive SAH: rapid and fatal course
■ MRI and CT confirm the diagnosis; ultrasonography is unreliable

Treatment/Management

■ Prevent or reduce the risk of trauma and hypoxia during the perinatal period.

■ Observe at-risk infants for seizures and other neurologic signs.

■ Perform general nursing care (Ditzenberger & Blackburn, 2020; Hong & Lee, 2018; Levene & deVries, 2009; Shah & Wusthoff, 2016; Volpe, 2008; Volpe et al., 2018).

Prognosis

■ Most survive

■ Asymptomatic/isolated seizure on day 2 to 3: usually do well developmentally

■ Symptomatic with severe SAH: up to one-half of infants with severe traumatic or hypoxic injury: neurologic sequelae; occasional hydrocephalus (Ditzenberger & Blackburn, 2020; Levene & deVries, 2009; Volpe, 2008; Volpe et al., 2018)

SUBDURAL HEMORRHAGE

Risk Factors

■ Precipitous, prolonged, or difficult delivery

■ Mid-forceps or high forceps

■ Prematurity

■ Cephalopelvic disproportion

■ Macrosomia

■ Breech presentation

Incidence

■ Most common hemorrhage seen in newborns

■ Incidence has declined markedly due to improvements in obstetrical care; higher incidence with vaginal deliveries over Cesarean deliveries (Ditzenberger & Blackburn, 2020; Hong & Lee, 2018; Levene & deVries, 2009; Shah & Wusthoff, 2016).

Pathophysiology

■ Unilateral or bilateral bleeding between dura and arachnoid with rupture of superficial cerebral veins or of "bridging" veins between superomedial aspect of the cerebrum and superior sagittal sinus (Ditzenberger & Blackburn, 2020; Fenichel, 2007; Levene & deVries, 2009; Volpe, 2008; Volpe et al., 2018)

Assessment

■ Perinatal history: precipitous, prolonged, or difficult delivery; use of midforceps or high forceps; prematurity; cephalopelvic disproportion; macrosomia; breech presentation

■ Recognition is important for immediate intervention for large subdural hemorrhage.

■ Associated with cephalohematoma; subgaleal, subconjunctival, and retinal hemorrhages; skull fractures; and brachial plexus or facial palsies (Ditzenberger & Blackburn, 2020; Fenichel, 2007; Hong & Lee, 2018; Levene & deVries, 2009; Shah & Wusthoff, 2016; Volpe, 2008; Volpe et al., 2018; Waller et al., 2012)

Clinical Manifestations

■ Most common: minor hemorrhage
  ● Asymptomatic or have signs such as irritability and hyperalertness; resolve without consequence
■ Symptoms may occur 24 to 48 hours after delivery; nonspecific: apnea; respiratory distress; altered neurologic state; seizures, which are primarily focal; occasional hemiparesis; unequal pupils with sluggish response to light; full or tense fontanelle; bradycardia; irregular respirations.
■ Late-onset symptoms (rare): appear at 4 weeks to 6 months of age: increasing head size due to continued hematoma formation, poor feeding, failure to thrive, altered level of consciousness, and occasionally, seizures caused by the chronic subdural effusion.

Diagnosis

■ MRI or CT confirms diagnosis (Ditzenberger & Blackburn, 2020; Fenichel, 2007; Hong & Lee, 2018; Shah & Wusthoff, 2016; Volpe, 2008; Volpe et al., 2018).

Treatment/Management

■ Observe for seizures and other neurologic signs.
■ Massive posterior fossa hemorrhage requires craniotomy and surgical aspiration of the clot (Ditzenberger & Blackburn, 2020; Fenichel, 2007; Hong & Lee, 2018; Levene & deVries, 2009; Shah & Wusthoff, 2016).

Prognosis

■ Varies with the location and severity of the hemorrhage
■ Asymptomatic/transient neonatal seizures: do well
■ Most infants with bleeding over the tentorium or falx cerebri die; severe hydrocephalus and neurologic sequelae usually develop in those that survive (Ditzenberger & Blackburn, 2020; Hong & Lee, 2018; Shah & Wusthoff, 2016; Volpe, 2008; Volpe et al., 2018).

PERINATAL STROKE

Ischemic strokes are more common in the perinatal period than at any other time of life and are the leading cause of hemiplegic cerebral palsy, yet until recently they have been poorly understood and oftentimes not diagnosed in the neonatal period.

Risk Factors

■ Poorly understood, likely multifactorial and still being identified

■ Maternal: thrombophilias (factor V Leiden, factor VIII, protein S deficiency, protein C deficiency, prothrombin mutation, and antiphospholipid antibodies) and/or preexisting conditions such as thyroid disease, diabetes mellitus, or gestational diabetes or history of infertility

■ Pregnancy/labor related: significant maternal trauma, primiparity, placental abnormalities, oligohydramnios, decreased fetal movement, prolonged rupture of membranes, chorioamnionitis, prolonged second stage of labor, or assisted delivery

■ Fetal or neonatal: fetal distress during labor, cord abnormalities (tight nuchal or body cord, true cord knot), thrombophilias, congenital cardiac defects, and corrective surgery

Incidence

■ Estimated to be from fairly rare (17–93 per 100,000 live births) to relatively common (one in 2,300–5,000 live births) (Benders et al., 2009; Chabrier et al., 2011; Cheong & Cowan, 2009; Ditzenberger & Blackburn, 2020; Kirton & deVeber, 2009; Mineyko & Kirton, 2011; Murias, 2014; Myers & Ment, 2012; Volpe et al., 2018)

Physiology/Pathophysiology

■ Result of a focal disruption of cerebral blood flow secondary to an arterial or venous thrombosis or embolism occurring between 20 weeks' gestation and the 28th postnatal day of life (Ditzenberger & Blackburn, 2020; Kirton & deVeber, 2009; Mineyko & Kirton, 2011; Myers & Ment, 2012; National Institute of Neurological Disorders and Stroke, 2006)

■ Perinatal strokes classified as fetal, neonatal, presumed perinatal ischemic

  ● Fetal stroke: occurred between 20 weeks' gestation and the onset of labor or Cesarean section

  ● Neonatal stroke: occurred between the onset of labor and actual delivery

  ● Presumed perinatal ischemic stroke: identified by neuroimaging in infants greater than 28 days of life as having had a focal infarction at some point between 20 weeks' gestation and postnatal day 28 (Chabrier et al., 2011; Ditzenberger & Blackburn, 2020; Kirton & deVeber, 2009; Lynch, 2009; Myers & Ment, 2012; Volpe et al., 2018)

Assessment

■ Maternal, pregnancy/labor, fetal, and neonatal history

■ May be a gender effect, occurs more frequently in male (Chabrier et al., 2011; Cheong & Cowan, 2009; Ditzenberger & Blackburn, 2020; Kirton & deVeber, 2009; Lynch, 2009; Mineyko & Kirton, 2011; Myers & Ment, 2012)

Clinical Manifestations

■ Determined by the timing of the initial insult

■ Bulging and/or pulsatile fontanelle, dilated head and neck veins, papilledema, asymmetrical movements, primitive reflexes, or seizure-like activity (Kirton & deVeber, 2009)

■ Transient hemiparesis or generalized tone anomalies in early newborn phase

■ Seizures occur in 85% to 92% of affected newborns

  ● Often the earliest manifestation for healthy appearing newborns

  ● Most occur within the first 72 hours of life

  ● Approximately 50% focal motor, 33% generalized motor, 17% subtle

■ If not diagnosed during the newborn stage, identified ~6 months.

  ● Asymmetry of reach and grasp

  ● Seizures occurring after 28 days of life; language delay also reported (Ditzenberger & Blackburn, 2020; Kirton & deVeber, 2009; Myers & Ment, 2012)

Diagnosis

■ EEG and neuroimaging to evaluate for diagnosis

■ Echocardiogram and electrocardiogram may be indicated to assess for cardiac dysfunction or rhythm disorders (Cheong & Cowan, 2009; Ditzenberger & Blackburn, 2020; Kirton & deVeber, 2009; Myers & Ment, 2012).

Treatment/Management

■ Supportive; directed at minimizing secondary brain injury

■ Avoid hyperthermia and hyperthermic environment

■ Document and aggressively treat seizures (Ditzenberger & Blackburn, 2020; Kirton & deVeber, 2009; Myers & Ment, 2012)

Prognosis

■ Varies with area of original insult

■ Estimated 20% to 70% of hemiplegic cerebral palsy associated with perinatal stroke, with spasticity more marked in upper extremities

■ Intelligence is within normal parameters for two-thirds of affected infants.

■ Neurologic deficits are usually associated with cerebral injury from original trauma and/or hypoxic event (Ditzenberger & Blackburn, 2020; Myers & Ment, 2012).

SPINAL CORD INJURY

Risk Factors

■ Breech delivery
■ Shoulder dystocia
■ Macrosomia
■ Cephalopelvic disproportion

Incidence

■ Uncommon

Physiology/Pathophysiology

■ Injury can occur at any point along the cord.
■ Caused by excessive traction, rotation, and torsion of the vertebral column and neck
■ Occurs from stretching of spinal cord; damage ranges from complete transection to laceration, edema, hemorrhage, and hematoma formation (Bonifacio et al., 2012; Ditzenberger & Blackburn, 2020; Fenichel, 2007; Madsen et al., 2005; Volpe, 2008; Volpe et al., 2018).

Assessment

■ Birth history: breech delivery, dystocia, macrosomia, cephalopelvic disproportion

Clinical Manifestations

■ Spinal cord shock: hypotonia, weakness, flaccid extremities, sensory deficits, relaxed abdominal muscles, diaphragmatic breathing, Horner syndrome (ipsilateral ptosis, anhidrosis, and miosis), distended bladder
■ Low cervical lesions: shallow, paradoxical respirations
■ Degree of neurologic insult often cannot be accurately evaluated until the infant has recovered from the initial period of spinal shock and any edema or hemorrhage has been reabsorbed.

Diagnosis

■ Spinal ultrasonography, CT, or MRI is used to determine level and extent of injury.

Treatment/Management

■ Stabilize.

■ Treat associated problems (e.g., asphyxia, hemorrhage, shock).

■ Maintain respiratory status.

● Midcervical to upper cervical or brainstem lesions require assisted ventilation.

■ Monitor for signs of respiratory infection and pneumonia.

■ Maintain skin integrity over the paralyzed area.

■ Require meticulous bowel and bladder care; regular glycerin suppositories, urinary catheterization

■ Follow-up care: multidisciplinary team: nursing, medicine, neurology, neurosurgery, physical therapy, orthopedics, urology, social work, and psychology

Prognosis

■ Depends on the level and severity of the injury; generally, poor

■ Many are stillborn or die shortly after birth.

■ Survivors have varying degrees of residual paralysis, respiratory problems, and bowel and bladder dysfunction depending on the level of the injury (Bonifacio et al., 2012; Ditzenberger & Blackburn, 2020; Fenichel, 2007; Madsen et al., 2005; Volpe, 2008; Volpe et al., 2018).

PERIPHERAL NERVE INJURIES

Peripheral nerve injuries result from stretching, compression, twisting, hyperextension, or separation of nerve tissue. Injury can occur before, during, or after birth and is seen predominantly in term and large for gestational age (LGA) infants.

The more common sites affected are the radial, median, sciatic, and phrenic nerves and the brachial plexus. Damage can range from swelling of the nerve to complete peripheral degeneration (with later total recovery) to complete division of all structures (Bonifacio et al., 2012; Ditzenberger & Blackburn, 2020; Fenichel, 2007; Levene, 2009; Volpe, 2008; Volpe et al., 2018).

RADIAL NERVE INJURY

■ Usually results from compression of the nerve caused by fracture of the humerus during a breech delivery or by intrauterine compression of the arm

■ Symptoms: wrist drop with a normal grasp reflex

■ Recovery: over the first few weeks to months

MEDIAN AND SCIATIC NERVE INJURIES

■ Typically, postnatal iatrogenic events

■ Median nerve injury can be a complication of brachial or radial arterial punctures

■ Symptoms: diminished pincer grasp and thumb strength; flexed fourth finger

■ Recovery is variable.

■ Sciatic nerve injuries: often permanent

■ Trauma from a misplaced intramuscular injection or from ischemia from an injection of hypertonic solutions into the gluteal muscle

■ Symptoms: diminished abduction and distal joint movement (Bonifacio et al., 2012; Ditzenberger & Blackburn, 2020; Levene, 2009; Missios et al., 2014; Volpe, 2008; Volpe et al., 2018)

FACIAL NERVE PALSY

Facial nerve palsy must be differentiated from nuclear agenesis (Möebius syndrome), a significant disorder characterized by congenital facial muscle paralysis (Ditzenberger & Blackburn, 2020; Levene, 2009; Terzis & Anesti, 2011; Volpe, 2008; Volpe et al., 2018).

■ Incidence: 0.23%

■ Caused by trauma from oblique application of forceps, prolonged pressure on the nerve during labor from the maternal sacral promontory, or pressure from an abnormal fetal posture

■ Most common on the left

■ Clinical manifestations vary depending on whether the injury is to the central nerve, the peripheral nerve, or the peripheral nerve branch.

  ● Complete peripheral nerve injury: unilateral inability to close the eye or open the mouth; lower lip on the affected side does not depress during crying, forehead does not wrinkle; affected side appears full and smooth, with obliteration of the nasolabial fold; dribble milk while feeding

  ● Central injury: spastic paralysis of the lower portion of the face contralateral to the side of central nervous system (CNS) injury without involvement of eyes or forehead

  ● Peripheral injury: varying degrees of paralysis of the forehead, eye, or lower face, depending on the branch involved; paralysis is apparent at birth or within 1 to 2 days after birth

Prognosis

■ Almost all infants recover completely by 1 to 4 weeks (Ditzenberger & Blackburn, 2020; Fenichel, 2007; Levene, 2009; Terzis & Anesti, 2011).

PHRENIC NERVE PALSY

Phrenic nerve palsy must be differentiated from CNS, cardiac, and pulmonary problems.

Risk Factors

■ Vaginal delivery of large-for-gestational-age (LGA) infants
■ Shoulder dystocia
■ Breech presentations
■ Prolonged labor
■ Difficult delivery

Incidence

■ Rare

Physiology/Pathophysiology

■ Paralysis of the diaphragm due to phrenic nerve damage
■ Usually unilateral, on the right side
■ Caused by injury of the cervical nerve roots at C3 to C5
  ● Results from tearing of the nerve sheath, accompanied by edema and hemorrhage
  ● May occur as an isolated event or in association with brachial nerve palsy

Assessment

■ Birth history: vaginal delivery of large-for-gestational-age (LGA) infants, shoulder dystocia, breech presentations, prolonged labor, or difficult delivery

Clinical Manifestations

■ Respiratory difficulty
■ Recurrent episodes of cyanosis and dyspnea
■ Primarily thoracic movement with minimal or no abdominal excursions, opposite of the normal newborn breathing pattern
■ If complete avulsion or bilateral injury: severe respiratory distress from birth

Diagnosis

■ Ultrasound of the diaphragm

Treatment/Management

■ Promote ventilation and oxygenation.

■ If severe distress: positive pressure ventilation or constant positive airway pressure for support until recovery occurs

■ Position on affected side

■ No enteral feeds until respiratory status improves; gavage; advance as tolerated to oral feeds

■ Surgical plication of the diaphragm may be needed if no improvement is noted or if the infant is still ventilator dependent at 4 to 6 weeks of age.

Prognosis

■ Recovery 6 to 12 months of age

■ Some infants recover clinically but have residual abnormalities of diaphragmatic movement on radiography (Ditzenberger & Blackburn, 2020; Fenichel, 2007; Volpe, 2008; Volpe et al., 2018).

BRACHIAL PLEXUS INJURY

Risk Factors

■ Vaginal delivery of LGA infants

■ Shoulder dystocia

■ Breech presentations

■ Prolonged labor

■ Difficult delivery

Incidence

■ Occurs in 0.5% to 2%; almost exclusively in term infant

■ May occur in multiparity as frequently as in nulliparity

Physiology/Pathophysiology

■ Injury of the C5 to T1 nerve roots

■ Degree of injury varies, ranging from edema and hemorrhage of the nerve sheath to avulsion of the nerve root from the spinal cord

Assessment

■ Birth history: vaginal delivery of LGA infants, shoulder dystocia, breech presentations, prolonged labor, or difficult delivery

■ Can occur in uncomplicated deliveries; after Cesarean birth

■ Usually unilateral, on left side; clavicle fracture may occur

Clinical Manifestations/Diagnosis

■ Vary with the location and severity of the injury

■ Usually apparent from birth; may be delayed for several days to a few weeks

■ Can be hereditary; autosomal-dominant inheritance (mapped to 17q25); should be considered with uncomplicated delivery and positive family history

■ Can be associated with phrenic nerve palsy with hemidiaphragm paralysis—consider if newborn also has increased respiratory rate and intermittent/continuous oxygen requirement

■ May be associated with clavicle fracture

Erb (Erb–Duchenne) Palsy (Most Common)

■ Upper plexus injury involving C5 to C7; shoulder and upper arm; denervation of the deltoid, supraspinous, biceps, and brachioradialis muscles

■ Passive arm, abducted and internally rotated; pronated forearm; flexed wrist and fingers; absent Moro reflex; biceps, radial reflexes diminished, or absent; normal grasp reflex

Klumpke Palsy

■ Lower plexus injury at C5 to T1; seen primarily in breech infants whose arm has been hyperabducted and delivered with the head affecting the flexors of the wrist and hand

■ Affected hand and arm without sensation; held passively to side; claw hand position; absent Moro, grasp reflexes; triceps reflex diminished or absent; biceps and radial reflexes present

Erb–Klumpke (Total) Palsy

■ Injury to the nerve roots of the brachial plexus from C5 to T1

■ Complete paralysis of the upper and lower arm and hand; flaccid; no sensation; absent deep tendon, Moro reflexes

■ MRI or CT: visualize the degree of injury

■ If improvement is not noted within the first few weeks to months, electromyography and nerve conduction studies to determine the extent of the damage, to follow recovery, and to determine whether surgical intervention are needed

Treatment/Management

■ Protect arm until localized edema and pain subsides.

■ Support arm in position of relaxation; no splints; do not immobilize.

■ Provide comfort measures to reduce pain.

■ Evaluate for associated problems: fractures; respiratory difficulty secondary to phrenic nerve paralysis.

■ After edema subsides, 7 to 10 days: physical therapy.

■ Continue massage and exercise over the first months until total or partial recovery occurs.

Prognosis

■ Depends on the level and severity of the injury

■ Approximately 65% to 95%: full recovery by 4 months to 3 years of age

■ Infants with total paralysis most likely for ongoing residual functional deficits: alterations in shoulder abduction and external rotation; restricted movement of the elbow and forearm; hand weakness; potential for abnormal muscle development and arm growth (Abzug & Kozin, 2014; Akangire & Carter, 2016; Alfonso, 2011; Clapp et al., 2016; Ditzenberger & Blackburn, 2020; Doumouchtsis & Arulkumaran, 2009; Fenichel, 2007; Govindan & Burrows, 2019; Levene, 2009; Volpe, 2008; Volpe et al., 2018)

REFERENCES

Abzug, J., & Kozin, S. (2014). Evaluation and management of brachial plexus birth palsy. *Orthopedic Clinics of North America, 45*, 225–232. https://doi.org/10.1016/j.ocl.2013.12.004

Akangire, G., & Carter, B. (2016). Birth injuries in neonates. *Pediatrics in Review, 37*(11), 451–461. https://doi.org/10.1542/pir.2015-0125

Alfonso, D. T. (2011). Causes of neonatal brachial plexus palsy. *Bulletin of the NYU Hospital for Joint Diseases, 69*(1), 11–16. https://hjdbulletin.org/files/archive/pdfs/237.pdf

Benders, M. J. N. L., Groenendaal, F., & deVries, L. S. (2009). Preterm arterial ischemic stroke. *Seminars in Fetal and Neonatal Medicine, 14*(5), 272–277. https://doi.org/10.1016/j.siny.2009.07.002

Billington, C. J., Jr., Schmidt, B., Marcucio, R. S., Hallgrimsson, B., Gopalakrishnan, R., & Petryk, A. (2015). Impact of retinoic acid exposure on midfacial shape variation and manifestation of holoprosencephaly in Twsg1 mutant mice. *Disease Models & Mechanisms, 8*(2), 139–146. https://doi.org/10.1242/dmm.018275

Bonifacio, S. L., Gonzalez, F., & Ferriero, D. M. (2012). Central nervous system injury and neuroprotection. In C. A. Gleason & S. Devaskar (Eds.), *Avery's diseases of the newborn* (9th ed., pp. 869–891). Saunders/Elsevier.

Chabrier, S., Husson, B., Dinomais, M., Landrieu, P., & Nguyen The Tich, S. (2011). New insights (and new interrogations) in perinatal arterial ischemic stroke. *Thrombosis Research, 127*(1), 13–22. https://doi.org/10.1016/j.thromres.2010.10.003

Cheong, J. L. Y., & Cowan, F. M. (2009). Neonatal arterial ischaemic stroke: Obstetric issues. *Seminars in Fetal and Neonatal Medicine, 14*(5), 267–271. https://doi.org/10.1016/j.siny.2009.07.009

Clapp, M., Basat, S., Zera, C., Smith, N., & Robinson, J. (2016). Relationship between parity and brachial plexus injuries. *Journal of Perinatology, 36*, 357–361. https://doi.org/10.1038/jp.2015.205

Ditzenberger, G. R., & Blackburn, S. T. (2020). Neurologic system. In C. Kenner, L. B. Altimier, & M. V. Boykova (Eds.), *Comprehensive neonatal nursing care* (6th ed., pp. 373–416). Springer Publishing Company.

Doumouchtsis, S., & Arulkumaran, S. (2009). Are all brachial plexus injuries caused by shoulder dystocia? *Obstetrical and Gynecological Survey, 64*(9), 615–623. https://doi.org/10.1097/OGX.0b013e3181b27a3a

Fenichel, G. M. (2007). *Neonatal neurology* (4th ed.). Churchill Livingstone/Elsevier.

Gabbay-Benziv, R., Reece, E. A., Wang, F., & Yang, P. (2015). Birth defects in pregestational diabetes: Defect range, glycemic threshold and pathogenesis. *World Journal of Diabetes, 6*(3), 481–488. https://doi.org/10.4239/wjd.v6.i3.481

Gilbert, M. T., Sulik, K. K., Fish, E. W., Baker, L. K., Dehart, D. B., & Parnell, S. E. (2016). Dose-dependent teratogenicity of the synthetic cannabinoid CP-55,940 in mice. *Neurotoxicology and Teratology, 58*, 15–22. https://doi.org/10.1016/j.ntt.2015.12.004

Govindan, M., & Burrows, H. (2019). Neonatal brachial plexus injury. *Pediatrics in Review, 40*(9). 494–496. https://doi.org/10.1542/pir.2018-0113

Hong, J., & Lee, J. (2018). Intracranial hemorrhage in term neonates. *Child's Nervous System, 34*, 1134–1143. https://doi.org/10.1007/s00381-018-3788-8

Hong, M., & Krauss, R. S. (2017). Ethanol itself is a holoprosencephaly-inducing teratogen. *PLoS One, 12*(4), e0176440. https://doi.org/10.1371/journal.pone.0176440

Kirton, A., & deVeber, G. (2009). Advances in perinatal ischemic stroke. *Pediatric Neurology, 40*(3), 205–214. https://doi.org/10.1016/j.pediatrneurol.2008.09.018

Levene, M. (2009). Disorders of the spinal cord, cranial and peripheral nerves. In M. Levene & F. A. Chervenak (Eds.), *Fetal and neonatal neurology and neurosurgery* (4th ed., pp. 778–791). Churchill Livingstone/Elsevier.

Levene, M., & deVries, L. S. (2009). Neonatal intracranial hemorrhage. In M. Levene & F. A. Chervenak (Eds.), *Fetal and neonatal neurology and neurosurgery* (4th ed., pp. 395–430). Churchill Livingstone/Elsevier.

Lynch, J. K. (2009). Epidemiology and classification of perinatal stroke. *Seminars in Fetal and Neonatal Medicine, 14*(5), 245–249. https://doi.org/10.1016/j.siny.2009.07.001

Madsen, J. R., Frim, D. M., & Hansen, A. R. (2005). Neurosurgery of the newborn. In M. G. McDonald, M. D. Mullett, & M. M. Seshia (Eds.), *Avrey's neonatology: Pathophysiology and management of the newborn* (6th ed., pp. 1410–1427). Lippincott, Williams and Wilkins.

Mineyko, A., & Kirton, A. (2011). The black box of perinatal ischemic stroke pathogenesis. *Journal of Child Neurology, 26*(9), 1154–1162. https://doi.org/10.1177/0883073811408312

Missios, S., Bekelis, K., & Spinner, R. J. (2014). Traumatic peripheral nerve injuries in children: Epidemiology and socioeconomics. *Journal of Neurosurgery: Pediatrics, 14*(6), 688–694. https://doi.org/10.3171/2014.8.PEDS14112

Murias, K. G. (2014). A review of cognitive outcomes in children following perinatal stroke. *Developmental Neuropsychology, 39*(2), 131–157. https://doi.org/10.1080/87565641.2013.870178

Myers, E., & Ment, L. R. (2012). Perinatal stroke. In J. Perlman (Ed.), *Neurology* (2nd ed., pp. 91–108). Saunders/Elsevier.

National Institute of Neurological Disorders and Stroke. (2006). Report and workshop on perinatal and childhood stroke. *Journal of Child Neurology, 21*, 415–418. https://doi.org/10.1177/0883073819866609

Schierholz, E., & Walker, S. R. (2010). Responding to traumatic birth: Subgaleal hemorrhage, assessment, and management during transport. *Advances in Neonatal Care, 10*(6), 311–315. https://doi.org/10.1097/ANC.0b013e3181fe9a49

Schierholz, E., & Walker, S. R. (2014). Responding to traumatic birth: Subgaleal hemorrhage, assessment, and management during transport. *Advances in Neonatal Care, 14*(Suppl. 5), S11–S15. https://doi.org/10.1097/ANC.0b013e3181fe9a49

Shah, N., & Wusthoff, C. (2016). Intracranial hemorrhage in the neonate. *Neonatal Network, 35*(2), 67–72. https://doi.org/10.1891/0730-0832.35.2.67

Terzis, J. K., & Anesti, K. (2011). Developmental facial paralysis: A review. *Journal of Plastic, Reconstructive & Aesthetic Surgery, 64*(10), 1318–1333. https://doi.org/10.1016/j.bjps.2011.04.015

Volpe, J. J. (2008). *Neurology of the newborn* (5th ed.). Saunders/Elsevier.

Volpe, J. J., Inder, T. E., Darras, B. T., de Vries, L. S., du Plessis, A. J., Neil, J., & Perlman, J. M. (2018). *Volpe's neurology of the newborn* (6th ed.). Saunders/Elsevier.

Waller, S. A., Gopalani, S., & Benedetti, T. (2012). Complicated deliveries: Overview. In C. A. Gleason & S. Devaskar (Eds.), *Avery's diseases of the newborn* (9th ed., pp. 146–158). Saunders/Elsevier.

Watchko, J. F. (2009). Identification of neonates at risk for hazardous hyperbilirubinemia: Emerging clinical insights. *Pediatric Clinics of North America, 56*(3), 671–687. https://doi.org/10.1016/j.pcl.2009.04.005

Weber, M. A., & Sebire, N. J. (2010). Genetics and developmental pathology of twinning. *Seminars in Fetal & Neonatal Medicine, 15*(6), 313–318. https://doi.org/10.1016/j.siny.2010.06.002

CONCLUSION

Infants with neurologic dysfunction present a significant challenge to the neonatal nurse. The nurse must respond to infants with life-threatening conditions, such as perinatal hypoxic–ischemic injury and intracranial hemorrhage; to those with transient problems, such as an isolated seizure; and to those with chronic problems, such as neural tube defects (NTDs). Nurses must also deal with their own responses and those of the families of infants who may die during the neonatal or early infancy periods or whose short- and long-term outcomes may be altered by the extent of neurologic insult. Nurses must understand the basis for and the implications of specific types of neurologic dysfunction; recognize the clinical manifestations of these types of dysfunction; and respond appropriately in concert with other healthcare professionals.

Nursing management of the infant involves activities to address alteration in level of consciousness, potential for injury related to trauma or infection, impairment of skin integrity, alterations in comfort, impaired mobility, alterations in thermoregulation, alterations in nutrition and fluid and electrolyte status, and promotion of neurobehavioral organization and development. Nurses must also assess family coping, interactive processes, knowledge, and grieving to assist the family in coping with the birth of an ill infant and, for many families, with the uncertainty or certainty of long-term neurologic deficits in their infant.

Gastrointestinal System

MICHELE KACMARCIK SAVIN AND ANN GIBBONS PHALEN

OVERVIEW

The primary functions of the gastrointestinal (GI) system are ingestion, absorption, and digestion of nutrients and elimination of waste products. These processes are dependent on a patent, structurally intact, and adequately functioning GI tract. Development, assessment, and nursing care along with selected issues of the GI system are discussed here. The interaction between the GI system, feeding, nutrition, and growth is discussed in Chapter 7.

GASTROINTESTINAL SYSTEM DEVELOPMENT

Anatomy and Physiology of the Gastrointestinal System

Anatomic Development of the Gastrointestinal Tract

The development of the human GI tract begins between the third and fourth fetal week and is essentially complete by the 20th fetal week. The GI tract develops in a cranial-to-caudal and ventral direction. The horseshoe-shaped tube that rises from the embryonic neural plate is divided into three distinct regions of the GI tract: the foregut, midgut, and hindgut.

The foregut forms the pharynx, esophagus, stomach, liver, gallbladder, pancreas, and the proximal duodenum, and blood is supplied to the foregut by the celiac artery. Common anomalies associated with a disruption in foregut development include:

- Atresia of the esophagus
- Tracheoesophageal fistula (TEF)
- Pyloric stenosis
- Duodenal atresia or stenosis
- Biliary atresia
- Annular pancreas

The midgut forms the lower (caudal) portion of the duodenum, jejunum, ileum, appendix, ascending colon, and first two-thirds of the transverse colon, and blood is supplied to the midgut by the superior mesenteric artery. Midgut development is characterized by rapid elongation of the gut and associated mesentery. Midgut development involves four stages:

- Herniation—loops of intestines protrude into the umbilical cord (around the seventh fetal week)

- Rotation—rotates in a counterclockwise fashion about 90° at the same time of herniation

- Retraction—after sufficient expansion of the abdominal cavity, the loops of intestines retract back into the abdomen and rotate again in a counterclockwise fashion another 180° (around the 10th fetal week)

- Fixation—once in proper placement, the mesentery attaches to the posterior abdominal wall

    Common anomalies associated with a disruption in midgut development include:

- Omphalocele

- Gastroschisis

- Umbilical hernia

- Intestinal stenosis, atresia, and malrotation

    The hindgut is the precursor of the distal one-third of the transverse colon, the descending colon, the rectum, and the urogenital sinus. Blood is supplied to the hindgut by the inferior mesenteric artery. Common anomalies associated with a disruption in hindgut development include:

- Urorectal septal defects

- Lower anorectal defects such as imperforate anus

- Anal agenesis

- Hirschsprung disease

Physiological Development of the Gastrointestinal System

Development of the digestive and liver enzyme systems, as well as the absorptive surfaces of the intestines, begins in fetal life and matures during the postnatal period. By 33 to 34 weeks' gestation, processes needed for adequate enteral nutrition are in place.

    During postnatal maturation of GI development and function, certain factors can influence development, which include:

- Genetic factors

- Intrinsic timing mechanisms

- Initiation of feeding

- Type of feeding

- Composition of diet

■ Hormonal regulatory mechanisms

■ Gut trophic factors such as nutrients, hormones, and peptides

Meconium

Meconium is first seen around 10 to 12 fetal weeks and moves into the colon around the 16th fetal week. It is found in amniotic fluid in small amounts during the second trimester until development of the anal sphincter function around 20 to 22 fetal weeks. In the postnatal period, meconium is an essential step in initiation of intestinal function. It consists of vernix, lanugo, squamous epithelial cells, occult blood, bile, and other intestinal secretions. Thought to be sterile, there is some newer evidence of bacteria present at birth; most definitely within 24 hours after birth bacteria is present. Most healthy full-term newborns will pass meconium within 48 hours of delivery, although premature infants without GI disease may not pass meconium for several days. In premature infants who are ill and not receiving enteral feedings, passage of meconium may be further delayed.

Swallowing

Swallowing begins around 10 to 14 fetal weeks; by the 16th fetal week, the fetus swallows 2 to 6 mL of amniotic fluid/day and increases to approximately 500 to 1,000 mL/day by term. Twenty percent of fluid swallowed during this period is lung fluid, not amniotic fluid. Swallowing helps regulate amniotic fluid volume and may contribute to programming of thirst and appetite. Swallowed amniotic fluid contributes to growth of the fetus as they receive 10% of their protein intake this way. Failure to adequately swallow amniotic fluid is associated with polyhydramnios and GI obstruction.

Swallowing is typically well developed by 28 to 30 weeks; however, premature infants born between 30 and 35 weeks do not have the endurance of the term infant for feeding. The gag reflex presents by 18 weeks but is not complete until around 34 weeks. Air and milk swallowed compete for space in the neonate's stomach, leading to regurgitation.

Sucking

All components of suck–swallow–breathe are present by 28 weeks; however, coordination of these activities is warranted for safe enteral feedings to occur. Maturation of sucking is related to gestational age and not postnatal age.

There are two types of sucking, nonnutritive sucking (NNS) and nutritive sucking (NS), which are most efficient after 32 to 34 weeks. Sucking stimulates secretion of GI regulatory peptides and enhances gastric emptying.

There are three stages of the suck–swallow pattern:

■ Mouthing—no effective suck

■ Immature pattern—short burst and not synchronized with swallowing

■ Mature pattern—long burst, coordinated swallowing, and propulsive peristaltic waves in the esophagus

Esophageal Motility

In the esophagus, food is moved by peristaltic waves initiated by impulses from autonomic nerves (enteric nervous system [ENS]) and coordinated by the swallowing center in the medulla. Esophageal motility and muscle tone are decreased during the first 3 postnatal days.

When esophageal contractions begin, the lower esophageal sphincter (LES) relaxes, allowing food to pass from the esophagus into the stomach. The LES forms a pressure barrier between the esophagus and stomach to prevent reflux. In neonates, the length of the LES is reduced and it is located primarily above the diaphragm, increasing the chance of reflux. LES tone develops rapidly during the first week of life, though the sphincter remains immature for 6 to 12 months. All infants have intermittent periods of LES relaxation.

Gastric Emptying

Gastric emptying is delayed in neonates, especially during the first 3 postnatal days. Coordination of peristaltic waves between the upper stomach and duodenum is decreased, especially in the preterm, delaying emptying. Other factors that influence gastric emptying include:

■ Muscle tone—low tone delays emptying
■ Mucus—delays emptying
■ Pyloric sphincter tone
■ Presence of amniotic fluid in the stomach
■ Elevated gastrin level
■ Hormones

Types of nutrients can also influence gastric emptying time as follows:

■ Carbohydrates—increase emptying time
■ Fats—decrease emptying time
■ Medium-chain triglycerides (MCTs) empty faster than long-chain triglycerides (LCTs)
■ Human milk empties twice as fast as formula
■ High-caloric formula—takes longer to empty than regular formula

Intestinal Motility

In the intestines, peristaltic waves continue to propel food from the stomach toward the small intestines. Once in the small intestines, contractions become more oscillatory to promote the absorptive and digestive processes.

In the premature neonate, both the intestinal musculature and motor mechanisms are immature, which result in irregular peristaltic activity and disorganized patterns. Disorganized movements of this nature lead to:

- Decreased ability to clear upper gut
- Decreased absorptive function
- Prolonged transit time in upper intestine
- More rapid emptying of the ileum and colon

The immature surface of small intestines of the premature infant reduces absorption of important nutrients; however, as gestational age increases, so does the number of intestinal villi and epithelial cells, improving absorption. Enteral feedings after birth promote epithelial hyperplasia, increase cell turnover, and stimulate production of digestive enzymes like pancreatic lipase, amylase, and trypsin. Colostrum and human milk also contain factors that stimulate cell turnover and maturation, whereas ischemia, anoxia, and infection have a negative impact on the surface area of small intestines blocking absorption of nutrients (Dingeldin, 2020).

THE GASTROINTESTINAL SYSTEM AND IMMUNITY

Although traditionally felt to be sterile at birth, there is some evidence of bacterial organisms in the first meconium. Normal bacterial flora has nutritional roles, such as the maturation of the intestinal lining and the synthesis of vitamin K, and immune roles, such as blocking pathogens and strengthening the mucosal lining. The microbiome of the infant is dependent on factors including type of birth, feeding, and interventions such as antibiotic use and feeding tubes. The neonate's gut is exposed to bacteria and antigens, and complex immune and nonimmune host defenses are present that serve to enhance the neonate's immune response. Factors that enhance GI immunity include:

- Efficient motility prevents colonization of pathologic bacteria in the lumen of the gut.
- Early enteral nutrition stimulates the release of gastric acid and pancreaticobiliary secretions that inhibit bacterial growth and activate proteolysis.
- Mucus lining of the gut provides a protective barrier to larger bacterial molecules.
- Cytokines stimulate chemotaxis of neutrophils and promotion of IgA (immunoglobulin A) expression after mucosal injury.
- Human milk contains substances such as oligosaccharides that protect the gut from infection and enhance maturation of the system.
- The acidic environment supported by breast milk favors healthy bacteria such as *Lactobacillus* and *Bifidobacterium*.
- Certain cells, immunonutrients, probiotics, and prebiotics also play a role in the immune defense of the neonatal gut (Lenfestey & Neu, 2018).

GASTROINTESTINAL ASSESSMENT

Prenatal Assessment of the Gastrointestinal Tract

In prenatal assessment of the GI tract, it is important to review family history for genetic or congenital anomalies. Some GI disorders are related to chromosomal and single-gene defects or exist as part of a multisystem syndrome. Examples include:

■ Apert syndrome—cleft palate, pyloric stenosis

■ Trisomy 13—cleft lip and/or palate, omphalocele, malrotation

■ Trisomy 18—cleft lip and/or palate, omphalocele, malrotation, pyloric stenosis

■ Trisomy 21—VACTERL association (V-vertebral defects, A-anal atresia, C-cardiac defects, T-tracheoesophageal fistula, E-esophageal defects, R-renal and radial-thumb side dysplasia, L-other limb defects) or VATER syndrome (Vertebral defects, Anal atresia, TracheoEsophageal fistula with esophageal atresia, and Radial and Renal dysplasia) association, duodenal atresia, TEF, Hirschsprung disease

■ Cystic fibrosis—occurs in greater than 90% of cases of meconium ileus.

In prenatal assessment of the GI tract, ultrasonography is best performed during the second and third trimester. Ultrasonography is of value in the following assessments:

■ To survey the abdominal wall

■ To observe insertion of the umbilical cord

■ To visualize the fluid-filled stomach

■ To observe for bowel dilation

■ To survey for abnormal echolucencies that resemble cysts but are abnormal collections of fluid within the bowel, secondary to obstruction

■ To evaluate for the presence of polyhydramnios—indicative of a high obstruction in the GI tract

Postnatal Assessment of the Gastrointestinal Tract

Postnatal assessment of the GI tract should include observation, auscultation, palpation, and occasionally percussion to determine liver size or look for ascites. It also may include diagnostic procedures to further a diagnostic conversation when abnormalities are observed prenatally or postnatally.

Physical Assessment of the Gastrointestinal Tract

In physical assessment of the GI tract, begin with direct visualization, as many GI defects are evident in the following:

■ Oral–facial structures: Inspect position; size; shape; symmetry; and integrity of the mouth, lips, palate, and uvula. Nares should be symmetric and patent.

■ Abdomen: Inspect the overall abdomen for contour, symmetry, and integrity as well as distention and surface color, as the presence of visible peristalsis accompanied by vomiting or distention can be a sign of obstruction. Inspect the umbilical cord for size, shape, and vessels (if still present), and the insertion site. Of concern for obstruction or liver disease would be visible loops, stretching and shiny skin, or prominent visible veins, especially in a term infant.

■ Anus: Examine the anus for presence and position and inspect the perineal area for fistulas. Do not insert a rectal thermometer to assess rectal patency, as this increases the risk of perforating the rectum. If indicated, a digital examination is performed using a gloved small finger. An anal wink should be elicited by stroking the perineal area next to the anus with a responsive pucker.

■ Bowel sounds: Bowel sounds are initially absent; however, as the neonate swallows air and peristaltic activity is initiated, bowel sounds become audible within the first 30 minutes of life. In assessing bowel sounds, note the following:

● Bowel sounds have a metallic tinkling quality and occur two to five times per minute.

● Bowel sounds can be hyperdynamic or absent in a normal examination.

● Bowel sounds are best heard in the right lower quadrant in normally oriented intestines due to turbulence at the ileocecal valve connecting small and large bowel.

● Note in the very preterm infant, bowel and breath sounds can be heard over each other; bowel sounds in the chest are suspicious for congenital diaphragmatic hernia.

● Hyperdynamic sounds along with distention and vomiting should be concerning signs and require further evaluation.

Palpation of the abdomen is best performed on a quiet infant lying in the supine position and within the first 24 hours. Holding an infant's knees and hips in a flexed position helps facilitate relaxation of the musculature. Palpation is best done gently with a warmed hand using the pads of the fingers; this helps to avoid stressing the infant, which would result in a transient elevation of systolic and diastolic pressures.

■ Liver: Palpate the liver by placing the index finger in the area of the right groin and advancing slowly upward until the liver edge is felt. Note normal/abnormal findings:

● Normal findings—the organ is firm, but not hard, and the sharp edge is 1 to 2 cm below the right costal margin and can be followed across the abdomen into the left upper quadrant.

● Abnormal findings—the organ is hard and enlarged. When the liver edge is greater than 3.5 cm in a newborn, this is considered hepatomegaly (Wolf & Lavine, 2000). In infants, the most common causes of hepatomegaly are infection and biliary obstruction.

■ Spleen: Palpate the spleen using the same technique as that used for the liver. In most instances, the spleen cannot be palpated. If palpable, one should feel only the size of a small fingertip.

■ Kidneys: Locate the kidneys in the flank areas above the level of the umbilicus; normally 4.5 to 5 cm in length in the term infant. Palpate the kidneys as follows:

- Bimanual palpation—one hand is placed posterior, supporting the flank area, while the thumb or a finger of the free hand moves anterior over the same area.

- Single-hand palpation—the fingers of one hand support the flank posterior, while the thumb of the same hand moves anterior over the same area. Kidneys are easiest to palpate in the first day of life when the bowels have less air and stool.

Related Findings in Assessment of the Gastrointestinal Tract

In postnatal assessment of the GI tract, it is particularly important to note three cardinal signs indicating a possible GI obstruction: persistent vomiting, abdominal distention, and failure to pass meconium. The ampulla of Vater is where the common bile duct and pancreatic duct join to empty into the small intestine.

With persistent vomiting, note the following:

■ The ampulla of Vater is where the common bile duct and pancreatic duct join to empty into the small intestine.

■ If there is bile-stained vomiting, this indicates the point of obstruction is distal to the ampulla of Vater.

■ Nonbilious vomiting can indicate the point of obstruction is proximal to the ampulla of Vater.

Failure to pass meconium within the first 48 hours (about 2 days) after birth can indicate obstruction of the large intestines.

■ Respiratory difficulties:

- Can occur secondary to the infant's inability to handle excessive oral secretions or aspiration of gastric content associated with a TEF.

- Abdominal distention can compromise diaphragmatic movement, resulting in respiratory distress.

- Airway obstruction can occur in an infant with a cleft palate as inspiratory pressures pull the tongue into the hypopharynx.

■ Jaundice: Occurs when the excretion of bilirubin is impeded from such problems as biliary atresia, Hirschsprung disease, intestinal atresias, and meconium ileus.

■ Systemic hypertension: Rare but occurs when a mass or significant distention increases intra-abdominal pressure.

■ Stool color: Yellow to brown is normal; bright red—bleeding likely from colon or anus; dark red—bleeding likely from small intestine or stomach; green—rapid transit; light or pale—suspicious for biliary atresia or cholestasis.

REFERENCES

Dingeldin, M. (2020). Development of the neonatal gastrointestinal tract. In R. J. Martin, A. A. Fanaroff, & M. C. Walsh (Eds.), *Fanaroff and Martin's neonatal-perinatal medicine* (pp. 1506–1512). Elsevier.

Lenfestey, M. W., & Neu, J. (2018). Gastrointestinal development implications for management of preterm and term infants. *Gastroenterol Clinics of North America, 47,* 773–791. https://doi.org/10.1016/j.gtc.2018.07.005

Wolf, A. D., & Lavine, J. E. (2000). Hepatomegaly in neonates and children. *Pediatrics in Review, 21*(9), 303–310. https://doi.org/10.1542/pir.21-9-303

DIAGNOSTIC PROCEDURES FOR EVALUATION OF THE GASTROINTESTINAL TRACT

Various diagnostic tools are used to evaluate a neonate when a GI problem is suspected, including radiographic studies, ultrasonography, testing of bodily substances, and others.

■ Radiography: Includes x-ray, upper GI series, and contrast enema.

■ X-ray: Useful in the diagnosis of an obstruction, since air serves as a naturally occurring contrast medium. Within 30 minutes of birth, air should be seen in the stomach; within 3 to 4 hours, air is seen in the small bowel; and by 6 to 8 hours, the entire colon and rectum should be filled with air. When an obstruction is present, air is not seen in the intestine distal to the obstruction. However, the infant continues to swallow air; therefore, the area proximal to the obstruction becomes distended and is seen as dramatic radiolucent (black) bubbles on x-ray.

- Esophageal and intestinal atresia are often diagnosed with anterior/posterior (AP) and lateral radiographic views of the chest and abdomen.

- Cross-table lateral views, whereby the infant is supine and the x-ray is shot across the baby from the side, are helpful in identifying air in the rectum or air/ fluid levels of infants with intestinal obstructions.

- A left lateral decubitus view, where the infant is placed on the left side and the x-ray shot from above, assists in determining the presence of free air in the peritoneal cavity, for example, in the case of necrotizing enterocolitis (NEC).

■ Upper GI series: Assists in the diagnosis of pyloric stenosis and malrotation, although it is not reliable in the diagnosis of gastroesophageal reflux (GER) as it only measures a brief window of time. In the upper GI series procedure:

- The infant receives nothing by mouth (NPO) for 4 to 6 hours prior to the study.

- The study uses contrast material, such as barium or a water-soluble agent such as Gastrografin. This is swallowed or administered via a naso/orogastric (NG/OG) tube and observed by fluoroscopy as it travels through the digestive tract. Gastrografin is preferred when perforation is suspected since it is a water-soluble solution (Kee, 2001).

- The procedure can take as long as 4 hours, depending on the motility of the small intestine.

■ Contrast enema: Assists in the diagnosis of malrotation, Hirschsprung disease, meconium ileus, and meconium plug syndrome. In the contrast enema procedure, the following occurs:

- The study uses contrast material, such as barium or Gastrografin, which is instilled through the rectum via a small catheter.

- No specific preparation is necessary.

- Gentle saline enemas post procedure may be used to help clear the barium and trapped air.

- Contrast enemas can be both diagnostic and therapeutic in the case of meconium plug.

■ Ultrasonography: Used in the diagnosis of pyloric stenosis, enteric duplication, and biliary atresia, if the intrahepatic or proximal extrahepatic tract is dilated. Ultrasonography uses sound waves from the tissues and transforms them into scans, graphs, or audible sounds. In the ultrasonography procedure, conducting gel and a transducer are placed on the abdomen to identify the sound waves.

■ Gastric aspirate: Gastric aspirate is a point-of-care testing procedure that measures the pH of gastric content, which is obtained by inserting a premeasured feeding tube into the stomach. At least 1 mL of gastric content is withdrawn for analysis.

■ Apt test: Differentiates neonatal blood loss from swallowed maternal blood. In this procedure:

- Bloody aspirate or bloody stool is collected and sent to the laboratory for analysis.

- The bloody aspirate or stool is centrifuged in 5 mL of water. One part 0.25% sodium hydroxide is added to five parts supernatants.

- If the fluid turns pink, it indicates fetal blood; if the fluid turns brown, it indicates maternal blood.

■ Stool culture: Used in cases of bloody diarrhea, where a stool culture helps to differentiate between an intestinal lining insult and an infection. In this procedure, a stool specimen is taken from a diaper, placed in a container, labeled, and sent to a laboratory for testing.

■ Stool hematest: This is a rapid and convenient test to detect fecal occult blood. In this procedure:

- Thin smear of stool is placed on guaiac paper and developer is applied over the smear. Results are read in 60 seconds.

- Any blue colorization on or at the edge of the smear indicates a positive occult blood result.

- Certain drugs can cause a false-positive result, such as iron preparations, indomethacin, potassium preparations, salicylates, and steroids.

- Large amounts of ascorbic acid may cause a false-negative result.

■ Stool-reducing substances: Stool-reducing substances help in the detection of carbohydrate intolerance. In this procedure:

● Stool specimen is taken from a diaper, placed in a container, labeled, and sent to a laboratory for testing.

● A Clinitest tablet is added to the test tube containing the prepared supernatant; after 15 seconds, it is gently shaken. The color of the liquid is compared with the color chart on the Clinitest bottle.

● More than 0.5% glucose in the stool indicates an abnormal amount of sugar, and carbohydrate intolerance should be suspected.

■ Twenty-four–hour pH monitoring:

● A thin, flexible pH probe is inserted into the distal esophagus for a 24-hour period.

● The test records the amount of time the esophagus is exposed to an acidic pH level. It measures the time, duration (should be <4 minutes of exposure), frequency of reflux, time of longest episode, and the percentage of time the infant was having reflux during the 24-hour period.

● An impedance probe can be combined with the pH probe to identify fluid bolus activity as well; these probes may also be clipped in place in the esophagus removing the need for a tube obstructing the nares.

● Formula feedings may obscure episodes of reflux by buffering the gastric acid.

● Results can be compromised by such factors as infant position during the study, activity, frequency, and composition of feedings and medications; infants should be off acid suppressors and prokinetic agents 24 to 28 hours before the test.

● The nursing role is to document time of feedings, feeding composition, and medications administered during the study, as well as the position and activity of the infant throughout the study.

■ Scintigraphy: Used to measure gastric emptying, aspiration with swallowing, and reflux with aspiration. In this procedure, the infant is fed a radionucleotide-tagged formula—a technetium radioisotope is added to formula and has relatively low radiation.

■ Endoscopy: Assists in the diagnosis of esophagitis. In this procedure, flexible endoscopy with biopsy of the distal esophagus can detect basal cell hyperplasia, increased stromal papillary length, and the presence of intraepithelial eosinophils. This can be performed at the bedside.

■ Fecal fat: Used to screen for the presence of malabsorption. Fecal fat content greater than 6 g/24 hours is predictive of malabsorption syndrome. It should be noted that small stool samples can cause false test results.

■ Suction rectal biopsy: Used to look for ganglion cells when Hirschsprung disease is suspected. Mucosal and submucosal layers are excised and sent to pathology. Ensure proper clotting times before and observe for bleeding and fever; watch vital signs closely after the biopsy.

■ Chromosomal studies: Such studies may be indicated if a GI anomaly is found with other multisystem abnormalities.

REFERENCE

Kee, J. L. (2001). *Laboratory and diagnostic tests with nursing implications* (4th ed.). Prentice Hall.

GENERALIZED NURSING CARE

Common Nursing Management Interventions Related to Gastrointestinal System Alterations

A variety of nursing procedures and interventions are used in the management and treatment of GI system alterations and include the following:

■ Gastric decompression: Prevents aspiration, respiratory compromise, and perforation.

- The OG/NG tube is connected to low intermittent suction.
- Tube patency should be maintained to ensure proper tube functioning.
- The tube should be irrigated with 2 mL of air every 2 to 4 hours.
- There are several types of OG/NG tubes including the eight or 10 French red rubber tube and the 10 French soft vinyl, double-lumen gastric sump tube. Replogle tubes have both holes on the end and may be preferred for draining esophageal pouches.

■ Fluid and electrolytes balance: Vomiting, diarrhea, gastric drainage, and the shifting of fluids from the vascular bed into the interstitial compartment can lead to dehydration, hypovolemia, hypoperfusion, and electrolyte abnormalities. Additionally, premature skin contributes to fluid loss. The treatment goal is to maintain fluid and electrolyte balance; this includes the following:

- Maintenance fluids: 60 to 80 mL/kg for the first 24 hours
- Increase daily by 10 mL/kg/day or as needed to 120 to 160 mL/kg/day
- Monitor urine output: Goal is 1 to 2 mL/kg/hr; adjust fluids to maintain urine output

In patients at risk for increased sodium and potassium losses, it is important to:

■ Provide sodium at approximately 2 to 3 mEq/kg/day.
■ Provide potassium at approximately 2 mEq/kg/day.

Increased gastric losses via NG/OG tube require replacement.

■ Measure drainage minimally every shift; with small infants or large losses, you may need to measure and replace more frequently.

■ Replace the total volume of gastric output with one-half normal saline with potassium chloride 10 to 20 mEq/L every 4 to 8 hours. Replacement fluids are in addition to maintenance fluids.

■ Metabolic alkalosis, metabolic acidosis, and respiratory acidosis can occur with gastric losses.

● Metabolic alkalosis is associated with pyloric stenosis or high jejunal obstruction due to a loss of acidic gastric juice.

● Metabolic acidosis occurs with obstructions in the distal segment of the small intestines because large quantities of alkaline fluids are lost.

● Respiratory acidosis develops when there is abdominal distention because of carbon dioxide retention from hypoventilation.

■ Thermoregulation: In patients with abdominal wall defects:

● Monitor for heat loss, especially with exposed bowel.

● Provide an external heat source and monitor temperature hourly.

● In defects with exposed bowel, apply sterile warm saline soaks over the defect and use a bowel bag or plastic wrap.

■ Positioning: Head elevation assists in reducing reflux of gastric content as follows:

● In neonates with a tracheal esophageal fistula, this position reduces reflux of gastric content into the trachea via the distal fistula.

● In ventilated infants, this may be part of a bundle to decrease infection.

● In neonates with isolated esophageal atresia (EA), the flat or head-down position assists in the gravity drainage of the esophageal pouch.

■ Prevention of infection: Newborns have increased susceptibility for infection; use broad-spectrum antibiotics for presumed infections cautiously, keeping antibiotic stewardship in mind.

■ Pain management: Preoperative and postoperative pain should be monitored. Pain should be assessed at regular intervals and interventions evaluated for effective relief.

● Nonpharmacologic pain measures include the following:

• Breastfeeding

• Containment when possible

• Positioning aids if age and diagnosis appropriate

• Pacifier

• Skin-to-skin (kangaroo mother) care when possible

• Sucrose

● Pharmacologic measures include paracetamol (Tylenol) or opioids such as morphine and fentanyl. Use of pharmacologic measures should be supported by a pain protocol based on expected severity of pain and limited with daily assessment of patient need for medication.

● Nutrition: Meeting the nutritional needs of neonates preoperatively and postoperatively is challenging. Enteral feeding is not ordered in the preoperative period and may be delayed by days or weeks in the postoperative period, depending on diagnosis. Parenteral nutrition with hyperalimentation is ordered to meet the caloric and metabolic needs and is administered via a peripherally inserted central catheter (PICC) or a surgically inserted central catheter. Once enteral feeds are introduced, gradual advancement is warranted, as follows:

  * Start with human milk; if unavailable or unable to be tolerated, consider elemental formula, complemented with parenteral nutrition.

  * Introduce small, frequent feedings or continuous feedings and gradually advance as tolerated.

  * The extent of bowel loss or severity of the defect will influence tolerance.

  * Signs of intolerance include vomiting, diarrhea or increased ostomy output, abdominal distention, or presence of reducing substances in the stool.

■ General preoperative management: Principles of preoperative management include the following:

  ● Replacement of fluid losses

  ● Decompression of the distended bowel

  ● Support failing organ systems

  ● Maintain thermoregulation to prevent cold stress

  ● Maintain adequate oxygenation, ventilation, and acid–base balance

  ● Provide nutrition with parenteral nutrition

  ● Prevent infection through antibiotic therapy, covering both aerobic and anaerobic infections

  ● Pain management

■ General postoperative management: Includes the same principles as preoperative management as well as the following:

  ● Maintaining skin integrity postoperatively

  ● Providing ostomy care for infants with ostomies: see the text that follows

  ● Monitoring for complications such as infections, respiratory distress, fluid and electrolyte imbalance, third spacing of fluids, skin breakdown, pain, short bowel syndrome, peritonitis, and intestinal obstructions related to adhesions, strictures, or volvulus

■ Ethical issues: Congenital malformations often have associated organ defects. Family-based care requires consideration of individual patient/family preferences as part of the care team. Advice, evaluation and input, treatment, and support come from an interprofessional team.

■ Family support: Family members of a neonate with a GI system disorder/anomaly experience grief, feelings of loss, guilt, and confusion. In these occurrences, communication is most important, in order to:

● Provide factual information about the disorder, prognosis, and plan of care.

● Ensure communication with family members is consistent among caregivers, frequent, and reinforced.

● Provide a supportive environment for parents to express their concerns.

● Encourage parents to participate in care activities such as skin-to-skin holding, diapering, and feedings.

● Prepare families for their infant's discharge early in the transition period and connect them with support services when indicated.

SELECTED COMMON GASTROINTESTINAL PROBLEMS IN THE NEONATE

Two significant GI problems in the neonate are GER and gastrointestinal reflux disease (GERD) as well as infantile hypertrophic pyloric stenosis (IHPS).

GASTROESOPHAGEAL REFLUX AND GASTROINTESTINAL REFLUX DISEASE

GER is defined as the physiologic retrograde of stomach content into the esophagus, whereas GERD is defined as the pathologic condition where this retrograde of fluid from the stomach into the esophagus causes medical complications, most of which are multifactorial (Hasenstab & Jadcherla, 2020; Hibbs, 2020, p. 1513). Due to lack of definitive tests and association with other nonspecific symptoms, GERD is hard to diagnose and manage (Chabra & Peeples, 2020); the global prevalence is unknown and variable, based on local characteristics of parents, providers, and policies (Badran & Jadcherla, 2020). In addition, empiric therapies are often not objective and practice variation is large (Hasenstab & Jadcherla, 2020). Examples of clinical signs suggestive of GERD include anemia, esophagitis, apnea, and aspiration events (Ngo & Shah, 2020, p. 187). Endoscopies should be considered to confirm underlying mucosal disease or before escalating therapy. Refractory GERD does not respond to optimal treatment after 8 weeks (Rosen et al., 2018) and may require surgical intervention.

Incidence

Incidence is higher in premature infants born at less than 32 weeks of age, although 50% of healthy term infants will have symptomatic reflux at 2 months of age. Incidence is also higher in infants diagnosed with a neurologic disorder or inborn errors of metabolism, small bowel obstruction, or other intestinal anomalies. Peak incidence is at 4 months decreasing to less than 5% at 1 year (Chabra & Peeples, 2020). Physiologic GER rarely begins before 1 week or after 6 months (Rosen et al., 2018). Preterm infants with GERD have longer and more expensive hospital stays than peers without GERD (Chabra & Peeples, 2020).

Pathophysiology

The esophagus enters the stomach at the angle of HIS (Ngo & Shah, 2020, p. 187).

In premature neonates, the angle is decreased, thereby increasing the chance for reflux of gastric content into the esophagus. The distal portion of the esophagus has higher pressure than the proximal esophagus and stomach. The pressure helps prevent reflux of gastric content into the esophagus. However:

■ Lower esophageal pressure below gastric pressure allows for the retrograde of gastric content. This is often seen in the immature neonate.

■ Transient LES relaxations are common in the premature neonate, leading to reflux.

Neonates born with structural abnormalities may have malposition of the esophagus or stomach and an increase of intra-abdominal pressure.

Clinical Presentation

The most common presentation with GER is vomiting. Regurgitation occurs with burping during a feeding or occurs 2 to 3 hours after feeding. The vomiting can be forceful. History should include feeding and dietary questions such as milk type, volume, additives, interval pattern of emesis, family history including allergens, and environmental contributors such as tobacco use and secondhand smoke (Rosen et al., 2018).

Symptoms seen in infants with GERD can be esophageal such as regurgitation, poor weight gain, and esophagitis or extraesophageal such as crying, arching, or aversion to feeding, stridor, worsening lung disease, cough, wheezing, or recurrent otitis media (Chabra & Peeples, 2020).

Preterm infants suffer from both GER and apnea; they are temporally but not clearly causally related. Insufficient evidence exists to confirm that GER causes apnea; in fact, apnea may trigger GER. Insufficient evidence also exists to support the causality between GERD and bronchopulmonary dysplasia (BPD; Hibbs, 2020, p. 1514). Caffeine and bronchodilators, which are often used in preterm infants, may worsen GER by increasing gastric secretions and decreasing LES tone (Hasenstab & Jadcherla, 2020). On the other hand, human milk has better gastric emptying time and may lead to less GER; term infants with cow's milk allergy may be mistaken for GER. These infants should be trialed on hydrolyzed formula if breast milk is not an option before escalating GERD treatment (Badran & Jadcherla, 2020).

Differential Diagnosis

GER should be suspected in an otherwise healthy infant with postprandial regurgitation.

Evaluate the neonate for other problems that cause reflux, such as sepsis, urea cycle defects, formula intolerance, increased intracranial pressure, drug toxicity, and hydronephrosis.

Consider an upper GI series to rule out other anatomic causes, such as esophageal stricture, esophageal webs, volvulus, meconium ileus/plug, peptic stricture, and esophageal dysmotility.

Diagnostic procedures include (Hibbs, 2020, p. 1515) contrast studies, esophageal pH studies, and nuclear medicine scintigraphy.

- Contrast studies: In general, these are not reliable and only measure a brief window of time, although they can be useful in ruling out anatomic abnormalities that mimic GERD.
- Esophageal pH studies: These require monitoring for 12 to 24 hours to provide data on the timing and frequency of GER events. Esophageal pH probes measure acid reflux, and a pH <4 indicates GER. Esophageal multichannel intraluminal impedance (MII-pH) detects the presence of fluid in the esophagus regardless of pH and assesses the direction of flow and the distance from the LES of each GER event. This can help determine the association between GER events and symptoms but cannot define causality. It is more useful to diagnose motility issues.
- Nuclear medicine scintigraphy: Identifies postprandial reflux and aspiration and quantifies gastric emptying time. Age-specific norms have not been established in infants and therefore are not recommended as routine testing but may be helpful in diagnosing microaspiration.

Treatment

Treatment for GER and GERD includes noninvasive/nonpharmacologic treatment options, pharmacologic options, and surgical options. The goal of therapy for GERD is to improve symptoms and complications, not only physiologic measures. "The most effective treatment is time and maturation. Routine use of anti-reflux medications for GERD or apnea and desaturation is to be avoided" (Hibbs, 2020, p. 1515). Additionally, it is important to look for conditions that mimic GERD, including hiatal hernia, malrotation, IHPS duodenal web or atresia, or esophageal strictures (Rosen et al., 2018).

- Noninvasive/nonpharmacologic treatment options: small volume, frequent feedings that may be thickened with oat as opposed to rice cereal or use of a commercially available thickened formula. Thickening of feeding reduces clinical vomiting but not necessarily the physiologic measures of GER. Note breast milk is the preferred food of choice, and the safety of thickening feeds in preterms is not established. Supine positioning is standard in the infant; upright has no benefit versus flat and placing in a car seat or swing will increase GER. Left lateral positioning will decrease GER but may not change symptoms. "Prone positioning decreases GER but is contraindicated because of the increased risk of sudden infant death (SIDS)" (Hibbs, 2020, p. 1516). A trial of hydrolyzed or amino acid–based formula for a minimum of 2 weeks is recommended before escalation of therapy when GERD is suspected (Rosen et al., 2018).

■ Pharmacologic options (Hibbs, 2020, pp. 1516–1518): Drug therapy may be considered in neonates with high-risk symptoms such as failure to meet milestones or failure to thrive. Presently, insufficient evidence exists for either the efficacy or safety of pharmacologic interventions in the treatment of GERD in the neonatal population. Any pharmacologic intervention should be attempted after failure of medical management and limited to a short (2–4 weeks) trial with regular assessment for the need to continue therapy.

Histamine-2 (H_2) receptor antagonists suppress HCl production and therefore decrease gastric acidity. This action may protect the esophageal mucosa from acid injury and the development of esophagitis. However, the majority of GER events are nonacid. Examples include ranitidine, cimetidine, and famotidine. Risks include late-onset sepsis, necrotizing enterocolitis (NEC), and bradyarrhythmia.

Proton pump inhibitors (PPIs) inhibit the action of the acid pump. Examples are omeprazole, lansoprazole, dexlansoprazole, esomeprazole, pantoprazole, and rabeprazole. PPIs have not been shown to be effective in infants, and no PPIs are currently labeled for use in infants younger than 1 year of age, though their use in infants has continued. PPIs are indicated if reflux-related esophageal erosion is documented (Rosen et al., 2018). However, there is increasing evidence that H_2 agonists and PPIs are associated with NEC (Lenfestey & Neu, 2018). Long-term use of PPIs is also associated with negative effects such as respiratory and GI infection, osteoporosis, and fractures, as well as calcium and magnesium deficiency (Lenfestey & Neu, 2018).

Drugs to improve GI motility are used based on the idea that if gastric emptying is increased or esophageal motility and LES are improved, then there is a decrease in GER. Examples are metoclopramide and erythromycin. Metoclopramide is not recommended in infants and children (Rosen et al., 2018). Cisapride and domperidone can cause serious cardiac arrhythmias and QT prolongation (Djeddi et al., 2008) and should not be used in infants. "Despite a seeming correlation, gastric motility and emptying time were not associated with preterm GER in one study" (Hibbs, 2020, p. 1514).

■ Surgical options: When optimal treatment has failed, life-threatening complications of GERD may exist. In this case, surgical treatment can be considered. Transpyloric or jejunal feeding should be trialed first (Rosen et al., 2018).

Several gastric fundoplication techniques can be considered for neonates with life-threatening GERD when other management therapies have failed. These include:

■ Nissen's fundoplication—stomach is wrapped 360° around the distal esophagus.

■ Thal's fundoplication—stomach is wrapped 270°, which may decrease gastric distention of the stomach.

The wrap increases the pressure in the lower esophagus and acts as a one-way valve. Often a gastrostomy tube is inserted to ensure adequate nutrition and provide a vent for gas. Procedures are performed laparoscopically, allowing for better recovery during the postoperative period and decrease in the length of hospitalization.

Importantly, medical and surgical treatments for GER and/or GERD should not be based solely on clinical signs or the perception of providers or parents (Badran & Jadcherla, 2020).

Prognosis

GER is a self-limiting diagnosis which most children outgrow in the first year of life. There are some risks associated with GERD, most notably the aspiration of gastric content into the lungs, which can cause pneumonia. Severe GERD can lead to failure to thrive, esophagitis, anemia, esophageal strictures, and inflammatory esophageal polyps.

Most GERD patients will recover with medical treatment though some will require long-term medical treatment. When symptoms are controlled by medical management, therapy should regularly be assessed to see if it can be discontinued. A small percentage of infants will require surgery; however, long-term surgical results are good (Salminen et al., 2012).

Summary of the Joint Taskforce Diagnostic Recommendations

■ Barium or ultrasound studies only to look for underlying anatomic defects

■ Endoscopies only to assess for GERD complications

■ Manometry only to assess motility issues

■ Scintigraphy, transpyloric feedings, and trial of PPIs should not be used for diagnosis of GERD

■ Thickened feeds may be used with visible regurgitation

■ A 2- to 4-week trial of hydrolyzed protein-based formula after failure of non-pharmacologic treatment

■ Modify feeding volume and frequency to not overfeed

■ There is no evidence for positioning, massage, probiotics and prebiotics, or herbal medications for the treatment of GER/GERD in infants.

REFERENCES

Badran, E. F., & Jadcherla, S. (2020). The enigma of gastroesophageal reflux disease among convalescing infants in the NICU: It is time to rethink. *International Journal of Pediatrics and Adolescent Medicine, 7,* 28–32. https://doi.org/10.1016/j.ijpam.2020.03.001

Chabra, S., & Peeples, E. (2020). Assessment and management of gastroesophageal reflux in the newborn. *Pediatric Annals, 49*(2), e77–e81. https://doi.org/10.3928/19382359-20200121-02

Djeddi, D., Kongolo, G., Lefaix, C., Mounard, J., & Leke, A. (2008). Effect of domperidone on QT interval in neonates. *Journal of Pediatrics, 153*(5), 663–666. https://doi.org/10.1016/j.jpeds.2008.05.013

Hasenstab, K. A., & Jadcherla, S. R. (2020). Gastroesophageal reflux disease in the neonatal intensive care unit neonate: Controversies, current understanding, and future directions. *Clinics in Perinatology, 47*, 243–263. https://doi.org/10.1016/j.clp.2020.02.004

Hibbs, A. M. (2020). Gastroesophageal reflux and gastroesophageal reflux disease in the neonate. In R. J. Martin, A. A. Fanaroff, & M. C. Walsh (Eds.), *Fanaroff and Martin's neonatal-perinatal medicine* (11th ed., pp. 1513–1521). Elsevier/Saunders.

Lenfestey, M. W., & Neu, J. (2018). Gastrointestinal development implications for management of preterm and term infants. *Gastroenterol Clinics of North America, 47*, 773–791. https://doi.org/10.1016/j.gtc.2018.07.005

Ngo, K., & Shah, M. (2020). Gastrointestinal system. In C. Kenner, L. B. Altimier, & M. V. Boykova (Eds.), *Comprehensive neonatal nursing care* (6th ed., pp. 190–192). Springer Publishing Company.

Rosen, R., Vandenplas, Y., Singendonk, M., Cabana, M., Di Lorenzo, C., Gottrand, F., Gupta, S., Langendam, M., Staiano, A., Thapar, S., Tipnis, N., & Tabbers, M. (2018). Pediatric gastroesophageal reflux clinical practice guidelines: Joint recommendations of the North American Society for Pediatric Gastroenterology, Hepatology, and Nutrition (NASPGHAN) and the European Society for Pediatric Gastroenterology, Hepatology, and Nutrition (ESPGHAN). *Journal of Pediatric Gastroenterology and Nutrition, 66*(3), 516–554. https://doi.org/10.1097/MPG.0000000000001889.

Salminen, P., Hurme, S., & Ovaska, J. (2012). Fifteen-year outcome of laparoscopic and open nissen fundoplication: A randomized clinical trial. *Annals of Thoracic Surgery, 93*(1), 228–233. https://doi.org/10.1016/j.athoracsur.2011.08.066

INFANTILE HYPERTROPHIC PYLORIC STENOSIS

Progressive hypertrophy of the muscle that surrounds the gastric pylorus may cause partial to complete blockage of the gastric outlet. Due to an increase in the number and size of the muscle cells, the pylorus becomes narrow and longer. The stomach will in turn become more peristaltic, trying to push against the enlarged pylorus muscle.

Incidence

Ranges from 2 to 3.5/1,000; four times higher in boys versus girls; higher in preterm, may be increasing over time, but the reason is unclear.

Pathophysiology

Unknown but may be related to a primary abnormality of the ENS; presumed genetic and environmental factors.

Genetic factors include male predominance and increased risk in babies whose mothers had IHPS; environmental factors include smoking and macrolide antibiotics (erythromycin), among others (Ngo & Shah, 2020).

Clinical Presentation

It is observed in the first 2 months of life, most often the third to sixth week, with nonbilious vomiting that may be bloody; baby seems hungry afterward; weight loss, dehydration, and unconjugated hyperbilirubinemia.

During the physical exam, vomiting may be persistent and forceful; pyloric olive sign–enlarged pylorus, best felt at the end of feeding, is noted in 23% of cases; decreased output, dry mucous membranes, and sunken fontanelle are possible signs of dehydration (Dingeldin, 2020; Gomella et al., 2020).

Differential Diagnosis

Other diagnoses to consider are overfeeding, GI reflux, malrotation, and small bowel atresia.

Ultrasound is the gold standard; the muscle layer will show a thickening of more than 3 mm; the pyloric canal will be greater than 12 mm in length—abnormally long (Gomella et al., 2020).

Treatment

Vomiting may lead to gastritis or esophagitis. If hematemesis is noted, the baby needs hydration and surgical (laparoscopic) pyloromyotomy; surgery is never an emergency.

Management: Start intravenous (IV) maintenance fluid to correct dehydration and electrolyte anomalies; follow intake and output (I&O), preoperative protocol, avoid nasogastric tube (NGT; preoperative may cause more bleeding, whereas postoperative may interrupt the internal wound site). Pain med requirement is minimal, routine wound care; can feed quickly on the same day. Some postoperative vomiting is expected (Bradshaw, 2021).

Prognosis

Discharge usually at 48 hours (about 2 days), no recurrence rate.

REFERENCES

Bradshaw, W. (2021). Gastrointestinal disorders. In M. T. Verklan, M. Walden, & S. Forrest (Eds.), *Core curriculum for neonatal intensive care nursing* (6th ed., p. 515). Elsevier.

Dingeldin, M. (2020). Selected gastrointestinal anomalies in the neonate. In R. J. Martin, A. A. Fanaroff, & M. C. Walsh (Eds.), *Fanaroff and Martin's neonatal-perinatal medicine* (pp. 1554–1556). Elsevier.

Gomella, T. L., Eyal, F. G., & Bany-Mohammed, F. (Eds.). (2020). *Gomella's neonatology management, procedures, on-call problems, diseases, and drugs*. Lange.

Ngo, K., & Shah, M. (2020). Gastrointestinal system. In C. Kenner, L. B. Altimier, & M. V. Boykova (Eds.), *Comprehensive neonatal nursing care* (6th ed., pp. 190–192). Springer Publishing Company.

OSTOMY CARE

An ostomy is a surgical opening created to divert movement of material to or from an organ.

These can include an opening in the intestine (enterostomy), stomach (gastrostomy), or urinary tract (urostomy). The opening itself, especially the portion of the organ at the surface, is the stoma.

Diagnoses which may require an ostomy include EA, TEF, NEC, volvulus, Hirschsprung disease, intestinal atresias, decompression of an organ, or neurologic/congenital anomalies.

Types of Ostomies

■ Ileostomy—opening in the ileum

■ Colostomy—opening in the colon

■ Mucous fistula/distal ostomy—nonfunctional part of the intestine connected to the abdominal skin

■ End ostomy/proximal ostomy—functioning end of the intestine brought external to the abdomen

■ Gastrostomy—opening in the stomach where a tube for feeding can be inserted

■ Urostomy—opening to divert urine from the urinary tract

■ Vesicostomy—opening from the bladder to the skin to divert urine such as with posterior urethral valves (Gomella et al., 2020, p. 376).

OSTOMY CARE: ILEOSTOMY AND COLOSTOMY OR GASTROSTOMY

For procedures, use universal precautions, identify infant, remember pain management, and offer family teaching whenever possible.

Equipment

■ One- or two-piece ostomy appliance, gloves, gauze, stoma powder or paste, scissors, water, skin barrier

Care

■ When initially postoperative, use petroleum or xeroform gauze; no bag is needed until output is noted.

The goal is always to contain stool and protect the skin. Regularly assess skin, stoma size, and position. Monitor intake and ostomy output; consider replacement fluid of saline with or without potassium if output is greater than 10 to 15 mL/kg/d.

Note that ileostomy output is usually greater in volume and more liquid than colostomy output.

Empty regularly when bag is half full; replace the bag if it is leaking or as needed if caustic effluent wears away the wafer.

To replace the appliance:

■ Changing bag is a clean procedure. Remove appliance gently using water or saline wipes.

■ Evaluate skin and clean with water. You do not need to remove all of the barrier layer; avoid excess rubbing. Keep in mind preterm skin is more permeable and sensitive than the skin of term infants.

■ Select pouch: One-piece versus two-piece (wafer and bag separate) appliance.

■ Measure 2 mm more than the stoma circumference and cut the wafer. Save the template for future appliance changes. Apply the wafer to the skin after using paste or stoma powder if the skin is broken down. You may use skin barrier or protectant under the bag. Paste will help the bag fit, and powder helps create a dry layer over damaged skin to aid bag adherence; apply both sparingly.

■ Apply bag to the wafer if using a twopiece appliance. Hold in place 1 to 2 minutes; you may use the warmth of your hand or a heel warming device to help mold the wafer to the skin.

■ Position the bag down and to the side using gravity to allow for drainage into the bag. The length of time the bag will last depends on the site, output (ileostomy has more enzymes and volume so shorter time), and "maturity" of stoma.

■ Check for leakage. Chart the date and time of appliance change along with stoma appearance.

Complications

■ Cutting hole too small constricts the stoma, whereas too big allows leakage and skin breakdown.

■ Watch stoma for bleeding, hernia, stenosis, retraction, necrosis, or prolapse.

■ Document size, shape, and color of the stoma, as well as quality and quantity of output, and notify the provider with any change or concern.

■ If difficulties ensue with skin breakdown or the baby requires frequent changes, consider a stoma team consult (Bauman & Bowles, 2019, pp. 141–143).

GASTROSTOMY CARE

Types of Feeding Tubes

■ Balloon tip

■ Mushroom tip

■ Percutaneous endoscopic
■ Button or low profile (Gomella et al., 2020, p. 377).

Equipment

■ Feeding supplies, slip tip syringe, gloves, sterile water, gauze, cotton tip swab, soap, and water

Care

■ Nurses need to know the type of tube, size and when it was placed, tube length, and balloon volume.
■ Tubes should be secured snug and perpendicular to the skin but not tight. Movement and tension allow leakage and granulomas to form.
■ Measure external length of tube, when applicable, to ensure tube remains in stable position.
■ Initial change is 3 to 5 days postoperatively, then daily and as needed.
■ The gastrostomy site care is initially with normal saline or mild soap and water once healed. Remove old dressing; measure tube, assess site.
■ Clean with saline and cotton tip swab until healed, then with water and gauze pad. Allow to dry and then apply any prescribed skin treatments.
■ Use a single layer of gauze at the base of the tube and secure tube to prevent movement, which can lead to granuloma; if using button tube, no gauze needed.
■ Once well healed, the site can be left open to air.

Feeding

■ Attach the correct size syringe, and allow feeding by gravity. Follow feeding and medications with 1 to 5 mL sterile water to rinse the tube. Flush with 3 mL of air every 4 hours if infant is on continuous feeds. Provide nonnutritive sucking (NNS) during feeds. Disconnect feeding and vent the tube with an open syringe if patient has had a Nissan fundoplication; otherwise, clamp. Keep skin dry.

Complications

■ Watch for skin breakdown, leaking, granulation tissue, tube occlusion, or accidental dislodgement. Note the site can close in as rapidly as 1 to 4 hours if the tube is dislodged.
■ Document any redness, leakage, or change in appearance of the ostomy and notify provider with changes or concerns.
■ Dislodgment: The tube should be replaced quickly with a Foley catheter of the same size using water-based lubricant and secured by an inflating balloon; notify provider immediately.

■ Documentation includes feeding, tolerance, site, skin, leaking, dressing and changes, tube measurement, and any provider notifications (Bauman & Bowles, 2019, pp. 255–256; Gomella et al., 2020, p. 378).

REFERENCES

Bauman, S. S., & Bowles, S. (Eds.). (2019). *Policies, procedures, and competencies for neonatal nursing care*. National Association of Neonatal Nurses.

Gomella, T. L., Eyal, F. G., & Bany-Mohammed, F. (Eds.). (2020). *Gomella's neonatology management, procedures, on-call problems, diseases, and drugs*. Lange.

ADDITIONAL READING

Blackburn, S. T. (2018). Gastrointestinal and hepatic systems and perinatal nutrition. In S. T. Blackburn (Ed.), *Maternal, fetal and neonatal physiology: A clinical perspective* (5th ed., pp. 387–434). Elsevier.

Bradshaw, W. (2021). Gastrointestinal disorders. In M. T. Verklan, M. Walden, & S. Forrest (Eds.), *Core curriculum for neonatal intensive care nursing* (6th ed., p. 515). Elsevier.

Desai, N. S., & Hacker, J. F. (2020). Ostomy Care. In T. L. Gomella, F. G. Eyal, & F. Bany-Mohammed (Eds.), *Gomella's neonatology: Management, procedures, on-call problems, diseases, and drugs* (8th ed., pp. 375–378). Lange.

Dingeldin, M. (2020a). Development of the neonatal gastrointestinal tract. In R. J. Martin, A. A. Fanaroff, & M. C. Walsh (Eds.), *Fanaroff and Martin's neonatal-perinatal medicine* (pp. 1506–1512). Elsevier.

Dingeldin, M. (2020b). Selected gastrointestinal anomalies in the neonate. In R. J. Martin, A. A. Fanaroff, & M. C. Walsh (Eds.), *Fanaroff and Martin's neonatal-perinatal medicine* (pp. 1554–1556). Elsevier.

Hibbs, A. M. (2020). Gastrointestinal reflux and motility in the neonate. In R. J. Martin, A. A. Fanaroff, & M. C. Walsh (Eds.), *Fanaroff and Martin's neonatal-perinatal medicine* (pp. 1513–1521). Elsevier.

Ngo, K., & Shah, M. (2020). Gastrointestinal system. In C. Kenner, L. B. Altimier, & M. V. Boykova (Eds.), *Comprehensive neonatal nursing care* (6th ed., pp. 190–192). Springer Publishing Company.

5

Renal System

LESLIE A. PARKER

OVERVIEW

The renal and urinary system consists of the kidneys, ureters, urinary bladder, and urethra. The kidney regulates fluid and electrolyte balance, maintains arterial blood pressure, and excretes toxic and waste substances. These regulatory mechanisms are intimately tied to formation of urine, which involves three basic processes: ultrafiltration of plasma by the glomerulus, reabsorption of water and solutes from the ultrafiltrate, and secretion of certain solutes into the tubular fluid.

ANATOMY AND PHYSIOLOGY

The nephron is the functional unit of the kidney and the site of urine formation. Nephrons consist of a glomerulus (Bowman's capsule and glomerular capillaries) and a renal tubule with three sections: a proximal convoluted tubule, the loop of Henle, and a distal convoluted tubule. After urine is produced, it drains from the nephron into the minor and major calyces, then into the renal pelvis, out through the ureter, and into the bladder.

As blood flows into the kidney via the renal artery, it is directed into the afferent arterioles and carried into the glomerulus. Plasma driven through the glomerular capillaries is filtered and the protein-free plasma (ultrafiltrate) is forced into the Bowman's capsule or leaves via the efferent arterioles and enters the renal vein. To produce ultrafiltrate, the glomerulus functions as a filtering site.

The glomerular filtration rate (GFR) is the rate at which fluid is filtered through the glomerulus and reflects kidney function. Oncotic and hydrostatic pressures (Starling forces) drive the ultrafiltration process. Oncotic pressure is osmotic pressure generated by large proteins or colloids while hydrostatic pressure is pressure exerted by fluids in equilibrium and depends on arterial pressure and vascular resistance. GFR is therefore, affected by changes in arterial blood pressure, vascular resistance, concentration of plasma proteins, and glomerular capillary permeability.

The kidneys control fluid and electrolyte balance by reabsorption and secretion of sodium and water. The four segments of the nephron—the proximal tubule, loop of Henle, distal tubule, and the collecting duct—determine the composition and volume of urine.

Tubular reabsorption, secretion, and excretion are closely tied together and function to maintain internal homeostasis and regulation of fluids and electrolytes.

Tubular reabsorption is the process where substances in the tubular lumen move into the capillary system through simple diffusion and active transport. Many of the body's nutrients, electrolytes, and 99% of the filtered water are reabsorbed. Tubular secretion moves substances including potassium and hydrogen from the epithelial lining of the tubules' capillaries into the interstitial fluid and finally into the tubular lumen. Tubular excretion is the process where substances enter the filtrate that will eventually exit the body as urine. Ions such as potassium, which are secreted in the distal tubule (a portion is also reabsorbed in the proximal tubule), find their way into the urine when the body has no need for higher concentration levels.

RENAL SYSTEM DEVELOPMENT

Development of the renal system begins around the fourth week of gestation, urine is produced by week 10, and renal anatomic development is complete by approximately 36 weeks, while functional development continues until 2 years. Formation of the renal system occurs within the nephrogenic cords in three stages which form three structures (pronephros, mesonephros, and metanephros).

■ The pronephros or primitive kidney develops during the first month of gestation and then gradually degenerates, contributing to the duct system for the next developmental stage. The pronephros has no excretory function.

■ Development of the mesonephros occurs during the fourth to sixth month of gestation and contains primitive but functional glomeruli and tubules which produce ultra-urine by 8 to 10 weeks. The mesonephric structure degenerates and leaves a duct system for the following stage. Failure of the mesonephric duct to develop may result in anomalies in both the urinary and genital systems.

■ The final stage begins in the fifth week of gestation and results in formation of the metanephros or definitive kidney. The ureteric bud is an outgrowth of the mesonephric duct, and the metanephrogenic blastema originates from the nephrogenic cord. The stalk of the ureteric bud becomes the ureter and the renal pelvis, major and minor calyces, and collecting tubes are formed through elongation and branching of the ureteric bud. Cells of the metanephric blastema stimulate formation of the glomerulus, proximal tubule, loop of Henle, and distal tubule.

■ Early in development, the kidneys are located in the pelvic region and make a gradual ascent into their final location in the flank. Failure of normal ascent of the kidneys results in abnormalities such as horseshoe kidneys or pelvic kidneys.

■ Fetal urine contributes significantly to amniotic fluid volume, especially during the third trimester. A reduction in fetal urine excretion results in oligohydramnios and can signify abnormalities of the urinary system.

RENAL ASSESSMENT

Renal assessment includes physical examination, urine analysis and chemistries, serum BUN and creatinine, and radiologic studies.

Physical Examination Findings

■ Examination for abdominal masses or bladder distention.

■ If possible, assess the urinary stream, which should be a continuous, straight stream.

■ Inspect for general characteristics suggesting renal abnormalities such as those consistent with Potter's sequence (flattened facies, beaklike nose, wide set eyes; micrognathia, abnormal positioning of the hands and feet, as well as pulmonary hypoplasia).

Urine Examination

Collection

■ Bagged specimen: Used for urinalysis; however, due to the high risk of contamination, it is not recommended for Gram stain or culture.

■ Suprapubic bladder aspiration: Uses a needle inserted above the symphysis pubis to obtain urine.

■ Urethral catheterization

Urinalysis

■ Includes color, pH, specific gravity, white blood cells, blood, and protein.

■ Leukocytes and nitrites can indicate a urinary tract infection (UTI).

■ pH should be 4.5 to 8 and should be evaluated in relation to serum bicarbonate levels. Alkaline urine with documented metabolic acidosis may indicate renal pathology.

■ Specific gravity indicates the kidney's ability to concentrate and dilute urine. Normal levels range from 1.001 to 1.015. High levels can indicate dehydration or high solute excretion.

Urine Chemistries

■ Helpful in determining fluid and electrolyte balance when evaluated in comparison to serum electrolyte levels.

■ Sodium excretion is very high in the fetus and premature infant and decreases with increasing gestational age.

■ Urinary potassium levels reflect the amount secreted by the collecting tubule.

Blood Urea Nitrogen and Creatinine

■ Creatinine levels are the most common indicator of GFR.

■ Creatinine levels at birth are high and reflect maternal levels, gestational age, and the infant's GFR.

■ Level may temporarily increase on day 1 but then begins to decrease over the first few weeks of life.

■ Serial levels are necessary to evaluate renal function.

■ Elevated blood urea nitrogen (BUN) levels can result from significant dehydration, ingestion of high protein loads, and renal dysfunction.

Urine Culture

■ Used to assess for a UTI.

Radiologic Evaluation

Renal Ultrasonography

■ Examines kidney structure and can identify renal obstruction, hydronephrosis, renal calculi, and, in some cases, advanced parenchymal disease.

■ Often combined with Doppler imaging to provide information on blood flow in the renal arteries and veins.

Prenatal Ultrasound

■ Seventy percent of renal anomalies are diagnosed with prenatal ultrasound.

■ Provides information regarding amniotic fluid volume; since it is predominantly produced by the kidneys, anhydramnios or severe oligohydramnios may indicate kidney disease.

Voiding Cystourethrogram

■ Contrast material is instilled through a catheter in the bladder and fluoroscopy is used to monitor bladder filling and voiding and to assess for vesicoureteric reflux as well as bladder and urethral function and anatomy.

Renal Scintigraphy With Dimercaptosuccinic Acid Scan

■ Assesses renal parenchyma and evaluates renal function through intravenous (IV) administration of a radioactive isotope which is taken up by the renal parenchyma and identifies regions of decreased uptake representing inflammation or renal scarring.

Diuretic Renography

■ A radionuclide test is used to differentiate between obstructive and nonobstructive uropathies and to assess renal function.

GENERALIZED NURSING CARE

Fluid, Electrolytes, and Nutrition

■ Frequent assessment of serum electrolytes, phosphorus, and calcium levels is used to prevent derangement.

■ Frequent monitoring of serum creatinine and BUN is used to monitor renal function.

■ Measure intake and output meticulously.

■ Carefully monitor for dehydration and overhydration.

■ Daily or twice-daily weights may be required.

■ Assess for edema, which may indicate overhydration in the periorbital area, as well as edema of the hands, feet, labia, and scrotum.

■ Presence of pitting edema may be assessed by gently depressing a fingertip into the site.

■ Assess for appropriate growth and nutrition, which may be compromised due to fluid and protein restriction.

Skin Management

■ Impaired skin integrity is common, especially if severe edema is present.

■ Change the infant's position every 2 to 3 hours.

■ Inspect operative sites for signs of irritation or infection and keep the area clean and dry.

■ Inspect any dressings for bloody drainage or secretions.

Overall Nursing Care

■ Meticulously monitor vital signs.

■ Frequently assess the infant's EKG monitor for cardiac arrhythmias, which may occur due to hyperkalemia.

■ Monitor for hypertension, which frequently occurs in infants with renal disorders.

■ Because infants with renal disorders may be prone to infections including UTIs, carefully monitor for signs and symptoms of infection.

■ Monitor for signs and symptoms of a UTI, including positive leukocytes, nitrites, blood, or protein in the urine and physical symptoms consistent with infection.

■ Assess for pain and provide pharmacologic and/or nonpharmacologic pain relief as indicated.

Parental Support

■ Individualized parental support, depending on disease severity and the family's needs, is essential.

■ Provide parents accurate and complete information regarding their infant's condition and allow the opportunity for them to express concerns and ask questions.

■ Care by an interdisciplinary team is essential and should include neonatologists, pediatric renal physicians and/or urologists, nurses, clergy, and social workers.

■ Discharge teaching is dependent on the specific renal disorder but should be clear and include specific instructions on follow-up appointments and signs and symptoms requiring further evaluation.

URINARY TRACT INFECTION

Incidence

■ Occurs in 0.1% to 2% of all newborns.

■ Occurs in 20% of preterm and high-risk infants.

■ More common in males, potentially due to an increased risk in uncircumcised males.

■ Increased risk exists in infants with a neurogenic bladder.

Physiology

A UTI is an infection of the kidney and/or bladder. Pyelonephritis refers to an infection of the kidney, and cystitis is an infection of the bladder. If not properly treated, UTIs can result in long-term sequelae including decreased renal function, renal scarring, and hypertension.

Pathophysiology

The bacteria most commonly responsible for UTIs include *Escherichia coli, Klebsiella, Pseudomonas, Proteus, Enterococcus, Staphylococcus,* and *Candida*. UTIs often occur in conjunction with systemic infection.

Assessment

While a UTI can be an isolated occurrence, it can also be associated with systemic infection or an underlying abnormality of the urinary tract system.

Clinical Manifestations/Diagnosis

The diagnosis of a UTI is based on history, physical examination, and laboratory findings, as well as urine Gram stain and culture.

Physical Examination

■ Symptoms may be nonspecific, especially during the first 1 to 2 months of life.

■ Temperature instability, lethargy, poor feeding, cyanosis, abdominal distention, poor weight gain, hepatomegaly, jaundice, and fever

■ Protein, blood, nitrites, or leukocytes on urine dipstick

Diagnostic Procedures/Tests

■ Elevated or decreased white blood cell count with a left shift

■ Elevated C-reactive protein (CRP)

■ Positive leukocytes or nitrites on urinalysis

■ Bacteria present on Gram stain and/or culture obtained by suprapubic aspiration or sterile bladder catheterization prior to initiation of antibiotics

- Never use a bagged urine specimen because of contamination risk.
- Any bacteria obtained from a suprapubic aspiration is diagnostic.
- More than 10^5 colony-forming units (CFUs) obtained from a catheterization are diagnostic.

■ Obtain a blood culture due to the high risk of systemic infection.

Treatment

■ Antibiotic therapy:

- Empiric broad-spectrum intravenous (IV) antibiotic therapy
- Adjust antibiotics as needed following identification of infective organisms on culture and specification of sensitivities.
- Continue antibiotic therapy for 7 to 14 days IV.
- Obtain repeat urine culture 48 to 72 hours following initiation of treatment.

■ Use renal ultrasound to assess for hydronephrosis, renal scarring, severe vesico-ureterral reflux, or obstructive uropathy.

■ A voiding cystourethrogram (VCUG) is performed after the first UTI if the ultrasound is abnormal or with any subsequent UTIs.

■ Nonpharmacologic interventions including sucrose nipples, swaddling, and nonnutritive sucking may be helpful for associated pain and discomfort.

■ Symptoms of a UTI should be included in the discharge instructions, and parents should be instructed to seek medical care immediately if symptoms occur.

Prognosis

Prompt treatment is imperative to prevent complications including renal scarring that can lead to hypertension or permanent kidney failure. With prompt diagnosis and treatment, the prognosis is generally excellent for isolated UTIs. The prognosis of UTIs associated with renal abnormalities is dependent on the severity and type of underlying abnormality.

ACUTE RENAL FAILURE

Incidence

■ Occurs in 24% of neonates admitted to the NICU.

■ May be underestimated.

■ It is associated with significant mortality and morbidity.

Physiology

Acute renal failure (ARF) occurs when the GFR abruptly decreases or completely ceases, leading to impairment in fluid and electrolyte regulation and acid–base homeostasis. Any condition that interferes with normal kidney function can cause acute kidney injury.

Pathophysiology

ARF can be classified as prerenal, intrinsic, or postrenal. Prerenal failure, the most common type, accounts for 75% to 80% of cases and is due to inadequate perfusion of a normal kidney. Failure to adequately treat prerenal failure can result in permanent kidney damage.

Intrinsic renal failure (IRF) results from damage to the renal parenchyma and can occur due to progression of either prerenal or postrenal failure, infection, renal vein thrombosis, and nephrotoxicity from medications. Acute tubular necrosis (ATN) is the most common cause of IRF and results from renal tubular cellular injury due to severe hypoxia, dehydration, sepsis, or blood loss. Other causes of IRF include structural abnormalities of the kidney such as renal dysplasia and polycystic or multicystic kidney disease.

Postrenal failure is caused by obstruction of the urinary tract. Obstruction can be caused by posturethral valves, ureteropelvic and UVJ obstruction, prune-belly syndrome, and neurogenic bladder. Backflow of urine into the kidney pelvis to these obstructive processes can cause damage to the renal parenchyma.

Assessment

Any infant with a history of asphyxia and those born prematurely should be considered at high risk for ARF and should undergo a thorough assessment. The severity of ARF is related to the underlying etiology.

Clinical Manifestations/Diagnosis

The diagnosis of ARF is based on history, physical examination, and laboratory analysis.

Physical Examination Findings

■ Urine output less than 1 mL/kg/hr is a cardinal sign.

■ Infants with nonoliguric renal failure may have a normal or high urine output.

■ Edema

■ Hypertension

■ Possible flank mass, abnormal genitalia, or other genitourinary (GU) abnormalities

Laboratory Findings

■ Elevated BUN and creatinine levels

■ Hyperphosphatemia, hyponatremia, metabolic acidosis, and hypocalcemia

■ Hematuria and proteinuria on urine dipstick and urinalysis

■ A urine-to-plasma osmolality ratio of ≤1:1

Diagnostic Procedures/Tests

■ Family, prenatal, perinatal, and postnatal history

  ● Prenatal ultrasound results

  ● Amniotic fluid measurements

  ● History of perinatal depression, conditions associated with decreased renal blood flow, and administration of nephrotoxic medications

■ Administration of 10 to 20 mg/kg of an IV isotonic solution may be used to differentiate between prerenal and IRF.

  ● Urine output of at least 1 mL/kg/hr within 2 hours suggests prerenal failure.

  ● Diuretic administration following the fluid challenge may be necessary.

■ A FeNa (fractional excretion of sodium) greater than 3% and a renal failure index less than 3% suggest prerenal failure.

  ● It is only accurate greater than 48 hours following birth.

■ Placement of a urinary catheter can diagnose postrenal failure.

■ Renal ultrasound is used to evaluate the etiology of intrinsic and postrenal failure.

Treatment

Prerenal Failure

■ Increase renal perfusion through administration of intravascular fluids and possibly low-dose dopamine.

Intrinsic Renal Failure

■ Limit fluid administration to replacement of insensible water losses, other fluid losses, and urine output.

■ Carefully calculate fluid intake and urine output.

■ Follow electrolytes closely.

■ Monitor for signs of infection.

■ Assess vital signs, including blood pressure.

■ Monitor for complications related to electrolyte abnormalities.

■ Treat hyponatremia with additional sodium administration.

■ Treat hyperphosphatemia.

- Phosphorus restriction

- Oral calcium carbonate binds phosphate and prevents absorption.

■ Treat hypocalcemia with calcium supplementation.

■ Treat hyperkalemia.

- Eliminate or severely limit potassium intake.

- Use sodium bicarbonate and a combination of insulin and dextrose to drive potassium from the intracellular into the extracellular space.

- Use IV calcium for cardiac protection.

- Use kayexalate to increase potassium elimination.

■ Treat metabolic acidosis.

- IV sodium acetate

- Oral or IV sodium bicarbonate

■ Treat anemia due to decreased production and release of erythropoietin.

■ Treat hypertension with sodium/fluid restriction and antihypertensives.

■ Limit renally excreted medication and monitor levels carefully.

■ Promote adequate nutrition.

- Limit protein to 1 to 2 g/kg/d.

- Restrict fluid administration.

- Consider Similac PM 60/40 (Ross Laboratories, Columbus, OH), SMA (Wyeth, Madison, NJ), or human milk to limit sodium, potassium, and phosphorous.

■ Dialysis may be indicated in the following situations:

- Continued clinical deterioration

- High BUN, creatinine, and ammonia levels

- Severe hyperkalemia, metabolic acidosis, hypocalcemia, and hyperphosphatemia

- Volume overload and malnutrition

Postrenal Failure

■ Relief of urinary obstruction

■ Correction of underlying condition

Prognosis

Early recognition and treatment of ARF may prevent further renal failure and improve outcome. Prognosis is related to severity of the underlying disease and the ability to treat the underlying problem. ARF increases mortality and is associated with short- and long-term complications including renal dysfunction and hypertension.

HYDRONEPHROSIS

Incidence

- The most common renal abnormality detected prenatally
- Present in 2.3% of all pregnancies

Pathophysiology

Hydronephrosis is the accumulation of urine within the renal pelvis and calices, causing overdistention which can result in irreversible kidney damage. Hydronephrosis is caused by obstruction of urine flow at the junction of the ureteropelvis, the uretero-vesical valve, or the urethrovesical valve. Nonobstructive abnormalities such as vesicourethral reflux and prune-belly syndrome as well as obstruction from kidney stones or tumors can also result in hydronephrosis. Severity is classified from grade I to grade V depending on the diameter of the renal pelvis.

Assessment

The severity of hydronephrosis is determined by the degree of hydronephrosis and whether renal failure is present. Severe hydronephrosis may cause signs of Potter's syndrome from severe antenatal oligohydramnios. Following delivery, infants with severe hydronephrosis can have signs of ARF including oliguria, hypertension, and fluid/electrolyte disturbances.

Clinical Manifestations/Diagnosis

The diagnosis of hydronephrosis is based on history and physical examination, as well as renal ultrasound and VCUG findings.

Physical Findings

- Decreased urine output and signs of ARF if hydronephrosis is bilateral and severe
- Features of Potter's syndrome from oligohydramnios
- Symptoms of a UTI
  - Hematuria, proteinuria, and white blood cells on urinalysis
  - Positive urine culture

■ Large, smooth, solid, palpable abdominal mass

■ Hypertension

Diagnostic Procedures and Tests

■ Presence of a dilated renal pelvis on prenatal ultrasound

■ Postnatal renal ultrasound

- Determines presence, severity, and etiology of the hydronephrosis

- Often delayed until 24 to 72 hours of age, since the newborn's physiologic dehydration may mask hydronephrosis

■ VCUG to assess for reflux of urine into the kidney

Treatment

■ Goal is preservation of renal function.

■ Dependent on severity.

■ If mild to moderate, management is usually conservative with close monitoring via ultrasound.

■ Severe cases are initially managed conservatively but may require pyeloplasty if renal function deteriorates.

■ Prophylactic antibiotics are used to prevent UTI if urinary reflux is present.

■ If severe, a prenatal vesicoamniotic shunt (catheter to drain urine from bladder into the amniotic fluid) may be indicated.

- Reduces oligohydramnios and its associated complications.

- Sustains kidney function.

■ Careful assessment of vital signs, including blood pressure, is performed.

■ Monitoring of fluid and electrolyte status, including serum creatinine and BUN, is conducted.

■ After birth, definitive surgery may be necessary to correct the obstructive defect or to provide a diversion for urine flow.

Prognosis

Prognosis depends on the underlying cause, severity, and presence of permanent renal damage. Outcome ranges from complete resolution to end-stage renal disease. Complications include hypertension, UTI, and progressive renal damage. Hydronephrosis secondary to vesicoureteral reflux generally spontaneously resolves. Antenatally diagnosed hydronephrosis can indicate obstruction or other serious abnormalities but can also represent a transient developmental change that resolves prior to birth.

CYSTIC KIDNEY DISEASE (POLYCYSTIC AND MULTICYSTIC KIDNEY DISEASE)

Incidence

The overall incidence of cystic kidney disease is 0.1% to 2%. Autosomal recessive polycystic kidney disease (ARPKD) has an incidence of 1 in 20,000 and while generally considered a sporadic anomaly has also been associated with genetic syndromes. Multicystic kidney disease (MKD) has an incidence of 1 in 4,300.

Physiology

Cystic disease of the kidney occurs when normal kidney tissue is replaced with nonfunctioning cysts. These cysts may occur unilaterally or bilaterally, and the amount of cystic formation within each kidney determines the severity of the disease. Severely affected kidneys often have associated ureteral agenesis.

Pathophysiology

Polycystic kidney disease (PKD) includes both kidneys and presents as micro- or macroscopic cysts throughout the renal parenchyma. While there are two types of PKD, only ARPKD generally presents in neonates. It is associated with significant liver disease, which does not occur in the neonatal period. MKD is usually a unilateral process where there is a collection of noncommunicating cysts resulting in lack of renal function, which occurs due to early ureter obstruction resulting in kidney maldevelopment.

Assessment

Cystic kidney disease should be on the differential diagnosis of infants presenting with an abdominal mass after birth.

Clinical Manifestations/Diagnosis

The diagnosis of cystic kidney disease is based on history, physical examination, and radiologic studies.

Physical Examination

■ PKD

- Bilateral abdominal masses and hypertension
- Hypertension
- Respiratory distress if enlarged kidneys press on the diaphragm or with pulmonary hypoplasia

▪ MKD
  - Abdominal mass (usually unilateral)

Diagnostic Procedures/Tests

▪ Often diagnosed on prenatal ultrasound.

▪ Postnatal ultrasound showing small cysts in the collecting ducts (polycystic) or multiple noncommunicating renal cysts (multicystic).

▪ Radionuclide renal scale will show no renal function (multicystic).

Treatment

Polycystic Kidney Disease

▪ Treatment of hypertension
▪ Treatment of renal failure if present
▪ Respiratory and ventilatory support as needed
▪ Nephrectomy if enlarged kidney is impeding respiration

Multicystic Kidney Disease

▪ Conservative with careful follow-up until involution of affected kidney.
▪ Follow for decreased kidney function in unaffected kidney.

Prognosis

Between 6% and 30% of infants with PKD will die in the neonatal period, usually as a result of respiratory failure from pulmonary hypoplasia. In those who survive the neonatal period, 70% to 87% are alive at 1 year and 70% to 88% are alive at 5 years. An additional 50% of infants will advance to end-stage renal disease. Multicystic kidneys general involute spontaneously.

OBSTRUCTIVE UROPATHY

▪ Includes ureteropelvic junction obstruction (UPJ), UVJ obstruction, and posturethral valves (PUVs).

Incidence

▪ The incidence of UPJ is one in 2,000 and is more common in males.
▪ PUVs occur in one in 3,000 to 8,000 infants and only occur in males.

Physiology

Occurs due to obstruction along the urinary tract which can be unilateral or bilateral. The most common cause is UPJ obstruction.

Pathophysiology

When there is obstruction to urinary flow, urine can reflux into the kidney and result in hydronephrosis and kidney failure. Obstruction can occur at the ureterovesical junction (UVJ), at the UPJ, or due to PUV. UPJ obstruction prevents the flow of urine from the kidney pelvis into the ureter, UVJ obstruction impedes urine flow from the ureter into the bladder, and PUV is obstruction at the bladder outlet due to enlarged valves. Severity ranges from mild obstruction to severe disease.

Clinical Manifestations/Diagnosis

The diagnosis of obstructive uropathy is based on history, physical examination, and radiologic studies.

Physical Examination

■ Symptoms of a UTI

■ Abdominal mass

■ Symptoms of renal failure

■ Palpable bladder (PUV)

■ Anuria, oliguria, or a weak urinary stream (PUV)

Diagnostic Procedures/Tests

■ Often diagnosed on prenatal ultrasound

■ Postnatal ultrasound

■ VCUG is the gold standard for PUV diagnosis.

Treatment

Ureterovesical Junction and Ureteropelvic Junction Obstruction

■ Depends on severity.

■ If mild, observation and conservative treatment are recommended.

■ If severe, surgical intervention may be needed to relieve obstruction.

Posturethral Valves

■ Immediate bladder catheterization or suprapubic diversion is used to relieve obstruction.

■ Definitive treatment is ablation of the enlarged valves.

Prognosis

Obstructive uropathy can result in chronic renal failure and is a common cause of pediatric kidney transplantations. In addition, PUVs are associated with bladder dysfunction and urethral strictures.

RESOURCES

American Academy of Pediatrics. (2011). Urinary tract infection: Clinical practice guidelines for the diagnosis and management of the initial UTI in febrile infants and children, 2 to 24 months. *Pediatrics, 128*(3), 595–610. https://doi.org/10.1542/peds.2011-1330

American Academy of Pediatrics. (2016). Reaffirmation of AAP clinical practice guidelines: The diagnosis and management of the initial urinary tract infection in febrile infants and young children 2–24 months of age. *Pediatrics, 138*(6), e20163026. https://doi.org/10.1542/peds.2016-3026.

Basu, R. K., Devarajan, P., Wong, H., & Wheeler, D. S. (2011). An update and review of acute kidney injury in pediatrics. *Pediatric Critical Care, 12*(3), 339–347. https://doi.org/10.1097/PCC.0b013e3181fe2e0b

Casella, D. P., Tomaszewski, J. J., & Ost, M. C. (2012). Posterior urethral valves: Renal failure and prenatal treatment. *International Journal of Nephrology, 2012*, 351067. https://doi.org/10.1155/2012/351067

Chiappinelli, A., Savanelli, A., Farina, A., & Settimi, A. (2011). Multicystic dysplastic kidney: Our experience in non-surgical management. *Pediatric Surgery International, 27*, 757–779. https://doi.org/10.1007/s00383-011-2910-8

Coulthard, M. G. (2016). The management of neonatal acute and chronic renal failure: A review. *Early Human Development, 102*, 25–29. https://doi.org/10.1016/j.earlhumdev.2016.09.004

Drumm, C. M., Siddiqui, J. N., Desale, S., & Ramasethu, J. (2019). Urinary tract infection is common in VLBW infants. *Journal of Perinatology, 39*(1), 80–85. https://doi.org/10.1038/s41372-018-0226-4

Durkan, A. M., & Alexander, R. T. (2011). Acute kidney injury post neonatal asphyxia. *Journal of Pediatrics, 158*(Suppl. 2), e29–e33. https://doi.org/10.1016/j.jpeds.2010.11.010

Goldstein, S. L. (2011). Continuous renal replacement therapy: Mechanism of clearance, fluid removal, indications and outcomes. *Current Opinions in Pediatrics, 23*, 181–185. https://doi.org/10.1097/MOP.0b013e328342fe67

Jelton, J. G., & Askenazi, D. J. (2012). Update on acute kidney injury in the neonate. *Current Opinions in Pediatrics, 24*(2), 191–196. https://doi.org/10.1097/MOP.0b013e32834f62d5

Khan, O. A., Hageman, J. R., & Clardy, C. (2015). Acute renal failure in the neonate. *Pediatric Annals, 44*(10), 251–253. https://doi.org/10.3928/00904481-20151012-10

Khare, A., Krishnappa, V., Kumar, D., & Raina, R. J. (2018). Neonatal renal cystic disease. *Journal of Maternal, Fetal, and Neonatal Medicine, 31*(21), 2923–2929. https://doi.org/10.1080/14767058.2017.1358263

Kibar, Y., Ashley, R. A., Roth, C. C., Frimberger, D., & Kropp, B. P. (2011). Timing of posterior urethral valve diagnosis and its impact on clinical outcome. *Journal of Pediatric Urology, 7*, 538–542. https://doi.org/10.1016/j.jpurol.2010.08.002

Koeppen, B., & Stanton, B. (2018). *Renal physiology* (6th ed.). Mosby.

Liu, D. B., Armstrong, W. R., & Maizels, M. (2014). Hydronephrosis: Prenatal and postnatal evaluation and management. *Clinics in Perinatology, 41*(3), 661–678. https://doi.org/10.1016/j.clp.2014.05.013

Maayan-Metzger, A., Lotan, D., Jacobson, J. M., Raviv-Zilka, L., Ben-Shlush, A., Kuint, J., & Mor, Y. (2011). The yield of early postnatal ultrasound scan in neonates with documented antenatal hydronephrosis. *American Journal of Perinatology, 28*(8), 613–617. https://doi.org/10.1055/s-0031-1276735

Mesrobian, H. G., & Mirza, S. P. (2013). Hydronephrosis: A view from the inside. *Pediatric Clinics of North America, 59*(4), 839–851. https://doi.org/10.1016/j.pcl.2012.05.008

Moore, K. L., & Persaud, T. V. N. (2019). *The developing human: Clinically oriented embryology* (11th ed.). Elsevier.

Nasir, A. A., Ameh, E. A., Abdur-Rahman, L. O., Adeniran, J. O., & Abraham, M. K. (2011). Posterior urethral valves. *World Journal of Pediatrics, 7*(3), 205–216. https://doi.org/10.1007/s12519-011-0289-1

Oliveira, E. A., Oliveira, M. C., & Mak, R. H. (2016). Evaluation and management of hydronephrosis in the neonate. *Current Opinions in Pediatrics, 28*(2), 195–201. https://doi.org/10.1097/MOP.0000000000000321

Sweetman, D. U., Riordan, M., & Molloy, E. J. (2013). Management of renal dysfunction following term perinatal hypoxia-ischaemia. *Acta Paediatrics, 102*(3), 233–241. https://doi.org/10.1111/apa.12116

Subramanian, S., Agarwal, R., Deorari, A. K., Paul, V. K., & Bagga, A. (2011). Acute renal failure in neonates. *Indian Journal of Pediatrics, 73*, 385–391. https://doi.org/10.1007/BF02759894

Verghese, P., & Miyashita, Y. (2014). Neonatal polycystic kidney disease. *Clinics in Perinatology, 41*(3), 543–560. https://doi.org/10.1016/j.clp.2014.05.005

Weems, M. F., Wei, D., Rananatha, R., Barton, L., Vachon, L., & Sardesai, S. (2015). Urinary tract infections in a neonatal intensive care unit. *American Journal of Perinatology, 32*(7), 695–702. https://doi.org/10.1055/s-0034-1395474

Hematologic and Immune System

CAROLE KENNER

OVERVIEW

The hematologic system is very complex as it involves the development of the body's blood cells and regulates the hemostatic system. The hematopoietic system is characterized by the presence of pluripotent stem cells that differentiate into three types of circulating blood cells: red blood cells (RBCs), white blood cells (WBCs), and thrombocytes (platelets). Hematopoiesis is an ongoing process of cell development and death. The liver is the main site of this activity (Bagwell & Steward, 2020). The maturation of the cells is dependent on gestational and postnatal age.

Hemostasis is dependent on blood coalition and fibrinolysis or the breakdown of a clot. The three components of the hemostatic system are procoagulants or clotting factors, anticoagulants or inhibitors, and fibrinolytics or clot dissolvers. The initial steps in hemostasis are vascular spasm, platelet plug formation, and coagulation (Bagwell & Steward, 2020).

HEMATOLOGIC AND IMMUNE SYSTEM DEVELOPMENT

The hematologic system begins development early in gestation around the fifth to sixth week as the liver starts hematopoiesis (Bagwell & Steward, 2020). Pluripotent stem cells are present. These cells are important as they can differentiate and become RBCs, WBCs, or platelets. Around 4 to 5 months' gestation, the liver becomes less involved in hematopoiesis as the bone marrow takes on this primary function aided by the spleen, lymph nodes, thymus, and kidneys.

The hematologic system is comprised of the RBCs, hemoglobin, WBCs, platelets, blood volume, and blood type. Fetal hemoglobin (hemoglobin F) has a higher affinity for oxygen than does an adult's; thus, it does not release the oxygen to the cells as easily. Erythropoietin is a hormone that stimulates the production of RBCs. Release occurs when tissue oxygenation is low (Bagwell & Steward, 2020). The RBCs exchange oxygen and carbon dioxide. Their life cycle is considerably shorter than an adult's, 60 to 90 days in the term infant, 35 to 50 days in the preterm, and 120 days in the adult. RBC count in a term infant is about 5.8 million/mL with a reticulocyte count of 3% to 7% while a preterm infant's RBC count is 4.6 to 5.3 million/mL with a reticulocyte count of 6% to 12% (Bagwell & Steward, 2020). Hemoglobin is produced by the RBCs. WBCs protect the infant from invading proteins such as those found in infectious diseases. They are an important part of the immune system. Platelets assist with clotting and coagulation.

Another hematologic factor is blood volume. The volume is influenced by the gestational age and the timing of cord clamping. Delayed cord clamping for 30 to 60 seconds to allow an intact placenta to empty can be beneficial in increasing not only blood volume but also the hematocrit and ferritin levels. The antigens, either immunoglobulins or Rh, found on the RBC's surface determine the infant's blood type. The four blood types are A, B, O, and AB. The Rh antigen is either positive or negative, and is the basis for Rh incompatibility if there is a difference between the mother and infant. Hemostasis occurs through a series of steps:

■ Vascular spasm

■ Platelet plug formation

■ Coagulation

The coagulation, in turn, consists of three phases:

■ Formation of prothrombin activator

■ Formation of thrombin

■ Fibrin clot formation (Bagwell & Steward, 2020)

The immune system, like the hemotologic system, develops early in gestation. The primary function is to protect the infant from invading organisms. The preterm infant is at risk for many infections simply because the immune system is immature. There are two main subsystems: the innate and adaptive components (Bodin & Hoffman, 2020). The innate refers to the first response to an encounter of a foreign substance or pathogen. This system consists of granulocytes—neutrophils, monocytes, and natural killer cells. When there is a preponderance of immature cells due to a pathogen exposure, this is referred to as a shift to the left (Bodin & Hoffman, 2020). The innate system responds by producing cytokines such as tumor necrosis factors and interleukin 6 (IL-6). These factors are limited in the neonate. The adaptive system occurs when memory cells are present. For the system to remember or recognize an invading substance, there has to have been a prior encounter. These memory cells are the basis for booster injections or a series of vaccinations. The second encounter results in an immune response that is higher and faster than the innate response. T lymphocytes provide cell-mediated immunity. The T lymphocytes are produced in the thymus. The two types of T lymphocytes are CD4 and CD8 T cells (Bodin & Hoffman, 2020). B lymphocytes provide humeral immunity and develop in the bone marrow. Both T and B lymphocytes circulate through the lymphatic system. Once the B lymphocytes enter the peripheral lymphatic system, they become plasma cells that in turn produce five types of immunoglobulins—IgA, IgD, IgE, IgG, and IgM (Bodin & Hoffman, 2020). IgG passes from the placenta to the fetus/neonate naturally. When IgM is in the neonate, it is indicative of an in utero infection (Bodin & Hoffman, 2020). The neonate's immune system is influenced by the mother's health and lifestyle.

HEMATOLOGIC AND IMMUNE ASSESSMENT

For both the hematologic and immune systems, it is important to have a complete maternal history that includes infections, prolonged rupture of membranes (PROM), use of substances including alcohol, tobacco, and other medications including over-the-counter and prescription drugs. When hematologic disorders are suspected, assess for hypoglycemia, hypocalcemia, temperature instability (especially hypothermia), apneic or bradycardic episodes, cyanosis, lethargy, poor feeding, prolonged bleeding, or jaundice (Bagwell & Steward, 2020).

Lab tests include complete blood count (CBC) with platelets, clotting studies, fibrinogen levels, D-dimer, fibrin split products, or fibrin degradation products (Bagwell & Steward, 2020). If jaundice is present, bilirubin levels should be drawn. Presence of hematomas, excessive bruising—ecchymosis, petechiae, plethora, pallor, hepatosplenomegaly, and abrasions can also indicate hematologic problems (Bagwell & Steward, 2020).

Neonatal risk factors for infection include antenatal or postpartal stress, congenital anomalies, male sex, one of a multiple gestational birth, prematurity, invasive procedures, antibiotic administration, perinatal asphyxia, or other comorbidities (Bodin & Hoffman, 2020). Signs of clinical infection must be considered. For the neonate, especially a premature one, infection may present as very diffuse, general symptoms—apnea, bradycardia, poor feeding, irritability, temperature instability, decreased peripheral perfusion, vomiting, diarrhea, abdominal distention, hypotonia, or even seizures. Unfortunately, many of these signs also are associated with prematurity. Lab values may show a decreased or increased WBC count and/or decreased platelet count; in addition, cerebrospinal fluid (CSF) may demonstrate the presence of protein or glucose in higher than expected amounts (Bodin & Hoffman, 2020). If infection is suspected, it is important to determine if this is early-onset sepsis (EOS), which occurs within the first 72 hours of life up to and through the first 6 days of life, or late-onset sepsis (LOS), after the first week of life (Bodin & Hoffman, 2020). A CBC with differential along with a C-reactive protein (CRP) may help in the diagnosis. If the neonate exhibits central nervous system (CNS) signs, then a lumbar puncture for CSF is warranted.

GENERALIZED NURSING CARE

Hematologic System

■ Assess for clinical signs of hematologic problems such as bruising, bleeding, pallor, plethora, jaundice.

■ Review the maternal history for risk factors.

■ Follow the diagnostic labs.

■ Support respiratory and circulatory functions.

■ Administer blood products as appropriate.

■ Use phototherapy as needed.

Immune System

■ Assess for clinical signs of infection.

■ Review the maternal history for risk factors, including during the delivery.

■ Follow the diagnostic labs.

■ Support respiratory and circulatory functions.

■ Administer antibiotics judiciously—these are selected based on the type of infection.

■ Protect from infection or further infection—good handwashing, gloves, and gowns as appropriate; minimize invasive procedures as possible and screen health professionals and family members for signs of infection.

BLOOD GROUP INCOMPATIBILITIES

Blood group incompatibilities were first recognized in the 1940s with the discovery of the Rh grouping and the first test for detection of antibody-coated RBCs, which was devised by Coombs in 1946. Before the introduction of Rh immune globulin in 1964 and its release for general use in 1968, Rh incompatibility accounted for one-third of all blood group incompatibilities. With the use of RhIgG, the frequency or Rh incompatibility dropped significantly. ABO has become the main blood group incompatibility, with sensitization occurring in 3% of all infants. Both of these conditions are related to maternal antibodies released in response to fetal antigens and passed to the fetus. The Rh antibody is only released upon an exposure to the antigen (Bagwell & Steward, 2020).

ABO INCOMPATIBILITY

Antigens or agglutinogens present on the RBC surface of each blood type (A, B, O, and AB) react with antibodies or agglutinins found in the plasma of opposing blood types. If the antibodies conflict, then RBCs can be destroyed or they can clump together due to an antibody binding to more than one RBC. This clump or agglutination can cause vessel blockage and impair circulation and tissue oxygenation (Bagwell & Steward, 2020). Hemolysis can also occur if there are high antibody titers (hemolysins) that stimulate release of proteolytic enzymes that cause the cell's membrane to rupture (Bagwell & Steward, 2020).

In a transfusion reaction, when opposing blood types are mixed, the donor's RBCs are agglutinated, whereas the recipient's blood cells tend to be protected. The plasma portion of the donor blood that contains antibodies becomes diluted by the recipient's blood volume, thus reducing donor antibody titers in the recipient's circulation. However, recipient antibody titers are adequate to destroy the donor RBCs by agglutination and hemolysis or by hemolysis alone. This is the situation in ABO incompatibility. In such cases, the maternal blood type usually is O, containing anti-A and anti-B antibodies in the serum, whereas the fetus or newborn is type A or B. Although incompatibility can occur between A and B types, it is not as frequent as AO or BO because of the globulin composition of the antibodies. When transplacental hemorrhage (TPH) occurs between an ABO-incompatible mother and fetus, fetal blood entering the maternal circulation undergoes agglutination and hemolysis by maternal antibodies (Bagwell & Steward, 2020).

Incidence

■ Between 40% and 50% of the occurrences are in a first pregnancy; however, only about 3% to 20% of the infants ever show symptoms.

■ A 1.5% to 2% risk is present with each pregnancy.

Assessment

Jaundice is the primary manifestation seen in the first 24 hours of life.

Peripheral blood smear may show spherocytes or RBCs that appear to lack the normal central pallor and biconcave disk-like shape that is expected.

■ Hepatosplenomegaly

■ Labs

■ Positive direct Coombs

■ Positive indirect Coombs

Treatment

In the fetus:

■ Amniocentesis and monitoring of amniotic fluid bilirubin levels

■ Intrauterine transfusions

■ Early delivery

In the newborn:

■ Phototherapy

■ Exchange transfusions (Bagwell & Steward, 2020)

Rh INCOMPATIBILITY

Incidence

■ There is a 16% chance with each pregnancy of Rh incompatibility problems when there is an Rh difference between the mother and fetus/newborn.

■ The maternal Rh antibody is slow to develop and initially may consist exclusively of IgM, which cannot cross the placenta due to its size. This is followed by the production of IgG, which can cross the placenta and enter fetal circulation. The maximum concentration of the IgG form of antibody occurs within 2 to 4 months after termination of the first pregnancy that sensitizes the mother's system. This sensitization can also occur from a small fetal bleed, often undetectable, or from an aminocentesis, or an abortion, ectopic pregnancy, or during labor. Whatever the cause, there is a release of fetal RBCs that triggers the mother's immune response, producing antibodies against the fetal blood that are not compatible (Hall, 2020). If the initial immunization occurs shortly before or at the time of delivery, the first Rh-positive infant born to such a mother may trigger the initial antibody response, with no effect on that infant. However, each subsequent pregnancy will carry a risk for the fetus/infant.

ERYTHROBLASTOSIS FETALIS

Erythroblastosis fetalis is caused by hemolysis in the fetus due to Rh incompatibility.

Assessment

The assessment is based on the expected clinical signs of incompatibility related to immature RBCs and hemolysis.

■ Clinical manifestations

- Anemia
- Hyperbilirubinemia
- Jaundice
- Hepatosplenomegaly
- Hydrops (hydrops fetalis is a severe, total body edema often accompanied by ascites and pleural effusions. This only occurs in 25% of the affected infants.)
- Altered hepatic synthesis, which can impair vitamin K and vitamin K–dependent clotting factors, leads to hemorrhage
- Petechiae or prolonged bleeding from the cord or blood sampling sites
- Hypoglycemia related to hyperplasia of the pancreatic islet cells (Bagwell & Steward, 2020)

Treatment

Antenatally

■ Screening for incompatibilities

■ Coombs' testing

■ Blood typing

■ Unsensitized Rh-negative mothers should receive RhIgG (use Kleihauer–Betke test for fetal cells to determine if this treatment should be used)

Postnatally

Assessment of cardiorespiratory status is important as ascites, pleural effusions, and circulatory collapse can occur, often requiring airway stabilization and mechanical ventilation.

Paracentesis or thoracentesis is recommended if there is peritoneal or pleural fluid that is compromising the infant.

Delivery of an infant shortly after intraperitoneal transfusion may not allow adequate time for absorption of blood from the peritoneal cavity. Lung expansion can be compromised and result in respiratory failure. Mechanical ventilation may be necessary. Blood may need to be removed via paracentesis.

Collaborative Management

■ Assess for adequacy of circulating blood volume.

■ If hydrops is present, anemia is treated with transfusion of packed RBCs. O-negative or type-specific Rh-negative blood cross-matched against the maternal blood should be used.

■ Single-volume or partial exchange may be needed.

■ Congestive heart failure (CHF) may occur during transfusion.

■ Damage to the liver can result in coagulation problems and hyperbilirubinemia.

■ Liver function tests need to be followed along with hematocrit and coagulation studies.

■ Position to reduce abdominal pressure to allow lung expansion.

■ Watch vital signs closely for cardiorespiratory changes.

■ Maintain PaO_2 without overexpansion of the lungs; lungs may be hypoplastic.

■ Administer intravenous immunoglobulin (IVIG) if there is a rapid rising bilirubin level.

■ Perform phototherapy as needed.

■ If bilirubin levels do not require immediate exchange, check levels every 4 to 8 hours, depending on the initial cord blood levels and subsequent rate of rise (Bagwell & Steward, 2020). In Rh incompatibility, exchange is imminent if the rate of rise exceeds 1 mg per hour for the first 6 hours of life. The interval of blood sampling may be increased to 6 to 12 hours after the infant is 48 hours old (Bagwell & Steward, 2020).

REFERENCES

Bagwell, G. A., & Steward, D. K. (2020). Hematologic system. In C. Kenner, L. B. Altimier, & M. V. Boykova (Eds.), *Comprehensive neonatal nursing care* (6th ed., pp. 315–354). Springer Publishing Company.

Bodin, M. B., & Hoffman, J. (2020). Immune system. In C. Kenner, L. B. Altimier, & M. V. Boykova (Eds.), *Comprehensive neonatal nursing care* (6th ed., pp. 257–280). Springer Publishing Company.

Hall, J. E. (2020). *Guyton and Hall textbook of medical physiology* (14th ed.). Elseiver.

BILIRUBIN

Overview

Neonatal hyperbilirubinemia is manifested by jaundice, the yellow-orange tint found in the sclera and skin of infants with a total serum bilirubin (TSB) level greater than 5 mg/dL (86 mcmol/L). It is estimated that 60% of term infants and 80% of preterm newborns will appear clinically jaundiced during the first weeks of life. Although this condition is generally a benign, transitional phenomenon, unconjugated bilirubin levels that can pose a direct threat of serious brain injury develop in a small proportion of neonates.

Bilirubin Metabolism

Bilirubin is the final by-product from the breakdown of RBCs. This "unbound" bilirubin will rapidly bind to the carrier protein albumin for transport to the liver, where it is conjugated. The binding of unconjugated bilirubin can be influenced by decreases in albumin, changes in binding capacity, or competition for binding sites by certain drugs (e.g., sulfisoxazole, salicylates, and sodium benzoate) or free fatty acids. A harmful effect can occur when there is insufficient binding that results in increased amounts of unbound or "free" bilirubin. Unconjugated bilirubin can be troublesome because it is not water soluble, it is difficult to excrete, and it can cross the intact blood–brain barrier causing acute bilirubin encephalopathy (ABE). Conjugated bilirubin is water soluble and is excreted via the biliary system to the small intestine and excreted into the stool.

Conjugated bilirubin is an unstable substance in the newborn's intestines. In the presence of an enzyme in the intestine called beta-glucuronidase, which is 10 times the adult concentration, conjugated bilirubin can be hydrolyzed back into unconjugated bilirubin. This unconjugated bilirubin re-enters the bloodstream via enterohepatic circulation. Delayed stooling, decreased intestinal motility, and starvation potentially increase exposure of conjugated bilirubin to beta-glucuronidase, necessitating repetition of the entire conjugation process.

Risk Factors for Hyperbilirubinemia

Risk factors that place an infant at increased risk of hyperbilirubinemia are as follows:

- Exclusively breastfed
- Infant-known hemolytic disease (e.g., glucose-6-phosphate dehydrogenase [G6PD] deficiency)
- Gestational age 35 to 37 weeks 6 days out of 7
- Infant of diabetic mother
- Previous sibling received phototherapy
- Weight loss greater than 10% of birth weight

■ Cephalohematoma or significant bruising at birth

■ Discharge less than 24 hours of age

■ Jaundice observed before discharge

■ ABO incompatibility with positive Coombs or direct antiglobulin test (DAT)

Two tools that can be used to identify the risk toward the development of hyperbilirubinemia in newborns over 35 weeks' gestational age are the Bhutani nomogram and the BiliTool™. The latter tool can be embedded into an electronic medical record (EMR).

Clinical Patterns of Neonatal Hyperbilirubinemia

"Physiologic jaundice" is a term to describe transient, mild unconjugated hyperbilirubinemia that occurs between 24 and 72 hours of life. The patient's TSB usually rises to a peak level of 12 to 15 mg/dL (204–257 mcmol/L) by day 3 and then falls. In preterm infants, the TSB peak level occurs on days 3 to 7 of age and can rise over 15 mg/dL. It can last up to 1 to 2 weeks in both term and preterm newborns.

Pathologic Jaundice

Elevated bilirubin levels within the first 24 hours of life and exceeding 15 mg/dL should be considered pathologic and deserve investigation. These pathologic conditions can be classified as follows:

1. Increase in RBC breakdown (e.g., Rh, ABO incompatibility, G6PD, sepsis, drug reactions, extravascular blood, and polycythemia)

2. A decrease in bilirubin clearance (e.g., bowel obstructions, hypoxia or asphyxia, inborn error of metabolism such as congenital hypothyroidism, and galactosemia)

3. Those that interfere with bilirubin conjugation (e.g., breast milk jaundice, drug interactions, hypothyroidism, acidosis, and hypoxia)

Premature infants develop more significant jaundice due to two factors: decreased oral intake and immaturity of the liver's conjugating system.

Jaundice and the Breastfed Neonate

Inadequate breastfeeding contributes to an increased incidence of newborn jaundice because of a decreased amount of breast milk along with a weight loss (>6% by the 3rd postnatal day) and a slow intestinal peristalsis, as well as an increase in the enterohepatic circulation of bilirubin. This type of early-onset jaundice is termed "breast milk jaundice" since it is not breastfeeding itself that determines jaundice but breastfeeding inadequacy. Successful breastfeeding will decrease the risk of hyperbilirubinemia. Newborns need to be fed at least 8 to 12 times in the first days after birth to improve the mother's milk supply. Monitoring urine output, stool output, and weight are the best ways to judge successful breastfeeding. Newborns should have four to six wet diapers and three to four yellow seedy stools per day by the fourth day after birth. Formula supplementation or intravenous (IV) fluids may be necessary if the newborn has significant weight loss, poor urine output, poor caloric intake, and lethargy.

Late-onset breast milk jaundice will typically appear between days 4 and 7 of life, reaching a peak around 2 to 3 weeks, and can take up to 3 months to resolve completely. The newborn will have a regular weight gain and a normal production of urine and stool. Although the exact mechanism is not completely clear, it is believed that certain substances present in breast milk cause a reduced intestinal motility and increased reabsorption of bilirubin. It is no longer recommended to stop breastfeeding for a brief time to identify breast milk jaundice. Even if breast-feeding withdrawal is short, it places the newborn at risk to return to exclusive breastfeeding and becomes a source of worry for the mother such as to discourage breastfeeding.

Bilirubin Encephalopathy

When the blood–brain barrier is intact, the rate of bilirubin uptake by the brain is determined by the following:

■ Concentration of unbound bilirubin

■ Vulnerability of the brain

■ Duration of exposure

■ Ability of bilirubin to bind to albumin

■ Local cerebral blood perfusion

The exact level of when unconjugated serum bilirubin becomes neurotoxic is unclear, but the effects can lead to ABE. The classic signs of ABE are increased hypertonia, varying degrees of drowsiness, poor feeding, hypotonia, alternating tone, and high-pitched cry. Prompt and effective interventions when ABE symptoms appear can usually prevent the chronic kernicteric sequelae. The classic clinical features of kernicterus are athetoid cerebral palsy, impairment of upward gaze, hearing loss, and enamel dysplasia of the teeth. Approximately one-third of infants with kernicterus develop intellectual impairment.

Nursing Assessment and Actions

Reviewing the neonate's family and birth history can indicate which neonates may have an increased risk for severe hyperbilirubinemia.

Visual assessment can be a noninvasive and easy way to identify jaundice. Jaundice is assessed by placing the neonate in a well-lit area, preferably in natural daylight. Apply gentle pressure to the skin, blanching it to reveal the underlying color of the skin and subcutaneous tissue. Mucous membranes should also be assessed. Jaundice progresses in a cephalocaudal direction from the face to the trunk and then to the lower extremities. The assessments should be made at least every 8 to 12 hours, preferably each time vital signs are measured. When jaundice is present in the first 24 hours or if jaundice seems excessive for the newborn's age in hours, a TSB or transcutaneous bilirubin (TcB) should be measured. It is difficult to accurately predict the TSB concentration based on caudal progression alone due to interobserver variability.

TSB is a diagnostic blood test that most accurately measures bilirubin levels. All bilirubin levels are to be interpreted according to the infant's age in hours.

TcB measurements are a noninvasive method of assessing bilirubin levels and may be used as a screening tool when the bilirubin level is less than 15 mg/dL (257 mcmol/L).

Treatment

In addition to nutritional support to ensure adequate hydration, milk intake, and gastrointestinal motility, common treatment strategies for severe hyperbilirubinemia include phototherapy, exchange transfusion, and drug therapy.

Phototherapy remains the mainstay of treating hyperbilirubinemia. It acts by converting insoluble unconjugated bilirubin into soluble isomers that can be excreted in urine and stool. It is typically used either prophylactically in preterm newborns or those with a known hemolytic process to prevent a significant rapid rise or therapeutically to reduce excessive bilirubin levels. It is important to be familiar with institutional policies, procedures, and manufacturer recommendations regarding care and use because of the wide range of phototherapy lighting equipment available. Nursing care of the infant receiving phototherapy should include the following:

■ Check the irradiance of the bulbs prior to use and then daily.

■ Place light sources as close to the infant as possible, with the exception of halogen-lamp phototherapy units.

■ Avoid assessing an infant's well-being solely by skin color because of the "blue hue" effect of the phototherapy lights.

■ Use opaque eye shields at all times; inspect the eyes for drainage, edema, and abrasions when the lights are turned off and eye shields are removed for infant feedings and parent visits.

■ Assess the infant's skin integrity with every diaper change to prevent breakdown due to loose stools, urinary excretion of bilirubin, and exposure to the phototherapy lights. In most cases, it is not necessary to remove the diaper or boundary materials while providing phototherapy unless the bilirubin levels are approaching the exchange transfusion range.

■ Monitor the infant's temperature every 4 hours for hypothermia and hyperthermia.

■ Maintain adequate hydration.

■ Promote parent–infant interactions. Phototherapy can be interrupted at feeding times to allow for breastfeeding, parental visits, and skin-to-skin care unless the bilirubin level is approaching the exchange level.

■ Monitor bilirubin levels every 6 to 24 hours depending on the rate of rise. Phototherapy lights must be turned off while drawing the blood samples for serum bilirubin testing.

Exchange transfusion is considered if the bilirubin levels start to approach those associated with kernicterus despite intensive phototherapy or signs of ABE (even if TSB is falling). A double-volume exchange transfusion (170 mL/kg) removes 85% to 90% of circulating RBC; however, because most of the infant's total bilirubin is in the extravascular compartment, only 25% of the total bilirubin is removed. This procedure may need to be repeated more than once before stabilization of the bilirubin level occurs. Significant morbidities include apnea, anemia, thrombocytopenia, electrolyte and calcium imbalance, necrotizing enterocolitis, hemorrhage, infection, and catheter-related complications.

Pharmacologic Agents

For infants with severe hyperbilirubinemia due to blood group incompatibilities, administration of IVIG (0.5–1 g/kg over 2 hours) is used if the TSB is rising despite intensive phototherapy or if the TSB is within 2 to 3 mg/mL of the exchange level. There is no proven evidence regarding the benefits of other drugs such as phenobarbital, steroids, or tin-mesoporphyrin to prevent or treat hyperbilirubinemia.

Sunlight is not a recommended source of light for phototherapy. The effect of heat and water loss/dehydration, the risk to skin and eyes, and the effect of exposure to unnecessary ultraviolet light from direct sunlight are potential side effects and complications of sunbathing.

NEONATAL INFECTION

The neonate, although born with an immature immune system, is still capable of responding to foreign antigens from the environment. This immaturity, however, does make the neonate—term and especially preterm—vulnerable to infections. These infections can be acquired in utero, intrapartally, or postnatally. The latter can be due to invasive procedures and exposure to pathogens in the neonatal intensive care units, resulting in nosocomial or hospital-acquired infections. Globally, infections in the form of pneumonia, sepsis, tetanus, meningitis, and diarrhea are the major causes of neonatal death. Most of these deaths are preventable (Healthy Newborn Network, 2021; Liu et al., 2014). Therefore, awareness of risk factors, early identification, and appropriate timely treatment are essential if infectious diseases are to be prevented or at least minimized.

Incidence

■ On a global scale, incidence varies widely according to the region of the world (Bodin & Hoffman, 2020; Liu et al., 2014). However, global data suggest that 26% of the neonatal deaths are due to severe infections (6% pneumonia; 17%

sepsis, meningitis, tetanus; and 1% diarrhea; Adatara et al., 2019; Healthy Newborn Network, 2021).

■ In the United States, the incidence in term newborns is two to four per 1,000 live births.

■ Incidence occurs more frequently in male and low-birthweight infants.

■ Maternal group B strep colonization, PROM, chorioamnionitis, and preterm delivery increase the risk of infection.

Physiology

During pregnancy, the infant is protected from many sources of infection by the uterus and the fetal membranes. The fetal immune system is immature and easily overwhelmed even when delivery occurs at term. Preterm infants are at an even greater risk of infection due to immaturity, the interruption in the passage of maternal antibodies, and the need for instrumentation. Rupture of membranes, exposure to the vaginal canal, and the external environment introduce a variety of microorganisms and put the newborn at risk for infection.

Pathophysiology

Neonatal infections can be categorized in several ways. These categories may help guide evaluation and management of infection in the newborn. Sepsis can be classified as early onset or late onset. Early-onset infections are generally recognized as those occurring in the first 7 days of life. Late-onset infections occur from day 7 to day 30. Late-onset infections can be further categorized as nosocomial or hospital acquired if the infection is related to care in a hospital. Infections can also be categorized by the site of the infection, such as pneumonia, bacteremia, or meningitis. The patterns of infection seen and outcomes are different for each of these categories.

The most frequent causes of early-onset neonatal infection are bacteria, including group B strep, *Escherichia coli* (*E. coli*), and *Listeria*, but neonates can also develop infections due to viruses, such as herpes.

Late-onset infections can be caused not only by these organisms but also by staph species and a broad spectrum of gram negatives. Hospital-acquired infections may also be caused by *Pseudomonas*, *Klebsiella*, *Serratia*, *E. coli*, and unit-specific species.

Assessment

The nurse must maintain a high index of suspicion for any newborn with an abnormal examination or behaviors. The neonate's immature immune system frequently can only provide nonspecific symptoms of infection.

Nursing assessment should include a complete maternal and neonatal history, a complete physical examination, glucose screening, and vital signs at frequent intervals. Any infant with even subtle signs of possible infection should be medically evaluated and receive increased nursing surveillance. Complications of infection may include signs of shock, problems with coagulation, and abnormalities in neurologic status. Nursing surveillance should include ongoing assessment for hypotension, bleeding, glucose, and changes in the patient's neurologic exams, including seizures.

Clinical Signs and Symptoms of Infection. Please see Box 6.1.

BOX 6.1 Signs and Symptoms of Neonatal Infection

Clinical

- General
- Poor feeding
- Irritability
- Lethargy
- Temperature instability

Skin

- Petechiae
- Pustulosis
- Sclerema
- Edema
- Jaundice

Respiratory

- Grunting
- Nasal flaring
- Intercostal retractions
- Tachypnea/apnea

Gastrointestinal

- Diarrhea
- Hematochezia
- Abdominal distention
- Emesis
- Aspirates

Central Nervous System

- Hypotonia
- Seizures
- Poor spontaneous movement

Circulatory

- Bradycardia/tachycardia
- Hypotension

(continued)

Box 6.1.   Signs and Symptoms of Neonatal Infection (*continued*)

■ Cyanosis

■ Decreased perfusion

Laboratory Values:

White Blood Cell Count

■ Neutrophils
  - <5,000 cells/mm^3, neutropenia
  - >25,000 cells/mm^3, neutrophilia
■ Absolute neutrophil count (neutrophil and bands)
  - <1,800 cells/mm^3 (during 1st week)
■ Immature: total neutrophil ratio
  - 0:2
■ Platelet count
  - <100,000, thrombocytopenia

Cerebrospinal Fluid

■ Protein
  - 150–200 mg/L (term)
  - 300 mg/L (preterm)
■ Glucose
  - 50%–60% or more of blood glucose level

Source: Adapted with permission from Lott, J. W., & Kilb, J. R. (1992). The selection of antibacterial agents for treatment of neonatal infection. *Neonatal Pharmacy Quarterly, 1*(1), 19–29.

Clinical Manifestations and Diagnosis

Evaluation may include:

■ Blood cultures

■ CBC, with platelet count and differential

■ Lumbar puncture with culture and chemistries performed on CSF if infant believed to be at risk for meningitis

■ Urine cultures (for late-onset infections)

■ Screening for acidosis

■ In the hospitalized patient, screening of any indwelling tubes should be considered if the infant is older than 7 days.

■ More specific testing may be required if the infant is suspected of an atypical infection or viral infection.

■ Other screens for inflammation: CRP, many other screening labs (IL-6, procalcitonin, neutrophil CD 64, RNA markers, etc.) are being developed and tested to identify the body's response to infection and monitor response to antimicrobial treatment. Availability of these screens is variable and site dependent.

An evaluation for coagulopathy should be performed if the infant has multisystem involvement or signs of bleeding (peripheral blood smear, prothrombin time, activated partial thromboplastin time, fibrinogen, fibrinogen split products, or d-dimer), a full sepsis workup including chest x-rays, urinalysis, urine culture, or CSF culture (Painter et al., 2020). Other tests to reveal leucocyte adhesion disorders may be needed (Painter et al., 2020).

Some screening can be performed on the placenta when possible; when infection is suspected, the placenta should be sent for pathologic evaluation.

Culture-negative sepsis may be diagnosed in the infant whose mother received antibiotics prior to delivery. Even if all cultures are negative, the infant may appear to have clinical signs and symptoms of infection and respond to the use of antimicrobials.

Treatment

Treatment of infection includes the support of airway, breathing, and circulation as needed; evaluation for complications; and the administration of appropriate antimicrobials. Newborn antimicrobials ideally should be provided by the IV route. If IV antibiotics are not possible in a low-resourced setting, oral antibiotics can be used, but this route is not ideal. The newborn should also be screened for the complications of infection, including shock and bleeding abnormalities.

Initial treatment of early-onset infection: Broad-spectrum antibiotics should be started before confirmatory testing is complete. The choice of antibiotics should be based on the most frequent pathogens seen in infants born in the specific region. For most infants, a combination of ampicillin and gentamicin is preferred. These antibiotics provide coverage for frequently seen bacterial pathogens and are synergistic against meningitis. A third-generation cephalosporin may be considered rather than gentamicin. Acyclovir should be added if herpes is suspected.

Initial treatment of late-onset infection: Broad-spectrum antibiotics should be started before confirmatory testing is complete. The choice of antimicrobials should be based on the infant's status, exam, and other medical care. Coverage for staph species should be considered. If the infant has been hospitalized, is older than 7 days, and has been receiving support, the possibility of nosocomial infection should be considered and coverage should be modified to cover suspected sources of infection.

Independent of the timing of infection, when a causative agent is identified the antimicrobials used should be narrowed to be specific to that pathogen.

Treatment should include ongoing surveillance for improvement in clinical status, any abnormal labs, abnormal vital signs, and signs of bleeding.

Nursing-specific care and treatment includes:

- Monitoring and support of airway, breathing, and circulation
- Infant comfort and pain control during procedures
- Administration of antimicrobials and screening for complications of infection
- Family support (Family support during this time cannot be overemphasized. Not only do families have the stress of a sick newborn but also perhaps the guilt of an infection that was potentially transmitted by the mother.)
- Breastfeeding support

Prognosis

Prognosis depends on the pathogen that infected the neonate and the presence of meningitis. Term infants with rapid recognition and treatment of infection seldom have long-term consequences. The incidence of neurologic sequelae may be as high as 15% to 30% if the infant has meningitis. The incidence of long-term sequelae is higher in the preterm infant, especially if shock was present (Bodin & Hoffman, 2020).

Prevention

Infection prevention is an integral part of nursing care. Good hand hygiene and aseptic technique has been shown to prevent many infections.

OMPHALITIS

Omphalitis is an infection of the umbilical stump. It usually presents as a cellulitis around the cord but may progress to necrotizing fasciitis and systemic disease. Omphalitis is rare in industrialized countries but remains a significant cause of neonatal death in areas with unhygienic delivery practices (Bugaje et al., 2020). In low-resourced countries, chlorhexidine is still used for cleansing (Mullany et al., 2017). The majority of omphalitis cases are polymicrobial (Gallagher, 2014), and this should be considered when antibiotics are being chosen. Suggested antibiotics are an antistaphylococcal penicillin or vancomycin and gentamicin. Many cases of omphalitis are culture positive for anaerobes; metronidazole or clindamycin can provide anaerobic coverage (Gallagher, 2014). Topical antimicrobials are also sometimes used, but their use is not well studied (Gallagher, 2014).

Local customs and care of the umbilical stump have been implicated in the incidence of omphalitis. Using clean equipment to cut the cord and assessment of local practices around care of the cord are of utmost importance. Dry cord care versus antiseptic treatment differs little in the risk of infections according to findings by Guen and colleagues (2017).

FUNGAL INFECTIONS

The neonate is at risk for infections from fungal pathogens as well. *Candida* species are frequently found in humans and are the most frequently occurring. Topical infections with *Candida* species such as thrush and monilial diaper rashes are not unusual in the newborn period and are easily treated with oral and topical medications. Invasive fungal disease is unusual, except in the premature infant with a history of invasive procedures, indwelling lines, parenteral nutrition, and multiple courses of broad-spectrum antibiotics. Prolonged antibiotic use may lead to fungal overgrowth in the gastrointestinal system and put the infant at risk for systemic disease. Fungal sepsis should be considered in any small, septic-appearing infant who is not responding to standard antimicrobial therapy. If an infant develops cultures positive for fungus, the infant will be screened to determine the extent of the disease and ultrasound may be used to look for vegetations in the eye, kidney, and heart. These infants can develop infections of the central nervous system with significant sequelae and even death.

Some neonatal units provide fungal prophylaxis with oral nystatin or IV fluconazole. The lowest dose (3 mg/kg) is generally suggested to reduce the chances of toxicity (Leonart et al., 2017).

Treatment of active systemic fungal infections generally uses the antifungal agent amphotericin B. Some other newer agents are available, but evidence to support its use in neonates is still limited. All of these drugs have significant potential nephrotoxic and bone marrow effects. Neonates need to be monitored carefully during the administration of antifungal agents.

CONGENITAL INFECTIONS

The microorganisms responsible for congenital infections have been traditionally grouped together as the TORCH infections; however, as the number of infections has grown, Maldonado et al. (2016) have recommended that the acronym be expanded to TORCHES CLAP.

TO: *TOxoplasma gondii*

R: Rubella

C: Cytomegalovirus (CMV)

H: HSV

E: Enteroviruses

S: Syphilis (*Treponema pallidum*)

C: Chicken pox (varicella-zoster virus)

L: Lyme disease (*Borrelia burgdoferi*)

A: AIDS/HIV

P: Parvovirus B9

The most effective treatment for most congenital infections is prevention. Good maternal prenatal care and immunizations can limit their prevalence. Outcomes can be highly variable and are dependent on the timing and severity of illness. A cursory review of a select group of these pathogens, their presentation, and their treatment can be found in Table 6.1. HIV will be addressed separately.

TABLE 6.1 Short Review of Selected Congenital Infections

CONDITION	TRANSMISSION	SYMPTOMS	TREATMENT/NURSING CONSIDERATIONS	OUTCOMES
Toxoplasmosis	Protozoa transmission to mother per uncooked meat or animal feces.	May be asymptomatic or mild symptoms in mother. Infant presentation is highly variable: from normal appearing at birth to hydrocephalus, retinitis, intracranial calcifications, and hydrops. New lesions may develop for years.	Prevention and early recognition are best treatments. Treatment: pyrimethamine + sulfonamides daily for 2–6 months, then 3 times weekly for 1 year Leucovorin may be given concurrently or after this therapy. Nursing care: supportive.	Dependent on the extent of disease and treatment. Deafness, microcephaly, and low IQ.
Rubella	Virus German measles infection during pregnancy.	Infection prior to 20 weeks' gestation may cause neonatal birth defects: auditory, ophthalmic (cataracts), cardiac, neurologic, and growth restriction Treatment of active infection after birth is rare. New symptoms may appear for years.	Prevention and immunization prior to pregnancy are the most effective treatments. Nursing care: supportive	Dependent on the severity of birth defects Persistent shedding of virus may occur for the 1st year of life; pregnant women should avoid contact.

TABLE 6.1 Short Review of Selected Congenital Infections (continued)

CONDITION	TRANSMISSION	SYMPTOMS	TREATMENT/NURSING CONSIDERATIONS	OUTCOMES
CMV	DNA virus	By adulthood, most people have been exposed to CMV and developed antibodies.	Evaluation: urine culture, IgG, and IgM titers.	Highly variable Generally, outcomes are worse if the primary infection occurred during pregnancy.
	Methods of transmission: transplacental, contact with blood and body fluids, including breast milk	Symptoms in the mother are usually fatigue, fever, and liver complications. Neonatal symptoms: IUGR, microcephaly, deafness, blindness, cataracts, profound intellectual deficits, hepatosplenomegaly, and jaundice. Classic pattern of petechiae "blueberry muffin syndrome."	Treatment: supportive, immunoglobulin therapy, vaccines, and chemotherapy are all under development. Valacyclovir, ganciclovir, and valganciclovir have been used in the treatment of neonates (Hamilton et al., 2014). Chemotherapy may be toxic, and there is limited data to demonstrate improvement in long-term outcomes. Nursing care: preventive and supportive	26% of severely infected infants die, 90% of symptomatic infected infants will have sequelae.

Herpes	DNA virus may be dormant for extended periods Transmission: ascending infection from vaginal vault or transmission from infected fluids during delivery.	Wide range of symptoms from asymptomatic to severe disseminated disease that presents with CNS problems, multisystem organ failure, and frequent death. Three categories: 1. Localized infections of skin, eyes, and mouth 2. Patients with encephalitis (may not have vesicles) 3. Disseminated disease (may not have vesicles)	Prevention is the best treatment strategy. Active HSV outbreak is a contraindication for vaginal delivery. It is not recommended that women with HSV have internal monitoring used. Acyclovir is the recommended mode of therapy; it is an inhibitor of viral replication. The recommended dosage is 30 mg/kg/day divided every 8 hours.	Outcome is dependent on category of disease and rapid detection and treatment. Infants who present with encephalitis have a rate of neurologic sequelae of approximately 50%.
	Rate of transmission is much higher during primary infections than during recurrent outbreaks. Transmission has also been documented from lesions on the breast or oral lesions.	Multiple laboratory tests can now identify HSV.	Nursing care: supportive and prevention education.	Infants who present with disseminated disease present with multisystem organ failure. The CNS is involved in 70%–90% of these infants.

(continued)

TABLE 6.1 Short Review of Selected Congenital Infections (*continued*)

CONDITION	TRANSMISSION	SYMPTOMS	TREATMENT/NURSING CONSIDERATIONS	OUTCOMES
Syphilis	Spirochete; vertical transmission may occur at any time during pregnancy.	Maternal history, snuffles, hepatosplenomegaly, jaundice, low birthweight, osteochondritis, and peeling of the palms of the hands and the soles of the feet.	Prevention of incomplete maternal treatment Evaluation: includes maternal and infant serologic screening, CSF analysis, and bone x-rays. Treatment is with aqueous penicillin G for 10–14 days.	Infection can be treated, but outcome is dependent on organ damage during development.

CMV, cytomegalovirus; CNS, central nervous system; CSF, cerebrospinal fluid; IUGR, intrauterine growth restricted.

Source: Unless otherwise noted, data was extracted from Bodin, M. B., & Hoffman, J. (2020). Immune system. In C. Kenner. L. B. Altimier, & M. V. Boykova (Eds.), *Comprehensive neonatal nursing care* (6th ed., pp. 257–280). Springer Publishing Company.

HUMAN IMMUNODEFICIENCY VIRUS

The incidence of HIV and AIDS varies by geography. Almost 100% of the neonatal cases are a result of mother to infant or vertical transmission and most are found in sub-Saharan Africa (Abbas et al., 2021). In the United States, the incidence of neonatal HIV has dropped from 42.8/100,000 live births in 1991 to 1.3/100,00 live births in 2015 (Abbas et al., 2021). There are still health disparities noted, with Black versus White infants' infectivity rate being five times higher (Abbas et al., 2021; Nesheim et al., 2019). If preventative maternal strategies are used such as antiretroviral therapies (ART), the transmission is less than 1% (Abbas et al., 2021; Nesheim et al., 2019).

Many countries have recommendations for screening pregnant women, prophylaxis during pregnancy, and neonatal prophylaxis. In the United States, the National Institutes of Health (NIH) has guidelines that recommend universal screening of pregnant women, prophylaxis during pregnancy, and zidovudine prophylaxis in the newborn. This prophylaxis should start soon after birth. Zidovudine with or without nevirapine is recommended for varying lengths of time depending on the mother's current treatment and disease. Current guidelines can be downloaded from https://clinicalinfo.hiv.gov/en/guidelines. The World Health Organization (WHO) has also developed guidelines for ART prophylaxis. Their recommendations take into consideration the resources available. WHO frequently reviews and revises these guidelines. The current recommendations include the use of zidovudine prophylaxis and other medications for the infant. WHO guidelines can be downloaded from www.who.int/health-topics/hiv-aids#tab=tab_1.

A growing concern in many parts of the world is that due to COVID-19 or coronavirus, many HIV clinics and the ART supplies have been reduced (The Lancet HIV, 2020).

Breastfeeding is contraindicated in HIV women. The only exception to this is if the woman and her infant live in an area with no safe water supply. If the risk of death from formula made with unclean water is higher than the risk of HIV transmission, maternal daily prophylaxis with nevirapine may reduce transmission (McLean & Wallace, 2020).

■ Maternal education should include:
- Importance of compliance with ART regimes
- Breastfeeding not recommended
- Mother not sharing food she has chewed with her infant
- Importance of compliance with infant ART and follow-up

■ Infants receiving ART should be assessed and monitored for anemia and neutropenia.

■ Infants at risk for HIV/AIDS should be monitored for unexplained fever, recurrent infections, yeast infections, diarrhea, hepatosplenomegaly, lymphadenopathy, and failure to thrive.

COVID-19

Coronavirus disease 2019 (COVID-19) is caused by severe acute respiratory syndrome coronavirus 2 (SARS-CoV-2) and is the worst pandemic since the 1918 Spanish Flu. There are many forms of coronaviruses including Middle East respiratory syndrome (MERS), but COVID-19 is a novel form that is mutating throughout various parts of the world. The appearance of this virus resulted in many countries locking down or shuttering business, including hospital units such as maternity services. The added stress of the pandemic has also taken its toll on pregnant women. The result is that in the United States, women are either electing for home births or having to travel a distance to deliver. More concerning is the lack of data to support best practices for neonatal/maternal care if the infant is born small or sick. WHO and the Global Alliance for Newborn Care (GLANCE) have advocated for Zero Separation of mothers and babies while in the NICU. Information on this initiative can be found at www.glance-network.org/news/details/zero-separation-global-campaign.

Pregnant women who have contracted COVID-19 tend to have more mild symptoms than the general population (Smith et al., 2020). These women do tend to have infants born prematurely requiring NICU stays (Smith et al., 2020). The virus has not been detected in breast milk so, in general, women, if well enough, can breastfeed (Mimouni et al., 2020). While there have been a few case reports of vertical transmission, the neonatal data are still inconclusive (Juan et al., 2020). To date, while vaccines are being distributed, clinical trials have not been done on pregnant women or newborns. Some pregnant women have elected to take the vaccine but that has to be an individual choice.

Much needs to be learned about this virus and its impact/transmission to neonates and children. For up-to-date information, please go to the Centers for Disease Control and Prevention (CDC) website: www.cdc.gov/coronavirus/2019-ncov/index.html. At this time the CDC recommends that neonates born to mothers who have tested positive for or are suspected of having COVID-19 should be tested (CDC, 2020). Testing includes SARS-CoV-2 RNA reverse transcription polymerase chain reaction (RT-PCR) or nasal or oral swabs (CDC, 2020).

CONCLUSION

The immature immune system of the neonate puts the infant at greater risk for acquiring almost every type of infection and offers a limited ability to respond to pathogens and localized infections. The signs and symptoms of infection in the neonate are nonspecific. The nurse has a critical role in identifying early, subtle signs of infection; assessing for complications; safely administering antimicrobials; and providing the family information and support.

REFERENCES

Abbas, M., Bakhtyar, A., & Bazzi, R. (2021). *COVID-19 information*. Neonatal HIV. https://www.ncbi.nlm.nih.gov/books/NBK565879/

Adatara, P., Afaya, A., Salia, S. M., Afaya, R. A., Konlan, K. D., Agyabeng-Fandoh, E., Agbinku, E., Ayandayo, E. A., & Boahene, I. G. (2019). Risk factors associated with neonatal sepsis: A case study at a specialist hospital in Ghana. *Scientific World Journal, 2019.* https://doi.org/10.1155/2019/9369051

Bodin, M. B., & Hoffman, J. (2020). Immune system. In C. Kenner, L. B. Altimier, & M. V. Boykova (Eds.), *Comprehensive neonatal nursing care* (6th ed., pp. 257–280). Springer Publishing Company.

Bugaje, M. A., McHoney, M., Ameh, E. A., & Lakhoo, K. (2020). Omphalitis. In E. A. Ameh, S. W. Bickler, K. Lakhoo, B. C. Nwomeh, & D. Poenaru (Eds.), *Pediatric surgery.* Springer Publishing Company. https://doi.org/10.1007/978-3-030-41724-6_20

Centers for Disease Control & Prevention. (2020). *Evaluation and management considerations for neonates at risk for COVID-19.* https://www.cdc.gov/coronavirus/2019-ncov/hcp/caring-for-newborns.html

Gallagher, P. G. (2014). *Omphalitis.* http://emedicine.medscape.com/article/975422-overview

Guen, C. G.-L., Caille, A., Launay, E., Boscher, C., Godon, N., Savagner, C., Descombes, E., Gremmo-Feger, G., Pladys, P., Saillant, D., Legrand, A., Caillon, J., Barbarot, S., Roze, J. C., & Biraudeau, B. (2017). Dry care versus antiseptics for umbilical cord care: A cluster randomized trial. *Pediatrics, 139*(1), 320161857. https://doi.org/10/1542/peds.2016-1857

Hamilton, S. T., van Zuylen, W., Shand, A., Scott, G. M., Naign, Z., Hall, B., Craig, M. E., & Rawlinson, W. D. (2014). Prevention of congenital cytomegalovirus complications by maternal and neonatal treatments: A systematic review. *Reviews in Medical Virology, 24,* 420–433. https://doi.org/10.1002/rmv.1814

Healthy Newborn Network. (2021). *Newborn numbers.* http://www.healthynewbornnetwork.org/page/newborn-numbers

Juan, J., Gil, M. M., Rong, Z., Zhang, Y., Yang, H., & Poon, L. C. (2020). Effect of coronavirus disease 2019 (COVID-19) on maternal, perinatal and neonatal outcome: Systematic Review. *Ultrasound in Obsterics & Gynecology, 56,* 15–27. https://doi.org/10.1002/uog.22088

Leonart, L. P., Tonin, F. S., Ferreira, V. L., Penteado, S. T. D. S., Motta, F. D. A., & Pontarolo, R. (2017). Fluconazole doses used for prophylaxis of invasive fungal infection in neonatal intensive care units: A network meta-analysis. *Journal of Pediatrics, 185,* 129–135. https://doi.org/10.1016/j.jpeds.2017.02.039

Liu, L., Ai, H. W., Wang, W. P., Chen, L., Hu, H. B., Ye, T., Zhu, X. H., Wang, F., Liao, Y. L., Wang, Y., Ou, G., Xu, L., Sun, M., Jian, C., Chen, Z. J., Li, L., Zhang, B., Tian, L., Wang, B., . . . Sun, Z. Y. (2014). Comparison of 16S rRNA gene PCR and blood culture for diagnosis of neonatal sepsis. *Archives de Pédiatrie, 21*(2), 162–169. https://doi.org/10.1016/j.arcped.2013.11.015

Liu, L., Oza, S., Hogan, D., Perin, J., Rudan, I., Lawn, J. E., Cousens, S., Mathers, C., & Black, R. E. (2015). Global, regional, and national causes of child mortality in 2000–13, with projections to inform post-2015 priorities: an updated systematic analysis. *Lancet, 385*(9966):430–440. https://doi.org/10.1016/S0140-6736(14)61698-6

Lott, J. W., & Kilb, J. R. (1992). The selection of antibacterial agents for treatment of neonatal infection. *Neonatal Pharmacy Quarterly, 1*(1), 19–29.

Maldonado, Y. A., Nizet, V., Klein, J. O., Remington, J. S., & Wilson, C. B. (2016). Current concepts of infections of the fetus and newborn infant. In C. B. Wilson, V. Nizet, Y. A. Maldonado, J. S. Remington, & J. O. Klein (Eds.), *Infectious diseases of the fetus and newborn* (8th ed., pp. 3–23). Elsevier.

McLean, K. R., & Wallace, T. (2020). Emerging infections. In C. Kenner, L. B. Altimier, & M. V. Boykova (Eds.), *Comprehensive neonatal nursing care* (6th ed., pp. 587–610). Springer Publishing Company.

Mimouni, F., Lakshminrusimha, S., Pearlman, S. A., Raju, T., Gallagher, P. G., & Mendlovic, J. (2020). Perinatal aspects on the COVID-19 pandemic: A practical resource for perinatal-neonatal specialists. *Journal of Perinatology, 40,* 820–826. https://doi.org/10.1038/s41372-020-0665-6

Mullany, L. C., Arifeen, S. E., Khatry, S. K., Katz, J., Shah, R., Baqui, A. H., & Tielsch, J. M. (2017). Impact of chlorhexidine cord cleansing on mortality, omphalistis, and cord separation time among facility-born babies in Nepal and Bangladesh. *Pediatric Infectious Disease Journal, 36*(1), 1011–1013. https://doi.org/10.1097/INF.0000000000001617

Nesheim, S. R., FitzHarris, L. F., Mahle Gray, K., & Lampe, M. A. (2019). Epidemiology of perinatal HIV transmission in the United States in the era of its elimination. *Pediatric Infectious Disease Journal, 38*(6), 611–616. https://doi.org/10.1097/INF.0000000000002290

Painter, K., Anand, S., & Phillip, K. (2020). Omphalitis. *StatPearls.* https://www.ncbi.nlm.nih.gov/books/NBK513338

Smith, V., Seo, D., Warty, R., Payne, O., Salih, M., Chin, K. L., Ofor-Asenso, R., Krishnan, S., Costa, F. D. S., Vollenhoven, B., & Wallace, E. (2020). Maternal and neonatal outcomes associated with COVID-19 infection: A systematic review. *PLoS One, 15,* e0234187. https://doi.org/10.1371/journal.pone.0234187

The Lancet HIV. (2020). Lockdown fears for key populations. *The Lancet HIV, 7*(6), e373. https://doi.org/10.1016/S2352-3018(20)30143-0

Special Care Considerations in Neonatal Nursing

11

7

Nutrition

BREASTFEEDING

MONA LIZA HAMLIN

OVERVIEW

IMPORTANCE OF BREAST MILK

Breast milk is the ideal food for most infants. It is safe, it is clean, and it contains antibodies that help protect against many common childhood illnesses. Breast milk provides all the energy and nutrients that the infant needs for the first months of life, and it continues to provide up to half or more of a child's nutritional needs during the second half of the first year and up to one-third during the second year of life (World Health Organization [WHO], 2020). There are several significant short- and long-term beneficial effects of feeding the preterm infant human milk. Lower rates of sepsis and necrotizing enterocolitis (NEC) indicate that human milk contributes to the development of the preterm infant's immature host defense (American Academy of Pediatrics [AAP], 2012). The potent benefits of human milk are such that all preterm infants should receive human milk. Mother's* own milk, fresh or frozen, should be the primary diet, and it should be fortified appropriately for the infant born weighing less than 1.5 kg. If mother's own milk is unavailable despite significant lactation support, pasteurized donor milk should be used (AAP, 2012). Premature milk is higher in protein and minerals, such as salt, and contains different types of fat that the infant can more easily digest and absorb. The fat in human milk helps to enhance the development of the baby's brain and neurologic tissues, which is especially important for premature infants (HealthyChildren.org, 2021). The use of formula should only occur in the absence of the mother's own milk or donor milk in most instances. Despite the overwhelming benefits of breastfeeding and human milk to neonates, there are barriers and disparities in achieving such feedings for all infants. All clinicians should be educated on the importance and

---

* We understand that all lactating individuals may not self-identify with the term "mother." It is important that clinicians and supporters are inclusive of pronouns and terminology that the parent chooses during any encounter, and specifically as it pertains to infant feeding.

benefits of breastfeeding and ways to support and promote breastfeeding and human milk feeding for all infants. The Baby-Friendly Hospital Initiative's Ten Steps to Successful Breastfeeding has recently been expanded to include guidance for NICUs, and all clinicians should be aware of these recommendations.

PHYSIOLOGY OF LACTATION

The normal physiology of lactation is a process that begins to take effect well before the initial latch of the newborn infant. It requires the breast to change in composition, size, and shape during each stage of female development. Development includes puberty, pregnancy, and lactation. These stages are influenced by a cascade of physiologic changes that are crucial to successful breastfeeding (Pillay & Davis, 2020). Changes that the breasts undergo to enable breast milk production and expression are commonly known as lactogenesis.

Lactogenesis is the process of developing the ability to secrete milk and involves the maturation of alveolar cells. It takes place in two stages: secretory initiation and secretory activation. Stage I lactogenesis (secretory initiation) takes place during the second half of pregnancy. The placenta supplies high levels of progesterone that inhibit further differentiation. In this stage, small amounts of milk can be secreted by week 16 gestation. By late pregnancy, some women can express colostrum. Stage II lactogenesis (secretory activation) starts with copious milk production after delivery. With the removal of the placenta at delivery, the rapid drop in progesterone, as well as the presence of elevated levels of prolactin, cortisol, and insulin, are what stimulate this stage. Usually, at days 2 or 3 postpartum, most women experience swelling of the breast along with copious milk production (Pillay & Davis, 2020). The two primary hormones that are needed for lactation are prolactin and oxytocin. Prolactin stimulates milk biosynthesis within the alveolar cells of the breast, and oxytocin stimulates contraction of the myoepithelial cells that surround the alveoli, causing the milk to be ejected into the ducts leading to the nipple (King, 2007).

Despite the ability to create milk as early as 16 weeks' gestation, mothers of NICU babies need support and guidance to optimize their milk production. Education and support provided immediately after delivery and throughout the NICU admission will help the mother provide breast milk to their premature infant and meet their breastfeeding goals. Early and frequent stimulation through hand expression and pumping will help to bring the milk in and build and maintain the milk supply. Support of the lactating mother should come from all clinicians and caregivers who encounter the dyad throughout the hospital admission.

SUPPORTING BREASTFEEDING IN THE NICU

Depending on the medical stability and age of the premature infant, most mothers in the NICU will have to initiate lactation by hand expression or pump, rather than by an infant feeding directly at their breast. Supporting lactation and breastfeeding in the NICU requires collaboration between NICU staff, maternal care staff, and the mother. Guidance on the importance of breast milk and how to build and maintain a milk supply for lactating mothers of infants who are not able to orally feed at birth is critical. Education and support should follow the Baby-Friendly Hospital Initiative's Ten Steps to Breastfeeding.

Implement strategies to support breast milk production and breastfeeding:

■ Educate lactating parents on the medical importance of their breast milk for their baby.

  ● Educate on hand expression that may optimize early milk production and expression.

  ● Educate on pumping and provide instruction on pumping techniques (hand expression, manual, and/or electric pump).

■ Initiate hand expression or pumping within 6 hours of birth.

■ Initiate skin-to-skin contact as soon as medically possible after birth and promote frequent sessions.

■ Milk expression should occur eight or more times every 24 hours.

■ Provide emotional support and acknowledge differences between breast pumping and direct breastfeeding an infant.

  ● Encourage mother no matter the amount she produces.

■ Initiate nonnutritive suckling or direct feeding from the breast when appropriate according to the infant's feeding readiness prior to bottles.

■ Support semidemand breastfeeding (infant put to breast whenever signs of waking or hunger and not fed according to a schedule).

Although breast milk provides the ideal nutrition for infants, it is recommended that fortification (especially of protein) is used in infants less than 1,500 g to support growth that is similar to intrauterine growth (AAP, 2012; Adamkin & Radmacher, 2014).

There are various ways to provide support to the breastfeeding mother beyond the clinical aspects as well. Breastfeeding peer counselors and mother-to-mother peer support should be used both during hospitalization and once home. Ongoing support can lead to improved self-efficacy, increased duration of breastfeeding, and provision of breast milk. Breastfeeding peer support is particularly valuable for the NICU mother, due to the unique experiences and challenges that a NICU stay may bring to the dyad. Additional ways to consider supporting the mother may be through the utilization of technology. The increasing popularity and use of social media platforms offers the opportunity to create more innovative, targeted mobile health interventions for infant feeding and breastfeeding promotion (Asiodu et al., 2015).

DISPARITIES IN BREASTFEEDING

Although breastfeeding is recommended to be the feeding norm by leading healthcare organizations, there are stark differences in breastfeeding rates when looking at race and ethnicity. African Americans continue to have the lowest rates of breast-feeding initiation (60%) and continuation at 6 months (28%) and 12 months (13%) compared with all other racial/ethnic groups in the United States. Although improvements in breastfeeding rates for African American women are evident from the 2000 to 2007 National Immunization Survey, African American mothers are still 2.5 times less likely to breastfeed than White women. A 16 percentage-point gap in the prevalence of continued breastfeeding for 6 months has been consistent since 1990 between African American and White women. African American women (32%) are also more likely than most minority groups to provide formula supple-mentation by 2 days of life (McKinney et al., 2016).

It is critical to address the ongoing disparities of breastfeeding, especially for the premature and NICU infant. Premature very low-birth-weight (VLBW; <1,500 g birth weight) infants are almost three times more likely to be born to non-Hispanic Black (Black) than to non-Black (non-Hispanic White [White], Hispanic, Asian, Native American) mothers in the United States (March of Dimes, 2020).

To address disparities in breastfeeding duration, continued efforts are needed to increase rates of breastfeeding initiation and support continuation of breastfeeding among Black women. Closing the Black–White gap in breastfeeding duration might require efforts of multiple groups. Families, hospitals, and employers can help Black women initiate and continue breastfeeding, thereby providing their infants with optimal nutrition (Beauregard et al., 2019).

Standardized practices, such as the Baby-Friendly Hospital Initiative's Ten Steps to Successful Breastfeeding, improve the opportunity to close the breastfeeding gaps. Standardized practices allow for all lactating mothers and infants to receive care without bias and can improve outcomes. Clinician training to disrupt implicit bias is aimed at improving the care provided to all patients, regardless of their race, ethnicity, or marital or economic status. Education of NICU staff and providing breastfeeding education and support to mothers is a cornerstone of many successful NICU breastfeeding quality improvement initiatives. NICUs should ensure that all mothers of NICU infants receive the same education and support with careful review of reports of inequity or variation in practice (Patel et al., 2020).

ORAL CARE WITH BREAST MILK

As soon as the infant is born and the lactating parent initiates pumping, oral care with human milk can commence. This should be done after each time the parent pumps around the clock until the infant can receive human milk by mouth. Oral care mimics what would occur with a healthy term infant feeding by breast. There are three primary rationales regarding the benefits of oral care for the infant: (a) Human milk is a powerful antimicrobial agent, and by coating the infant's mouth with milk, a front-line defense is provided (Edwards & Spatz, 2010; Gephart & Weller, 2014); (b) human milk is a rich source of cytokines, and these cytokines may be absorbed through the infant's buccal mucosa, thus positively impacting the infant's immune system (Rodriguez et al., 2008); and (c) human milk has a sweet flavoring, therefore, oral care with human milk provides a positive oral experience

(Edwards & Spatz, 2010; Gephart & Weller, 2014). In addition, recent research by Froh and colleagues demonstrated that maternal and family participation in human milk oral care was a strong motivator for mothers to keep pumping to build their milk supply for their infant (Froh et al., 2015).

BENEFITS OF DIRECT BREASTFEEDING

When medically able, breastfeeding infants should receive their first oral feeding at the breast, with support of continued direct breastfeeding during hospitalization. Most premature infants will require assistance in transitioning to the breast for feedings. Continuation of gavage feeds while the infant practices nonnutritive suckling before attempting partial at-breast feeds may be beneficial. Breastfeeding readiness is dependent on gestational age and the medical needs of the infant. Feeding infants directly at the breast (direct breastfeeding) has additional benefits over feeding expressed breast milk in a bottle. Direct breastfeeding provides a more stable feeding environment with infants more likely to maintain appropriate oxygenation levels (Buckley & Charles, 2006). In addition, direct breastfeeding provides the freshest breast milk, skin-to-skin contact, and better infant oral development (Buckley & Charles, 2006). Close support by the NICU staff and lactation team and a realistic feeding plan can help the lactating parent achieve their breastfeeding goals.

TRANSITIONING TO DIRECT BREASTFEEDING AND DISCHARGE

If infants have not achieved exclusive direct breastfeeding before discharge, the following strategies should be used to support the transition after discharge:

■ Continued encouragement of skin-to-skin contact at home

■ Clear discharge plan for breastfeeding and supplementation guided by input from the mother and family

■ Education and participatory guidance on "triple feeding" during the transition (direct breastfeeding followed by pumping and bottle feeding); consider the recommendations of Meier et al. (2013)

■ Consistent breastfeeding follow-up and support at home with access to skilled clinical support as needed

BREASTFEEDING AND DRUGS

The concerns regarding the effects of drugs are different in pregnancy than with breastfeeding. Advising a breastfeeding mother on the compatibility of her medications and breastfeeding can often be a source of confusion. Clinicians must consider several factors: the benefit the medication will give to the mother; the risk of discontinuation of breastfeeding, even temporarily, to the baby; the risk of the medication to the baby; and the risk of the medication to the maternal milk supply. Unfortunately, the typical sources of information on medications and breast milk, such as Epocrates, Clin-eguide, Lexi-Comp, and the Physicians Desk Reference (PDR), are often inaccurate and may lead to unnecessary interruption or weaning from breastfeeding.

The most accurate sources of information to aid clinicians about medications in breastfeeding mothers are the National Library of Medicine's Drugs and Lactation Database (LactMed) (https://www.ncbi.nlm.nih.gov/books/NBK501922/), a searchable database of drugs and other chemicals to which breastfeeding mothers may be exposed, and Dr. Thomas Hale's "Medications and Mother's Milk" and his website forums (https://www.springerpub.com/hale-s-medications-mothers-milktm-2021 -9780826189257.html). LactMed is peer reviewed, fully referenced, and continually updated, and is a free service. The data given for each drug include maternal and infant levels of drugs, possible effects on breastfed infants and on lactation, and alternate drugs to consider (Sachs, 2013).

Most drugs are considered compatible with breastfeeding. However, there are certain drugs or medications that may be contraindicated. One of the more popular methods for estimating risk is to determine the relative infant dose (RID). The RID is calculated by dividing the infant's dose via milk (mg/kg/day) by the mother's dose in mg/kg/day. The RID gives the clinician a feeling for just how much medication the infant is exposed to on a weight-normalized basis. However, many authors calculate the infant dose without normalizing for maternal and infant weight, so be cautious (Hale, 2021). Clinicians should compare the RID with the pediatric dose of the medication if known. Hale suggests that clinicians try to use medications with shorter half-lives as they are generally eliminated from the maternal plasma rapidly, thus exposing the milk compartment (and the infant) to reduced levels of medication (Hale, 2021).

Additionally, Hale suggests clinicians choose drugs that have higher protein binding because they are generally sequestered in the maternal circulation and do not transfer readily into the milk compartment or the infant. Remember, it is the free drug that transfers into the milk compartment. The most important parameter that determines drug penetration into milk is plasma protein binding. Anticonvulsants, antidepressants, and antipsychotics are found to be centrally active and likely to penetrate milk at higher levels (Hale, 2021). With CNS-active drugs, one should always check the data available in resources such as those mentioned earlier. Obtaining input from the pharmacist and lactation team may also be beneficial when determining medication safety and risk versus infant benefit when it comes to medications and breast milk.

REFERENCES

Adamkin, D. H., & Radmacher, P. G. (2014). Fortification of human milk in very low birth weight infants (VLBW < 1500 g birth weight). *Clinical Perinatology, 41*(2), 405–421. https://doi.org/10.1016/j.clp.2014.02.010

American Academy of Pediatrics. (2012). Breastfeeding and the use of human milk. *Pediatrics, 129*(3), e827–e841. https://doi.org/10.1542/peds.2011-3552

Asiodu, I. V., Waters, C. M., Dailey, D. E., Lee, K. A., & Lyndon, A. (2015). Breastfeeding and use of social media among first-time African American mothers. *Journal of Obstetric, Gynecologic, and Neonatal Nursing, 44*(2), 268–278. https://doi.org/10.1111/1552-6909 .12552

Beauregard, J. L., Hamner, H. C., Chen, J., Avila-Rodriguez, W., Elam-Evans, L. D., & Perrine, C. G. (2019). Racial disparities in breastfeeding initiation and duration among U.S. infants born in 2015. *MMWR Morbidity and Mortality Weekly Report, 68,* 745–748. https://doi.org/10.15585/mmwr.mm6834a3

Buckley, K. M., & Charles, G. E. (2006). Benefits and challenges of transitioning preterm infants to at-breast feedings. *International Breastfeeding Journal, 1,* 13. https://doi .org/10.1186/1746-4358-1-13

Edwards, T. M., & Spatz, D. L. (2010). An innovative model for achieving breast-feeding success in infants with complex surgical anomalies. *Journal of Perinatal and Neonatal Nursing, 24*(3), 246–253. https://doi.org/10.1097/JPN.0b013e3181e8d517

Froh, E. B., Hallowell, S., & Spatz, D. L. (2015). The use of technologies to support human milk and breastfeeding. *Journal of Pediatric Nursing, 30*(3), P521–P523. https://doi.org/10.1016/ j.pedn.2015.01.023

Gephart, S. M., & Weller, M. (2014). Colostrum as oral immune therapy to promote neonatal health. *Advances in Neonatal Care, 14*(1), 44–51. https://doi.org/10.1097/ANC.0000000 000000052

Hale, T. W. (2021). *Hale's medications & mothers' milk.* Springer Publishing Company.

HealthyChildren.org. (2021). *Providing breastmilk for premature and ill newborns.* https:// www.healthychildren.org/English/ages-stages/baby/breastfeeding/Pages/Providing -Breastmilk-for-Premature-and-Ill-Newborns.aspx

King, J. (2007). Contraception and lactation. *Journal of Midwifery and Women's Health, 52*(6), 614–620. https://doi.org/10.1016/j.jmwh.2007.08.012

March of Dimes. (2020). *Peristats: 2020 March of Dimes Report Card.* https://www .marchofdimes.org/peristats/tools/reportcard.aspx

McKinney, C., Hahn-Holbrook, J., Chase-Lansdale, L., Ramey, S., Krohn, J., Reed-Vance, M., Raju, T., & Shalowitz, M. (2016). Racial and ethnic differences in breastfeeding. *Pediatrics, 138*(2), e20152388. https://doi.org/10.1542/peds.2015-2388

Meier, P., Patel, A. L., Wright, K., & Engstrom, J. L. (2013). Management of breastfeeding during and after the maternity hospitalization for late preterm infants. *Clinical Perinatology, 40*(4), 689–705. https://doi.org/10.1016/j.clp.2013.07.014

Patel, A. L., Johnson, T. J., & Meier, P. P. (2020). Racial and socioeconomic disparities in breast milk feedings in US neonatal intensive care units. *Pediatric Research , 89,* 344–352. https://doi.org/10.1038/s41390-020-01263-y

Pillay, J., & Davis, T. J. (2020). Physiology, lactation. In *StatPearls.* StatPearls Publishing. https://www.ncbi.nlm.nih.gov/books/NBK499981/

Rodriguez, N. A., Meier, P. P., Groer, M. W., & Zeller, J. M. (2008). Oropharyngeal administration of colostrum to extremely low birth weight infants: Theoretical perspectives. *Journal of Perinatology, 29*(1), 1–7. https://doi.org/10.1038/jp.2008.130

Sachs, H. C. (2013). Committee on drugs. The transfer of drugs and therapeutics into human breast milk: An update on selected topics. *Pediatrics, 132,* e796–809. https://doi.org/10 .1542/peds.2013-1985

World Health Organization. (2020). *Health topic: Breastfeeding.* https://www.who.int/health -topics/breastfeeding#tab=tab_1

ORAL FEEDINGS

KSENIA ZUKOWSKY, CHRISTINE CATTS, AND MICHELE KACMARCIK SAVIN

OVERVIEW

Human breast milk is the food of choice for all infants—term and preterm—rather than formula. Research has demonstrated that infants have better outcomes in the areas of development, immunology, infectious disease, and childhood obesity when fed human milk. Additionally, there are also better maternal outcomes noted for mothers who feed their infants human milk (American Academy of Pediatrics [AAP], 2012).

The enteral caloric recommendations for healthy newborn infants vary according to sources. Recommendations may range from 98 to 120 kcal/kg/day for adequate growth and development (AAP Committee on Nutrition, 1985; Merves, 2012). Enteral caloric recommendations for premature infants are a little higher—110 to 135 kcal/kg/day for growth (Agostoni et al., 2010). These enteral nutrition recommendations are based on the goal of duplicating the rates of intrauterine accretion of the fetus (Pointdexter & Schanler, 2012). The goal of nutritional intake for this population is for the premature infant to grow in extrauterine life at the same rate and composition as the fetus of the same gestational age. This extrauterine goal is difficult to attain for the premature low-birth-weight infant.

PREMATURE NEONATES

Premature low-birth-weight neonates generally have one or more comorbidities to contend with that may compromise their growth. These may include one or more diseases such as bronchopulmonary dysplasia, severe intraventricular hemorrhage, necrotizing enterocolitis (NEC), or sepsis, which may contribute to additional caloric demands that impact the premature infant's ability to grow (Pointdexter & Schanler, 2012). Preterm infants also have limited nutrient stores, an increase in energy expenditure, and/or an immaturity and inability to tolerate enteral feedings. These issues all affect the preterm infant's ability to grow sufficiently over time. Therefore, parenteral nutrition is given immediately after birth to create positive nitrogen balance for growth. Enteral feedings are introduced to preterm infants in small amounts over time (Pointdexter & Schanler, 2012).

Small volumes of feedings, trophic feedings, given early to preterm low-birth-weight infants lead to the neonate's increased ability to tolerate and advance to full volume feedings. Importantly, beginning with early trophic enteral feedings can lead to fewer days on total parenteral nutrition (Pointdexter & Schanler, 2012; Slagle & Gross, 1988). Neonatal enteral feedings when initiated will increase slowly and steadily over time as parenteral nutrition can be decreased to accommodate for total fluid volume for the neonate (total cc/kg/day). This acceleration of enteral feeding may occur over a period of several days and/or weeks. The initiation of trophic feedings may begin with 5 to 20 mL/kg/day, depending on gestational age, and advance by 10 to 20 mL/kg/day until total enteral intake is equal to 150 mL/kg/day (Ehrenkranz, 2007). Early trophic feeds have been found to decrease days to reach full enteral feedings in very low-birth-weight infants (Specht et al., 2020).

The total caloric intake goals of enteral feedings for premature infants may range between 110 and 135 kcal/kg/day (Agostoni et al., 2010). These caloric requirements are derived from the preterm low-birth-weight infant's energy expenditure. Within the energy expenditure, the infant's resting metabolic rate is the largest component of the total estimated energy requirement. Other energy expenditures that contribute to energy requirements are movement, activity, thermoregulation, and growth. However, the preterm infant has limited energy storage of fat and lean mass. The preterm also has energy losses that are due to incomplete absorption of nutrients and immature body organs (Pointdexter & Schanler, 2012). Enteral nutrition and preterm low-birth-weight infant feeding may be increased over time as the neonate tolerates. A mean weight gain for the preterm infant is approximately 15 g/kg/day, with a goal of regaining the neonate's birth weight by the seventh to 14th day of life (Cloherty et al., 2012). As with all nutrition, the major components of enteral nutrition are protein, fat, and carbohydrates. Due to the immature gastrointestinal and enzyme systems, the preterm low-birth-weight infant is at a disadvantage when trying to feed and absorb these nutrients.

Protein

Gastric acid is required for protein breakdown. The preterm infant's gastric acid levels are lower than those of term infants (Anderson, 2020). Protein requirements for very-low-birth-weight and premature infants are 4 g/kg/day. A recommended intake of enteral protein by fortified human milk and/or premature formula would need to supply 3.2 to 4.1 g protein/100 kcal. Fortified human milk and/or premature formula is derived to yield an increased protein accretion and improved weight gain without causing toxicity to the infant (AAP, 2012; Pointdexter & Schanler, 2012).

Fat

Human milk contains fat, a major energy source. Fat comprises nearly 50% of breast milk's calories, although the fat content varies from mother to mother. Fat may adhere to collection containers, feeding tubes, and/or syringes when administering or storing human milk. Because of this, human milk administration is performed judiciously. Times and dates are noted when it is being administered to premature low-birth-weight infants (Pointdexter & Schanler, 2012). Fats are broken down into triglycerides and fatty acids by enzymes located in the infant's lingual secretions, from the pancreas, and in the intestines (Anderson, 2020). A recommended intake of fat for enteral-fed premature low-birth-weight infants ranges between 4.8 and 6.6 g/kg/day. Medium-chain triglycerides are the major source of fat in formula (Agostoni et al., 2010; Pointdexter & Schanler, 2012). Fat makes up 40% to 50% of total caloric intake of either human milk or formula (Anderson, 2020).

Carbohydrates

Lactose is the primary carbohydrate in human milk. Lactase (*beta-galactosidase*) is an intestinal enzyme that hydrolyzes lactose to glucose and galactose in the small intestine. The preterm infant, due to their immaturity, has a lower level of lactase yet will tolerate lactose in human milk well (Pointdexter & Schanler, 2012). Glucose polymers are the source of carbohydrate in premature formula. Glucose polymers have an advantage in that they increase caloric density without a rise in osmolality. Recommended carbohydrate intake for premature infants is 11.6 to 13.2 g/kg/day (Agostoni et al., 2010; Pointdexter & Schanler, 2012).

Calcium and Phosphorus

Calcium and phosphorus are essential for all neonates. The premature infant requires greater quantities of calcium and phosphorus than the term infant; these quantities are not available in human milk. Calcium and phosphorus are necessary for 99% and 85%, respectively, of bone mass. Human milk contains calcium and phosphorus that is ionized easily; thus, it is better absorbed than the calcium and phosphorous that is contained in formula (Pointdexter & Schanler, 2012).

Although the calcium and phosphorous in human milk are better absorbed by neonates, in the preterm infant the amount of calcium and phosphorus in human milk is not adequate to attain the intrauterine accretion growth rates. This is exhibited in low serum and urine phosphorous concentrations, elevated serum alkaline phosphatases, and elevated urine calcium concentrations (Pointdexter & Schanler, 2012).

Human milk supplementation with calcium and phosphorus improves retention of these minerals in the preterm infant. Preterm formulas are fortified with greater amounts of calcium and phosphorous than term infant formulas (Pointdexter & Schanler, 2012).

PARENTERAL NUTRITION

The largest component of the total estimated energy requirement is that needed for the resting metabolic rate. When nourished parenterally, the premature infant has less fecal energy loss, generally fewer episodes of cold stress, and somewhat lesser activity so that the actual energy needs for growth are lowered to 80 to 100 kcal/kg/day for the first week of life (Schanler, 2015).

Parenteral nutrition initiated early in this population minimizes weight loss, improves growth and neurodevelopmental outcome, and appears to reduce the risk of mortality and morbidity. There is literature to support better neurodevelopmental outcomes with initiation of higher protein intake (Christmann et al., 2013; Ehrenkranz et al., 2011; Moyses et al., 2013).

Protein

Recommendations are that 1.5 g/kg/day of protein be started within the first 24 hours after birth and then increased to 3.5 to 4 g/kg/day by 0.5 to 1 g/kg/day increments. There are not significant increases in blood urea nitrogen (BUN) and/or acidosis with this higher protein initiation (Burattini et al., 2013; Clark et al., 2007; Klein, 2002; Porcelli & Sisk, 2002; Schanler, 2015; Schanler et al., 1994; Tan & Cooke, 2008). Essential and nonessential amino acids are necessary to attain a positive nitrogen balance leading to attainment of growth (Malloy et al., 1984).

Studies have shown that administering protein of ≥4 g/kg/day was well tolerated and yielded an association of lower rates of bronchopulmonary dysplasia when compared with lower protein (Malloy et al., 1984). Currently, recommendations are to start protein/amino acids administration immediately after birth with an infusion rate of 3.5 g/kg/day. There is an improved nitrogen balance and stable serum BUN or glucose concentrations with these higher doses (te Braake et al., 2005; Thureen et al., 2003). Infants who receive protein on the first day of life have a positive nitrogen balance with no side effects from the amino acids (Ibrahim et al., 2004; Poindexter & Ehrenkranz, 2015).

As for toxicity, there are no differences between 3 g/kg/day compared with 1 g/kg/day in serum BUN (Paisley, 2000). Estimated parenteral protein requirements for premature infants who are low birth weight are 3 to 3.5 g/kg/day. Estimates for term infants are 2.5 to 3 g/kg/day (Poindexter & Denne, 2012).

TrophAmine (B. Braun Medical, Inc, Bethlehem, Pennsylvania) is a brand of amino acid solution that yields normal amino acid plasma concentrations (Thureen et al., 2003). TrophAmine and Premasol (Baxter, Deerfield, Illinois) supply amino acids L-tyrosine and N-acetyl-L-Tyrosine. Aminosyn-PF (Hospira, Inc., Lake Forest, Illinois) and Primene (Baxter, Deerfiedl, Illinois) do not supply substantial tyrosine. Cysteine is not in most parenteral amino acid solutions. The ideal intravenous amino acid is not known for parental nutrition (Poindexter & Ehrenkranz, 2015).

Glucose

As with enteral nutrition, carbohydrates and fat primarily provide the calories for energy. The percentages of nonprotein calories are carbohydrates 40% and lipids 45% (Schanler, 2015). Others have noted the fat-to-glucose ratio of 60:40 can mimic human milk (Poindexter & Ehrenkranz, 2015). Glucose is the source of carbohydrate used in parenteral nutrition. Exogenous glucose is often needed initially until the infant can begin to mobilize glycogen stores and produce glucose.

The primary source of energy for the neonatal brain is glucose (Poindexter & Ehrenkranz, 2015). Term infants, due to their utilization and glucose production, need 3 to 5 mg/kg/minute of glucose. Preterm infants' demands are greater—approximately 8 to 9 mg/kg/minute. Preterm infants may start at a glucose infusion rate of 6 mg/kg/day and increase as high as 10 to 12 mg/kg/minute as long as hyperglycemia does not occur. Glucose infusion rates of 5 to 8 mg/kg/minute may be needed. Very-low-birth-weight infants who weigh 1,000 g or more will usually tolerate 10% glucose–dextrose solution. Infants that weigh less than 1,000 g may require 5% glucose–dextrose solution (Poindexter & Ehrenkranz, 2015).

Fat

Fat emulsions are important to prevent essential fatty acid deficiency and serve as a nonprotein energy source. These emulsions are from soybean oil, olive oil, medium-chain triglycerides, and fish oil. The fish oil emulsions contain very long-chain omega-3 fatty acids, docosahexaenoic acid, and eicosapentaenoic acid (Mayer & Schafer, 2006; Poindexter & Ehrenkranz, 2015). Lipids can be given 3 mg/kg/day. Plasma lipid clearance improves when intravenous lipids are given continuously over 24 hours (Poindexter & Ehrenkranz, 2015).

READINESS FOR ORAL FEEDING

The ability for an infant to feed orally is dependent on their attainment of coordination of sucking, swallowing, and breathing, a highly organized behavior (Lau, 2015; Medoff-Cooper et al., 1993). This is affected by gestational age, neurodevelopmental maturity, behavioral state organization, and physiologic stability (Shaker, 2017a, 2017b). This coordination occurs around 32 to 34 weeks' gestational age (Delaney & Arvedson, 2008; Jones, 2012). The coordination of swallowing and breathing matures around 37 weeks corrected gestational age (Amaizu et al., 2008; Lau, 2015). Nasogastric or orogastric feeding alone or in conjunction with partial oral feeding is used until full oral feedings are achieved (Viswanathan & Jadcherla, 2019). Supporting readiness for oral feeding may occur as early as 28 weeks with nonnutritive sucking (DeMauro et al., 2011; Kirk et al., 2007).

Assessment of oral feeding readiness is done with consideration of physiologic stability, alert behavioral states, and prefeeding cues (Griffith et al., 2017, Shaker, 2017a, 2017b). There are validated scales that focus on the assessment of feeding readiness to initiate oral feeding based on readiness cues (Griffith et al., 2017; Kirk et al., 2007). These scales measure defined standards to assess each infant's cues to initiate oral feeding. They also drive stopping oral feeding with signs of stress. The goal is for the infant to develop positive feeding experience to facilitate desired neurodevelopmental outcome (Griffith et al., 2017; Shaker, 2017a, 2017b).

Bottle Feeding

There are many types of nipples and bottle systems to use for feeding the premature infant. Some systems have nipples that regulate the flow of milk when the infant compresses the nipple (Pados et al., 2019). Changes to a different type of nipple within a system are based on assessment of the infant's ability to self-regulate coordination of sucking bursts, swallowing, and rest periods based on the flow of milk the infant obtains (Pados et al., 2019). Side-lying is the optimal positioning during feeding (Shaker, 2017a, 2017b).

Nasogastric/Orogastric Tube Feeding

Nasogastric or orogastric enteral feeding is used to provide enteral feeding until oral feeding skills have developed or in infants who are unable to orally feed (Beauman

& Bowles, 2019). Intermittent bolus feeds are given by gravity. Transpyloric feeds are used in infants with persistent feeding intolerance, emesis, and gastric residuals (Watson & McGuire, 2020). Placement of the gastric tube should be confirmed once placed and before feedings or medications as indicated. Stomach aspiration is the preferred method of tube placement. The injection of air is unreliable and should not be used (Beauman & Bowles, 2019). In a Cochrane review (2019) of routine monitoring of gastric aspirates for the prevention of NEC, the authors found insufficient evidence that the routine practice of checking residuals decreased NEC. There was low-level evidence that checking aspirates leads to episodes of feeding interruption, increased time to reach full volume feeds, and longer time to regain birthweight (Abiramalatha et al., 2019).

The preterm infant has immature organs that contribute to enteral feeding issues. There is a relaxation of the lower esophageal sphincter, which leads to reflux. A delay in gastric emptying and a decrease in intestinal motility also are present. Intestinal motility usually starts to improve around 32 weeks' gestation (Anderson, 2020; Beauman & Bowles, 2019; Griffith et al., 2017). The ileocecal valve, which acts as a barrier between the small and large intestine, has a relative incompetence that allows free movement of fluid. There is also an impaired retro sphincter reflux that can be noted in a delay in stool evacuation (Anderson, 2020).

CLEFT LIP AND PALATE

MICHELE KACMARCIK SAVIN

A cleft lip is a congenital fissure in the upper lip, whereas a cleft palate is a congenital fissure in either the soft palate alone or in both the hard and soft palate. The two conditions can occur as separate defects or together. They can be unilateral or bilateral. The most severe form is bilateral cleft lip and palate occurring together.

Incidence

Cleft lip with or without an associated cleft palate occurs at a rate of approximately one in 700 varying by different populations and geographic location (National Birth Defects Prevention Network, 2014; Vieira, 2008). The occurrence is higher in males and in Asians. Isolated cleft palate has a lower incidence rate and occurs more frequently in females. Seventy percent of neonates with unilateral cleft lip and 85% of neonates with bilateral cleft lip will also have a cleft palate (Merritt, 2005). Ten percent of neonates with cleft lip and cleft palate will have an associated syndrome. In parents with a cleft lip/palate, the offspring has a 3% to 5% risk of being born with a cleft lip/palate. Upper lip clefts are usually lateral. Midline clefts are rare and highly associated with other midline central nervous system defects including those of the pituitary-adrenal axis, thyroid issues, and holoprosencephaly. No single gene has been identified to explain clefts, but various mutations of at least 14 genes have been associated. Environmental factors also contribute to the development of clefts.

Pathophysiology

Cleft lip and cleft palate are considered distinct embryologic disorders. Cleft lip occurs when the maxillary process fails to merge with the medial nasal elevation on one or both sides; cleft palate occurs when the lateral palatine processes fail to meet and fuse with each other, the primary palate, or the nasal septum. When both cleft lip and palate occur together, the failure of the secondary palate to close may be a developmental consequence of the abnormalities in the primary palate associated with the cleft lip rather than an intrinsic defect in the secondary palate.

Maternal conditions associated with clefting include advanced maternal age, smoking, alcohol use, diabetes, hypo/hypervitaminosis, and influenza and fever (National Birth Defects Prevention Network, 2014; Spritz, 2001). Antenatal exposure to certain medications is associated with clefting; these include benzodiazepines, phenytoin, opiates, penicillin, salicylates, cortisone, and high doses of vitamin A. Mothers taking folic acid reduce the risk of orofacial clefts by one-third (Wilcox et al., 2007).

Physical Examination

A cleft lip can be diagnosed prenatally by ultrasound, which can assist the family in preparation and management. As many as 25% of children with cleft lip and/or palate may have associated syndromes. Up to 15% of children with cleft lip and palate in one study had cardiac anomalies, the most common of which was ventricular septal defects (Kasatwar et al., 2018). Palatal differences are varied; physical examination including both palpation and visual inspection is necessary.

Treatment

Treatment of clefts includes an interprofessional team of healthcare providers and incorporates emotional support for parents, thorough history to identify etiology, and surgical repair.

Goals of surgical repair include minimizing maxillary growth retardation, limiting dental deformity, and allowing normal speech development. Cleft lip repair can occur around 3 months of age, although cleft palate repair is delayed allowing for medial movement of the palatal shelves. The palatal repairs begin after 6 months of life; some sites repair the soft and hard palates together and some prefer two-stage repairs with the hard palate later to aid mid-facial development. If further cosmetic repair of the lip is required, this occurs later as well. Coordination of care between family and specialists including surgery and dentistry is paramount (Alonso & Raposo-Amaral, 2018).

Oral Feedings

Oral feedings require patience and attention to technique, as infants with a cleft are often unable to create a vacuum for adequate sucking. In such instances, several techniques are identified to be successful.

■ Infant's cheeks are grasped to close the cleft.

■ Frequent burping occurs due to excessive amounts of air being swallowed.

■ Infant is positioned in an upright or semi-upright position to avoid choking.

■ The flow of milk is directed to the side of the mouth.

■ Breastfeeding is possible and encouraged; the support of a lactation counselor is helpful (Boyce et al., 2019).

■ Modified breastfeeding positions, chin support, and manual expression into babies' mouth may help.

■ Use of a "squeeze" bottle, "preemie" nipple, or a special cleft palate nipple has been helpful.

■ Small volume and frequent feedings are used to prevent exhaustion and frustration.

■ Some prosthetic devices are available to occlude the cleft; they are molded to the shape of the infant's mouth. The device is rinsed with water after feedings.

■ Milk does collect around the cleft. To prevent infection and excoriation, offer a small amount of sterile water after oral feedings.

■ Oral microbiota may show a marked presence of pathogenic bacteria such as methicillin-resistant *S. aureus* (Machorowska-Pienidhek et al., 2017).

■ Auditory evaluations, speech, and language development as well as growth patterns must be closely followed.

Prognosis

An excellent prognosis for survival is expected, although infants with clefts are at risk for and require close follow-up for language and speech delays, an associated hearing impairment, and dental problems such as malocclusions, irregularity of teeth, and dental caries. Over 300 syndromes include cleft lip, cleft palate, or both, and may not be recognized in the early neonatal period. The prognosis can vary for infants with an associated anomaly; therefore, thorough physical examination is important and genetic screening via microarray or whole-exome sequencing should be considered.

REFERENCES

Abiramalatha, T., Thanigainathan, S., & Ninan, B. (2019). Routine monitoring of gastric residual for prevention of necrotizing enterocolitis in preterm infants (Review). *Cochrane Database of Systematic Reviews, 7*(7), CD012937. https://doi.org/10.1002/14651858.CD012937

Agostoni, C., Buonocore, G., Carnielli, V. P., De Curtis, M., Darmaun, D., Decsi, T., Domellöf, M., Embleton, N. D., Fusch, C., Genzel-Boroviczeny, O., Goulet, O., Kalhan, S. C., Kolacek, S., Koletzko, B., Lapillonne, A., Mihatsch, W., Moreno, L., Neu, J., Poindexter, B., … ESPGHAN Committee on Nutrition. (2010). Enteral nutrient supply for preterm infants: Commentary from the European Society for Paediatric Gastroenterology, Hepatology, and Nutrition (ESPGHAN) committee on nutrition. *Journal of Pediatric Gastroenterology Nutrition, 50*(1), 85–91. https://doi.org/10.1097/MPG.0b013e3181adaee0

Alonso, N., & Raposo-Amaral, C. E. (2018). *Cleft lip and palate treatment.* Springer Publishing Company.

Amaizu, N., Shulman, R. J., Schanler, R. J., & Lau, C. (2008). Maturation of oral feeding skills in preterm infants. *Acta Paediatrica, 97*(1), 61–67. https://doi.org/10.1111/j.1651 -2227.2007.00548.x

American Academy of Pediatrics. (2012). Breastfeeding and the use of human milk section on breastfeeding. *Pediatrics, 129*(3), e837–e841. https://doi.org/10.1542/peds.2011-3552

American Academy of Pediatrics Committee on Nutrition. (1985). Nutritional needs of low-birth-weight infants. *Pediatrics, 75*(5), 976–986. https://pediatrics.aappublications.org/content/pediatrics/75/5/976.full.pdf

Anderson, D. (2020). Nutrition management of the premature infants. In C. Kenner, L. Altimier, & M. Boykova (Eds.), *Comprehensive neonatal nursing care* (6th ed., pp. 497–514). Springer Publishing Compay.

Beauman, S., & Bowles, S. (2019). *Policies, procedures, and competencies for neonatal nursing care.* National Association of Neonatal Nurses.

Boyce, J., Reilly, S., Skeat, J., Cahir, P., & the Academy of Breastfeeding Medicine. (2019). ABM Clinical Protocol #17: Guidelines for breastfeeding infants with cleft lip, cleft palate, or cleft lip and palate—Revised 2019. *Breastfeeding Medicine, 14,* 7. https://doi.org/10.1089/bfm.2019.29132.job

Burattini, I., Bellagamba, M. P., Spagnoli, C., D'Ascenzo, R., Mazzoni, N., Peretti, A., Cogo, P. E., Carnielli, V. P., & Marche Neonatal Network. (2013). Targeting 2.5 versus 4 g/kg/day of amino acids for extremely low birth weight infants: A randomized clinical trial *Journal of Pediatrics, 163*(5), 1278–1282. https://doi.org/10.1016/j.jpeds.2013.06.075

Christmann, V., Visser, R., Engelkes, M., de Grauw, A. M., van Goudoever, J. B., & van Heijst, A. F. J. (2013). The enigma to achieve normal postnatal growth in preterm infants–using parenteral or enteral nutrition? *Acta Paediatrica, 102*(5), 471–479. https://doi.org/10.1111/apa.12188

Clark, R. H., Chace, D. H., & Spitzer, A. R. (2007). Pediatrix amino acid study group. Effects of two different doses of amino acid supplementation on growth and blood amino acid levels in premature neonates admitted to the neonatal intensive care unit: A randomized, controlled trial. *Pediatrics, 120*(6), 1286–1296. https://doi.org/10.1542/peds.2007-0545

Cloherty, J. P., Eichenwald, E. C., & Stark, A. R. (Eds.). (2012). *Manual of neonatal care* (7th ed.). Wolters Kluwer/Lippincott Williams & Wilkins.

Delaney, A. L., & Arvedson, J. C. (2008). Development of swallowing and feeding: Prenatal through first year of life. *Developmental Disability Research Review, 14*(2), 105–117. https://doi.org/10.1002/ddrr.16

DeMauro, S. B., Patel, P. R., Medoff-Cooper, B., Posencheg, M., & Abbasi, S. (2011). Postdischarge feeding patterns in early- and late-preterm infants. *Clinic in Pediatrics, 50*(10), 957–962. https://doi.org/10.1177/0009922811409028

Ehrenkranz, R. A. (2007). Early, aggressive nutritional management for very low birth weight infants: What is the evidence? *Seminar Perinatology, 31*(2), 48–55. https://doi.org/10.1053/j.semperi.2007.02.001

Ehrenkranz, R. A., Das, A., Wrage, L. A., Poindexter, B. B., Higgins, R. D., Stoll, B. J., & Oh, W. (2011). Early nutrition mediates the influence of severity of illness on extremely LBW infants. *Pediatric Research, 69,* 522–529. https://doi.org/10.1203/PDR.0b013e318 217f4f1

Griffith, T., Rankin, K., & White-Traut, R. (2017). The relationship between behavioral states and oral feeding efficiency in preterm infants. *Advances in Neonatal Care, 17*(1), 1–19. https://doi.org/10.1097/ANC.0000000000000318

Ibrahim, H. M., Jeroudi, M. A., Baier, R. J., Dhanireddy, R., & Krouskop, R. W. (2004). Aggressive early total parenteral nutrition in low birth weight infant. *Journal of Perinatology, 24*(8), 482–486. https://doi.org/10.1038/sj.jp.7211114

Jones, L. R. (2012). Oral feeding readiness in the neonatal intensive care unit. *Neonatal Network, 31*(3), 148–155. https://doi.org/10.1891/0730-0832.31.3.148

Kasatwar, A., Borle, R., Bhola, N., Rajanikanth, K., & Anendd Jadhav, P. (2018). Prevalence of congenital cardiac anomalies in patients with cleft lip and palate—Its implications in surgical management. *Journal of Oral Biology and Craniofacial Research, 8,* 241–244. https://doi.org/10.1016/j.jobcr.2017.09.009

Kirk, A. T., Alder, S. C., & King, J. D. (2007). Cue-based oral feeding clinical pathway results in earlier attainment of full oral feeding in premature infants. *Journal of Perinatology, 27*(9), 572–578. https://doi.org/10.1038/sj.jp.7211791

Klein, C. J. (2002). Nutrient requirements for preterm infant formulas. *Journal Nutrition, 132*(6), 1295S–1577S. https://doi.org/10.1093/jn/132.6.1395S

Lau, C. (2015). Development of suck and swallow mechanisms in infants. *Annals of Nutrition and Metabolism, 66*(05), 7–14. https://doi.org/10.1159/000381361

Machorowska-Pienidhek, A., Mertas, A., Skucha-Nowak, M., Tanasiewicz, M., & Morawiec, T. (2017). A comparative study of oral microbiota in infants with complete cleft lip and palate or cleft soft palate. *BioMed Research International, 2017,* 1460243. https://doi.org/10.1155/2017/1460243

Malloy, M. H., Rassin, D. K., & Richardson, C. J. (1984). Total parenteral nutrition in sick preterm infants: Effects of cysteine supplementation with nitrogen intakes of 240 and 400 mg/kg/day. *Journal of Pediatric Gastroenterology and Nutrition, 3*(2), 239–244.

Mayer, K., & Schafer, M. B. (2006). Fish oil and the critically ill: From experiment to clinical data. *Current Opinion Clinical Nutrition Metabolic Care, 9*(2), 140–148. https://doi.org/10.1097/01.mco.0000214573.75062.0a

Medoff-Cooper, B., Verklan T., & Carlson, S. (1993). The development of sucking patterns and physiologic correlates in very-low-birth-weight infants. *Nursing Research, 42*(2), 100–105. https://journals.lww.com/nursingresearchonline/abstract/1993/03000/the_development_of_sucking_patterns_and.7.aspx

Merritt, L. (2005). Part 1: Understanding the embryology and genetics of cleft lip and palate. *Advances in Neonatal Care, 5*(2), 64–71. https://doi.org/10.1016/j.adnc.2004.12.006

Merves, M. H. (2012). Newborn assessment. In M. Tschudy & M. Jones (Eds.), *Harriet lane* (19th ed.). Elsevier.

Moyses, H. E., Johnson, M. J., Leaf, A. A., & Cornelius, V. R. (2013). Early parenteral nutrition and growth outcomes in preterm infants: A systematic review and meta-analysis. *American Journal Clinical Nutrition, 97*(4), 816–826. https://doi.org/10.1002/14651858.CD002777.pub2

National Birth Defects Prevention Network. (2014). Birth defects data from population-based birth defects surveillance programs in the United States, 2007 to 2011: Highlighting orofacial clefts. *Birth Defects Research A: Clinical and Molecular Teratology, 100*(11), 895–904. https://doi.org/10.1002/bdra.23329

Pados, B. F., Park, J., & Dodrillm, P. (2019). Know the flow: Milk flow from bottle nipples used in the hospital and after discharge. *Advances in Neonatal Care, 19*(1), 32–41. https://doi.org/10.1097/ANC.0000000000000538

Paisley, J. E. (2000). Safety and efficacy or low versus high parental amino acids in extremely low birth weight neonates immediately after birth. *Pediatric Research, 47*(4), 293A.

Poindexter, B., & Ehrenkranz, R. (2015). Nutrient requirements and provision of nutrition supporting the preterm infant. In R. J. Martin, A. A. Fanaroff, & M. C. Walsh (Eds.), *Fanaroff and Martin's neonatal-perinatal medicine: Diseases of the fetus and infant* (10th ed.). Saunders/Elsevier.

Poindexter, B. B., & Denne, S. C. (2012). Parenteral nutrition. In C. S. Gleason & S. Devaskar (Eds.), *Avery's diseases of the newborn* (9th ed., pp. 963–972). Elsevier Health Science.

Pointdexter, B. B., & Schanler, R. J. (2012). Enteral nutrition for the high risk neonate. In C. S. Gleason & S. Devaskar (Eds.), *Avery's diseases of the newborn* (9th ed., pp. 952–962). Elsevier Health Science.

Porcelli, P. J., & Sisk, P. M. (2002). Increased parenteral amino acid administration to extremely low-birth-weight infants during early postnatal life. *Journal of Pediatric Gastroenterology Nutrition, 34*(2), 174–179. https://doi.org/10.1097/00005176-200202000-00013

Schanler, R. J. (2015). *Parenteral nutrition in premature infants.* http://www.uptodate.com/contents/parenteral-nutrition-in-premature-infants?source=search_result&search=Parenteral+Nutrition+in+premature&selectedTitle=1~150

Schanler, R. J., Shulman, R. J., & Prestridge, L. L. (1994). Parenteral nutrient needs of very low birth weight infants. *Journal of Pediatrics, 125*(6), 961–968. https://doi.org/10.1016/s0022-3476(05)82016-5

Shaker, C. (2017a). Infant-guided, co-regulated feeding in the neonatal intensive care unit. Part I: Theoretical underpinnings for neuroprotection and safety. *Seminars in Speech and Language, 38*(2), 96–105. https://doi.org/10.1055/s-0037-1599107

Shaker, C. (2017b). Infant-guided, co-regulated feeding in the neonatal intensive care unit. Part II: Interventions to promote neuroprotection and safety. *Seminars in Speech and Language, 38*(2), 106–115. https://doi.org/10.1055/s-0037-1599108

Slagle, T. A., & Gross, S. J. (1988). Effect of early low-volume enteral substrate on subsequent feeding tolerance in very low birth weight infants. *Journal of Pediatrics, 113*(3), 526–531. https://doi.org/10.1016/s0022-3476(88)80646-2

Specht, R., Barroso, L., Machado, R., Dos Santos, M. S., Ferreira, A. A., Chacon, I., & de Carvalho Padilha, P. (2020). Enteral and parenteral nutrition for neonates at a neonatal unit: A longitudinal retrospective study. *Journal of Maternal Fetal and Neonatal Medicine, 19*, 1–7. https://doi.org/10.1080/14767058.2020.1818212

Spritz, R. (2001). The genetics and epigenetics of orofacial clefts. *Current Opinions in Pediatrics, 13*(6), 556–560. https://doi.org/10.1097/00008480-200112000-00011

Tan, M. J., & Cooke, R. W. (2008). Improving head growth in very preterm infants—A randomised controlled trial I: Neonatal outcomes. *Archives Disease Child Fetal & Neonatal Education, 93*, F337–F341. https://doi.org/10.1136/adc.2007.124230

Te Braake, F. W., van den Akker, C. H., Wattimena, D. J., Huijmans, J. G., & van Goudoever, J. B. (2005). Amino acid administration to premature infants directly after birth. *Journal of Pediatrics, 147*(4), 457–461. https://doi.org/10.1016/j.jpeds.2005.05.038

Thureen, P. J., Melara, D., Fennessey, P. V., & Hay, W. W., Jr. (2003). Effect of low versus high intravenous amino acid intake on very low birth weight infants in the early neonatal period. *Pediatric Research, 53*(2), 24–32. https://doi.org/10.1203/00006450-200301000-00008

Vieira, A. R. (2008). Unraveling human cleft lip and palate research. *Journal of Dental Research, 87*(2), 119–125. https://doi.org/10.1177/154405910808700202

Viswanathan, S., & Jadcherla, S. (2019). Transitioning from gavage to full oral feeds in premature infants: Where should we discontinue the nasogastric tube? *Journal of Perinatology, 39*, 1257–1262. https://doi.org/10.1038/s41372-019-0446-2

Watson, J., & McGuire, W. (2020). Nutrition management of premature infants. In C. Kenner, L. Altimier, & M. Boykova (Eds.), *Comprehensive neonatal nursing care* (6th ed.). Springer Publishing Company.

Wilcox, A. J., Lie, R. T., Solvoll, K., Taylor, J., McConnaughey, D. R., Abyholm, F., Vindenes, H., Vollset, S. E., & Drevon, C. A. (2007). Folic acid supplements and risk of facial clefts: National population-based case-control study. *British Medical Journal, 25*(3), 334–464. https://doi.org/10.1136/bmj.39079.618287.0B

Surgical Care for the Neonate

MICHELE DEGRAZIA

OVERVIEW

This section reviews special considerations in the care of newborns with surgical needs. It begins by providing essential information nurses need to know about consenting parents or guardians, the delivery of family-centered care, and fluid, electrolyte, and pain management. Nurses will also find detailed information related to management of tubes and drains followed by guidance on contemporary preoperative/postoperative management of commonly observed noncardiac surgical conditions of the neonate. Since care of these neonates changes frequently, the information provided is intended for use in conjunction with institutional policies and procedures.

GENERAL CONSIDERATIONS IN THE MANAGEMENT OF THE SURGICAL NEONATE: CONSENT, FAMILY-CENTERED CARE, FLUID AND ELECTROLYTE, AND PAIN MANAGEMENT

DENISE CASEY

OVERVIEW

The care of the surgical neonate requires considerable skill and expertise. To care for a surgical neonate, nurses must possess the skills to provide routine well-newborn care and deliver care to those with isolated surgical conditions as well as those with multiple, complex medical, and surgical diagnoses (Kelly et al., 2008). Nurses must advocate, monitor, and identify concerns related to the surgical neonate and provide holistic, family-centered care to the family. This section will touch briefly on the topics of consent, family-centered care, fluid and nutrition management, and pain management.

CONSENT

Informed consent is the initial process of educating the patient or surrogate who is responsible for the care of the patient.

■ In the case of a neonate, the responsible person is usually the parent(s), but sometimes it is another family member or surrogate. For simplicity, we will use parent(s) throughout this section, knowing that in some situations a family member or surrogate may be substituted (Sudia & Catlin, 2021).

Education of the parent should include specific information about the surgical procedure that is to be performed. This education should be delivered in the form of a discussion where families feel comfortable asking questions to enhance their understanding. This will ensure parents remain engaged and involved in the decision-making process. During informed consent, the provider must use clear language and minimize the use of medical terminology that can be misinterpreted or misunderstood by the parent(s).

Prior to the consent process, consider the following:

■ Primary language of the person receiving the information

● Is an interpreter needed?

■ Education level of the individual

● Language used to explain the procedure should be done at the individual's educational level.

Obtaining surgical procedure informed consent includes:

■ Indications for the procedure
■ Potential benefits, risks, side effects
■ Likelihood of achieving the goals of the procedure
■ Reasonable alternatives to the procedure (if any)
■ Risks and benefits associated with not receiving the procedure (if any)
■ What is involved in the procedure?

Obtaining anesthesia informed consent includes:

■ Obtaining a separate consent for anesthesia
■ Discussing the indication, type of anesthesia, and method of administration; in addition, the consent for anesthesia should include potential benefits, risks, side effects, and reasonable alternatives to the procedure (if any)

Nursing responsibilities during informed consent:

■ Understand institutional policies and procedures for obtaining informed consent.
■ Identify and document the name of the person responsible for giving informed consent and their contact information in the chart.

■ Confirm that the person giving consent fully understands what they are consenting to.

● If the information is not understood, it is the responsibility of the nurse to notify the provider that more education regarding the procedure is needed.

FAMILY-CENTERED CARE

When a newborn infant is admitted to a NICU and needs to undergo surgery, it can be very scary and overwhelming to parents. Family-centered care focuses not only on the patient but the entire family. The family takes an active role in participating, decision-making, and advocating, which has been shown to improve safety as well as outcomes (Gephart & McGrath, 2012; McGrath & Vittner, 2020).

ENCOURAGING A FAMILY-CENTERED CARE ENVIRONMENT

■ Orient the patient and family to the hospital and NICU surroundings.

● Waiting room

● Self-care facilities (bathrooms, parents' rooms, laundry)

● Dining options, lactation services, rooms, and supplies

■ Orient them to available support services.

● Social worker

● Lactation

● Chaplain

● Center for families

■ Develop and maintain open and honest communication.

● Assist the family with establishing realistic expectations and goals about their infant's hospitalization as well as surgery. You may want to ask them, "What is your understanding of the surgical procedure and what will it achieve?"

● Describe the operating room (OR) procedures and postoperative course (cardiorespiratory needs, pain control, goals/expectations, expected time frame for the procedure; Curley et al., 2012, pp. 1133–1139).

● Empower parents to be involved as advocates for their infant.

* Involve the parents in decision-making for their newborn.

* Encourage the parents' presence on rounds.

— Rounding with the patient care team

* Encourage the parents' presence during procedures.

— Have a dedicated team member (family facilitator) available to explain what is taking place as it is happening.

— If parents are unable to stay or if they choose not to be present, then provide regular updates during the procedure.

■ Hold routine family meetings.

   ● Give scheduled updates.

   ● Include patient's current status, plan, or goals for the day, week, or month.

■ Use a team approach in meetings; include (if applicable):

   ● Surgeon

   ● Neonatologist

   ● Nurse practitioner

   ● Fellow or resident physicians

   ● Nurse

   ● Social worker

   ● Appropriate consulting team representatives

■ Allow time for questions.

   ● Describe what is known and not known.

   ● Encourage family members to voice concerns they have regarding their newborn.

■ Involvement and learning new skills

   ● On admission and throughout the hospitalization, assess the parents' readiness to learn new skills.

   ● Identify how the parents learn best.

      • Written information

      • Demonstration

      • Hands on

      • Reinforcement of new skills

   ● Anticipate which skills parent(s) will need when caring for their newborn following surgery.

      • Teach parent(s) in the care of their newborn and, when possible, have them participate in their infant's care (taking temperature, changing diaper, bathing/dressing, and feeding; Sprull, 2021).

FLUID AND ELECTROLYTE MANAGEMENT

Approximately 75% of the total body weight of the term infant consists of water and approximately 80% to 85% of the preterm infant's total body weight is water (O'Brien & Walker, 2014). The more premature the infant is, the greater the percentage of total body weight is water. Within the first week of life, the infant experiences a postnatal diuresis. During this diuresis, the term infant will typically lose 5% to 10% of their birthweight while the preterm infant will lose 10% to 20% (Lorenz, 1997). This diuresis consists of water and electrolyte losses, mainly sodium, potassium, and glucose (Snyder, 2015).

Demands on the infant transitioning to extrauterine life will affect fluid hemostasis and necessitate close monitoring of their fluid status. The need for surgery within this time frame will further complicate fluid and electrolyte management. Fluid homeostasis status is necessary to maintain good perfusion, prevent cellular damage, and avoid acidosis. Nurses must be vigilant with close monitoring of their patients' fluid balance in order to maintain homeostasis (Koletzko et al., 2005).

PERIOPERATIVE MAINTENANCE OF FLUID HOMEOSTASIS

■ Strictly monitor total fluid intake and output.

■ Consider the gestational age of the infant when determining their fluid needs (Davies et al., 2008).

● Premature infants experience increased insensible water losses (IWLs).

■ Assess risks for IWL.

● Decreased gestational age

● Environmental losses

● Body temperatures

● Skin breakdown or open wounds

● Congenital defects (tracheoesophageal fistula/esophageal atresia [TEF/EA], abdominal wall defects, bowel perforation)

● Open warmer (choose an isolette or similar containment to decrease IWL)

● Phototherapy

● Ventilator

• Humidity (decreases IWL)

● Maintain detailed calculation of all fluid losses.

• Urine

• Stool (diarrhea/ostomy)

• Nasogastric/orogastric (NG/OG) drainage

• Cerebrospinal fluid (CSF; ventricular drainage)

• Blood

POSTOPERATIVE ASSESSMENT OF FLUID AND ELECTROLYTE STATUS

Vigilant monitoring of fluid status should be done for every postoperative patient, inclusive of the following assessments:

■ Physical examination

■ Vital signs

■ Acid–base balance

■ Respiratory

  ● Inadequate oxygenation and ventilation can lead to a respiratory acidosis; monitor for:

    • Abdominal distention

    • Ascites

    • Fluid overload

■ Cardiac

  ● Poor tissue perfusion may cause acidosis; monitor for:

    • Low cardiac output

    • Sepsis

■ Renal

  ● Impaired renal function may lead to metabolic acidosis; monitor for:

    • Decreased output

    • Acute tubular necrosis (ATN)

    • Premature kidney

■ Weight

  ● Assess fluid gains/losses.

  ● Obtain daily weights for all stable postoperative patients (consider twice daily weights for infant with excessive fluid changes, especially premature infants).

■ Skin/mucosa

  ● Evaluate for dry mucous membranes, altered turgor, sunken fontanelle, and edema.

■ Cardiovascular

  ● Assess for tachycardia from too little extracellular fluid (hypovolemia) and/or anemia.

  ● Check for delayed capillary refill from low cardiac output.

    • Monitor for hypotension (later sign).

    • Use inotropes to support blood pressure with excessive losses.

■ Blood loss

  ● Estimate blood loss during procedure to assess for anemia.

    • Was it replaced in the OR?

    • Does the patient require further blood products?

    • Bleeding—is the patient continuing to bleed?

    • Monitor hematocrit and bleeding studies; transfuse as needed.

- Packed red blood cells (PRBCs)
- Platelets
- Fresh frozen plasma (FFP)
- Cryoprecipitate

■ Intake and output

● Perform close monitoring of maintenance fluid and total output.

● Conduct close monitoring of tube output from surgically placed drain(s).

  • Consider replacement of surgical drain/tube output if excessive (>2 mL/kg/hr).

  • Replacement fluids are given in addition to maintenance fluids.

    - Gastric losses: NG tube output, vomiting, gastrointestinal (GI) bleed

    - Drain losses: chest tube, Jackson–Pratt

    - Urinary losses

    - Stool output: dumping syndrome, diarrhea

    - Insensible losses: open wounds, exposed abdominal organs

  • Replacement fluid chosen is based on the type of fluid losses.

  • Fluid is typically replaced milliliter for milliliter, or a fraction of the total volume lost over a certain time period (4 or 8 hours).

  • Fluids typically used:

    - Normal saline (NS)

    - One half NS

    - Lactated Ringer's (caution must be taken because it does contain electrolytes but does not contain glucose)

      ○ Typically, fluid with potassium is not used due to the potential for hyperkalemia.

■ Nutritional requirements

● If the enteral feedings are delayed (for >48–72 hours), initiate parenteral nutrition and lipids as soon as possible (Koletzko et al., 2005).

● Determine feeding advancement plan if feeding via the enteral route.

■ Lab evaluation

● Serum electrolytes

● Urine output

● Urine electrolytes

● Blood urea/serum creatinine

● Arterial blood gas (ABG; low pH and bicarbonate may indicate poor perfusion)

● Develop routine schedule for laboratory studies (i.e., every 4, 8, or 24 hours).

- Notify prescriber of abnormal values (see Table 8.1 for normal values and causes of electrolyte imbalances) so that a treatment plan can be implemented.
  - Consider institutional variations among normative lab values.
  - Obtain a repeat sample if aberrant values do not fit with the patient's clinical status.
- Blood sampling of electrolytes and glucose
  - If laboratory values are abnormal, take the following into consideration:
    - A slow return of blood can yield false labs due to hemolysis or breakdown of red blood cells and release of electrolytes into serum.
    - Dextrose in the tubing of the line may cause a false elevation in blood glucose level

DOCUMENTATION

- Vital signs
- Accurate intake and output
- Tissue perfusion

TABLE 8.1 Electrolyte Abnormalities

Sodium	Normal Range	Hyponatremia	Hypernatremia
	135–145 mEq/mL	<135 mEq/mL Fluid losses Inadequate intake Third spacing	>145 mEq/mL Excessive fluid intake Sepsis Paralysis
Potassium	Normal Range	Hypokalemia	Hyperkalemia
	3.5–5.5 mEq/mL	<3.5 mEq/mL Fluid losses Nasogastric losses Inadequate supplementation	>5.5 mEq/mL Acidosis Excessive intake Renal failure
Glucose	Normal Range	Hypoglycemia	Hyperglycemia
	60–100 mg/dL	<60 mg/dL Inadequate intake Low glycogen stores (premature and intrauterine growth restricted [IUGR] infants) Diabetic mother (excessive production of insulin)	>100 mg/dL Extreme prematurity IUGR Stress Sepsis Steroids Excessive intake

■ Laboratory values and management of aberrant values
■ Symptoms of electrolyte depletion and abnormality

PAIN MANAGEMENT

Neonatal pain management has evolved tremendously over the past two decades. Pain assessment is now considered the fifth vital sign for all patients, including premature infants and neonates. Pain management for all infants requires a multimodal approach. The combination of nonpharmacologic and pharmacologic measures should be utilized to optimize the benefits to the patient while decreasing the total amount of opioids the patient will receive.

Nonpharmacologic Measures

■ Minimize exposure to painful or stressful procedures.
■ Provide opportunities for nonnutritive sucking.
■ Offer oral sucrose (24% solution).
■ Swaddle infant when condition permits.
■ Arrange for skin-to-skin contact (SSC) care sessions with parents.

Pharmacologic Measures

■ Nonnarcotic analgesics: acetaminophen, administered alone or as adjunct treatment
■ Opioids: such as morphine or fentanyl
■ Sedatives: for example, midazolam is a useful adjunct treatment; however, there are age restrictions on use, and prescribers are recommended to always address pain first

GOAL OF POSTOPERATIVE PAIN MANAGEMENT AND ASSESSMENT

The goal of postoperative pain management is to utilize the lowest amount of analgesia necessary to provide adequate pain relief while also minimizing the side effects of the agents (Walker, 2014). Pain management is a collaborative process that involves the nurse, anesthesiologist, surgeon, neonatologist, and the parents. Management of postoperative pain should begin preoperatively with a thoughtful discussion from all services and with the development of a pain management plan. When developing the pain management plan, consider the type of procedure, airway management, desired sedation, pain estimate, and previous opioid or benzodiazepine exposure. Establishment of the pain plan preoperatively allows for seamless pain management as soon as the patient returns from surgery.

PAIN ASSESSMENT SCALES

There are several reliable and valid pain assessment scales for the neonatal population (McNair et al., 2004; Suraseranivongse et al., 2006). The nurse should use the appropriate scale based on the age of the infant and the hospital's standard:

■ PIPP: premature infant pain profile (Stevens et al., 1996)
■ CRIES: crying, requires increased oxygen administration, increased vital signs, expression, and sleeplessness (Krechel & Bildner, 1995)
■ FLACC: face, legs, activity, cry, and consolability (Merkel et al., 1997)

POSTOPERATIVE PAIN PROTOCOLS

Standardized postoperative pain protocols should be established at institutions caring for the surgical infant. These protocols should include select opioids for minor surgical procedures or interventions as well as those for moderate-to-major surgical procedures. Minor surgical procedures may be treated with nonpharmacologic measures (i.e., sucrose, swaddling) to intermittent opioids (i.e., fentanyl or morphine). Major surgical procedures may be treated with intermittent or continuous opioids as well as sedatives depending on the extent of surgery and postoperative recovery required. (i.e., morphine, fentanyl, and midazolam infusion). More recently, there is a trend of utilizing benzodiazepine more sparingly and utilizing dexmedetomidine for increased sedation needs. Minor and major surgical procedures should be defined to standardize treatment for surgical procedures.

■ It is recommended that routine postoperative pain assessment occur with relative frequency, at a minimum every 1 to 4 hours.
■ If pharmacologic agents are used, reassessment should be completed within a short time of administration to ensure adequate pain relief is achieved (within 1 hour).
■ Epidurals are defined as regional anesthesia that numbs or blocks pain sensation/feeling in a certain part of the body.
■ Epidurals are managed by the anesthesia or pain team in the institution.
■ Common epidural anesthetics include:
  ● Chloroprocaine
■ Rarely used epidural anesthetics for patients who are younger than 1 month:
  ● Bupivacaine (rarely used in patients under a month of age)
  ● Ropivacaine (rarely used in patients under a month of age)
■ The addition of small amounts of fentanyl or clonidine has proven effective in enhancing the anesthetic effects in the epidural agents; however, use with caution due to their potential toxic effects (Krane, 2005)

TABLE 8.2 Medications Commonly Used in the Postoperative Phase

MEDICATION		ROUTE AND DOSING (LEXICOMP ONLINE, 2020)	PRIMARY SIDE EFFECTS CONSULT MEDICATION REFERENCE FOR FULL LIST OF SIDE EFFECTS	SPECIAL CONSIDERATIONS
CLASSIFICATION	NAME			
Sedative	Midazolam	**IV Bolus** 0.05–0.2 mg/kg **IV Continuous** 0.03–0.06 mg/kg/hr	Hypotension Respiratory insufficiency Bradycardia Tolerance and dependency	*Reversal agent:* Flumazenil *Avoid use of midazolam in premature infants <35 weeks* due to reduced clearance of the metabolites and seizure-like myoclonus
Analgesics	Morphine	**IV Bolus** 0.05–0.2 mg/kg/dose every 4 hours **IV Continuous** 0.01–0.02 mg/kg/hr	Urinary retention Seizures Tolerance and dependency	*Reversal agent:* Naloxone
	Fentanyl	**IV Bolus** 0.5–4 mcg/kg/dose every 2–4 hours **IV Continuous** 0.5–5 mcg/kg/hr	Chest wall rigidity (rapid administration)	*Reversal agent:* Naloxone Give IV slow push to avoid chest wall rigidity

(continued)

TABLE 8.2 Medications Commonly Used in the Postoperative Phase *(continued)*

MEDICATION		ROUTE AND DOSING (LEXICOMP ONLINE, 2020)	PRIMARY SIDE EFFECTS CONSULT MEDICATION REFERENCE FOR FULL LIST OF SIDE EFFECTS	SPECIAL CONSIDERATIONS
CLASSIFICATION	NAME			
	Acetaminophen	*Oral:* 10–15 mg/kg/dose every 4–6 hours *Rectal:* 10–20 mg/kg/dose every 4–6 hours		Adjunct for low to moderate pain to decrease total amount of overall opioids
	Sucrose	*Oral:* 1–10 dips on pacifier or 2 mL		Use for heel sticks, with starting IVs
Local anesthetic	LMX4 (lidocaine topical)	*Topical:* Apply 1 × 1 inch to intact skin 30 minutes prior to venipuncture or injection		Cover with bio-occlusive dressing Analgesia lasts 1 hr Do not exceed 2 g/24 hour

Source: Data from Lexicomp Online. (n.d.). *Welcome to Lexicomp Online.* Lexicomp Online Login. Accessed November 2020; Neofax®. 2021. https://www.micromedexsolutions.com/micromedex2/librarian/CS/115E30/ND_PR/evidencexpert/ND_P/evidencexpert/DUPLICATIONSHIELDSYNC/A8C00D/ND_PG/evidencexpert/ND_B/evidencexpert/ND_AppProduct/evidencexpert/ND_T/evidencexpert/PFActionId/evidencexpert.GoToNeofaxPediatricsAction?navitem=topNeoFaxID&isToolPage=true

■ Paravertebral catheters are thin catheters placed near the surgical incision site to provide continuous local anesthetic to the surgical area (i.e., thoracotomy).

● These catheters may remain in place for several days to optimize pain management and relief for the patient.

● Typically, these catheters are used in conjunction with other opioid and sedative medications to optimize the patients' comfort; this could decrease the total amount of opioid a patient receives postoperatively (Liu et al., 2006).

POSTOPERATIVE NURSING ASSESSMENT

■ Close monitoring of vital signs: Respiratory depression can be a common side effect (Table 8.2).

■ Monitor for toxicity.

■ Close monitoring of insertion site

■ Monitor for drainage: Leaking from the epidural catheter is common with epidurals.

■ Monitor comfort level of patient.

REFERENCES

Curley, M. A. Q., Meyer, E. C., Scoppettuolo, L. A., McGann, E. A., Trainor, B. P., Rachwal, C. M., & Hickey, P. A. (2012). Parent presence during invasive procedures and resuscitation. *American Journal of Respiratory and Critical Care Medicine, 186*(11), 1133–1139. https://doi.org/10.1164/rccm.201205-0915OC

Davies, P., Hall, T., Ali, T., & Lakhoo, K. (2008). Intravenous postoperative fluid prescriptions for children: A survey of practice. *BMC Surgery, 8*, 10. https://doi.org/10.1186/1471-2482-8-10

Gephart, S., & McGrath, J. (2012). Family-centered care of the surgical neonate. *Newborn Infant Nurse Review, 12*(1), 5–7. https://doi.org/10.1053/j.nainr.2011.12.002

Kelly, A., Liddell, M., & Davis, C. (2008). The nursing care of the surgical neonate. *Seminars in Pediatric Surgery, 17*(4), 290–296. https://doi.org/10.1053/j.sempedsurg.2008.07.008

Koletzko, B., Goulet, O., Hunt, J., Krohn, K., Shamir, R., Parenteral Nutrition Guidelines Working Group, European Society for Clinical Nutrition and Metabolism, European Society of Paediatric Gastroenterology, Hepatology and Nutrition, & European Society of Paediatric Research. (2005). Guidelines on paediatric parenteral nutrition of the European Society of Paediatric Gastroenterology, Hepatology and Nutrition (ESPGHAN) and the European Society for Clinical Nutrition and Metabolism (ESPEN), supported by the European Society of Paediatric Research (ESPR). *Journal of Pediatric Gastroenterology and Nutrition, 41*(Suppl. 2), S1–87. https://doi.org/10.1097/01.mpg.0000181841.07090.f4

Krane, E. (2005). *Pediatric pain management in children.* http://pedsanesthesia.stanford.edu/downloads/guideline-pain.pdf

Krechel, S. W., & Bildner, J. (1995). CRIES: A new neonatal postoperative pain measurement score. Initial testing of validity and reliability. *Paediatric Anaesthesia, 5*(1), 53–61. https://doi.org/10.1111/j.1460-9592.1995.tb00242.x

Lexicomp Online. (n.d.). *Welcome to Lexicomp Online.* Lexicomp Online Login, Last updated November 2020.

Liu, S. S., Richman, J. M., Thirlby, R. C., & Wu, C. L. (2006). Efficacy of continuous wound catheters delivering local anesthetic for postoperative analgesia: A quantitative and qualitative systematic review of randomized controlled trials. *Journal of the American College of Surgeons, 203*(6), 914–932. https://doi.org/10.1016/j.jamcollsurg.2006.08.007

Lorenz, J. (1997). Assessing fluid and electrolytes status in the newborn. *Clinical Chemistry, 43*(1), 205–210. https://doi.org/10.1093/clinchem/43.1.205

McGrath, J. M., & Vittner, D. (2020). Family: Essential partner in care. In C. Kenner, L. B. Altimier, & M. V. Boykova (Eds.), *Comprehensive neonatal nursing care* (6th ed., pp. 753–784). Springer Publishing Company.

McNair, C., Ballantyne, M., Dionne, K., Stephens, D., & Stevens, B. (2004). Postoperative pain assessment in the neonatal intensive care unit. *Archives of Disease in Childhood–Fetal and Neonatal Edition, 89*(6), F537–F541. https://doi.org/10.1136/adc.2003.032961

Merkel, S. I., Voepel-Lewis, T., Shayevitz, J. R., & Malviya, S. (1997). The FLACC: A behavioral scale for scoring postoperative pain in young children. *Pediatric Nursing, 23*(3), 293–297.

O'Brien, F., & Walker, I. A. (2014). Fluid hemostasis in the neonate. *Pediatric Anesthesia, 24,* 49–59. https://doi.org/10.1111/pan.12326

Snyder, C. (2015). *Fluid management for the pediatric surgical patient.* http://emedicine .medscape.com/article/936511-overview

Sprull, C. T. (2021). Developmental support. In M. T. Verklan, M. Walden, & S. Forrest (Eds.), *Core curriculum for neonatal intensive care nursing* (6th ed., pp. 172–190). Elsevier Saunders.

Stevens, B., Johnston, C., Petryshen, P., & Taddio, A. (1996). Premature infant pain profile: Development and initial validation. *Clinical Journal of Pain, 12*(1), 13–22. https://doi .org/10.1097/00002508-199603000-00004

Sudia, T., & Catlin, A. (2021). Ethical issues. In M. T. Verklan, M. Walden, & S. Forest (Eds.), *Core curriculum for neonatal intensive care nursing* (6th ed., pp. 714–719). Elsevier Saunders.

Suraseranivongse, S., Kaosaard, R., Pornsiriprasert, S., Karnchana, Y., Kaopinpruck, J., & Sangjeen, K. (2006). A comparison of postoperative pain scales in neonates. *British Journal of Anaesthesia, 97*(4), 540–544. https://doi.org/10.1093/bja/ael184

Walker, S. (2014). Neonatal pain. *Paediatric Anaesthesia, 24*(1), 39–48. https://doi .org/10.1111/pan.12293

SURGICAL DRAINS, TUBES, LINES, AND AIRWAY SECUREMENT

CAITLIN BRADLEY

ABDOMINAL DRAINS

Abdominal drains are soft, flexible drains inserted into the peritoneal space for evacuation of pneumoperitoneum, excess fluids, and/or infectious material identified on one or more radiographic studies.

Clinical Indications

Designed to drain the peritoneal cavity of free air, excess fluids, and infectious material; abdominal drains can be used for infants of all gestations. These tubes can be used in very premature infants that are too unstable for transport to the operating room (OR), or for infants with significant ascites or abscesses.

Critically ill very preterm infants with spontaneous intestinal perforation (SIP) or necrotizing enterocolitis (NEC) may benefit from drain placement either as the only treatment or a temporizing intervention to stabilize the infant until they can be taken to the OR for a surgical intervention (Nandivanda & Puder, 2016).

Preoperative Assessment and Nursing Care

■ Perform abdominal radiograph and/or ultrasound (US) prior to drain placement.

■ Ensure infants receive no enteral feedings for 4 to 6 hours prior to placement.

■ Place peripheral IV line.

■ Begin maintenance IV fluids.

■ Confirm the parent or guardian has given informed consent.

■ Obtain blood type, crossmatch, complete blood count (CBC), coagulation studies, and serum electrolytes.

Placement

■ Abdominal drains are placed by surgeons or interventional radiologists (IRs).

● They can be placed at the bedside, which is an advantage for an unstable infant.

Postoperative Assessment and Nursing Care

■ Collecting drainage

● If a penrose type drain is placed for management of SIP or NEC, allow drainage to flow into the gauze or a diaper.

● Other types of peritoneal drains must have a drainage system attached that ensures sterility of the drain, drainage system, and peritoneal cavity.

■ Describe and measure drainage for accurate intake and output.

■ Monitor the appearance and position of the drain and alert surgeons if the drain moves in position.

■ No enteral feedings should be given in the immediate postoperative period; the recommended time for holding enteral feedings depends on the condition being treated.

■ Administer antibiotic treatment for coverage of known or suspected intra-abdominal processes and skin flora.

■ Consider providing parenteral nutrition after an evaluation of nutritional needs based on the infant's gestational age and the length of time that enteral feedings are going to be held.

● Preterm infants should receive parenteral nutrition if the infant does not receive enteral nutrition ≥3 days (Hansen & Belfort, 2016).

● Term infants should receive parenteral nutrition if the infant does not receive enteral nutrition ≥5 days (Hansen & Belfort, 2016).

Documentation

■ Location of the drain(s)

■ Appearance of the skin integrity around the drain site

■ Presence and integrity of sutures, if applicable

■ Presence and integrity of the sterile, transparent dressing, if applicable

■ Appearance and quantity of drainage at the drain site or from the drain

CENTRAL VENOUS CATHETERS

Central venous catheters (CVCs) are IV catheters placed in large veins, such as the internal and external jugular, saphenous, femoral, and subclavian. CVCs should be considered in the following patient scenarios: need for long-term IV access (>1–2 weeks), infusion of hyperosmolar solutions (such as dextrose 25% and/or dopamine), poor vascular access, ongoing hemodynamic monitoring, and failed placement of peripheral-inserted central catheter (PICC; Hansen et al., 2016).

Clinical Indications

■ A vascular access decision-making algorithm can be an objective aid when determining the most appropriate CVC.

■ Consider the patient's condition, duration of therapy, specific procedure requirements, and history of vascular access challenges when choosing the appropriate CVC device.

Preoperative Assessment and Nursing Care

■ Confirm the parent or guardian has given consent.

  ● Obtain surgical and/or anesthesia team consent(s).

■ Secure peripheral IV access for infusion of maintenance fluids and medications prior to and during the procedure.

■ Assess CBC and coagulation tests for risk of bleeding.

■ Evaluate the patient for signs of infection.

  ● Blood cultures should be negative for at least 48 hours if the infant is being treated for an infection; this decreases the risk of seeding the new CVC with infectious material or infectious debris.

■ Ensure no enteral feedings have been given 4 to 6 hours prior to CVC placement.

Surgical Procedure

■ Common CVCs used in the NICU include lines placed in the upper chest, neck, or femoral area.

- Decisions around the location of CVC placement are complex and depend on the infant, their condition, the indications for the CVC, and more.

- Some sources suggest avoiding femoral vein placement due to a higher risk for infection (Young & You, 2020).

■ When deciding on a single, double, or triple lumen CVC, consider the size of the vessel and the patient's needs (infusions, medications, etc.).

■ CVCs may be nontunneled or tunneled (Hansen et al., 2016):

- Nontunneled CVCs are placed percutaneously and often sutured into place.

  - Nontunneled CVCs are meant for short-term access (typically <2 weeks); these types of catheters tend to be less flexible and lack the decreased thrombogenicity that tunneled CVCs offer.

- Tunneled CVCs follow a subcutaneous tunnel between the catheterized veins to the exit site located on the skin and are frequently placed in the upper chest or neck.

  - Tunneled CVCs are typically used for longer term access, as they are more pliable, are at decreased risk for infection, and have less thrombogenicity.

  - In addition to the external sutures remaining in place, the internal cuff of the CVC becomes fixated into the infant's subcutaneous tissue, thus enhancing the line's stability (Hansen et al., 2016).

Postoperative Assessment and Nursing Care

Confirmation of Placement

■ Confirm placement of the CVC with a prescriber, using a chest radiograph, prior to use.

- Ensure the transparent dressing is occlusive and intact.

  - Secure the CVC with a chevron loop.

■ Ideal positioning:

- A CVC placed in the upper body is considered central if the tip resides at the distal superior vena cava (SVC) or the SVC and the right atrium junction (Hansen et al., 2016).

- A CVC placed in the lower body is considered central if it resides within the inferior vena cava (IVC; Hansen et al., 2016).

- Caution should be exercised when CVCs terminate in the right atrium, as significant complications such as pericardial effusion may arise.

■ Repositioning of CVCs that terminate in the right atrium is recommended.

Dressing the Central Venous Catheter

■ CVC dressings

- A sterile, occlusive, transparent dressing is required to minimize the risk for infection and to allow for visualization of the insertion site.

■ Continually assess the insertion site for swelling, drainage, leakage, and erythema.

■ Change the dressing weekly or more frequently if it becomes nonocclusive or soiled.

- Nonsutured PICC dressings do not need to be changed regularly; these are only changed when soiled or nonocclusive (Hansen et al., 2016).

■ Assess for pain, dislodgement, and other complications (discussed later in this section) hourly or more frequently.

Blood Sampling

■ Follow individual, institutional evidence-based policies for accessing the CVC for blood sampling.

■ General procedures for accessing the CVC for blood sampling include:

- Consider the CVC infusion to determine if they can be interrupted to obtain the blood sample and also if the infusion will impact the sample results.

- Pause infusion(s) for 1 minute prior to obtaining a blood sample to ensure accuracy of the specimen, if the line has a continuous infusion.

- Perform hand hygiene and don clean gloves.

- Clean the hub with an approved antiseptic agent such as alcohol or chlorhexidine pads, scrubbing the hub for 15 (for alcohol) or 30 seconds (for chlorhexidine), and allow to dry.

- Flush the CVC with 1 to 3 mL normal saline (NS) or ½ NS in a pulsating manner.

  - The solution used for flushing is dependent on the gestational age and serum sodium level of the infant.

  - The volume of the flush is dependent upon the size of the catheter and fluid goals for the patient.

  - Withdraw 1 to 3 mL of blood (referred to as waste).

    − Depending on the catheter size and hospital policy, you may or may not return this waste.

    − If returning the waste, ensure the sterility of the syringe during the blood draw and throughout the procedure.

- Slowly withdraw your sample, removing the minimum amount of blood needed for the desired laboratory study(s).
  - Return waste (when applicable) after cleaning the hub (as mentioned earlier) and allow it to dry.
  - Return the waste to the infant slowly.
- Clean the hub again, and allow it to dry.
- Flush the tubing with ½ NS or NS in a pulsating manner.
- Reconnect to IV tubing and resume infusions, if applicable.

Complications

CVC line days, sedation/paralysis, and exposure to multiple surgical procedures all increase the incidence of CVC complications (Bairdain et al., 2014). Patients should be continually assessed for readiness to remove CVCs.

Infection

■ Bacterial infection is a major risk of CVC placement; it requires vigilant monitoring for signs and symptoms.

● Cellulitis: Continually assess the insertion site for signs of localized infection, including erythema, swelling, and drainage.

● Central line-associated bloodstream infection (CLABSI): Continually assess the patient for signs of systemic infection that include escalation in respiratory support, pallor, increase in apnea/bradycardia/desaturations, fever, feeding intolerance, and other changes in vital signs such as temperature instability and hypotension.

■ If local/skin infection (cellulitis) or CLABSI is suspected:

● Obtain a CBC.

● Determine the infection source by obtaining both peripheral and CVC line cultures.

■ Other specimens are collected based on the infant's signs and symptoms of infection (tracheal, urine, cerebral spinal fluid, and wound, for example).

● Carefully label specimens for precise diagnostics.

● Administer prescribed broad-spectrum antibiotics after cultures are drawn for symptomatic infants.

● Narrow or revise antibiotic coverage when cultures yield an organism.

● Discontinue antibiotics if infection is ruled out.

▪ Minimize infection risk by securing the CVC hub and IV tubing directed toward the head of the patient and never secure the CVC tubing in or around the diaper area (Hansen et al., 2016).

Malposition

▪ Malposition is defined as the accidental entrance or migration of the CVC into an anatomical area it was not intended to enter.

● Malposition can lead to pneumothorax, hemothorax, and/or cardiac tamponade depending on the location of the migrated catheter.

● Diagnose with chest radiograph, echocardiogram, and/or US.

● Removal of the line may be needed along with treatment for related complications.

• Treatment of related complications depends on the clinical scenario and infant's condition.

• Assess for symptoms of malposition, including pain when infusing, tachypnea, bradycardia, respiratory distress, hypoxia, ventilation/perfusion (VQ) mismatch, and hypotension.

Hemothorax

▪ Hemothorax is caused by atrial trauma during insertion leading to a blood collection in the pleural space.

▪ Assess for and report symptoms of respiratory distress.

Cardiac Tamponade

▪ Cardiac tamponade occurs when blood or fluid accumulates around the pericardium; this collection prevents effective contraction of the ventricles and leads to lack of proper oxygen delivery to tissues.

▪ Signs include findings of tachypnea, bradycardia, respiratory distress, hypoxia, VQ mismatch, and hypotension, along with venous engorgement of the face and neck, paradoxical pulse, and cardiac arrest.

Arrhythmia

▪ Arrythmia is an abnormal heart rhythm caused by malposition, typically in the atria.

▪ Reposition the CVC and obtain x-ray confirmation.

▪ Perform hemodynamic monitoring until the arrhythmia subsides and the line is repositioned or removed.

Venous Thrombosis

■ A venous thrombosis results from a fibrin clot formation surrounding the tip of the CVC.

■ Removal of the line and anticoagulation may be necessary depending on the size of the clot, the risks associated with dislodgement, and organs/tissues impacted by the clot.

Superior Vena Cava Syndrome

■ This syndrome results from an obstruction to venous drainage from the SVC, due to thrombosis or a CVC that fills the vessel.

■ Treat by raising the head of the bed, monitoring respiratory status, and considering/alleviating the cause such as removal of the CVC or exchanging for a smaller lumen CVC.

Catheter Occlusion

■ Cather occlusion occurs from blockage of fluids from infusing and inability to withdraw blood from the CVC.

■ Ensure that the entire length of the CVC tubing external to the patient is not kinked or clamped.

■ Restore patency of the occluded CVC lumen:

  ● Utilize a sterile technique, remove the injection cap, and try gently flushing the line with a small amount of NS.

■ Consult the prescriber if patency cannot be restored with these measures.

  ● Type of solution instilled to restore patency may depend on the type of fluids and/or medications infusing.

  ● Tissue plasminogen activator (TPA) is one of the medications instilled in the event of an occlusion.

  ● Instill this solution using sterile technique:

    • Use only enough to fill the volume of the catheter, as more would lead to undesired systemic effects.

    • Leave the solution to dwell in the catheter for the prescribed time (usually 30–60 minutes).

    • Aspirate the solution following the desired dwell time.

  ● Check for patency by attempting to flush the line (Hansen et al., 2016).

■ Consider removing the CVC if attempts to establish patency are not successful.

Documentation

- Size of the catheter and priming volume (this should be recorded in the operative note)
- Hourly site assessments for erythema, drainage, and swelling
- Dressing integrity (should be occlusive, clean, dry, and intact)
- Length of external visible catheter to recognize migration of the catheter during routine daily assessments

CHEST TUBES

Chest tubes can be made of silicone or polyvinyl chloride (PVC); they come in varying sizes, including the small-bore pigtail catheter type. Chest tubes are used during surgical procedures to treat isolated pneumothoraces and to drain the chest of fluids such as chylous fluid, blood, esophageal leakage, and many more conditions.

- The benefits to pigtail catheters include reduced pain; however, their small bore makes drainage of viscous or proteinaceous fluids difficult.

Clinical Indications

There are many clinical indications for chest tube placement, including drainage of both air and fluids from the pleural and extrapleural cavities. Chest tubes are often placed during operative procedures involving the chest and esophagus, including patent ductus arteriosus (PDA) ligation, esophageal atresia (EA), tracheoesophageal fistula (TEF), congenital diaphragmatic hernia (CDH), chylothorax, and pneumothoraces that occur as a result of the operative procedure.

The size and type of the chest tube used are dependent on the patient size, goals of treatment, and anticipated drainage. For example, a 10 or 12 French catheter may be placed for a full-term patient with a chylothorax. A smaller chest tube, such as 8 French, can be used to drain pneumothoraces for a preterm infant following PDA ligation (Ringer, 2016).

Preoperative Assessment and Nursing Care

- Conduct a complete respiratory assessment.
- Develop a plan for pain management.
- Perform other preoperative assessments and nursing care relevant to the infant's clinical condition and diagnosis.
- Select the chest drainage system to be used postoperatively.

Surgical Procedure

- Chest tubes are placed by trained providers under sterile conditions.
- The infant should be given an opioid prior to and during placement, for pain control.

■ A lidocaine injection may also be given for local analgesia

■ The infant should be positioned with the side of placement up and the head of the bed elevated to 30° to 45° to facilitate evacuation of air.

■ The entire area should be cleaned by the provider according to institutional policies and procedures.

■ To avoid injury to the nipple, muscle, and major blood vessels, the chest tube is placed at the anterior axillary line, fourth intercostal space.

■ US may be used for placement guidance, and a radiograph confirms placement.

■ The chest tube must be immediately connected to the drainage system to prevent backflow of air or fluid into the pleural space (see text that follows for the postoperative placement instructions; Ringer, 2016).

■ Confirmation of chest tube placement is via a chest radiograph.

Drainage of Air

■ The smallest possible chest tube size should be used to evacuate air; 8 French is used for extremely low-birthweight infants and 10 or 12 French for near-term or term infants.

■ If the chest tube is inserted to relieve a pneumothorax, there will potentially be a rush of air.

■ The intended positioning of the chest tube is anterior to facilitate air drainage.

Drainage of Fluid

■ Large bore chest tubes are used for evacuation of fluid (blood, chylous, or other forms of fluid exudate).

■ There potentially will be fluid material in the chest tube upon insertion.

■ If the chest tube is inserted to remove fluid, the intended positioning may be posterior to draining fluid material (Ringer, 2016).

Chest Tube Securement and Dressing

■ Chest tubes are sutured in place for stabilization.

■ The use of a petroleum gauze dressing forms a secure seal around the tube insertion site.

■ The site is then covered with dry gauze.

■ A transparent, occlusive dressing is placed to cover the entire site.

Postoperative Assessment and Nursing Care

■ Secure the chest tube, immediately following placement, with tape just outside of the dressing for stabilization using a chevron-style method.

■ Use a small piece of tape (about 2 inches long) wrapped around the tubing to form a tab or anchor.

■ Utilize a pin or another securement to attach the anchor to the patient's bedding to prevent accidental dislodgement.

■ Moving methodically, in order from the patient to the drainage system, ensure connection of the chest tube to the drainage system.

● Inspect the chest tube at the site: For proper drainage of air or fluid, ensure the holes for drainage are not protruding from the incision.

● Inspect the dressing; petroleum gauze should encircle the chest tube at the incision site, and the dressing should be occlusive.

● Ensure the chest tube is connected securely to the drainage system.

● A Christmas tree–style adaptor is sometimes needed to form a secure attachment between the chest tube and tubing from the drainage apparatus.

● Evaluate for any escape of air, fluid, or other drainages at all connections.

■ Consult with the provider to determine the level of suction; generally, it is set between 15 and 20 cm H_2O, negative pressure (Ringer, 2016).

● For postoperative patients and patients on extracorporeal membrane oxygenation (ECMO), less negative pressure may be used to avoid damage and/or hemorrhage.

■ Provide adequate pain management.

● For silicone or PVC catheters:

• Consider administering continuous opioid drips (morphine or fentanyl).

• If properly managed, low doses can be effective.

• Bolus doses of opioids should be administered during hands-on care.

● For pigtail catheters

• Each patient's pain should be evaluated and addressed on an individual basis.

• Continuous drips may be used, but they may not be needed for the entire length of time the pigtail is indwelling.

■ Removal of the chest tube

● A trained provider removes the chest tube.

● Removal should be considered when there is no further air or fluid evacuated for approximately 24 to 48 hours (Ringer, 2016).

• An exception is with EA repairs (see section on "Surgical Disorders of the Trachea and Esophagus" for details regarding management of chest tubes with this patient population).

- When no air or fluid is drained, the chest tube will remain in place, but the suction is turned to 0 cm H_2O; this is called placing the chest tube to water seal.
  - If the patient demonstrates respiratory distress or other symptoms of re-accumulation of air or fluid, a chest radiograph should be obtained and the negative pressure suction may be resumed.
- Obtain a chest radiograph prior to removal of the chest tube to ensure there has been no re-accumulation of air or fluid.
- Administer an opioid prior to chest tube removal to ensure proper pain control.
- Remove the chest tube upon inspiration if the patient is on continuous positive airway pressure (CPAP) or intubated on a ventilator.
- Remove the chest tube upon expiration if the patient is spontaneously breathing and not intubated or on CPAP (Ringer, 2016).
- Close a large wound with a single suture (Ringer, 2016) or sterile adhesive strips.
- Place a petroleum gauze dressing over the incision site immediately after removal, followed by a gauze sponge and transparent occlusive dressing.
  - This dressing is left in place for at least 24 hours, as instructed by the provider.

Documentation

- Respiratory assessment
- Chest tube site and dressing integrity
- Goals of the chest tube and progress toward removal
- Specific characteristics
  - Type and amount of drainage
  - Amount of suction
- Patient tolerance to the chest tube
- Pain medication requirements and response
- Untoward respiratory symptoms prior to, during, and following removal

FEEDING TUBES

Surgically placed gastric or gastrointestinal feeding tubes are utilized when patients are unable to feed orally, and nasal or oral feeding tubes are not an option or adequate to meet the patient's needs. The patient's diagnosis, clinical condition, and feeding tolerance are taken into consideration when deciding to place a feeding tube surgically. This section describes the care and management of surgically placed gastrostomy (G-tubes) and gastrojejunal (GJ) feeding tubes for the delivery of enteral nutrition.

GASTROSTOMY TUBES

Surgically placed gastrointestinal feeding tubes are used for a variety of purposes, but generally are meant to provide enteral nutrition, fluids and/or medications, and gastric decompression for infants with a variety of clinical conditions (i.e., risk of aspiration, including vocal cord paralysis; discoordination in suck, swallow, and breathe; muscle weakness; airway or gastrointestinal [GI] anomalies [microgastria]; oral aversion; neurologic or metabolic conditions; congenital heart disease; congenital syndromes EA and TEF; and prolonged ileus; Duro et al., 2016).

Clinical Indications

■ Inability to orally consume sufficient calories for growth and hydration
■ Inability to safely feed or take medications orally

Preoperative Assessment and Nursing Care

Obtain History

■ Obtain a complete history of the presenting problem from the parent(s) or caregivers.

● Document a history of vomiting/reflux.

■ Assess growth (anthropometric measurements, including weight, head circumference, and length).

● In general, infants should be more than 2 kg before having their gastric or gastrointestinal tube surgically placed; this will decrease the potential for surgical complications.

■ Evaluate ability to orally feed at bedside and/or via swallow study.

● There are two types of swallow studies: conventional and modified barium swallow (MBS).

● Both are fluoroscopic evaluations of the infant's swallow, as well as presence or absence of aspiration (Duro et al., 2016).

● The conventional swallow study provides additional information about the esophageal and gastric anatomy and should be chosen when there is concern for TEF and/or EA, or an obstruction (Duro et al., 2016).

■ Obtain a chest radiograph if there is a new suspected case of aspiration or in the event of chronic aspiration.

■ Assess the adequacy of home resources and supports.

Perform Examination

■ Evaluate the gag reflex in neurologically compromised and hypotonic infants.

■ Assess signs and symptoms consistent with lung or heart disease.

■ Appraise primitive reflexes prior to any oral feeding, including rooting and sucking.

■ Monitor coordination of suck, swallow, and breathe during feedings.

● If there are concerns and/or signs of discoordinated feeding and/or aspiration, speech therapists or occupational therapists can be of great assistance in evaluating an infant's feeding skills and safety.

Secure Laboratory Evaluation

■ Obtain nutrition labs: CBC with differential, electrolytes, calcium, phosphorous, albumin/total protein, and liver function tests (LFTs) and assess for abnormalities.

● Laboratory studies may reveal a specific disorder.

● Genetic and neurologic studies are sent when there is a suspicion for a specific disorder.

Preoperative Readiness

■ Choose the correct feeding tube in consultation with neonatology, nursing, surgery, gastroenterology, radiology, and speech therapy as applicable.

■ No enteral feedings should be given for 4 to 6 hours prior to placement of the feeding tube; consult institutional policies regarding when to hold feeds preoperatively.

■ The infant will need IV access, either peripheral IV (PIV), PICC, or CVC.

■ Infuse maintenance IV fluids.

■ Ensure that informed consents have been signed.

Surgical Procedure

G-Tube

There are several techniques used in placing a G-tube. Techniques include percutaneous endoscopic gastrostomy (PEG) placement, Stamm (open) gastrostomy, laparoscopic gastrostomy, or Seldinger technique (placed by interventional radiology).

The Seldinger and PEG procedures are the least invasive, the laparoscopic slightly more invasive, and the Stamm is the most invasive G-tube placement method (Duro et al., 2016).

■ G-tubes are placed by surgeons, gastroenterologists, and/or interventional radiologists who have training in surgical feeding tube placement.

■ G-tubes will have two ports: one for feeding and the other to inflate and deflate the balloon.

● Depending on the brand and type of the G-tube, there may also be a port for medication administration.

Postoperative Assessment and Nursing Care

G-Tube Management

■ Place the G-tube to drain while any postoperative ileus resolves.

● Minimal drainage may be expected and is typically serosanguinous or clear.

● Some bilious drainage may be observed if there is a temporary ileus.

● If there is no drainage after 4 to 6 hours, clamp or disconnect from drainage for several hours prior to enteral feeding.

■ Irrigate the G-tube with NS or sterile water to ensure patency; if unable to withdraw the irrigant, notify a nurse practitioner (NP), medical doctor (MD), or surgeon.

■ Achieve pain control through the use of opioids in conjunction with acetaminophen.

■ Prophylactic antibiotics may be prescribed and given for 24 hours.

■ Ensure securement of the G-tube to facilitate normal healing of the G-tube tract.

● There are two types of G-tube securement: external and internal.

• External securement on the abdomen with medical tape is done for at least 6 weeks to avoid tract enlargement and dislodgement (from movement of the tube).

– If a flange or disk is present, external securement is achieved by stabilizing the flange or disk onto the abdomen.

• Internal securement such as a balloon or bolster is used for internal stabilization on some G-tubes.

■ Place a hydrocolloid wound dressing between skin and tape, taking care to avoid excessive traction if there is skin breakdown or irritation.

● Excessive traction can affect the healing and may cause leakage around the G-tube site.

■ Check balloon inflation weekly, on a consistent day of the week.

- Balloons may have different volumes; during each check, aspirate the fluid from the balloon and ensure it is the correct amount (found in the operative note).
- If there is a discrepancy in volume, there may be a mechanical issue with the tube and the surgeon should be notified.

■ Assess for gastric content or feeding residuals by gently aspirating stomach contents via the G-tube.

■ Flush the G-tube.

- This maintains patency and ensures proper delivery of feedings, fluids, and medications.
- Flush both ports, twice daily and as prescribed.
- Use warm water (sterile water is used with immune-compromised infants).

■ Vent the G-tube between feedings to decrease the risk for reflux and/or aspiration, and to alleviate gastric distention when infants are on noninvasive ventilation.

Feedings

■ Administer bolus or continuous feedings via G-tubes after a period of observation following surgery and approved by the surgeon.

- If the infant has tolerated bolus feedings, they should be resumed after G-tube placement.

Dressings, Bathing, and Skin Care

■ Change dressings once or twice per day depending on drainage, redness, and irritation at the site.

■ Inspect the peristomal site, noting the site's integrity, erythema, and drainage.

■ Cleanse skin with saline, water, or mild soap and warm (not hot) water to clear drainage or crusting.

■ Dry the skin before reapplying the dressing.

■ Apply a split 2- × 2-inch gauze around the insertion site.

- Small amounts of drainage are appropriate.
- Consider using an absorbent dressing to wick moisture away from the skin.
- Drainage and skin irritation may indicate leakage of gastric contents onto skin.
- Reassess tube stabilization and the balloon inflation if leakage occurs.
  - Leakage could be due to inadequate balloon volume.
  - Check balloon volume and add appropriate fluid if needed and consider replacing the tube if balloon leakage is noted.

■ Resume tub baths for stable infants on postoperative day (POD) 7 if the site is healing well.

■ Notify providers of complications.

● Complications that occur within 2 weeks of placement include cellulitis, colonic perforation, duodenal hematoma, bleeding necrotizing fasciitis, and gastric outlet obstruction.

● Late complications include cellulitis, gastrocolic fistula, worsening reflux, perforation, granulation tissue, excessive leaking at the site, and buried bolster within the ostomy tract or gastric mucosa (Duro et al., 2016).

Dislodgement

■ Never try to reinsert the G-tube that dislodges.

● Without proper training, the individual attempting to replace the G-tube may incorrectly place the G-tube outside of the stomach or disrupt the tract.

■ A well-lubricated, flexible catheter (such as a red rubber tube or Foley catheter) that is either the same or smaller diameter as the dislodged G-tube can be placed in the tract to maintain patency (Duro et al., 2016).

● Less than 12 weeks postoperatively: Care must be sought promptly as the site may constrict quickly.

● Greater than 12 weeks postoperatively: Care must be sought quickly, but the risk of site constriction is less likely.

Occlusion

■ Milk or flush the tubing with 5 to 10 mL warm water or NS tubing if occlusion in the tubing is noted.

■ Establish patency by contacting a prescriber to order an enzymatic solution to manage an obstruction not relieved with an NS or water flush.

■ Replace the tube if patency is not achieved via flush or the administration of an enzymatic solution.

■ Consider causes (incompatibility, flushing frequency, thick formula) of occlusion when patency is reestablished.

■ Prevent future occlusion through anticipatory guidance.

Skin Breakdown

■ Check for leakage at the site.

● Application of a colloidal oatmeal soak or acetic acid–aluminum acetate solution can decrease moisture at the site.

■ Infection (cellulitis) is treated with antibiotics specific to the organism.

Worsening Reflux

■ G-tube placement may result in worse symptoms of reflux.

■ If reflux worsens following G-tube placement, lengthening the feeding time may improve symptoms.

■ Conversion to a postpyloric feeding tube can be considered if reflux is severe and noninvasive methods do not alleviate the symptoms.

Bleeding

■ Assess for granulation tissue and skin integrity.

● Ensure there is not excessive traction on the tube.

● Manage granulomas as described in the text that follows.

Granulation

■ Movement of the G-tube can lead to development of granulation tissue.

■ Treatment of granulation tissue

■ If small, consider preventative care through minimizing tube movement.

● Triamcinolone cream 0.5% applied three times daily for 7 to 10 days has been shown to decrease the granuloma size.

● If large and bleeding, cauterization of the granuloma is performed daily with silver nitrate sticks until granuloma is flat.

 * Apply a petrolatum ointment barrier to protect surrounding skin when treating with silver nitrate.

 * Cauterized granuloma tissue will turn gray or black during treatment.

Other Rare Complications

■ Early onset but less prevalent G-tube complications include colonic perforation, duodenal hematoma, and necrotizing fasciitis (Duro et al., 2016).

● These would manifest as abdominal distention, tenderness, discoloration of the abdomen, and other signs consistent with sepsis.

● A surgeon should be notified if these complications are suspected.

■ Late onset, less prevalent complications include gastrocolic fistula (Duro et al., 2016).

● Presenting symptoms include abdominal pain, diarrhea, and vomiting.

● A surgeon should be notified if this condition is suspected.

Documentation

■ Include G-tube type, length, and diameter

■ Type of securement(s)

■ Dressing applied

■ Amount of fluid to fill the balloon

■ Date balloon is due for a fluid check

■ Peristomal and stomal appearance

■ Presence of leakage

■ Presence of granuloma, including size and location in clock hours and treatment

GASTROJEJUNAL TUBES

Surgically placed GJ tubes are used for a variety of purposes but generally are meant to provide enteral nutrition, fluids and/or medications, and gastric decompression for infants with certain clinical conditions (i.e., due to risk of aspiration, including vocal cord paralysis, discoordination of suck, swallow, and breathe, and muscle weakness; and airway or GI anomalies [microgastria], oral aversion, neurologic or metabolic conditions, congenital heart disease, congenital syndromes EA and TEF, and prolonged ileus) who are unable to tolerate gastric feeding (Duro et al., 2016).

Clinical Indications

Postpyloric feedings are indicated for infants with the following situations:

■ Unable to tolerate nasogastric (NG), orogastric (OG), or G-tube feedings

■ High risk of aspiration

■ Delayed gastric emptying

■ Dysmotility with risk of reflux and aspiration

■ Anatomic abnormalities, such as microgastria

Preoperative Assessment and Nursing Care

Many preoperative evaluations take place to determine the necessity and appropriateness of a GJ tube. Consultation with neonatology, nursing, surgery, gastroenterology, radiology, and speech therapy is needed. Discussion with family or guardians throughout the process must take place, as well as evaluation of home resources.

Prior to placement, infants should have no enteral feedings for 4 to 6 hours, a peripheral IV should be placed, maintenance fluids should be infusing, and consents should be signed.

Evaluation frequently includes similar components such as described in the G-tube placement section. The preoperative assessment and care presented here are specific for management of GJ tubes.

History

■ Assess growth and ability to orally feed and tolerate gastric feedings.

● Anthropometric measurements (weight, head circumference, and length)

● In general, infants should be more than 2 kg before having their surgical feeding tube placed to decrease the potential for surgical complications.

■ Obtain a chest radiograph if there are new suspected aspiration events or in the event of chronic aspiration.

■ Evaluate for a history of vomiting/reflux.

Examination

■ Evaluation of a gag reflex is critical in neurologically compromised and hypotonic infants.

● Infants with a lack of a gag reflex are at extremely high risk for aspiration and have limited or no ability to coordinate suck/swallow/breathe.

■ Assess for the presence of signs consistent with lung or heart disease, especially if exacerbated by reflux and aspiration.

■ Evaluate for uncoordinated feeding ability and risk for reflux/aspiration using a modified barium swallow study.

■ Measure stomach clearance with a gastric emptying study when concerned for delayed emptying.

■ Perform an evaluation of an infant's feeding skills using experts from speech or occupational therapy.

Laboratory Evaluation

■ Obtain ordered labs for genetic and neurologic studies (specific to suspected disorder) and nutritional labs: CBC with differential, electrolytes, calcium, phosphorous, albumin, total protein, and LFTs.

● Laboratory studies will most likely be normal, but in the event of a specific disorder, they can help establish the etiology of the infant's oral feeding ability or inability.

Surgical Procedure

■ GJ tube placement is done after the G-tube is placed.

■ The J-portion is advanced through the G-tube, under fluoroscopy, and into the jejunum.

● Placement is confirmed with contrast imaging in the OR or in interventional radiology.

Postoperative Assessment and Nursing Care

GJ Tube Management

Surgically placed GJ tubes have a G, J, and balloon port.

■ Leave the gastric port to gravity and clamp the jejunal portion for 6 to 8 hours in the immediate postoperative period.

● This is done to avoid vomiting and aspiration due to temporary ileus.

■ Monitor for drainage from the G-tube port.

● Minimal drainage is expected.

● Drainage is typically serosanguinous or clear.

● Some bilious drainage may be observed if there is a temporary ileus or due to consistent stenting of the pylorus.

• Report bilious drainage to the surgeon; this may be expected, but comprehensive assessment is required to rule out an intestinal obstruction.

• Excessive bilious drainage may need to be replaced in the setting of electrolyte abnormalities, diminished urine output, or other signs of fluid and electrolyte imbalance.

■ Irrigate the G-tube port with NS (sterile water should be used with immunocompromised patients) to ensure patency.

● If unable to withdraw irrigation solution, notify the NP, MD, or surgeon.

■ Clamp the G-tube port when there is no drainage, or not a large amount of drainage, to prevent removal of normal gastric secretions.

● Begin enteral feeds if the infant can tolerate clamping the G-tube port and there is no vomiting of gastric secretions.

■ Manage postoperative pain control using opioids in conjunction with acetaminophen.

■ Administer prescribed antibiotics prophylactically for 24 hours or longer if there is a concern for infection.

■ Communicate the type of GJ tube to all care providers.

■ Securement is similar to the G-tube securement, but not all GJ tubes will have internal securement.

● When applicable, internal securement may be accomplished with a balloon or bolster.

● Apply external securement on the abdomen for at least 6 weeks to facilitate healing of the tract, avoid tract enlargement, and avoid dislodgement.

● Avoid excessive traction with securement as it can interfere with healing and may cause leakage.

- Stabilize the dressing onto the abdomen with tape, and stabilize the flange if an external flange or disk is present.
- Place a hydrocolloid wound dressing between the skin and tape if there is skin breakdown or irritation.

■ Balloon management is similar to management with a G-tube balloon (see earlier).

■ Vent the G-port to decrease the risk of reflux and aspiration, and alleviate gastric distention when infants are on noninvasive ventilation.

■ Flush the G and J ports before and after a feeding or medication administration.

- Warm water is used for flushing the ports (sterile water for immunocompromised patients).
- Flushing of unused ports:
  - Flush the G-port twice daily if not being used.
  - Flush the J-port every 4 hours if not being used.

Feeding

■ Administer jejunum feedings continuously.

- Never give feedings by bolus into the jejunum due to discomfort, the risk of intestinal perforation, and malabsorption/dumping syndrome.
  - Dumping syndrome is a condition where stool output is greater than 2 mL/kg/hr and can lead to abdominal discomfort, weight loss, dehydration, and electrolyte imbalances (Hansen & Modi, 2016).

Dressing, Bathing, and Skin Care

■ Change dressings once or twice per day.

■ Inspect the peristomal site: Note integrity, erythema, and drainage.

- Small amounts of drainage are appropriate.
- Drainage and skin irritation indicate leakage of gastric contents onto the skin.
  - Reassess for adequate tube stabilization and balloon inflation.

■ Cleanse skin with saline or water.

- If there is crust at the site, use mild soap and water.
- Rinse with saline or water.

■ Dry skin prior to reapplying dressing:

- Use a split 2- × 2-inch gauze placed around the insertion site if there is drainage.

- If there is significant drainage, use an absorbent dressing to wick moisture away from the skin.
■ Resume tub baths on POD 7 if the site is healing well and the infant is stable.

Dislodgement

■ Management of the G-tube tract is described earlier under G-tube dislodgement.
■ Do not reinsert the GJ tube that dislodges.
- GJ tubes that dislodge must be replaced by experienced personnel with fluoroscopic guidance (Hamilton et al., 2016).

Occlusion

■ Milk or flush with 5 to 10 mL NS or warm water if occlusion in the tubing is noted.
■ Establish patency by contacting a prescriber to order an enzymatic solution to manage an obstruction that is not relieved with an NS or water flush.
■ Replace the tube if patency is not achieved with the previously noted methods.
■ Consider causes (incompatibility, flushing frequency, thick formula) of occlusion when patency is reestablished, to prevent future occlusion.

Skin Breakdown

■ Check for leakage at the site, which can lead to skin breakdown.
- Apply a colloidal oatmeal soak or acetic acid–aluminum acetate solution to decrease moisture at the site.
■ Infection (cellulitis) is treated with systemic antibiotics for a specific organism.
■ Localized treatment of cellulitis involves targeting a specific organism.

Bleeding

■ Assess for granulation tissue and skin integrity that can lead to bleeding.
- Prevent excessive traction on the tube.
- Limit movement of the G-tube to preclude development of granulation tissue.

Granulation

■ See G-tube section for management of granulomas.

Residual Checks

■ Do not perform residual checks via the J-tube port.

  ● The narrow lumen of the J-port precludes residual checks as suction cannot be applied to the J-port.

■ Residual checks can be performed on the G-tube portion.

Complications

■ Early and late complications can be observed (Duro et al., 2016).

■ Early-onset rare complications that can occur (in the first 2 weeks) include colonic perforation, duodenal hematoma, and necrotizing fasciitis (Duro et al., 2016).

  ● A surgeon should be notified if these are suspected.

■ A late-onset complication, gastrocolic fistula, is a significant complication.

  ● A surgeon should be notified if this is suspected.

Documentation

■ Include tube type, length, and diameter

■ Type of securement(s)

■ Dressing applied

■ Amount of fluid to fill the balloon

■ Date the balloon check is due

■ Peristomal and stomal appearance

■ Presence of leakage

■ Presence of granuloma, including size and location in clock hours and treatment

TRACHEOSTOMY

Tracheostomy is a procedure that exposes, incises, and cannulates the trachea to create a surgical airway. The size and type of tracheostomy depend on the infant's anatomy and size. When matched for gestational age, infants with tracheostomies have a higher risk for morbidity and mortality (Walsh & Rastatter, 2018). Discussion with family around these risks is necessary prior to tracheostomy placement.

Clinical Indications

■ Conditions that may require treatment with tracheostomy include airway obstruction, bronchopulmonary dysplasia, vocal cord paralysis, chronic aspiration, congenital airway anomalies, laryngomalacia, tracheomalacia, respiratory failure, congenital central hypoventilation syndrome, and neuromuscular weakness.

■ Tracheostomies can reduce the risk of subglottic and tracheal stenosis in infants requiring long-term intubation and mechanical ventilation, as well as decrease complications related to long-term intubation.

■ Tracheostomies may be used for airway suctioning and also administration of aerosolized medications (Ohlms, 2016).

■ The tracheostomy tube must be attached to a ventilator or a system for humidification.

Preoperative Assessment and Nursing Care

■ No enteral feedings should be given for 4 to 6 hours prior to the procedure (follow institutional policies), and up to 8 hours may be needed if fortified feedings are being administered.

■ Confirm surgical and anesthesia team consents are obtained.

■ Secure peripheral IV access for infusion of maintenance fluids and medications.

■ Determine the goal level of sedation and plan for postoperative comfort.

General Assessment

■ Assess respiratory status, tolerance to ventilator support and weaning, and blood gas measurement for all patients undergoing a tracheostomy.

■ Communicate symptom management and respiratory status to the entire care team.

■ Evaluate for appropriate somatic weight gain that is critical for infants requiring a tracheostomy.

Testing

■ Diagnose suspected airway anomalies with flexible and direct laryngoscopy.

■ Perform diagnostic tests, including airway imaging, such as dynamic airway CT.

■ Assess for genetic anomalies or syndromes, neuromuscular problems, and difficulties swallowing (Ohlms, 2016).

Medications

■ Manage respiratory status with systemic medications, including diuretics, methylxanthines, and steroids.

■ Use inhaled bronchodilators and steroids as adjunct respiratory management therapy.

Reduce Infection Risk

■ Minimize risk for aspiration and pneumonia through the use of ventilator-associated pneumonia (VAP) bundles.

● Respiratory bundles include elevation of the head of the bed, frequent mouth care, and in-line tracheal suctioning, or sterile suctioning techniques when in-line suctioning is not feasible (Klompas et al., 2014).

Surgical Procedure

■ The infant's airway is secured prior to the operative procedure, typically with an endotracheal tube (ETT).

■ The infant is then positioned with a shoulder roll and head ring to expose the neck. The neck is incised, and subcutaneous fat is removed.

■ Incisions to the second and third tracheal rings are made.

■ The tracheostomy tube, with predetermined diameter and length, is placed by the surgeon (or most qualified provider if placed emergently).

■ Bilateral air entry is confirmed at the end of the procedure (Ohlms, 2016).

Postoperative Assessment and Nursing Care

Immediate Postoperative Period

■ Obtain chest radiograph to ensure proper placement, as well as lung expansion postoperatively.

■ Minimize infant movement postoperatively through PODs 5 to 7 to allow for the stoma and tract to heal.

● Movement of the head and neck during the first 5 to 7 days will increase stoma size, resulting in tissue damage, leakage of air, and bleeding.

● Excessive movement will encourage the formation of granulomas, which can bleed and cause leakage around the stoma.

● Limit manipulation of the tracheostomy to the surgeon and/or otolaryngology (ORL) team until the initial tracheostomy change on PODs 5 to 7.

■ Document the tracheostomy inner diameter and length.

■ Dislodgement of the tracheostomy may occur in the first 5–7 PODs.

● Contact the surgeon and/or ORL team emergently.

● "Stay sutures" are sutures secured to the chest and are covered with a transparent dressing.

- They must be intact and secured in the immediate postoperative period, first 5 to 7 days, in the case of tracheostomy tube dislodgement.
    - In the event of an early postoperative dislodgement, the dressings are removed and traction is applied to the "stay sutures" to spread the stomal opening, facilitating placement of a new tracheostomy tube.
- Keep a spare tracheostomy tube of the same size (length and diameter) and another that is one size smaller, scissors, oxygen, suction and suction catheters, and a syringe for cuffed tubes at the bedside in the event the tube needs to be replaced emergently.

Sedation

■ Control pain, decrease agitation, and limit movement using a combination of medications to achieve adequate pain control and sedation.

■ Maintain moderate sedation until the initial tracheostomy tube change on PODs 5 to 7.

Mechanical Ventilation

■ Support breathing postoperatively while patient is sedated.

■ Wean from mechanical ventilation if able to, depending on the infant's diagnosis and degree of lung disease.

■ Humidify air entering the trachea, even after infant is weaned from mechanical ventilation, since the air now bypasses the nares.

Suctioning

■ Clear the airway with routine care and as needed to ensure patency.

   - Scant bloody secretions may be noted in the immediate postoperative period.

■ Minimize infection by suctioning with an in-line catheter or open suction using sterile technique (sterile gloves and sterile catheter).

■ Minimize airway trauma and irritation by advancing the suction catheter to the appropriate depth (to the end of the tracheostomy tube, and not beyond) as determined by the surgeon/ORL team and respiratory therapy.

Nutrition

■ Do not give enteral feedings and maintain on parenteral nutrition or dextrose/electrolyte-containing IV fluids until bowel activity (bowel sounds and passage of gas) resumes.

   - Restart or begin enteral feedings and advance as tolerated once bowel activity returns.

■ Until safety with oral feeding is established, feedings should be administered through a nasal, oral, or surgically placed feeding tube.

  ● Surgically placed feeding tubes may be placed at the same time as the tracheostomy if the infant is not expected to orally feed.

■ A feeding team evaluation and modified barium swallow should be done to evaluate the safety of oral feedings for infants with a tracheostomy with a perceived ability to orally feed.

Routine Tracheostomy Site Care Is Started After Initial Tracheostomy Change

■ Gather supplies, perform hand hygiene, and don gloves before loosening the tracheostomy ties and cleaning the site.

■ Have appropriate providers at the bedside for tracheostomy changes, per institutional policy.

■ Clean secretions or drainage from the stoma site using cotton-tip applicators dampened with sterile water, sterile NS, and/or hydrogen peroxide/water solution (50/50 solution; optional).

■ Allow the site to briefly air dry.

■ Observe site for redness or cellulitis.

■ Apply prescribed treatments (such as local antibiotic or antifungal ointments) in a thin layer, as prescribed, followed by the dressing.

  ● Apply a split-gauze dressing to the stoma if there is scant drainage and the site is intact.

  ● Use a moisture-wicking dressing if there is significant drainage to prevent breakdown of the site.

Change Tracheostomy Ties

■ Have a minimum two healthcare providers present for the procedure.

  ● One provider is responsible for securing the tracheostomy flanges while the second provider manages the tracheostomy ties.

■ Cut the new tracheostomy ties so the Velcro straps do not overlap.

■ Taper the edges to 45° to make threading through the flanges easier.

■ Loosen the old ties and cleanse skin underneath.

■ Allow the skin to dry.

■ Apply medication if prescribed to treat fungal/yeast rash or cellulitis.

■ Thread the ends of the new tracheostomy ties, one at a time.

■ The free ends of the tracheostomy ties should be brought to the back of the neck.

■ Fasten Velcro ends of each tracheostomy tie, one at a time.

■ Ensure correct tightness; check to see if one small finger fits between the neck and ties.

■ Readjust if too loose or too tight.

■ Assess the patient throughout and document findings.

Complications

Initial:

■ Hemorrhage manifests as bleeding at the site, blood during suctioning, and respiratory distress.

■ Pneumothorax and pneumomediastinum manifest as respiratory, and potentially cardiovascular, instability and distress.

■ Loss of airway from dislodgement of the tracheostomy manifests as respiratory distress and oxygen desaturation that is not relieved by bag-mask ventilation.

■ Local cellulitis is observed at the site.

Later:

■ Granulation tissue, suprastomal collapse, subglottic stenosis, erosion, and tracheocutaneous fistula are long-term complications that will manifest as difficulty weaning from the ventilator and the need for increased ventilator support.

■ Speech delay is a long-term complication that must be assessed using speech therapy.

● Ideally, speech therapy should begin as early as possible to avoid this delay.

Documentation

■ Tracheostomy type, size, and presence or absence of a cuff

■ Inflation or deflation of cuff

● Quantity of fluid with cuff inflation (to assess for leakage)

■ Date of tracheostomy change

■ Respiratory examination and toleration of weaning

■ Stoma site assessment and drainage

■ Presence, appearance, and quantity of secretions

■ Parental response

■ Parental education

REFERENCES

Bairdain, S., Kelly, D., Tan, C., Dodson, B., Zurakowski, D., Jennings, R., & Trenor, C. (2014). High incidence of catheter-associated venous thromboembolic events in patients with long gap esophageal atresia treated with the Foker process. *Journal of Pediatric Surgery, 49*(2), 370–373. https://doi.org/10.1016/j.jpedsurg.2013.09.003

Duro, D., Santos, C., Puder, M., Smithers, J., & Sztam, K. (2016). Feeding tubes. In A. Hansen & M. Puder (Eds.), *Manual of neonatal surgical intensive care* (3rd ed., pp. 474–497). People's Medical Publishing House.

Hamilton, T., Smithers, J., & Nurko, S. (2016). Gastroesophageal reflux. In A. Hansen & M. Puder (Eds.), *Manual of neonatal surgical intensive care* (3rd ed., pp. 496–514). People's Medical Publishing House.

Hansen, A., & Belfort, M. (2016). Medical considerations. In A. Hansen & M. Puder (Eds.), *Manual of neonatal surgical intensive care* (3rd ed., pp. 27–43). People's Medical Publishing House.

Hansen, A., & Modi, B. (2016). Necrotizing enterocolitis. In A. Hansen & M. Puder (Eds.), *Manual of neonatal surgical intensive care* (3rd ed., pp. 375–397). People's Medical Publishing House.

Hansen, A., O'Reilly, D., Puder, M., & Chandonnet, C. (2016). Vascular access. In A. Hansen & M. Puder (Eds.), *Manual of neonatal surgical intensive care* (3rd ed., pp. 91–108). People's Medical Publishing House.

Klompas, M., Branson, R., Eicenwald, E., Greene, L., Howell, M., Lee, G., Magill, S., Maragakis, L., Priebe, G., Speck, K., Yokoe, D., & Berenholtz, S. (2014). Strategies to prevent ventilator-associated pneumonia in acute care hospitals: 2014 update. *Infection Control and Hospital Epidemiology, 35*(8), 915–936. https://doi.org/10.1086/677144

Nandivanda, P., & Puder, M. (2016). Surgical considerations. In A. Hansen & M. Puder (Eds.), *Manual of neonatal surgical intensive care* (3rd ed., pp. 44–56). People's Medical Publishing House.

Ohlms, L. (2016). Laryngeal and tracheal anomalies. In A. Hansen & M. Puder (Eds.), *Manual of neonatal surgical intensive care* (3rd ed., pp. 131–176). People's Medical Publishing House.

Ringer, S. (2016). Pneumothorax and air leak. In A. Hansen & M. Puder (Eds.), *Manual of neonatal surgical intensive care* (3rd ed., pp. 203–212). People's Medical Publishing House.

Walsh, J., & Rastatter, J. (2018). Neonatal tracheostomy. *Clinics in Perinatology, 45*(4), 805–816. https://doi.org/10.1016/j.clp.2018.07.014

Young, M., & You, T. (2020, May). Overview of complications of central venous catheters and their prevention. *UpToDate.* https://www.uptodate.com/contents/overview-of-complications-of-central-venous-catheters-and-their-prevention

SURGICAL DISORDERS OF THE BRAIN AND SPINAL CANAL

EILEEN C. DEWITT AND NOEL DWYER

HYDROCEPHALUS

Hydrocephalus is a disorder in which an excessive amount of cerebrospinal fluid (CSF) accumulates within the cerebral ventricles and/or subarachnoid spaces, which are dilated (Carey et al., 1994). In infants and children, hydrocephalus is almost always associated with increased intracranial pressure (ICP). In most cases, this is caused by excess CSF accumulation in the cerebral ventricles due to disturbances of CSF circulation. This is known as obstructive or noncommunicating hydrocephalus. Hydrocephalus results from an imbalance between the intracranial CSF inflow and outflow. It is caused by obstruction of CSF circulation, by inadequate absorption of CSF, or, rarely, by over-production of CSF (Beni-Adrani et al., 2006). Regardless of the etiology, excessive volume of CSF causes increased ventricular pressure and leads to cerebral ventricular dilatation.

Presentation

Hydrocephalus can be congenital or acquired. Congenital forms can result from central nervous system malformations such as neural tube defects, infection, intra-ventricular hemorrhage, genetic defects, trauma, and teratogens (Jeng et al., 2011). Acquired forms include infections, tumors, and posthemorrhagic hydrocephalus. Regardless of etiology, the signs and symptoms of hydrocephalus can be nonspecific and result from increased ICP and dilatation of the ventricles. Pain results from distortion of the meninges and blood vessels and can be intermittent or persistent (Kirkpatrick et al., 1989). Affected patients often have changes in behavior such as irritability. As hydrocephalus worsens, midbrain and brainstem dysfunction can result in lethargy. Increased ICP in the posterior fossa often leads to nausea, vomiting, and decreased appetite.

Diagnosis

Physical examination findings are due to the effects of increased ICP.

- Distortion of the brainstem can result in vital sign changes such as bradycardia, hypertension, and altered respiratory rate.
- Excessive head growth may be noted on serial measurements of head circumference.
  - Effects of hydrocephalus on the head are most common in infants while the cranial sutures are still open:
    - The anterior fontanelle may become full or distended.
    - The sutures become more widely split due to an enlarging head circumference.
    - The scalp veins may appear dilated and prominent.
    - Pressure on the midbrain may result in impairment of upward gaze, known as sun-setting sign because of the appearance of the sclera visible above the iris.
    - Stretching of the fibers from the motor cortex around the dilated ventricles may result in spasticity of the extremities, especially the legs (Kirkpatrick et al., 1989).

■ Along with the physical examination, the diagnosis of hydrocephalus is confirmed with neuroimaging.

 ● Ultrasonography is the preferred technique in the newborn because it is portable and avoids ionizing radiation.

 ● Serial head ultrasound (US) tests should be performed because signs of evolving hydrocephalus such as rapid head growth, full anterior fontanelle, and separated cranial sutures do not appear for days to weeks after ventricular dilatation has commenced.

■ In older infants with suspected hydrocephalus, MRI is generally the modality of choice; it provides superior visualization of pathologic processes in the CSF pathway, including CSF flow dynamics.

■ MRI helps to distinguish obstructive or noncommunicating hydrocephalus from absorptive or communicating hydrocephalus.

 ● This distinction informs treatment decisions about shunting versus third ventriculostomy.

Preoperative Assessment and Nursing Care

■ Conduct a thorough physical examination to assess for signs of hydrocephalus and increasing ICP.

■ Obtain a daily occipital frontal circumference (OFC) measurement just above the infant's ear.

■ Conduct weekly growth assessment of the head (Ditzenberger, 2021).

■ Assist with serial head USs.

■ Facilitate neurosurgical consultation.

■ Support the infant by decreasing noxious stimuli.

■ Position head to avoid pressure points.

■ Provide family support/education.

■ Obtain preoperative lab work, complete blood count (CBC), coagulation studies, type, and screen.

Surgical Procedure

■ Lumbar puncture (LP) is an invasive but nonsurgical therapeutic approach to decreasing CSF in the early stages of communicating hydrocephalus (Horinek et al., 2003).

 ● The nurse has a key role in positioning the patient and monitoring oxygen saturations, heart rate, respiratory rate, and color.

 ● The nurse notes opening and closing pressures and monitors the puncture site for CSF leakage.

■ If the LP proves to be inefficient, an external ventricular drain (EVD) is the next invasive step in the management of hydrocephalus.

External Ventricular Drain

■ A catheter is inserted into the dilated anterior horn of the right lateral ventricle.

■ The proximal end of the catheter is subcutaneously tunneled to a site on the scalp and connected to a drainage system (Horinek et al., 2003).

■ The amount of CSF drained can be adjusted by elevating or lowering the level of the drip chamber.

● A subcutaneous reservoir is another frequently used option in the management of hydrocephalus.

● Reservoirs can be tapped up to two to three times per day.

● A drawback with the reservoir is that the removal of CSF is intermittent.

● The fluid buildup and resulting rise in ICP between taps could be problematic to the infant.

Endoscopic Third Ventriculostomy

■ Endoscopic third ventriculostomy (ETV) is a procedure in which a perforation is made to connect the third ventricle to the subarachnoid space (Chumas et al., 2001).

● Warf (2005) first reported results combining ETV with bilateral endoscopic lateral ventricle choroid plexus cauterization (CPC) to treat hydrocephalus in infants. Stone and Warf (2014) demonstrated that more than half of all infants presenting for initial treatment of hydrocephalus can be successfully treated in this way. Expectations should be tempered for those with hydrocephalus secondary to neonatal meningitis, those with prepontine cistern scarring, and those who have previously undergone shunt treatment.

■ ETVs have been successful in the treatment of obstructive hydrocephalus and as an alternative to shunt placement.

■ When successful, an ETV provides a treatment that is relatively low cost, durable, and involves no surgically placed hardware.

Ventriculoperitoneal Shunt

■ A ventriculoperitoneal (VP) shunt is a permanent solution to managing excess CSF.

■ A VP shunt is a mechanical shunt system that is placed in order to prevent the excessive accumulation of CSF.

■ A catheter is placed into one of the lateral cerebral ventricles.

■ The catheter is connected to a one-way valve system that opens when the pressure in the ventricle exceeds a certain value.

■ The distal end of the system is connected to a catheter that is placed in the peritoneal cavity where the fluid is absorbed.

Postoperative Assessment and Nursing Care

■ Monitor vital signs and respiratory status.

■ Observe fontanelle and head circumference; changes can be critical and need to be reported immediately.

■ Observe and document neurologic vital signs to include pupillary reflex, motor and sensory reflexes, and primitive reflexes.

■ Observe and document physical examination.

■ Reestablish feedings once return of bowel function occurs following anesthesia.

■ Follow head USs for adequate CSF management.

Care Specific to External Ventricular Drain

■ Maintain clean, dry, and intact scalp dressing.

■ Every time the patient is repositioned, the system should be clamped and leveled.

■ Watch for changes in CSF flow, volume, and patency of the system (minimum every hour).

Care Specific to Endoscopic Third Ventriculostomy

■ Monitor surgical site and maintain clean, dry, and intact scalp dressing if present.

■ Assess head circumference and fontanelle daily or more frequently if ordered.

■ Evaluate for signs of increasing hydrocephalus such as changes in neurologic examination, including lethargy and irritability as well as changes in feeding.

Care Specific to Ventriculopertioneal Shunt

■ Monitor for shunt malfunction.

■ Assist with obtaining shunt series (often by MRI) to assess for shunt malfunction from mechanical failure such as obstruction of the catheter resulting in overdrainage or underdrainage:

- Overdrainage will result in a sunken anterior fontanelle.
- Underdrainage will result in symptoms associated with elevated ICP.

■ Perform close assessment for symptoms of infection such as fever, erythema at the insertion site, lethargy, and poor feeding.

- Symptoms of infection should prompt an immediate sepsis evaluation.
- Shunt infection is a common complication, occurring in 5% to 15% of procedures (Simon et al., 2009).

■ Careful positioning is crucial in order to prevent skin breakdown.

- Gel pillows may diminish skin breakdown and provide a source of comfort.

■ Provide postoperative pain management guided by unit-based scoring systems or tools to assess comfort.

Documentation (Applicable to External Ventricular Drain, Endoscopic Third Ventriculostomy, and Ventriculoperitoneal Shunt)

■ Head circumference

■ Neurologic assessment, including description of fontanelles and suture position

■ Respiratory assessment

■ Feeding irregularities, including vomiting

■ Assessment of skin at defect site and wound healing

■ Pain assessment and management postoperatively

MYELOMENINGOCELE

Myelomeningocele (a congenital neural tube defect) is the saclike protrusion of the spinal meninges through an opening in the spinal column. This defect is also known as spinal dysmorphism or spina bifida aperta. The majority of myelomeningoceles occur in the lumbar region (Mclone & Bowman, 2014). Findings associated with this defect can include frontal bone scalloping, cerebellum abnormalities, Chiari II malformation, hydrocephaly, microcephaly, and encephalocele. A majority of patients with myelomeningocele have hydrocephalus. Hydrocephalus results from an obstruction of the fourth ventricular outflow, or the flow of CSF through the posterior fossa, called Chiari II malformation.

Presentation

Standard of care is to screen for an elevation in the maternal serum alpha-fetoprotein (AFP) at 16 weeks' gestation. Elevated AFP is an indication for further diagnostic testing via US to evaluate for a neural tube defect. In-utero surgery may be an option although it is associated with increased risk of premature birth (Ditzenberger & Blackburn, 2020). A scheduled Cesarean section is the preferred delivery method to reduce the risk of rupturing the meningeal sac.

Diagnosis

■ Confirmation of the neural tube defect is made during the physical examination at birth.

■ A head US is usually indicated to diagnose Chiari II malformation (a smaller-than-normal space between the bones at the lower base of the skull, leading to downward protrusion of the cerebellum and brainstem into the foramen magnum and into the upper spinal canal; Soul & Madsen, 2016).

■ A thorough neurologic examination will show variations in motor control and reflexes from hip to foot, depending on the level of the lesion.

● Keep in mind that the neurologic system is derived from ectoderm; therefore, one should pay particular attention to the examination of the skin (Yang, 2004).

● Assess for associated anomalies, including clubfeet, cleft lip and palate, imperforate anus, and cryptorchidism.

Preoperative Assessment and Nursing Care

■ Monitor for hydrocephalus (and resulting ICP) by assessing head circumference, fontanelles, and sutures.

■ Position the infant prone with the lesion covered with wet sterile dressings (to protect the lesion as well as minimize insensible water losses [IWLs]).

■ Place a roll between the legs at hip level to maintain abduction of the legs.

■ Reposition frequently to help prevent skin breakdown and contractures.

■ Protect the defect from contamination with stool and urine.

■ Administer prophylactic IV antibiotics as prescribed.

■ Clean intermittent catheterization (CIC) should be practiced until renal and urologic functions are understood.

■ Use nonlatex gloves and equipment to prevent development of latex allergy.

■ Obtain a head US soon after birth to assess for obstructed CSF flow and hydrocephalus.

■ Monitor for seizures.

■ Perform regular neurologic examinations to assess upper and lower extremity motor and sensory function, as well as anal wink.

Surgical Procedure

Repair of the lesion within 24 to 48 hours is optimal. The abnormal end of the spinal cord, called the placode, is dissected from any possible adhesions, and the surrounding skin that is too thin to use in the repair is removed. The placode is formed into a more normal shape and sutured. The area around the placode and within the spinal canal is assessed for tethers. The dural edge is separated from the lumbar fascia, rolled around the dura, and closed watertight. Subcutaneous and cutaneous layers are closed with the goal of having a well-vascularized and watertight closure (Soul & Madsen, 2016). A VP shunt may be placed at the time of first surgery but is often postponed pending further monitoring for hydrocephalus.

Postoperative Assessment and Nursing Care

■ Keep in prone or side-lying position with occlusive dressing in place until wound is healed.

■ Monitor head circumference daily.

■ Assess for ICP, including irritability, bulging fontanelles, vomiting, feeding difficulties, stridor, and apnea.

■ Monitor urologic function and renal status closely.

 ● Consider a renal US, voiding cystourethrogram (VCUG), urinalysis, and serum creatinine.

■ Perform CIC every 4 hours to assess for postvoid residuals.

 ● CIC may be continued long term, depending on urologic function.

■ Reestablish feedings once return of bowel function occurs following anesthesia.

■ Provide postoperative pain management guided by unit-based scoring systems or tools to assess comfort.

Documentation

■ Head circumference
■ Neurologic assessment, including description of fontanelles and suture position
■ Respiratory assessment
■ Feeding irregularities, including vomiting
■ Assessment of skin at defect site and wound healing
■ Urine output via catheterization and diaper voids
■ Pain assessment and management postoperatively

TETHERED CORD

A tethered cord is characterized by a prolonged conus (or lower end of the spinal cord) and abnormal filum; fixation of the caudal end of the cord is by fibrous bands (Inder et al., 2018).

Presentation

In the newborn period, the physical characteristics (of an occult dysraphic state) such as abnormal collections of hair, subcutaneous mass, superficial cutaneous abnormalities, or cutaneous dimples or tracts raise suspicion of a disorder of caudal neural tube formation, including tethered cord (Inder et al., 2018).

Diagnosis

Noninvasive evaluation by US is preferred over plain radiograph given the poor ossification of the posterior spinal elements. Visualization of the spinal cord, subarachnoid space, conus medullaris, and filum terminale, along with real-time observation of the mobility of the cord, has allowed identification of a variety of occult dysraphic states. If US is normal and no neurologic signs exist, further radiologic study is not necessary in the neonatal period and clinical follow-up is appropriate. If an abnormality is present, proceed to MRI for better sagittal and coronal topography of the intravertebral and extravertebral components.

Preoperative Assessment and Nursing Care

■ Observe and document the neurologic examination to include overall muscle tone as well as lower limb movement and reflexes.

■ Observe and document the physical examination.

Surgical Procedure

Surgical release of the tethered cord combined with removal of any cysts can prevent deterioration or reverse deficits. Surgery is performed primarily to prevent development of neurologic deficits. Neurologic deficits may present suddenly from vascular insufficiency produced by tension on the tethered cord.

Postoperative Assessment and Nursing Care

■ Assess the surgical site for signs of infection and drainage.

■ Evaluate bladder function in the newborn.

■ Assess neurologic function.

● Follow the movement of the lower extremities and muscle tone closely.

■ Carefully position the infant to include side-to-side and prone positioning in the immediate postoperative period.

■ Reestablish oral feedings once return of bowel function occurs following anesthesia.

■ Provide postoperative pain management guided by unit-based scoring systems or tools to assess comfort.

Documentation

■ Evaluation of surgical site

■ Routine neurologic evaluation to include pupillary reflex, motor and sensory reflexes, along with primitive reflexes

■ Urine output

■ Pain assessment and management postoperatively

REFERENCES

Beni-Adrani, L., Biani, N., Ben-Sirah, L., & Constantini, S. (2006). The occurrence of obstructive v. absorptive hydrocephalus in newborns and infants: Relevance to treatment choices. *Childs Nervous System, 22*(12), 1543–1563. https://doi.org/10.1007/s00381-006-0193-5

Carey, C. M., Tullous, M. W., & Walker, M. L. (1994). Hydrocephalus: Etiology, pathologic effects, diagnosis, and natural history. In W. R. Cheek (Ed.), *Pediatric neurosurgery* (3rd ed., pp. 185–201). WB Saunders.

Chumas, P., Tyagi, A., & Livingston, J. (2001). Hydrocephalus, what's new. *Archives of Disease in Childhood, Fetal Neonatal Edition, 85*(3), F149–F154. https://doi.org/10.1136/fn.85.3.f149

Ditzenberger, G. (2021). Neurological disorders. In M. T. Verklan, M. Walden, & S. Forest (Eds.), *Core curriculum for neonatal intensive care nursing* (6th ed., pp. 629–653). Elsevier Saunders.

Ditzenberger, G. R., & Blackburn, S. T. (2020). Neurologic system. In C. Kenner, L. B. Altimier, & M. V. Boykova (Eds.), *Comprehensive neonatal nursing care* (6th ed., pp. 373–416). Springer Publishing Company.

Horinek, D., Cihar, M., & Tichy, M. (2003). Current methods in the treatment of posthemorrhagic hydrocephalus in infants. *Therapy, 104*(11), 347–351.

Inder, T. E., Darras, B. T., de Vries, L. S., du Plessis, A. J., Neil, J. J., & Perlman, J. M. (2018). *Neurology of the newborn* (6th ed.). Elsevier Saunders.

Jeng, S., Gupta, N., Wrensch, M., Zhao, S., & Wu, T. W. (2011). Prevalence of congenital hydrocephalus in California, 1991–2000. *Pediatric Neurology, 45*(2), 67–71. https://doi.org/10.1016/j.pediatrneurol.2011.03.009

Kirkpatrick, M., Engelman, H., & Minns, R. A. (1989). Symptoms and signs of progressive hydrocephalus. *Archives of Disease in Childhood, 64*(1), 124–128. https://doi.org/10.1136/adc.64.1.124

Mclone, D. G., & Bowman, R. (2014). *Overview of the management of myelomeningocele (spina bifida).* Wolters-Kluwer Health.

Simon, T. D., Hall, M., Riva-Cambrin, J., Albert, J. E., Jeffries, H. E., LaFleur, B., Dean, J. M., Kestle, J. R. W., & Hydrocephalus Clinical Research Network. (2009). Infection rates following initial cerebrospinal fluid shunt placement across pediatric hospitals in the United States. *Journal of Neurosurgical Pediatrics, 4*(2), 156–165. https://doi.org/10.3171/2009.3.PEDS08215

Soul, J., & Madsen, J. R. (2016). Neurological disorders, part 9.1 neonatal hydrocephalus. In A. R. Hansen & M. Puder (Eds.), *Manual of neonatal surgical intensive care* (3rd ed., pp. 521–533). BC Decker.

Stone, S. D., & Warf, B. C. (2014). Combined endoscopic third ventriculostomy and choroid plexus cauterization as primary treatment for infant hydrocephalus: A prospective North American series. *Journal of Neurosurgery Pediatrics, 14*, 439–446. https://doi.org/10.3171/2014.7.PEDS14152

Warf, B. C. (2005). Comparison of endoscopic third ventriculostomy alone and combined with choroid plexus cauterization in infants younger than 1 year of age: A prospective study in 550 African children. *Journal Neurosurgery, 103*, 475–481. https://doi.org/10.3171/ped.2005.103.6.0475

Yang, M. (2004). Newborn neurologic examination. *Neurology, 62*, E15–E17. https://doi.org/10.1212/wnl.62.7.e15

SURGICAL DISORDERS OF THE BRONCHOPULMONARY TREE AND DIAPHRAGM

KATIE ROY, ETHAN SCHULER, AND MARY-JEANNE MANNING

BRONCHOPULMONARY SEQUESTRATION

KATIE ROY AND ETHAN SCHULER

Bronchopulmonary sequestration (BPS) is a rare congenital thoracic malformation consisting of a mass of extraneous, nonfunctioning lung tissue that is separated from the tracheobronchial tree. BPS has an anomalous arterial blood supply from the systemic circulation, typically the aorta, rather than the pulmonary circulation. Multiple feeding vessels may be present. The primary forms of pulmonary sequestration are intralobar or intrapulmonary sequestration (ILS) and extralobar or extrapulmonary sequestration (ELS). In ILS, the mass is embedded in the normal lung parenchyma and shares the same visceral pleura. In ELS, the mass is located outside the lung and is enclosed within its own visceral pleura. In the hybrid form, ILS or ELS occurs in combination with congenital pulmonary airway malformation (CPAM; Oermann, 2019a).

BPS represents approximately 0.1% to 6% of all congenital pulmonary malformations. ILS is the most common form, with 60% occurrence in the posterior basal segment of the left lower lobe (LLL). Bilateral involvement is uncommon. ELS is frequently located between the LLL and hemidiaphragm, though it may occur below the diaphragm. Rare cases of ILS and ELS present with a connection to the gastrointestinal tract. ELS is more likely to be associated with other congenital anomalies such as congenital diaphragmatic hernia (Amano et al., 2017; DeParedes et al., 1970; Flye et al., 1976; Oermann, 2019a).

Presentation

■ BPS may present in the newborn with respiratory distress, particularly if the lesion is large; most newborns are asymptomatic.

■ ILS generally presents in childhood with recurrent pulmonary infections; ILS occurs equally between the sexes.

■ ELS generally presents in infancy with cough and respiratory compromise; infection is uncommon; ELS occurs more typically in males.

■ Rarely, high-output cardiac failure may result if the sequestration consumes a significant amount of the systemic arterial flow.

■ Additional signs and symptoms that may be seen with BPS include wheezing, dyspnea, chronic cough, hemoptysis, cyanosis, pleural effusion, prolonged respiratory infections, feeding difficulties, and poor weight gain.

Diagnosis

■ Chest radiography, CT/CT angiography, and MRI/MR angiography serve as the primary tools for diagnosing and defining BPS, as well as for surgical planning.

■ BPS may be detected on prenatal US, though it can be difficult to distinguish from CPAM.

Preoperative Assessment and Nursing Care

■ Provide supportive respiratory care as clinically indicated, ranging from supplemental oxygen to mechanical ventilation.

■ Establish a hydration and nutrition plan.

■ Administer prescribed antibiotics in children with associated respiratory infections.

Surgical Procedure

■ Open or thoracoscopic surgical resection is indicated for symptomatic patients, though asymptomatic patients may be observed or electively treated at a later time.

● Asymptomatic patients may benefit from repair to prevent future respiratory symptoms, recurrent infections, and complications such as heart failure.

● Resection is recommended for asymptomatic patients with large lesions.

■ ILS often requires lobectomy or segmentectomy to achieve complete excision; the margins of the sequestration may not be clearly defined.

● Complete thoracoscopic resection of pulmonary lobes in infants and children has been described with low mortality and morbidity (Albanese & Rothenberg, 2007).

■ ELS can usually be excised without loss of normal lung tissue.

■ Embolization of the systemic arterial supply may be an alternative option for initial therapy.

Postoperative Assessment and Nursing Care

Postoperative care depends on the surgical technique utilized.

Thoracoscopic Repair

■ Requires a short hospital stay, generally 2 to 3 days.

■ Assess chest tube for evacuation of air and fluid as the lung heals, including evidence of air leak.

■ Maintain clean, dry, and intact bioocclusive dressings over the chest incision(s) and the chest tube sites; these may be removed after 48 hours.

■ Resume the infant's normal diet once recovered from anesthesia.

■ Begin bathing the infant on postoperative day 5, or as prescribed by the operating surgeon.

● Gently clean the incision and its closures with soap and water, then pat dry; do not submerge in water for at least 1 week postoperatively.

● If incisional sterile strips are present, they will fall off on their own in 7 to 14 days.

■ Administer analgesia as indicated.

Thoracotomy

■ Requires a longer hospital stay, generally >3 days.

■ Assess chest tube for evacuation of air and fluid as the lung heals, including evidence of air leak.

■ Maintain clean, dry, and intact bioocclusive dressings over the chest incision(s) and the chest tube sites; these may be removed after 48 hours.

■ Monitor the surgical wound for drainage and evidence of infection.

■ Monitor for signs and symptoms of systemic infection.

■ Change the primary dressing according to the surgeon's instructions.

■ Assess postoperative analgesia routinely to ensure adequate depth of respirations and patient movement.

● Pain management options may include:

• Paravertebral block

- Epidural catheters
- IV nurse-controlled analgesia with intermittent or continuous infusion
- Oral analgesics (upon withdrawal of continuous pain control) for duration of time until pain free; oral analgesics may include acetaminophen, nonsteroidal anti-inflammatory drugs (NSAIDs), and narcotic agents.

■ Encourage oral feeding as soon as possible; engage parental participation to facilitate establishment of feedings.

■ Prevent postoperative respiratory insufficiency by maintaining a clear airway, frequent repositioning of the infant, gentle chest physiotherapy, and the prevention of edema.

Documentation

■ Vital signs
■ Ventilation or respiratory requirements
■ Thoracostomy tube output
■ Intake and output
■ Serum electrolytes, complete blood counts (CBCs), blood gas measurements, and other laboratory values
■ Sedation, state and pain scores

CONGENITAL DIAPHRAGMATIC HERNIA IN THE NEONATE

MARY-JEANNE MANNING

Congenital diaphragmatic hernia (CDH) is a developmental defect of the diaphragm in which the abdominal viscera herniate into the chest through an abnormal opening in the diaphragm. The presence of the abdominal organs in the thoracic cavity leads to pulmonary hypoplasia and pulmonary hypertension. The most common location is the left posterolateral side (Bochdalek hernia). This occurs in approximately 90% of cases. Right-sided lesions (Morgagni hernia) occur in approximately 9% of cases (McHoney, 2015). Despite advances in treatment, mortality remains high (Keller et al., 2010; McHoney, 2015).

■ It is one of the most common major congenital anomalies.

■ The incidence is reported as one in 3,000 live births worldwide (Wynn et al., 2013).

■ Infants with CDH can have lung hypoplasia and increased pulmonary vascular resistance (Kleinman & Wilson, 2016).

- Between 5% and 30% of cases are associated with chromosomal abnormalities (McHoney, 2015).

- Between 25% and 57% of cases have other structural defects such as congenital heart defects, as well as renal, neurologic, or gastrointestinal defects (Kosiński & Wielgoś, 2017).

■ Survival varies; permissive hypercapnia and treatment at a facility that has a standard approach to the management of CDH and sufficient patient volume are associated with improved survival (Kleinman & Wilson, 2016).

- Various characteristics are linked to poor prognosis; these include right-sided lesions, large lesions requiring patch repair, liver herniation into the chest, cardiac anomalies, and other congenital or chromosomal abnormalities (Kleinman & Wilson, 2016; Kosiński & Wielgoś, 2017; Snoek et al., 2017).

- The most common prognostic factor used prior to birth is the observed-to-expected lung-to-head ratio (O/E LHR). This measurement is done via prenatal US between 22- and 32-week gestation (Puligandla et al., 2018; Snoek et al., 2017).

Presentation

Respiratory distress or failure and cyanosis are seen shortly after birth with CDH. The degree of respiratory compromise is related to the severity of the defect and often the side of the defect (right side, less common, and often thought to be worse; Kosiński & Wielgoś, 2017; McHoney, 2015; Wynn et al., 2013). A large defect allows for more organs to enter the chest, including the bowel, stomach, and liver. Pulmonary hypoplasia and pulmonary hypertension are more severe in cases where more organs herniate into the chest during fetal development.

Diagnosis

■ Can be identified on prenatal ultrasound (US).

■ A postnatal chest radiograph confirms the CDH.

■ An abdominal radiograph confirms that bowel and other abdominal organs have herniated into the chest cavity.

■ Echocardiogram is used to determine the presence of congenital heart defects and to assess for, and follow, pulmonary hypertension and left and right ventricular function.

■ Fetal MRI is often used in CDH centers because it offers better contrast of the soft tissue, allowing differentiation of lung tissue from liver tissue in the chest.

- MRI also allows for diagnosis of cardiac and other structural defects (Kosiński & Wielgoś, 2017).

■ Physical examination reveals signs of respiratory distress, barrel-shaped chest, scaphoid-appearing abdomen, and the absence of breath sounds on the ipsilateral side.

- Left-sided defects may lead to displacement of the heart and heart sounds; the point of maximal intensity (PMI) is shifted to the right (Kleinman & Wilson, 2016; McHoney, 2015).

Preoperative Assessment and Nursing Care

- Avoid conditions that increase pulmonary vascular resistance, including hypoxemia, acidosis, hypothermia, and hypoglycemia, as well as environmental stressors, noise, excessive light, and invasive procedures (Kleinman & Wilson, 2016).
- Provide support such as intubation, gentle ventilation, permissive hypercapnia, high-frequency oscillatory ventilation, and/or extracorporeal membrane oxygenation (ECMO) depending on the severity of the defect and the resulting pulmonary hypoplasia and pulmonary hypertension.
- Maintain permissive hypercapnia (maintain pH <7.35, but >7.25) to avoid barotrauma, decrease pulmonary vascular resistance, and attain cardiovascular stability (Kleinman & Wilson, 2016).
- Consider pulmonary vasodilators such as inhaled nitric oxide, treprostinil, prostaglandin E1, and sildenafil, which have been used with some success in patients who exhibit severe, refractory pulmonary hypertension (Haroon & Chamberlain, 2012; Keller et al., 2010; McHoney, 2015; Olson et al., 2015).

Nursing assessment includes the following:

- Monitor preductal and postductal oxygen saturation, frequent blood gases to monitor for acidosis, and hypoxia and hypercarbia to evaluate respiratory function.
- Provide minimal effective sedation in order to preserve native respiratory function.
  - Deep sedation and muscle relaxation are reserved for patients who have greater ventilation and oxygenation needs and those with severe pulmonary hypertension (Puligandla et al., 2018).
- Obtain four extremity blood pressures and EKG to rule out cardiac anomalies.
- Monitor perfusion.
  - Provide inotropic support to maintain adequate peripheral perfusion.
- Maintain umbilical venous catheter/umbilical arterial catheter (UVC/UAC) or other central lines.
- Assess pupillary response, fontanelle size/tension, seizure activity, and signs of intraventricular/intraparenchymal bleeding.
  - Patients requiring ECMO will be at greatest risk for bleeding due to heparinization of the circuit.
- Maintain a quiet environment and cluster cares.

■ Assess hematologic status.

  ● Report and respond to signs of bleeding, due to anticoagulation if on ECMO.

■ Measure accurate intake and output.

■ Monitor electrolytes and diuretic treatment closely.

■ Obtain chest and abdominal x-rays, arterial blood gas (ABG), electrolytes, complete blood count (CBC), lactic acid.

■ Treat with narcotics and sedatives to achieve desired pain control and activity level.

■ Administer parenteral nutrition.

Surgical Procedure

If the patient remains unstable despite maximal ventilatory measures, the use of ECMO may be necessary (Kleinman & Wilson, 2016; McHoney, 2015). Repair is delayed until the patient's cardiovascular status is stabilized. No strong evidence exists showing advantages of early or delayed surgery (McHoney, 2015; Puligandla et al., 2018). The decision is often determined on a case-by-case basis. A primary closure is performed for small defects, and a patch closure is performed for larger or more complicated defects. Surgical repair is done by either the conventional abdominal approach or minimally invasive approach, as well as either the laparoscopic or thoracoscopic approach (McHoney, 2015; Qin et al., 2019).

Postoperative Assessment and Nursing Care

■ Monitor preductal and postductal oxygen saturation.

■ Follow frequent blood gases to monitor for acidosis, hypoxia, and hypercarbia to evaluate respiratory function.

■ Monitor perfusion.

  ● Normal saline or 5% albumin fluid boluses (5–10 mL/kg) and inotropic support to maintain adequate peripheral perfusion (Kleinman & Wilson, 2016)

■ Assess pupillary response, fontanelle size/tension, seizure activity, and signs of intraventricular/intraparenchymal bleeding.

■ Maintain a quiet environment and cluster care.

■ Measure accurate intake and output.

■ Monitor electrolytes and diuretic treatment closely.

■ Obtain chest x-ray (CXR), ABG, electrolytes, CBC, lactic acid.

■ Provide surgical wound assessment and care.

■ Maintain chest tube(s).

■ Assess comfort.

● Treat with narcotics and sedatives to achieve desired pain control and activity level.

■ Administer parenteral nutrition until enteral feedings can be reestablished.

Documentation

■ Vital signs

■ Preductal and postductal oxygen saturations

■ Perfusion

■ Accurate intake and output

■ Patient response to care and treatments

■ Daily weights

■ Wound assessment and management, including signs of infection

CONGENITAL PULMONARY AIRWAY MALFORMATION

KATIE ROY AND ETHAN SCHULER

The most common congenital malformation of the respiratory tract is the congenital pulmonary airway malformation (CPAM). Previously known as congenital cystic adenomatoid malformation (CCAM), CPAM is classically described as a cystic mass of abnormal lung tissue that does not function as normal lung. Unlike bronchopulmonary sequestration (BPS), CPAMs are connected to the tracheobronchial tree and arterial blood supply usually arises from pulmonary circulation (Oermann, 2019b).

CPAMs are typically unilateral and can arise in any lobe (Oermann, 2019b). They most commonly develop during the pseudoglandular phase of lung development, between 5 and 17 weeks of gestation (Baral et al., 2015). The reported incidence of CPAM is variable, ranging from one in 7,200 to one in 35,000 live births (Lau et al., 2017; Oermann, 2019b). There are five main types of CPAMs, which are classified based on the embryologic level of origin, characteristics, and histologic and pathologic features (Oermann, 2019b; Sfakianaki & Copel, 2012; Stocker, 2009):

■ Type 0 = tracheobronchial origin; diffuse involvement of the entire lung severely impairing gas exchange; rarest type of CPAM and incompatible with life

■ Type 1 = bronchial/bronchiolar origin; most common type; typically involves only one lobe; associated with very small risk of malignancy (bronchoalveolar carcinoma); favorable outcome

■ Type 2 = bronchiolar origin; associated with other congenital anomalies such as BPS, congenital diaphragmatic hernia (CDH), renal agenesis, or esophageal atresia; outcome may be dependent on the severity of the co-occurring anomalies

■ Type 3 = bronchiolar/alveolar origin; often appears as a large mass that may involve an entire lobe or several lobes; may cause mass effect within the mediastinum; poor prognosis when associated with hydrops

■ Type 4 = distal acinar origin; associated with malignancy and may be difficult to distinguish from pleuropulmonary blastoma (PPB)

Presentation

Prenatal

■ Infants with CPAM are often identified on prenatal US.

■ Large lesions may be associated with the development of hydrops fetalis (severe edema in the fetus or newborn), a poor prognostic sign.

● Hydrops typically develops by 28-week gestation and is the most critical predictor of poor outcome; antenatal intervention and premature delivery may be attempted to save the fetus (Davenport et al., 2004).

● Fetal echocardiography can help identify hydrops by assessing for cardiac compression, restricted ventricular filling, and reversal of inferior vena cava flow; this may lead to pleural effusion, pericardial effusion, skin edema, ascites, and polyhydramnios (Egloff & Bulas, 2020).

Neonatal/Childhood

■ Approximately 75% of patients diagnosed with CPAM prenatally are asymptomatic at birth.

■ Respiratory distress is present in most newborns with symptomatic CPAM.

● Respiratory distress may range in severity from grunting, retractions, tachypnea, and mild hypoxia to respiratory failure requiring aggressive ventilator support or extracorporeal membrane oxygenation (ECMO).

■ Pulmonary hypoplasia may result when a large CPAM compresses lung tissue and limits normal growth and development.

■ Mediastinal shift may occur due to air trapping and mass effect of the lesion, leading to cardiac and respiratory dysfunction.

■ Spontaneous pneumothorax may occur and is typically associated with type 4 CPAM.

● Dyspnea and chest pain may be symptoms of pneumothorax.

● Those presenting with CPAM and pneumothorax should be evaluated for PPB (Oermann, 2019b).

■ Recurrent pulmonary infections may develop due to bronchial compression, air trapping, and inability to clear secretions.

■ Hemoptysis has occasionally been described as a manifestation of CPAM in the older child.

■ Cough, fever, and failure to thrive have all been reported in the presentation of CPAM (Parikh & Samuel, 2005).

■ Presence of other congenital anomalies may be indicative of CPAM.

Diagnosis

■ Prenatal ultrasound (US) and MRI assist with prenatal diagnosis.

■ Chest radiography typically identifies CPAM of sufficient size to cause clinical problems (Stone, 2015).

● The usual appearance is characterized by air-filled cysts, though it may also contain air-fluid levels; type 3 CPAM may appear as a large solid mass with mediastinal shift and type 4 CPAM may demonstrate pneumothorax (Oermann, 2019b; Stone, 2015).

■ CT scan with angiography of the thorax provides a rapid means of defining the extent of the CPAM as well as associated blood supply.

■ MRI permits increased definition of the lesion and assists with surgical planning.

■ Additional imaging studies:

● Renal and cerebral ultrasonography should be performed in newborns with CPAM to exclude coexisting anomalies (Stone, 2015).

● Echocardiography should be performed in newborns with CPAM to rule out coexisting cardiac lesions and identify pulmonary hypertension (Stone, 2015).

Preoperative Assessment and Nursing Care

■ Provide supportive respiratory care as clinically indicated, ranging from supplemental oxygen to mechanical ventilation.

■ Establish a hydration and nutrition plan.

■ Administer prescribed antibiotics in children with associated respiratory infections.

Surgical Procedure

■ CPAMs may regress spontaneously in utero, decreasing the need for intervention.

● Fetal intervention is considered with CPAMs complicated by hydrops as the prognosis is otherwise poor (Egloff & Bulas, 2020).

■ Surgical resection, including segmentectomy or lobectomy, is the primary treatment for postnatal symptomatic patients and those with high-risk features; resection of CPAM in asymptomatic infants and children without high-risk features is at the discretion of the operating surgeon.

- High-risk features include large lesions, bilateral or multifocal cysts, pneumothorax, or family history of PPB-associated conditions (Oermann, 2019b).

- Elective resection may decrease risk of future complications, including recurrent infection, pneumothorax, and malignant transformation.

- Recommended timing of elective resection is after the neonatal period but before age 12 months as early intervention is thought to enhance compensatory lung growth.

- Studies have not uniformly confirmed differences in long-term lung function by age at the time of surgical resection (Kotecha et al., 2012).

■ Surgery is typically curative with few complications.

■ If observation is elected, the patient should have close follow-up with annual routine imaging (Oermann, 2019b).

■ Excised lesions should be sent for pathology review to confirm diagnosis and exclude potential malignancy (Sfakianaki & Copel, 2012).

Postoperative Assessment and Nursing Care

■ See "Postoperative Assessment and Nursing Care" for bronchopulmonary sequestration

Documentation

■ Vital signs

■ Ventilation or respiratory requirements

■ Thoracostomy tube output

■ Intake and output

■ Serum electrolytes, complete blood counts (CBCs), blood gas (0 measurements and other laboratory values)

■ Sedation, state, and pain scores

REFERENCES

Albanese, C. T., & Rothenberg, S. S. (2007). Experience with 144 consecutive pediatric thoracoscopic lobectomies. *Journal of Laparoendoscopic Advanced Surgical Techniques A,* *17*(3), 339–341. https://doi.org/10.1089/lap.2006.0184

Amano, H., Fujishiro, J., Hinoki, A., & Uchida, H. (2017). Intralobar pulmonary sequestration expanding toward the contralateral thorax: Two case reports. *BMC Surgery, 17*(1), 110–114. https://doi.org/10.1186/s12893-017-0313-z

Baral, D., Adhikari, B., Zaccarini, D., Dongol, R. M., & Sah, B. (2015). Congenital pulmonary airway malformation in an adult male: A case report with literature review. *Case Reports in Pulmonology, 2015,* 743452. https://doi.org/10.1155/2015/743452

Davenport, M., Warne, S. A., Cacciaguerra, S., Patel, S., Greenough, A., & Nicolaides, K. (2004). Current outcome of antenally diagnosed cystic lung disease. *Journal of Pediatric Surgery, 39*(4), 549–556. https://doi.org/10.1016/j.jpedsurg.2003.12.021

DeParedes, C. G., Pierce, W. S., Johnson, D. G., & Waldhausen, J. A. (1970). Pulmonary sequestration in infants and children: A 20-year experience and review of the literature. *Journal of Pediatric Surgery, 5*(2), 136–147. https://doi.org/10.1016/0022-3468(70)90269-1

Egloff, A., & Bulas, D. I. (2020). Congenital pulmonary airway malformation: Prenatal diagnosis and management. *UpToDate.* https://www.uptodate.com/contents/congenital-pulmonary-airway-malformation-prenatal-diagnosis-and-management

Flye, M. W., Conley, M., & Silver, D. (1976). Spectrum of pulmonary sequestration. *Annals of Thoracic Surgery, 22*(5), 478–482. https://doi.org/10.1016/s0003-4975(10)64457-8

Haroon, J., & Chamberlain, R. S. (2012). An evidenced-based review of the current treatment of congenital diaphragmatic hernia. *Clinical Pediatrics, 52*(2), 115–124. https://doi.org/10.1177/0009922812472249

Keller, R. L., Tacy, T. A., Hendricks-Munoz, K., Xu, J., Moon-Grady, A. J., Neuhaus, J., Moore, P., Nobuhara, K. K., Hawgood, S., & Fineman, J. R. (2010). Congenital diaphragmatic hernia; endothelin-1, pulmonary hypertension, and disease severity. *American Journal of Respiratory and Critical Care Medicine, 182,* 555–561. https://doi.org/10.1164/rccm.200907-1126OC

Kleinman, M., & Wilson, J. (2016). Diaphragmatic hernia and diaphragmatic eventration. In A. Hansen & M. Puder (Eds.), *Manual of neonatal surgical intensive care* (3rd ed., pp. 260–282). People's Medical Publishing House.

Kosiński, P., & Wielgoś, M. (2017). Congenital diaphragmatic hernia: Pathogenesis, prenatal diagnosis and management-literature review. *Ginekologia Polska, 88*(1), 24–30. https://doi.org/10.5603/GP.a2017.0005

Kotecha, S., Barbato, A., Bush, A., Claus, F., Davenport, M., Delacourt, C., Duprest, J., Eber, E., Frenckner, B., Greenough, A., Nicholson, A. G., Anton-Pacheco, J. L., & Midulla, F. (2012). Antenatal and postnatal management of congenital cystic adenomatoid malformation. *Paediatric Respiratory Reviews, 13*(3), 162–171. https://doi.org/10.1016/j.prrv.2012.01.002

Lau, C. T., Kan, A., Shek, N., Tam, P., & Wong, K. K. (2017). Is congenital pulmonary airway malformation really a rare disease? Result of a prospective registry with universal antenatal screening program. *Pediatric Surgery International, 33*(1), 105–108. https://doi.org/10.1007/s00383-016-3991-1

McHoney, M. (2015). Congenital diaphragmatic hernia, management in the newborn. *Pediatric Surgery International, 31,* 1005–1013. https://doi.org/10.1007/s00383-015-3794-9

Oermann, C. M. (2019a). Bronchopulmonary sequestration. *UpToDate.* https://www.uptodate.com/contents/bronchopulmonary-sequestration

Oermann, C. M. (2019b). Congenital pulmonary airway (cystic adenomatoid) malformation. *UpToDate.* https://www.uptodate.com/contents/congenital-pulmonary-airway-cystic-adenomatoid-malformation

Olson, E., Lusk, L. A., Fineman, J. R., Robertson, L., & Keller, R. L. (2015). Short-term treprostinil use in infants with congenital diaphragmatic hernia following repair. *Journal of Pediatrics, 167*(3), 762–764. https://doi.org/10.1016/j.jpeds.2015.06.016

Parikh, D., & Samuel, M. (2005). Congenital cystic lung lesions: Is surgical resection essential? *Pediatric Pulmonology, 40*(6), 533–537. https://doi.org/10.1002/ppul.20300

Puligandla, P. S., Skarsgard, E. D., Offringa, M., Adatia, I., Baird, R., Bailey, J. A. M., Brindle, M., Chiu, P., Cogswell, A., Dakshinamurti, S., Flageole, H., Keijzer, R., McMillan, D., Oluyomi-Obi, T., Pennaforte, T., Perreault, T., Piedboeuf, B., Riley, S. P., Ryan, G., Synnes, A., Traynor, M., & Canadian Congenital Diaphragmatic Hernia Collaborative. (2018). Diagnosis and management of congenital diaphragmatic hernia: a clinical practice guideline. *CMAJ, 190*(4), E103–E112. https://doi.org/10.1503/cmaj.170206

Qin, J., Ren, Y., & Ma, D. (2019). A comparative study of thoracoscopic and open surgery of congenital diaphragmatic hernia in neonates. *Journal of Cardiothoracic Surgery, 14*, 118. 10.1186/s13019-019-0938-3

Sfakianaki, A. K., & Copel, J. A. (2012). Congenital cystic lesions of the lung: Congenital cystic adenomatoid malformation and bronchopulmonary sequestration. *Reviews in Obstetrics & Gynecology, 5*(2), 85–93. https://www.ncbi.nlm.nih.gov/pmc/articles/PMC3410507

Snoek, K. G., Peters, N. C. J., van Rosmalen, J., Van Heijst, A. F. J., Eggink, A. J., Sikkel, E., Wijnen, R. M., IJsselstijn, H., Cohen-Overbeek, T. E., & Tibboel, D. (2017). The validity of the observed-to-expected lung-to-head ratio in congenital diaphragmatic hernia in an era of standardized neonatal treatment; a multicenter study. *Prenatal Diagnosis, 37*, 658–665. https://doi.org/10.1002/pd.5062

Stocker, J. T. (2009). Cystic lung disease in infants and children. *Fetal Pediatric Pathology, 28*(4), 155–184. https://doi.org/10.1080/15513810902984095

Stone, A. E. (2015). Cystic adenomatoid malformation workup. *Medscape.* https://emedicine.medscape.com/article/1001488

Wynn, J., Krishnan, U., Aspelund, G., Zhang, Y., Duong, J., Stolar, C. J., Hahn, E., Pietsch, J., Chung, D., Moore, D., Austin, E., Mychaliska, G., Gajarski, R., Foong, Y., Michelfelder, E., Potolka, D., Bucher, B., Warner, B., Grady, M., . . . Arkovitz, M. S. (2013). Outcomes of congenital diaphragmatic hernia in the modern era. *Journal of Pediatrics, 163*(1), 114–119. https://doi.org/10.1016/j.jpeds.2012.12.036

SURGICAL DISORDERS OF THE TRACHEA AND ESOPHAGUS

ETHAN SCHULER AND KATIE ROY

ESOPHAGEAL ATRESIA WITH OR WITHOUT TRACHEOESOPHAGEAL FISTULA

Esophageal Atresia (EA) is the interruption in the continuity of the esophagus (El-Gohary et al., 2010). EA with tracheoesophageal fistula (TEF) occurs from an abnormal septation between the trachea and esophagus. EA with TEF presents in several variants. EA with distal TEF is the most common (85%), followed by isolated EA without TEF (8%), TEF without EA (4%), EA with proximal TEF (3%), and EA with proximal and distal TEF (<1%; Parolini et al., 2017).

Presentation

The incidence of EA, combining all types, is 2.43 cases per 10,000 births (Parolini et al., 2017). Prenatal diagnosis of EA is suspected when US reveals a small or absent stomach bubble and polyhydramnios. Most prenatal cases remain undiagnosed as the positive predictive value for these US findings ranges between 44% and 56%. When suspected, fetal echocardiogram and chromosomal analysis are indicated given associations with other congenital anomalies. Up to 25% of EA/TEF patients may have three or more congenital VACTERL (vertebral, anorectal, cardiac, tracheo-esophageal, renal, limb) abnormalities (Kunisaki & Foker, 2012). Other notable genetic syndromes associated with EA/TEF include CHARGE (coloboma, heart defects, atresia choanae, retarded growth, genital hypoplasia, ear anomalies), DiGeorge syndrome, and tisomy 13, 14, and 18 (Parolini et al., 2017).

Diagnosis

▪ The infant with EA with or without TEF may be well appearing at delivery or exhibit symptoms, including:

- Excessive salivation or inability to manage secretions
- Feeding intolerance
- Respiratory distress due to aspiration of secretions or reflux of gastric contents via distal TEF

▪ EA should be suspected in patients who fail to pass an oroesophageal (OE) tube to the expected length of gastric tip location of 11 to 12 cm.

- A chest radiograph may show the OE tube coiled in a dilated proximal esophageal pouch.
- Radiographic presence of air in the intestines does not eliminate the diagnosis of EA because a distal TEF may exist.

▪ For suspected prenatal diagnosis of EA/TEF, delivery at a high-risk center should be arranged.

Preoperative Assessment and Nursing Care

▪ Conduct a full head-to-toe physical examination to identify other potential congenital anatomical abnormalities with superficial phenotypes (see Table 8.3).

▪ Insert a 10 to 12 French double-lumen OE tube in the upper esophageal pouch and place it to prescribed continuous low-wall suction (20–40 mmHg) for secretion management (Parolini et al., 2017)

- One lumen will apply suction for drainage removal while the other serves as an air vent (Replogle, 1963).
- The OE tube should be advanced to a predetermined length or until it meets resistance, and then pulled back 1 cm and secured with tape or occlusive dressing.
- Make a notation of the exit marking for the tube in the medical record.
- Maintain OE tube patency via intermittent irrigation of the drainage removal port with 1 to 2 mL of air every 2 to 4 hours and as needed as secretions may be tenacious.

TABLE 8.3 Evaluation of Associated Anomalies With EA/TEF

	EVALUATION	KEY ELEMENTS
VACTERL		
Vertebral anomalies	Radiographs, US	Butterfly or hemivertebrae
Anus to anal atresia	Physical examination	Anal position, vaginal fistula, imperforate anus
Congenital heart defects	Echocardiogram, chest CT	Situs, arch position, ASD, VSD, AV canal, TOF, pulmonary vein stenosis
TEF	Bronchoscopy	Proximal or distal fistula, tracheomalacia
EA	Radiograph, contrast study	Distance between proximal and distal segments determines gap
Renal anomalies	Abdominal US	Laterality, collecting system abnormalities, horseshoe kidney, hydronephrosis
Limb deformities	Physical examination, radiographs	Absent radius
CHARGE		
Coloboma	Ophthalmologic examination	Keyhole pupils
Choanal atresia	Physical examination, CT face/sinus	Blockage of posterior nasal passages
Retarded growth	Biometric measurement	Small for gestational age in parameters of weight, head circumference, and length
Genital anomalies	Physical examination	Hypospadias, microphallus, labial hypoplasia, rectovaginal fistula
Ear abnormalities	Physical examination	Microtia, auricular appendages, sinus

ASD, atrial septal defect; AV canal, atrioventricular canal; CT, computed tomography; EA, esophageal atresia; TEF, tracheoesophageal fistula; TOF, tetralogy of Fallot; US, ultrasound; VSD, ventricular septal defect.

■ Place infant on full aspiration precautions and maintain these at all times if TEF is suspected or diagnosed.

- Consider these precautions for patients diagnosed with EA without TEF, as the proximal pouch may fill with secretions if the OE tube malfunctions, increasing risk for aspiration.

- Raise the head of the bed to minimum 45° (Kunisaki & Foker, 2012).

  • If TEF is present, crying or bag-mask ventilation may force air into the stomach causing progressive abdominal distention, decreased lung excursion, and increased respiratory effort (Gupta & Sharma, 2008).

■ Avoid noninvasive positive pressure ventilation to prevent gastric distention

- Only intubate as medically necessary to avoid risk of iatrogenic perforation of the upper esophageal pouch or stomach from distention (Parolini et al., 2017).

■ Initiate antacid prophylactic therapy.

- Keep the infant nothing by mouth and administer intravenous fluids.

- Consider parenteral nutrition until enteral access can be surgically obtained.

■ Monitor BGs, electrolytes, complete blood counts (CBCs); obtain blood type and crossmatch in preparation for surgery.

■ Obtain echocardiogram to determine arch position for surgical approach and to identify congenital cardiac abnormalities found in up to 25% of cases (Parolini et al., 2017).

■ Complete evaluation with fluoroscopy, endoscopy, and tracheobronchoscopy (TBS) to thoroughly evaluate the defects.

- Upper gastrointestinal (UGI) with fluoroscopy and endoscopy are performed to identify the length of the upper esophageal pouch, as well as a potential proximal TEF.

- TBS is recommended to evaluate for TEF, laryngeal cleft, tracheobronchomalacia, and bilateral vocal cord mobility.

- Risk of injury to the recurrent laryngeal nerve exists during thoracic surgery, possibly leading to vocal cord paralysis, complicating the postoperative course (Lawlor et al., 2020; Mortellaro et al., 2011).

■ Encourage oral stimulation and nonnutritive sucking to promote successful oral feedings postoperatively.

■ Encourage parental participation in care to facilitate maternal–infant attachment.

Surgical Procedure

■ Goals of surgical repair are to place the esophagus in continuity and ligate the TEF if present.

- Commonly performed via right posterolateral thoracotomy with primary repair end-to-end anastomosis for short-gap EA (Kunisaki & Foker, 2012)

■ If the distance between the upper and lower esophageal pouches is greater than three vertebral bodies, a delayed primary repair is the preferred method for surgical repair (see following section on "Long-Gap Esophageal Atresia").

- Cervical esophagostomy, or creation of a spit fistula, is not recommended in these cases to preserve upper pouch integrity for future surgical procedures.

- Consider transfer to a center of expertise if long-gap EA is suspected or if first attempts at primary repair fail (van der Zee et al., 2017).

■ The patient typically returns to an intensive care setting with a thoracostomy tube in place to facilitate postoperative drainage.

Postoperative Assessment and Nursing Care

■ Maintain the head in a flexed position to minimize tension on the anastomosis site and mitigate risk of anastomotic site leak or stricture.

- Neuromuscular blockade may be used to achieve the desired position and to facilitate healing.

■ Ensure adequate analgesia.

■ Conduct frequent respiratory assessments while sedated and paralyzed.

■ Keep intubated until extubation readiness is established.

■ Maintain vigilance toward mouth care; positioning and closed suctioning may reduce risk of ventilator-associated pneumonia and iatrogenic injury to surgical repair sites.

■ Monitor thoracostomy tube drainage and consider removal when drainage is minimal, and radiograph reveals no evidence of air leak or anastomotic leak.

- Excessive frothy tube output, tachycardia, or escalation in respiratory requirements may indicate anastomotic leak.

■ Provide gastric decompression via surgically placed nasogastric tube.

- Avoid manipulation of tube and risk of injury to the anastomotic site.

■ Continue antacid prophylactic therapy.

■ Perform a fluoroscopic UGI contrast study at 1 to 2 weeks, or as prescribed by the surgical team, to ensure continuity of the esophagus prior to initiating oral feedings.

■ Good nutrition is essential for growth and healing.

- Feed using a surgically placed nasogastric or postpyloric feeding tube until the infant can receive oral feedings (Ngo & Shah, 2020).

- Optimize parenteral nutrition as needed until enteral feeds are established.

- Establish oral feedings when deemed ready by the surgical team and base readiness for oral feedings on cues, gestational age, and maturity.

■ Monitor for symptoms of postrepair esophageal stricture formation such as dysphagia, vomiting, choking with feeds, excessive drooling, and oral secretions.

● Strictures develop from scar formation at the repair site, leading to intraluminal narrowing.

● They may occur in up to 80% of EA repair cases; if suspected, consider UGI fluoroscopic study or endoscopy to identify (Manfredi, 2016).

Documentation

■ Vital signs

■ Ventilation requirement

■ Thoracostomy tube output

■ Nasogastric (NG) tube placement and output

■ Intake and output

■ Serum electrolytes, CBCs, blood gas measurements, and other laboratory values

■ Sedation, state, and pain scores

LONG-GAP ESOPHAGEAL ATRESIA

ETHAN SCHULER AND KATIE ROY

Referred to as "Pure EA," the definition of long-gap esophageal atresia (LGEA) remains vague. LGEA is suspected when the initial radiograph demonstrates no intestinal air and subsequent workup reveals a greater than three vertebral bodies, or 2 to 3 cm gap, between the upper and lower esophageal pouches. This significant distance makes primary anastomosis difficult to perform with acceptable tension (Shieh & Jennings, 2017). Advanced surgical techniques are required when early primary repair is not possible.

Presentation

The clinical presentation of LGEA mirrors that of esophageal atresia/tracheoesophageal fistula (EA/TEF) as previously described. While no distal bowel gas may be visualized on initial radiographs, a proximal TEF should be ruled out. A recent consensus statement recommends referral of all LGEA patients, or those in whom primary EA repair has failed, to a center of expertise (CoE). CoEs are pediatric surgical institutions equipped and experienced in the treatment of complex EA through a multidisciplinary approach between pediatric and neonatal ICU providers and specialists within pediatric surgery, anesthesiology, pulmonology, otolaryngology, gastroenterology, cardiology, radiology, neurology, neurosurgery, urology, registered dieticians, physical and occupational therapy, speech language pathology, and social work (van der Zee et al., 2017).

Diagnosis

■ After the diagnosis of EA is established, the distance between the upper and lower esophageal pouches must be measured via fluoroscopic gapogram (Shieh & Jennings, 2017).

- ● Water-soluble contrast is administered in the upper esophageal pouch via oroesophageal (OE) tube and stomach via surgically placed gastrostomy tube (GT).

Preoperative Assessment and Nursing Care

■ Perform a full head-to-toe physical examination to identify other potential congenital anatomical abnormalities as in the EA/TEF preoperative assessment.

■ Insert a 10 to 12 French double-lumen OE tube in the upper esophageal pouch and place it to continuous low-wall suction (20–40 mmHg) for secretion management (Parolini et al., 2017). One lumen will apply suction for drainage removal while the other serves as an air vent (Replogle, 1963).

- ● The catheter should be advanced to a predetermined length or until it meets resistance and then pulled back 1 cm and secured with tape or occlusive dressing.
- ● Make a notation of the exit marking for the tube in the medical record.
- ● Maintain tube patency via intermittent irrigation of the drainage removal port with 1 to 2 mL of air every 2 to 4 hours and as needed as secretions may be tenacious.

■ Implement full aspiration precautions and maintain at all times if TEF is suspected.

- ● Raise the head of the bed to minimum 45°.
- ● If TEF is present, crying or bag-mask ventilation may force air into the stomach causing progressive abdominal distention, decreased lung excursion, and increased respiratory effort (Gupta & Sharma, 2008).
  - • Avoid noninvasive positive pressure ventilation as able to prevent gastric distention
  - • Only intubate as medically necessary to avoid risk of iatrogenic perforation of the upper esophageal pouch or stomach from distention (Parolini et al., 2017).

■ Initiate antacid prophylactic therapy.

■ Keep the infant nothing by mouth and administer intravenous fluids.

■ Consider parenteral nutrition until enteral access can be surgically obtained.

■ Monitor blood gases, electrolytes, complete blood counts (CBCs); obtain blood type and crossmatch in preparation for surgery.

■ Obtain echocardiogram to determine arch position for surgical approach and to identify congenital cardiac abnormalities found in up to 25% of cases (Parolini et al., 2017).

■ Complete evaluation for defects with fluoroscopy, endoscopy, and tracheobronchoscopy (TBS).

● Identification of the upper esophageal pouch length and a potential proximal TEF is accomplished through radiologic evaluation, consisting of UGI with fluoroscopy and endoscopy.

● Evaluation for TEF, laryngeal cleft, tracheobronchomalacia, and bilateral vocal cord mobility is accomplished via TBS.

• Injury to the recurrent laryngeal nerve is a risk during thoracic surgery, possibly leading to vocal cord paralysis, complicating the postoperative course (Lawlor et al., 2020; Mortellaro et al., 2011).

■ Encourage oral stimulation and nonnutritive sucking to promote successful oral feedings postoperatively.

■ Encourage parental participation in care to facilitate maternal–infant attachment.

Surgical Procedure

■ Surgical techniques for LGEA repair depend on several factors, including CoE experience and infrastructure as well as patient characteristics such as gap length, quality of the upper and lower pouch tissue, strictures, and vascular or other associated congenital anomalies (Shieh & Jennings, 2017).

■ The goal of surgical repair is to preserve and utilize the native esophagus for primary anastomosis; when primary anastomosis is not achievable through traction/growth techniques, esophageal replacement is required.

Delayed Primary Anastomosis

■ With OE tube decompression and surgical G-tube placement, delayed primary anastomosis may be achieved as the gap decreases with spontaneous growth.

■ Serial gapograms obtained over 1 to 3 months monitor for surgical candidacy evidenced by a distance of less than two vertebral bodies apart.

■ Increase risk of prolonged hospitalization and long-term oral aversion.

Foker Process

■ Two-stage process involving placement of the esophageal pouches on static internal traction or external traction (Foker Stage I), followed by serial tension adjustments to decrease gap length over 1 to 2 weeks, concluded with primary anastomosis of the native esophagus (Foker Stage 2; Foker et al., 2005).

■ May require prolonged period of sedation, analgesia, and neuromuscular blockade with mechanical ventilation.

Gastric Transposition (Pull-Up)

■ The stomach is mobilized and transposed into the chest in place of the esophagus.

■ Technically less problematic due to adequate blood supply, minimally invasive techniques, and a single gastroesophageal anastomosis.

■ Long-term sequelae include severe gastroesophageal reflux (GER) that increases risk of esophageal cancer and pulmonary manifestations such as aspiration and restrictive lung disease.

Jejunal Interposition

■ Combined intra-abdominal and thoracic procedure to bring a jejunal conduit into the chest in place of the native esophagus (Kunisaki & Foker, 2012); can be performed via true interposition or Roux-en-Y configuration (Shieh & Jennings, 2017).

■ Jejunum mimics esophageal motility, minimizes GER, and grows with the patient over time.

■ Technically challenging procedure requiring a multidisciplinary approach between pediatric surgery, gastroenterology, otolaryngology, cardiothoracic surgery, and plastic surgery.

■ May require additional microvascular anastomoses to ensure adequate blood supply and graft health over time (Firriolo et al., 2019).

Postoperative Assessment and Nursing Care

■ Maintain the head in a flexed position to minimize tension on the anastomosis site and mitigate risk of anastomotic site leak or stricture.

● Neuromuscular blockade may be used to achieve the desired position and to facilitate healing.

■ For patients between Foker Stages I and II on externalized traction, do not slide or rub the patient's posterior surfaces as friction may disrupt external sutures; patients can be lifted to reposition.

■ Ensure adequate analgesia (see "Goal of Postoperative Pain Management and Assessment" section).

■ Conduct frequent respiratory assessments while sedated and paralyzed.

■ Keep intubated until extubation readiness is established.

■ Vigilance toward mouth care, positioning, and closed suctioning may reduce risk of ventilator-associated pneumonia and iatrogenic injury to surgical repair sites.

■ Monitor thoracostomy tube drainage and consider removal when drainage is minimal, and radiograph reveals no evidence of air leak or anastomosis leak.

- ● Excessive frothy tube output, tachycardia, or escalation in respiratory requirements may indicate anastomotic leak.
- ● Depending on the surgical technique, abdominal and mediastinal drains may be placed.
- ■ Provide gastric decompression via surgically placed nasogastric (NG) tube or G-tube.
  - ● Avoid manipulation of tube and risk of injury to the anastomosis.
- ■ Perform a fluoroscopic UGI contrast study at 1 to 2 weeks, or as prescribed by the surgical team, to ensure continuity of the esophagus or conduit prior to initiating oral or enteral feedings.
- ■ Feed using a surgically placed nasogastric, G-tube, or postpyloric feeding tube until the infant can receive oral feedings (Ngo & Shah, 2020).
- ■ Establish oral feedings based on oral feeding cues, gestational age, and maturity.
  - ● Good nutrition is essential for growth and healing.
  - ● Optimize parenteral nutrition as needed until enteral feeds are established.
- ■ Monitor for symptoms of postrepair esophageal stricture formation such as dysphagia, vomiting, choking with feeds, excessive drooling, and oral secretions.
  - ● Strictures result from scar formation at the repair site, leading to intraluminal narrowing.
  - ● They may occur in up to 80% of EA repair cases; if suspected, consider UGI fluoroscopic study or endoscopy to identify (Manfredi, 2016).

Documentation

- ■ Vital signs
- ■ Ventilation requirement
- ■ Thoracostomy tube output
- ■ NG tube placement and output
- ■ Intake and output
- ■ Serum electrolytes, CBCs, blood gas measurements, and other laboratory values
- ■ Sedation, state, and pain scores

REFERENCES

El-Gohary, Y., Gittes, G. K., & Tovar, J. A. (2010). Congenital anomalies of the esophagus. *Seminars in Pediatric Surgery, 19*, 186–193. https://doi.org/10.1053/j.sempedsurg.2010.03.009

Firriolo, J., Nuzzi, L., Ganske, I., Hamilton, T., Smithers, C., Ganor, O., Upton, J., Taghinia, A., Jennings, R., & Labow, B. (2019). Supercharged jejunal interposition: A reliable esophageal replacement in pediatric patients. *Plastic and Reconstructive Surgery, 143*(6), 1266e–1276e. https://doi.org/10.1097/PRS.0000000000005649

Foker, J., Kendall, T. C., Catton, K., & Khan, K. M. (2005). A flexible approach to achieve a true primary repair for all infants with esophageal atresia. *Seminars in Pediatric Surgery, 14*, 5–8. https://doi.org/10.1053/j.sempedsurg.2004.10.021

Gupta, D. K., & Sharma, S. (2008). Esophageal atresia: The total care in a high-risk population. *Seminars in Pediatric Surgery, 17*, 236–243. https://doi.org/10.1053/j.sempedsurg.2008.07.003

Kunisaki, S. M., & Foker, J. (2012). Surgical advances in the fetus and neonate: Esophageal atresia. *Clinics in Perinatology, 39*(2), 349–361. https://doi.org/10.1016/j.clp.2012.04.007

Lawlor, C., Smithers, C., Hamilton, T., Baird, C., Rahbar, R., Choi, S., & Jennings, R. (2020). Innovative management of severe tracheobronchomalacia using anterior and posterior tracheobronchopexy. *The Laryngoscope, 130*(2), E65–E74. https://doi.org/10.1002/lary.27938

Manfredi, M. A. (2016). Endoscopic management of anastomotic esophageal strictures secondary to esophageal atresia. *Gastrointestinal Endoscopy Clinics of North America, 26*(1), 201–219. https://doi.org/10.1016/j.giec.2015.09.002

Mortellaro, V. E., Pettiford, J. N., St. Peter, S. D., Fraser, J. D., & Wei, J. (2011). Incidence, diagnosis, and outcomes of vocal fold immobility after esophageal atresia (EA) and/or tracheoesophageal fistula (TEF) repair. *European Journal of Pediatric Surgery, 21*, 386–388. https://doi.org/10.1055/s-0031-1291269

Ngo, K. D., & Shah, M. (2020). Gastrointestinal system. In C. Kenner, L. B. Altimier, & M. V. Boykova (Eds.), *Comprehensive neonatal care* (6th ed., pp. 179–210). Springer Publishing Company.

Parolini, F., Bulotta, A. L., Battaglia, S., & Alberti, D. (2017). Preoperative management of children with esophageal atresia: Current perspectives. *Pediatric Health, Medicine and Therapeutics, 8*, 1–7. https://doi.org/10.2147/PHMT.S106643

Replogle, R. (1963). Esophageal atresia: Plastic sump catheter for drainage of the proximal pouch. *Surgery, 54*, 296–297.

Shieh, H., & Jennings, R. (2017). Long-gap esophageal atresia. *Seminars in Pediatric Surgery, 26*(2), 72–77. https://doi.org/10.1053/j.sempedsurg.2017.02.009

van der Zee, D. C., Bagolan, P., Faure, C., Gottrand, F., Jennings, R., Laberge, J., Ferro, M., Hernan, M., Parmentier, B., Sfier, R., & Teague, W. (2017). Position paper of INoEA working group on long-gap esophageal atresia: For better care. *Frontiers in Pediatrics, 5*(63), 1–3. https://doi.org/10.3389/fped.2017.00063

GASTROINTESTINAL SURGICAL CONDITIONS IN THE NEONATE

JULIE BRIERE AND MICHELLE LABRECQUE

GASTROINTESTINAL SURGERY GENERAL CONSIDERATIONS

Any segment of the gastrointestinal (GI) tract may have an obstruction in the neonate, either due to a structural anomaly or a functional etiology (Table 8.4).

General symptoms that raise concern for a bowel obstruction in the neonate include:

■ History of polyhydramnios

■ Abdominal distension

■ Emesis, often bilious

■ Failure to pass meconium within 24 to 48 hours after birth

TABLE 8.4 Common Types of Bowel Obstructions in Neonates

STRUCTURAL ANOMALIES: ANATOMICAL CONDITION AFFECTING BOWEL CONTINUITY	FUNCTIONAL CONDITIONS: MECHANICAL CONDITION EITHER DUE TO ALTERED PERISTALSIS OR A BLOCKAGE
Esophageal atresia Duodenal atresia Malrotation/midgut volvulus Ileal/jejunal atresia Imperforate anus	Hirschsprung disease Meconium ileus Meconium plug syndrome Necrotizing enterocolitis

Advances in neonatology, neonatal surgery, and anesthesia have led to increased survival and overall decreased morbidity in neonates with GI issues. Prompt assessment, stabilization, and surgical intervention are essential in the management of a neonate with suspected bowel obstruction. Initial stabilization of a neonate with a suspected bowel obstruction includes:

■ Cessation of enteral feeds

■ Gastric decompression with a sump tube and replacement of excess gastric losses

■ IV hydration

■ Correction of fluid, acid–base, and electrolyte derangements

■ Antibiotic therapy (in most situations)

■ Fluid resuscitation if fluid shifts occur from the vascular space into the bowel lumen, leading to shock

These therapies occur concurrently with surgical consultation and evaluation for a bowel obstruction with the following:

Radiologic Studies

■ Abdominal x-ray (anteroposterior and left lateral decubitus or cross-table lateral views)

■ Upper GI contrast series

■ Contrast enemas

■ Ultrasonography (less often) based on presenting symptoms and patient history

Laboratory Studies

■ Complete blood count (CBC) and differential, electrolytes, blood gas, blood culture, coagulation panel, and blood type and crossmatch (if surgery is anticipated)

Genetic Evaluation

■ Consult the genetic service for evaluation of associated congenital anomalies or syndromes (as is often the case), following stabilization of the infant.

Documentation

■ Bowel perfusion and color preoperatively (for gastroschisis and omphalocele)

■ Strict input and output measurement, including gastric drainage

■ Vital signs and abdominal girth

■ Physical assessment with specific attention to abdominal assessment and bowel function

■ Pain assessment and interventions

■ Medication administration

■ Stoma appearance and drainage (if applicable)

■ Peritoneal drain site appearance and drainage (if applicable)

DUODENAL ATRESIA

Duodenal atresia is a congenital structural obstruction of the small intestine, typically distal to the ampulla of Vater. One of the more common areas of a bowel atresia, this condition is thought to result from a failure of recanalization of the bowel lumen during the first trimester when the midgut begins to form. The obstruction can be partial, such as a membranous web, or complete. Duodenal atresia has a reported incidence of one in 5,000 to 10,000 live births and is often, more than 50% occurrence, associated with other anomalies such as trisomy 21, congenital heart defects, and VACTERL (Choudhry et al., 2009; Flynn-O'Brien et al., 2018).

Presentation

Newborns with duodenal atresia almost always have a maternal history of polyhydramnios. Shortly after birth, the infant presents with evidence of feeding intolerance, gastric distension, and emesis, which may be bilious depending on the location of the atresia. The majority of neonates with duodenal atresia will have the obstruction distal to the ampulla of Vater where the biliary ducts drain into the bowel, thus resulting in bilious emesis.

Diagnosis

Duodenal atresia is diagnosed by history, clinical presentation, and abdominal x-ray (anteroposterior and left lateral decubitus). Duodenal atresia is typically seen on x-ray as a "double bubble" pattern: dilated air-filled stomach and proximal duodenum.

Preoperative Assessment and Nursing Care

■ Discontinue enteral feedings.

■ Provide gastric decompression to decrease gastric distension and risk of aspiration of bilious emesis.

■ Establish IV access.

■ Collect laboratory studies, including a CBC, chemistries, coagulation studies, and blood type and crossmatch (in anticipation of surgery and subsequent blood loss).

■ Initiate IV hydration and correct any fluid and electrolyte abnormalities due to gastric losses.

■ Perform a cardiac evaluation, including a chest radiograph, electrocardiogram, and echocardiogram (due to the high incidence of associated cardiac anomalies).

■ Administer perioperative antibiotics.

■ Obtain genetic service consultation to evaluate for trisomy 21 and other associated genetic abnormalities.

  ● This is not urgent and may be delayed until postoperatively, including obtaining genetic studies.

Surgical Procedure

■ Goal of surgical repair is to restore duodenal continuity.

■ Most often this surgery is a laparotomy, although some centers are now performing this as a laparoscopic procedure with experienced surgeons (Chung et al., 2017).

■ The affected segment of duodenum is resected and an end-to-end anastomosis, a duodenoduodenostomy, is completed.

Postoperative Assessment and Nursing Care

■ Continue gastric decompression until return of bowel function, which may occur over several days.

■ Monitor for excessive amounts of gastric drainage and the need for fluid replacement if excessive.

■ Continue maintenance IV fluids with electrolytes and begin parenteral nutrition as soon as possible to optimize nutritional status.

■ Administer perioperative antibiotics, completing prescribed course.

■ Manage postoperative pain with regional analgesia and opioid therapy; standardized postoperative pain protocols are recommended.

Documentation

See the Documentation section under General Considerations.

GASTROSCHISIS

Gastroschisis is a full-thickness defect in the abdominal wall through which the uncovered intestines protrude (Ledbetter et al., 2018).

Presentation

Apparent at birth, this defect is not encapsulated in a sac often located to the right of the umbilical ring. The exposed bowel appears edematous, matted, and covered in a fibrous peel. The abdominal cavity is small and underdeveloped (Leeman & Puder, 2016a).

Diagnosis

Gastroschisis is usually prenatally diagnosed with elevated alpha-fetoprotein (AFP) level or found on a second-trimester fetal ultrasound (US) (Leeman & Puder, 2016a). The defect appears most often in young mothers and those of low gravidity. Incidence of gastroschisis is one in 4,000 to 20,000 live births (Jones et al., 2016; Leeman & Puder, 2016b).

Preoperative Assessment and Nursing Care

■ Use careful handling to avoid injury to the bowel wall.

■ Place the lower two-thirds of the infant in a bowel bag with 20 mL of warmed sterile saline.

■ Place the infant on their side to prevent injury to the bowel or kinking of mesenteric vessels.

■ Monitor for insensible water loss (IWL).

■ Assess the bowel frequently for adequate perfusion.

  ● The bowel should be pink throughout; report any areas on the bowel that are dusky or discolored.

■ Provide gastric decompression, fluid resuscitation, and antibiotic prophylaxis.

Surgical Procedure

■ Primary repair—This method involves stretching the abdominal cavity to return the contents and close the peritoneum and abdominal wall.

■ Staged repair—This occurs when the infant's abdominal contents are too large, or the infant is too unstable or premature, to tolerate a primary repair with full return of bowel into the abdominal cavity.

  ● An extra-abdominal prosthetic sac, that is, silo, is utilized that supports the defect at a 90° angle and assists with reduction of the defect by gravity.

  ● Various techniques are available to achieve the return of bowel to the abdomen; these include a silo with a spring-loaded ring placed under the fascia or a mesh sac that is sutured.

  ● Gradual reduction of the defect occurs over several days; optimal timing of the closure is 5 to 7 days to decrease the risk of infection.

Postoperative Assessment and Nursing Care

Primary Repair

■ For risk of increased intra-abdominal pressure, assess for adequate lung volumes and blood gases to assure sufficient ventilation.

■ For abdominal compartment syndrome risk, monitor for adequate urine output and distal pulses.

  ● With abdominal compartment syndrome, there is a concern for increased abdominal pressure causing decreased renal perfusion as well as decreased perfusion and blood flow to distal extremities.

Staged Repair

■ Assess the silo for dislodgement during daily reduction of the bowel back into the abdominal cavity.

■ Care should be taken to maintain a moist base at the level where the silo enters the abdominal wall, which can be achieved with a petroleum or Xeroform™ gauze dressing.

■ To measure for additional drainage and fluid losses, so that IV fluids can be adjusted, collect and measure fluid on the gauze dressing placed around the base of the silo.

For Primary and Staged Repairs

■ Conduct frequent assessments of respiratory and cardiovascular status since intra-abdominal pressure rises in both primary and staged repairs.

■ Maintain constant vigilance over the infant since there are major concerns of venous stasis, respiratory compromise, infection, and nutrition.

■ Report signs of increased respiratory distress.

■ Report decreased perfusion to the legs and decreased urine output, which is indicative of compromised perfusion related to increased abdominal pressure.

■ Provide ventilatory support, antibiotic prophylaxis, and central line for parenteral nutrition since enteral feedings are held until bowel function is restored.

■ Manage postoperative pain with regional analgesia and opioid therapy; standardized postoperative pain protocols are recommended.

■ Most patients with gastroschisis have good long-term survival; however, many will have ongoing morbidity such as abdominal pain and require additional surgery for strictures or scarring, growth delay in infancy, and prolonged intestinal dysmotility (Harris et al., 2014; Minutillo et al., 2013).

Documentation

See the Documentation section under General Considerations.

HIRSCHSPRUNG DISEASE

Hirschsprung disease, also called congenital aganglionic megacolon, is a functional bowel obstruction caused by a lack of ganglion cells in the intestine. It typically involves the sigmoid colon and rectum. Hirschsprung disease results from a failure of development in neural cell migration along the bowel lumen and results in aganglionosis, an absence of ganglion cells (neurons necessary for bowel function). This occurs in a cranial-to-caudal direction; the point of cessation of neural cell development results in a transition zone. Peristalsis below this level is ineffective; the affected colon and rectum cannot relax, which results in obstruction of stool. Hirschsprung disease occurs in one in approximately 5,000 to 8,000 live births and in males more often than females. The majority involves the rectum or sigmoid colon region, although 10% have total colonic aganglionosis. Most cases are sporadic, but 10% to 20% have a familial history (Flynn-O'Brien et al., 2018; Gallagher et al., 2020; Pursley et al., 2016). There is an approximate 18% incidence of multiple anomalies and 12% association with major chromosomal variants (Tilghman et al., 2019).

Presentation

An infant with Hirschsprung disease presents with a failure to pass meconium in the first 48 hours, feeding intolerance, and/or abdominal distension. The infant may present with constipation or diarrhea, depending on the length of intestine involved. Paradoxical diarrhea is due to liquid stool passing around obstipated stool. Hirschsprung-associated enterocolitis (HAEC), a rare and potentially life-threatening complication, can occur in the perioperative period, years after repair or in delayed diagnosis. HAEC presents as an enterocolitis with fever, emesis, abdominal distension, foul-smelling stool, and septic shock (Gallagher et al., 2020; Soh et al., 2018).

Diagnosis

A contrast enema shows a transitional zone between proximal dilated bowel and the contracted colon and rectum. Definitive diagnosis is made by suction rectal biopsy. A positive biopsy shows an absence of ganglion cells.

Preoperative Assessment and Nursing Care

■ Discontinue enteral feedings.

■ Provide gastric decompression to decrease gastric distension and risk of aspiration of bilious emesis.

■ Establish IV access.

■ Collect laboratory studies, including a CBC, chemistries, coagulation studies, and blood type and crossmatch (in anticipation of surgery and subsequent blood loss).

■ Initiate IV hydration and correct any fluid and electrolyte abnormalities due to gastric losses.

■ Administer antibiotics.

■ Assist in preparation for suction rectal biopsy, often performed at the patient's bedside.

■ Conduct rectal irrigations; if irrigations maintain an adequate stooling pattern and examination is stable, then enteral feeds may be restarted until evaluation is complete and surgery occurs.

Surgical Procedure

■ Surgical correction is based on the clinical condition of the infant and the level of intestinal involvement; if stable, a laparoscopic-assisted endorectal pull-through is performed.

■ A primary trans-anal pull-through or staged reconstruction is performed in some cases; this involves creation of a colostomy with delayed reanastomosis in 3 to 6 months.

■ Emergent colostomy is performed if enterocolitis presents.

■ Serial intraoperative biopsies occur to identify the level of intestine with functioning ganglion cells.

Postoperative Assessment and Nursing Care

■ Continue gastric decompression.

■ Maintain nothing by mouth (NPO).

● Continue maintenance IV fluids with electrolytes and begin parenteral nutrition as soon as possible to optimize nutritional status until the return of bowel function.

● Bowel function typically resumes 24 hours following pull-through procedures.

● In severe cases where there is significant bowel loss resulting in short bowel syndrome (SBS), long-term nutritional management may be indicated.

■ Administer perioperative antibiotics, completing the prescribed course.

■ Manage postoperative pain with regional analgesia and opioid therapy; standardized postoperative pain protocols are recommended.

■ Continue gastric decompression until the return of bowel function, which may occur over several days.

■ Rectal dilations may continue for several months.

■ Assess stoma and perform stoma care if indicated.

Documentation

See the Documentation section under General Considerations.

IMPERFORATE ANUS

Imperforate anus is a condition of anorectal malformation in which the anus is not patent. This condition often occurs with urogenital or rectal fistula. It occurs in one of every 2,500 to 5,000 live births and is slightly more common in males. The positioning of the rectum may be low, intermediate, or high; a high-placed rectum has a greater chance of associated anomalies. Occasionally a correlation exists with VACTERL association or trisomy 21 (Gallagher et al., 2020; Pursley et al., 2016).

Presentation

Imperforate anus is identified on physical examination as the absence of an anus.

Diagnosis

The abdominal x-ray may show dilated bowel loops consistent with a distal obstruction. A perianal US is performed to evaluate where the rectum terminates. In males, a contrast study of the urethra is performed to evaluate for a rectourethral fistula.

Preoperative Assessment and Nursing Care

■ Discontinue enteral feedings.

■ Provide gastric decompression to decrease gastric distension and risk of aspiration of bilious emesis.

■ Establish IV access.

■ Collect laboratory studies, including a CBC, chemistries, coagulation studies, and blood type and crossmatch in anticipation of surgery and subsequent blood loss.

■ Initiate IV hydration and correct any fluid and electrolyte abnormalities.

■ Administer antibiotics until presence of a fistula is ruled out.

Surgical Procedure

■ Varies depending on the level of rectum and presence of fistula.

● Anoplasty or repair of the rectum

● Dilation of fistulas

● Colostomy with reanastomosis in 3 to 6 months

Postoperative Assessment and Nursing Care

■ Continue gastric decompression until the return of bowel function, which may occur over several days.

■ Hold enteral feedings until bowel function is restored.

■ Continue maintenance IV fluids with electrolytes and begin parenteral nutrition as soon as possible to optimize nutritional status until the return of bowel function.

● Bowel function typically resumes 24 hours following a surgical procedure.

■ Administer perioperative antibiotics, completing the prescribed course.

■ Manage postoperative pain with regional analgesia and opioid therapy; standardized postoperative pain protocols are recommended.

■ Assess stoma and perform stoma care if indicated.

Documentation

See the Documentation section under General Considerations.

INTESTINAL ATRESIA

Intestinal atresia, which occurs in up to 3.4 per 10,000 live births (Lupo et al., 2017), is a congenital structural obstruction of the intestine. The defect typically occurs in the jejunum but may also occur in the ileum, or in both (Stollman et al., 2009). Unlike duodenal atresia that occurs early in gestation, ileal and jejunal atresia are believed to occur later in gestation as the result of ischemic necrosis and bowel resorption due to a mesenteric vascular accident or segmental volvulus. Intestinal atresia defects are usually not associated with other non-GI anomalies, although they sometimes occur with abdominal wall defects and malrotation. Intestinal atresia has been reported in some neonates with cystic fibrosis (Stollman et al., 2009).

Presentation

Polyhydramnios occurs frequently in proximal atresia but is rare in distal atresia. Atresia presents with early feeding intolerance, bilious emesis typically in the first 48 hours after birth, abdominal distention (more significant with distal atresia), and visible bowel loops on examination. Neonates with intestinal atresia tend to be small for gestational age.

Diagnosis

Abdominal x-rays show distended loops of bowel and a paucity of air distal to the obstruction. Contrast enemas may demonstrate a microcolon since that portion of bowel has been unused. Several classifications of intestinal atresias occur with varying degrees of mesentery involvement and bowel length that greatly affect morbidity and mortality.

Preoperative Assessment and Nursing Care

■ Discontinue enteral feedings.

■ Provide gastric decompression to decrease gastric distension and risk of aspiration of bilious emesis.

■ Establish IV access.

■ Collect laboratory studies including a CBC, chemistries, coagulation studies, and blood type and crossmatch in anticipation of surgery and subsequent blood loss.

■ Initiate IV hydration and correct any fluid and electrolyte abnormalities due to gastric losses.

Surgical Procedure

■ The goal of surgical repair is to restore intestinal continuity.

■ The segment of atresia is resected and, when possible, an end-to-end anastomosis is performed.

■ There is often a size disparity in the bowel ends due to dilation of the proximal end, which limits immediate anastomosis as an option.

■ Bowel resection of the dilated portion or temporary creation of a stoma may occur.

Postoperative Assessment and Nursing Care

■ Continue gastric decompression until the return of bowel function, which may occur over several days.

■ Monitor for excessive amounts of gastric drainage and the need for fluid replacement if excessive.

■ Continue maintenance IV fluids with electrolytes and begin parenteral nutrition as soon as possible to optimize nutritional status.

■ Administer perioperative antibiotics, completing the prescribed course.

■ Manage postoperative pain with regional analgesia and opioid therapy; standardized postoperative pain protocols are recommended.

■ Assess stoma appearance if applicable, including color and drainage.

■ Perform stoma care; typically a stoma is covered with moist dressing (i.e., Xeroform®-Cardinal Health, Dublin, OH-gauze) during the initial postoperative days and then is transitioned to an ostomy appliance once the output increases.

Documentation

See the Documentation section under General Considerations.

MALROTATION/VOLVULUS

Malrotation is the failure of rotation and fixation of the midgut during early gestation. Malrotation predisposes the bowel to twist, resulting in a volvulus, a condition that may acutely decrease enteric blood supply and result in bowel ischemia and infarction.

Presentation

Malrotation symptoms are present in approximately 50% of infants during the first months of life (Flynn O'Brien et al., 2018; Pursley et al., 2016). Early signs of malrotation are feeding intolerance and bilious emesis; however, the infant may be asymptomatic. Symptoms indicative of a volvulus are more acute and may include abdominal distension, bilious emesis, bloody emesis or stools, and abdominal erythema. As the condition progresses, infants often have symptoms of systemic signs of shock, hypotension, anuria, acidosis, and leukocytosis. A volvulus is a surgical emergency; failure to provide prompt medical and surgical intervention may result in significant bowel loss or death.

Diagnosis

Abdominal x-ray in the patient with a malrotation, with or without volvulus, demonstrates evidence of bowel obstruction, typically a dilated duodenum and stomach. The gold standard radiographic study is an upper GI that will demonstrate the malrotation and obstruction. Neonates with systemic signs consistent with a volvulus require immediate surgical intervention; the procedure is not delayed for the completion of an upper GI study.

Preoperative Assessment and Nursing Care

■ Discontinue enteral feedings.

■ Provide gastric decompression to decrease gastric distension and risk of aspiration of bilious emesis.

■ Establish IV access.

■ Collect laboratory studies, including a CBC, chemistries, coagulation studies, and blood type and crossmatch in anticipation of surgery and subsequent blood loss.

■ Initiate IV hydration and correct any fluid and electrolyte abnormalities due to gastric losses.

■ Provide volume resuscitation.

■ Administer antibiotic therapy.

Surgical Procedure

■ A laparotomy and Ladd's procedure, involving the division of Ladd's bands to relieve the duodenal obstruction, is performed to reposition the bowel and correct the malrotation.

■ During the procedure, there is widening of the mesenteric base to allow improved blood flow to the bowel.

● An appendectomy is also performed at the same time.

■ With a volvulus, any necrotic bowel is resected and a stoma is created.

Postoperative Assessment and Nursing Care

■ Continue gastric decompression until the return of bowel function, which may occur over several days.

■ Hold enteral feedings until bowel function is restored.

● Continue maintenance IV fluids with electrolytes and begin parenteral nutrition as soon as possible to optimize nutritional status until the return of bowel function.

■ Administer perioperative antibiotics, completing the prescribed course.

■ Manage postoperative pain with regional analgesia and opioid therapy; standardized postoperative pain protocols are recommended.

■ In severe cases, the infant may have significant bowel loss resulting in SBS; long-term nutritional management may be indicated.

■ Assess the stoma and perform stoma care if indicated.

Documentation

See the Documentation section under General Considerations.

MECONIUM ILEUS

Meconium ileus is the functional obstruction of the small intestine due to excessively thick meconium from abnormally viscous intestinal secretions and a lack of pancreatic enzymes. Ninety percent of neonates with meconium ileus have cystic fibrosis.

Presentation

Symptoms of meconium ileus include abdominal distension, bilious emesis, and failure to pass meconium. In severe cases, symptoms may worsen to include abdominal erythema, edema, and respiratory distress due to abdominal distension. Occasionally, intrauterine perforation has occurred.

Diagnosis

Meconium ileus most frequently occurs in the ileum. The abdominal radiograph demonstrates an echogenic abdominal mass, "soap-bubble" appearance of air trapped in meconium with dilated loops of bowel. A contrast enema typically shows a microcolon and pellets of thickened meconium at the distal end of the obstruction. Occasionally, a meconium ileus may lead to intrauterine perforation, which would be seen as microcalcifications.

Preoperative Assessment and Nursing Care

■ Discontinue enteral feedings.

■ Provide gastric decompression to decrease gastric distension and risk of aspiration of bilious emesis.

■ Establish IV access.

■ Collect laboratory studies, including a CBC, chemistries, coagulation studies, and blood type and crossmatch (in anticipation of surgery and subsequent blood loss).

■ Initiate IV hydration and correct any fluid and electrolyte abnormalities due to gastric losses.

■ Administer antibiotic therapy.

■ Assist with administering a hyperosmolar enema (i.e., Gastrografin), which draws fluid into the bowel lumen to dilute viscous meconium and ease passage of the meconium.

Surgical Procedure

■ Surgical repair typically includes an enterotomy (small incision in bowel) through which saline or acetylcysteine is instilled.

■ In severe cases, resection of the obstructed bowel segment and creation of stoma is performed.

Postoperative Assessment and Nursing Care

■ Continue gastric decompression until the return of bowel function, which may occur over several days.

■ Hold enteral feedings until bowel function is restored.

● Continue maintenance IV fluids with electrolytes and begin parenteral nutrition as soon as possible to optimize nutritional status until the return of bowel function.

■ In severe cases where there is significant bowel loss resulting in SBS, long-term nutritional management may be indicated.

■ Administer perioperative antibiotics, completing the prescribed course.

■ Manage postoperative pain with regional analgesia and opioid therapy; standardized postoperative pain protocols are recommended.

■ Assess the stoma and perform stoma care if indicated.

■ Administer rectal or ostomy irrigation with saline or acetylcysteine if indicated.

Documentation

See the Documentation section under General Considerations.

MECONIUM PLUG SYNDROME

Meconium plug syndrome is the failure to pass stool, resulting in a meconium plug. The plug often forms in the distal segment of the colon or rectum. It results from excessively thick meconium causing a functional obstruction of the bowel. Immature ganglion cells are the likely etiology. Newborns with meconium plug syndrome are occasionally associated with Hirschsprung disease (Dingeldein, 2020; Gallagher et al., 2020).

Presentation

Symptoms of meconium plug syndrome include bilious emesis, hyperactive bowel sounds, abdominal distension, and failure to pass stool, although they may pass a small amount of gray meconium. In severe cases, this condition may progress to perforation and the infant may develop systemic symptoms of sepsis.

Diagnosis

The plug most frequently occurs in the distal segment of the colon or rectum. Abdominal x-ray demonstrates multiple distended bowel loops. An intraluminal plug is often visualized by a water-soluble enema, which often dislodges the plug. Affected infants are evaluated for Hirschsprung, cystic fibrosis, and hypothyroidism.

Preoperative Assessment and Nursing Care

■ Discontinue enteral feedings.

■ Provide gastric decompression to decrease gastric distension and the risk of aspiration of bilious emesis.

■ Establish IV access.

■ Collect laboratory studies, including a CBC, chemistries, coagulation studies, and blood type and crossmatch (in anticipation of surgery and subsequent blood loss).

■ Initiate IV hydration and correct any fluid and electrolyte abnormalities due to gastric losses.

Surgical Procedure

■ A majority of infants will pass the plug spontaneously without surgical intervention.

■ Rectal dilation or contrast enema may be a curative treatment.

■ In rare instances of bowel perforation, the infant will require surgical repair and the creation of a stoma.

Postoperative Assessment and Nursing Care

■ Continue gastric decompression until the return of bowel function, which may occur over several days.

■ Maintain NPO.

■ Continue maintenance IV fluids with electrolytes and begin parenteral nutrition as soon as possible to optimize nutritional status until the return of bowel function.

■ In severe cases where there is significant bowel loss resulting in SBS, long-term nutritional management may be indicated.

■ Administer perioperative antibiotics, completing the prescribed course.

■ Manage postoperative pain with regional analgesia and opioid therapy; standardized postoperative pain protocols are recommended.

■ Assess the stoma and perform stoma care if indicated.

Documentation

See the Documentation section under General Considerations.

NECROTIZING ENTEROCOLITIS

Necrotizing enterocolitis (NEC) is an acquired disorder characterized by hemorrhage, ischemia, and sometimes necrosis of the mucosal and submucosal layers of the intestinal tract.

Presentation

Infants present with abdominal distention, increased gastric residuals, emesis, hypotension, and bloody stools. Infants may also present with symptoms of sepsis, including lethargy, temperature instability, apnea, and poor feedings. NEC commonly presents in extremely low-birthweight (ELBW) infants during the first couple of weeks after birth and before the initiation of enteral feedings (Caplan, 2020; Gordon et al., 2009). According to a recent Cochrane review, there is a 2.8-fold increase in risk of NEC in premature infants fed with formula, compared with those fed with human milk (Cristofalo et al., 2013; Quigley & McGuire, 2014).

Occasionally, a spontaneous intestinal perforation (SIP) may occur without evidence of NEC. Etiology of this event may be related to an immature intestinal barrier, increased gastric pH, use of umbilical artery catheters, and administration of medications for closure of the patent ductus arteriosis (indomethacin or ibuprofen).

The age at onset of NEC is inversely related to gestational age, with a mean age of 3 to 4 days for term infants and 3 to 4 weeks for infants born at less than 28 weeks' gestation (Caplan, 2020). The incidence of developing NEC for infants born weighing less than 1,500 g ranges between 7% and 10%. The mortality rate of affected infants ranges from 25% to 30%, and up to 50% for those that receive surgical intervention (Javid et al., 2018; Moss et al., 2008). One-third of the patients present with a milder form of disease that resolves with medical therapy alone, and approximately 50% of cases require surgical intervention (Javid et al., 2018; Moss et al., 2008). Initial injury to the intestinal mucosa is multifactorial with the combination of impaired intestinal perfusion, abnormal bacterial colonization, impaired gut barrier function, and an immature, overactive immune response leading to intestinal inflammation, ischemia, and eventual necrosis (Javid et al., 2018; Patel et al., 2015).

Diagnosis

Initial laboratory findings of metabolic and respiratory acidosis, electrolyte abnormalities, neutropenia, and thrombocytopenia are likely. Radiologic diagnosis is also reliable. Abdominal x-ray of the abdomen and left lateral decubitus x-rays need to be obtained to assess for small bubbles of gas in the lumen of the intestine (pneumatosis). If those bubbles of gas rupture into the mesenteric vascular bed, a pneumoperitoneum will be found on radiographic images. US is increasingly being used to diagnose NEC due to its increased sensitivity to assessing fluid collections and the ability to visualize bowel wall thickness, peristalsis, and perfusion (Cuna et al., 2018).

Preoperative Assessment and Nursing Care

◼ Assessment and documentation of apnea episodes, abdominal girths, emesis, or other subtle signs of sepsis need to be evaluated closely for etiology.

◼ Check for increased gastric residuals if indicated (Torrazza et al., 2015).

◼ Decompress the stomach with low intermittent suction through a sump tube.

◼ Promptly initiate antibiotic therapy as this is crucial to the treatment of NEC.

◼ Intubate and support the infant's respiratory status.

● Infants can experience apnea or increasing respiratory distress due to compression of the diaphragm from abdominal distension.

◼ Assess for hypotension.

● Support blood pressure and maintain adequate perfusion with the use of fluid resuscitation and vasoactive infusions.

◼ Insert a central line to allow adequate nutrition while the infant is unable to receive enteral feeds during the period the bowel heals.

◼ Follow serial abdominal x-rays every 6 to 8 hours (or more frequently) to assess for progression of the pneumatosis to intestinal perforation.

◼ Consider use of US to help in diagnosis of NEC.

■ Monitor blood work frequently to assess for anemia, thrombocytopenia, and abnormal coagulation.

■ Send the blood clot for blood type and crossmatch since infants with NEC frequently need treatment for bleeding or blood loss and sometimes a coagulopathy (with packed red blood cells [PRBCs], fresh frozen plasma [FFP], and cryoprecipitate).

Surgical Procedure

■ The most common surgical interventions performed on infants with NEC are laparotomies and placement of peritoneal drains (Hansen & Modi, 2016).

● The type of operation performed for perforated NEC does not influence survival or other clinically important early outcomes in preterm infants (Moss et al., 2006; Raval et al., 2013).

■ Placement of a peritoneal drain may be the best choice as either a temporary measure or definitive treatment in smaller or more unstable neonates (Han et al., 2020).

● The drain is less invasive, does not require the infant to be placed under anesthesia, and can be placed at the bedside.

■ During a laparotomy, necrotic bowel is resected, and an ostomy is created.

Postoperative Assessment and Nursing Care

■ Ensure the infant receives adequate parenteral nutrition to facilitate healing.

■ Maintain gastric decompression until the return of bowel function.

■ Monitor fluid status closely.

● Infant may require aggressive fluid resuscitation to maintain adequate blood pressure and perfusion due to fluid losses during surgery.

■ Assess the abdomen's appearance and girth; report changes in discoloration and girth.

■ Assess the peritoneal drain site or ostomy bud for color and adequate perfusion; report changes to the drain site or ostomy bud as soon as they are noted.

■ Manage postoperative pain with regional analgesia and opioid therapy; standardized postoperative pain protocols are recommended.

■ Resume enteral feedings once the infant has received 10 to 14 days of bowel rest, treatment with antibiotics, and bowel function has recovered.

■ Educate providers and parents that although more than 70% of patients with NEC survive, long-term GI complications include intestinal strictures and SBS.

Documentation

See the Documentation section under General Considerations.

OMPHALOCELE

An omphalocele is an abdominal wall defect most commonly found at the level of the umbilicus (Leeman & Puder, 2016b).

Presentation

This defect occurs from failure of the abdominal organs to completely return to the abdomen during week 10 of development, causing incomplete closure of the anterior abdominal wall. The defect is covered with a peritoneal sac that may be intact or have ruptured in utero. Bowel is trapped within the umbilical ring; larger defects may include the liver and bowel. The incidence of omphalocele is estimated to be between 1.5 and 3 per 10,000 births and the association of congenital heart disease with a diagnosed omphalocele is as high as 50% (Marshall et al., 2015). Multiple and often life-threatening syndromes and anomalies occur greater than 50% of the time with an omphalocele diagnosis (Ngo & Shah, 2020).

Diagnosis

Omphaloceles are usually prenatally diagnosed with elevated AFP level or found on second-trimester fetal US.

Preoperative Assessment and Nursing Care

■ Protect the eviscerated organs, decompress the gut, and provide hydration to account for IWL.

■ If the sac is intact, moisten sterile gauze with warmed sterile saline and loosely wrap around the defect.

■ Apply a dry gauze dressing around the outside over the moist dressing.

■ If the sac has ruptured, place the infant in a bowel bag, a clear polyurethane sac that provides a barrier, thus decreasing loss of fluid and heat.

Surgical Procedure

■ Primary repair—For small defects, the contents of the omphalocele are returned into the abdominal cavity and there is closure of the defect via a skin flap.

■ Staged repair—A silo (see "Gastroschisis" section for information on silos) is used to suspend the contents of large defects above the patient.

- Reduction maneuvers are then carried out daily to return the organs to the small abdominal cavity.
- Complete return of the organs into the abdominal cavity is generally achieved over 7 to 10 days.

■ Delayed repair—Performed when the infant is extremely premature, there is a giant omphalocele, or when respiratory failure makes a primary repair not feasible.

- The sac is treated with a drying antiseptic agent (to prevent infection); examples include povidone-iodine and silver sulfadiazine.
- Application of these agents dries the sac, creating an eschar covering that protects the abdominal contents.
- Tissue granulates and skin eventually cover the entire defect.
- With growth and stabilization of the infant, surgical repair is accomplished with an abdominal wall closure.

Postoperative Assessment and Nursing Care

■ Monitor for major concerns, including respiratory compromise, infection, and nutrition.

■ Conduct frequent assessments of respiratory and cardiovascular status for changes associated with increased intra-abdominal pressure.

■ Manage postoperative pain with regional analgesia and opioid therapy; standardized postoperative pain protocols are recommended.

■ Increase ventilator settings as needed to compensate for increased intra-abdominal pressure and monitor blood gases.

■ Administer antibiotic prophylaxis.

■ Place a central line for parenteral nutrition since enteral feedings are held until bowel function is restored.

Documentation

See the Documentation section under General Considerations.

REFERENCES

Caplan, M. (2020). Necrotizing enterocolitis. In A. Fanaroff & J. Fanaroff (Eds.), *Klaus and Fanaroff's care of the high-risk neonate* (7th ed., pp. 115–117). Elsevier.

Choudhry, M. S., Rahman, N., Boyd, P., & Lakhoo, K. (2009). Duodenal atresia: Associated anomalies, prenatal diagnosis and outcome. *Pediatric Surgery International, 25,* 727–730. https://doi.org/10.1007/s00383-009-2406-y

Chung, P. H., Wong, C. W., Ip, D. K., Tam, P. K., & Wong, K. K. (2017). Is laparoscopic surgery better than open surgery for the repair of congenital duodenal obstruction? A review of the current evidences. *Journal of Pediatric Surgery, 52*(3), 498–503. https://doi.org/10.1016/j.jpedsurg.2016.08.010

Cristofalo, E. A., Schanler, R. J., Blanco, C. L., Sullivan, S., Trawoeger, R., Kiechl-Kohlendorfer, U., Dudell, G., Rechtman, J., Lee, M. L., Lucas, A., & Abrams, S. (2013). Randomized trial of exclusive human milk versus preterm formula diets in extremely premature infants. *Journal of Pediatrics, 163*(6), 1592–1595. https://doi.org/10.1016/j.jpeds.2013.07.011

Cuna, A. C., Reddy, N., Robinson, A. L., & Chan, S. S. (2018). Bowel ultrasound for predicting surgical management of necrotizing enterocolitis: A systematic review and meta-analysis. *Pediatric Radiology, 48*(5), 658. https://doi.org/10.1007/s00247-017-4056-x

Dingeldein, M. (2020). Selected disorders of gastrointestinal tract. In A. Fanaroff & J. Fanaroff (Eds.), *Klaus and Fanaroff's care of the high-risk neonate* (7th ed., pp. 108–115). Elsevier.

Flynn-O'Brien, K. T., Rice-Townsend, S., & Ledbetter, D. J. (2018). Structural anomalies of the gastrointestinal tract. In C. A. Gleason & S. E. Juul (Eds.), *Avery's diseases of the newborn* (10th ed., pp. 1039–1053). Elsevier.

Gallagher, M. E., Pacetti, A. S., Lovvern, H. N., & Carter, B. S. (2020). Neonatal surgery. In S. L. Gardner, B. S. Carter, M. Enzman-Hines, & J. A. Hernandez (Eds.), *Merenstein & Gardner's handbook of neonatal intensive care* (9th ed., pp. 996–1038). Mosby Elsevier.

Gordon, P., Christensen, R., Weitkamp, J.-H., & Maheshwari, A. (2009). Mapping the new world of necrotizing enterocolitis (NEC): Review and opinion. *e-Journal of Neonatology Research, 2*(4), 145–172. https://www.ncbi.nlm.nih.gov/pmc/articles/PMC3666872

Han, S. M., Hong, C. R., Knell, J., Edwards, E. M., Morrow, K. A., Soll, R. F., Modi, B. P., Horbar, J. D., & Jaksic, T. (2020). Trends in incidence and outcomes of necrotizing enterocolitis over the last 12 years: A multicenter cohort analysis. *Journal of Pediatric Surgery, 55*(6), 998. https://doi.org/10.1016/j.jpedsurg.2020.02.046

Hansen, A. R., & Modi, B. P. (2016). Necrotizing enterocolitis. In A. R. Hansen & M. Puder (Eds.), *Manual of neonatal surgical intensive care* (3rd ed., pp. 273–290). People's Medical Publishing House.

Harris, E. L., Minutillo, C., Teresa, S. H., Warner, M., Ravikumara, M., Nathan, E. A., & Dickinson, J. E. (2014). The long term physical consequences of gastroschisis. *Journal of Pediatric Surgery, 49*(10), 1466–1470. https://doi.org/10.1016/j.jpedsurg.2014.03.008

Javid, P. J., Riggle, K. M., & Smith, C. (2018). Necrotizing enterocolitis and short bowel syndrome. In C. A. Gleason & S. E. Juul (Eds.), *Avery's diseases of the newborn* (10th ed., pp. 1090–1097). Elsevier.

Jones, A. M., Isenburg, J., Salemi, J. L., Arnold, K. E., Mai, C. T., Aggarwal, D., Arias, W., Carrino, G. E., Ferrell, E., Folorunso, O., Ibe, B., Kirby, R. S., Krapfl, H. R., Marengo, L. K., Mosley, B. S., Nance, A. E., Romitti, P. A., Spadafino, J., Stock, J., & Honein, M. A. (2016). Increasing prevalence of gastroschisis—14 States, 1995–2012. *Morbidity and Mortality Weekly Report, 65*(2), 23–26. https://doi.org/10.15585/mmwr.mm6502a2

Ledbetter, D. J., Chabra, S., & Javid, P. J. (2018). Abdominal wall defects. In C. A. Gleason & S. E. Juul (Eds.), *Avery's diseases of the newborn* (10th ed., pp. 1068–1078). Elsevier.

Leeman, K. T., & Puder, M. (2016a). Gastroschisis. In A. R. Hansen & M. Puder (Eds.), *Manual of neonatal surgical intensive care* (3rd ed., pp. 253–264). People's Medical Publishing House.

Leeman, K. T., & Puder, M. (2016b). Omphalocele. In A. R. Hansen & M. Puder (Eds.), *Manual of neonatal surgical intensive care* (3rd ed., pp. 265–272). People's Medical Publishing House.

Lupo, P. J., Isenburg, J. L., Salemi, J. L., Mai, C. T., Liberman, R. F., Canfield, M. A., Copeland, G., Haight, S., Harpavat, S., Hoyt, A. T., Moore, C. A., Nembhard, W. N., Nguyen, H. N., Rutkowski, R. E., Steele, A., Alverson, C. J., Stallings, E. B., Kirby, R. S.,

& The National Birth Defects Prevention Network. (2017). Population-based birth defects data in the United States, 2010–2014: A focus on gastrointestinal defects. *Birth Defects Research, 109*(18), 1504. https://doi.org/10.1002/bdr2.1145

Marshall, J., Salemi, J. L., Tanner, J. P., Ramakrishnan, R., Feldkamp, M. L., Marengo, L. K., Meyer, R. E., Druschel, C. M., Rickard, R., Kirby, R. S., & National Birth Defects Prevention Network. (2015). Prevalence, correlates, and outcomes of omphalocele in the United States, 1995–2005. *Obstetrics and Gynecology, 126,* 284–293. https://doi.org/10.1097/AOG .0000000000000920

Minutillo, C., Rao, S. C., Pirie, S., McMichael, J., & Dickinsone, J. E. (2013). Growth and developmental outcomes of infants with gastroschisis at one year of age: A retrospective study. *Journal of Pediatric Surgery, 48*(8), 1688–1696. https://doi.org/10.1016/j.jpedsurg.2012.11.046

Moss, R. L., Dimmitt, R. A., Barnhart, D. C., Sylvester, K. G., Brown, R. L., Powell, D. M, Islam, S., Langer, J. C., Sato, T. T., Brandt, M. L., Lee, H., Blakely, M. L., Lazar, E. L., Hirschl, R. B., Kenney, B. D., Hackam, D. J., Zelterman, D., & Silverman, B. L. (2006). Laparotomy versus peritoneal drainage for necrotizing enterocolitis and perforation. *New England Journal of Medicine, 354*(21), 2225–2234. https://doi.org/10.1056/NEJMoa054605

Moss, R. L., Kalish, L. A., Duggan, C., Johnston, P., Brandt, M. L., Dunn, J. C. Y., Ehrenkranz, R. A., Jaksic, T., Nobuhara, K., Simpson, B. J., McCarthy, M. C., & & Sylvester, K. G. (2008). Clinical parameters do not adequately predict outcome in necrotizing enterocolitis: A multi-institutional study. *Journal of Perinatology, 28,* 665–674. https://doi .org/10.1038/jp.2008.119

Ngo, K. D., & Shah, M. (2020). Gastrointestinal systems. In C. Kenner, L. B. Altimier, & M. V. Boykova (Eds.), *Comprehensive neonatal nursing care* (6th ed., pp. 179–210). Springer Publishing Company.

Patel, R. V., Kandefer, S., Walsh, M. C., Bell, E. F., Carlo, W. A., Laptook, A. R., & Stoll, B. J. (2015). Causes and timing of death in extremely premature infants from 2000 through 2011. *New England Journal of Medicine, 372*(4), 331–340. https://doi.org/10.1056/NEJMoa1403489

Pursley, D., Hansen, A. R., & Puder, M. (2016). Obstruction. In A. R. Hansen & M. Puder (Eds.), *Manual of neonatal surgical intensive care* (3rd ed., pp. 291–312). People's Medical Publishing House.

Quigley, M., & McGuire, W. (2014). Formula versus donor breast milk for feeding preterm or low birth weight infants. *Cochrane Database of Systematic Reviews, 2014*(4), CD002971. https://doi.org.10.1002/14651858.CD002971.pub3

Raval, M. V., Hall, N. J., Pierro, A., & Moss, R. L. (2013). Evidence-based prevention and surgical treatment of necrotizing enterocolitis: A review of randomized controlled trials. *Seminars in Pediatric Surgery, 22,* 117–121. https://doi.org/10.1053/j.sempedsurg.2013.01.009

Soh, H. J., Nataraja, R. M., & Pacilli, M. (2018). Prevention and management of recurrent postoperative Hirschsprung's disease obstructive symptoms and enterocolitis: Systematic review and meta-analysis. *Journal of Pediatric Surgery, 53*(12), 2423–2429. https://doi .org/10.1016/j.jpedsurg.2018.08.024

Stollman, T. H., de Blaauw, I., Wijnen, M. H., van der Staak, F. H., Rieu, P. N., Draaisma, J. M., & Wijnen, R. M. (2009). Decreased mortality but increased morbidity in neonates with jejunoileal atresia; a study of 114 cases over a 34-year period. *Journal of Pediatric Surgery, 44,* 217–221. https://doi.org/10.1016/j.jpedsurg.2008.10.043

Tilghman, J. M., Ling, A. Y., Turner, T. N., Sosa, M. S., Krumm, N., Chatterjee, S., Kapoor, A., Coe, B. P., Nguyen, K. H., Gupta, N., Gabriel, S., Eichler, E. E., Berrios, C., & Chakravarti, A. (2019). Molecular genetic anatomy and risk profile of Hirschsprung's disease. *New England Journal of Medicine, 380,* 1421–1432. https://doi.org/10.1056/NEJMoa1706594

Torrazza, R. M., Parker, L. A., Li, Y., Talaga, E., Shuster, J., & Neu, J. (2015). The value of routine gastric residuals in very low birth weight infants. *Journal of Perinatology, 35,* 57–60. https://doi.org/10.1038/jp.2014.147

SURGICAL DISORDERS OF THE LOWER ABDOMEN AND GENITALS

TRICIA GRANDINETTI AND AVERY FORGET

HYDROCELE

TRICIA GRANDINETTI

Hydrocele occurs when a collection of fluid moves from the abdomen to the scrotal sac.

Presentation

Surgery is rarely required. A majority of hydroceles will resolve spontaneously as the processus vaginalis closes, generally between 1 and 2 years of age (Clarke, 2010; Nandivada et al., 2016).

Diagnosis

Transillumination of the scrotum will reveal a fluid-filled sac when a hydrocele is present.

Preoperative Assessment and Nursing Care

■ Evaluate hydroceles daily to differentiate between the presence of fluid (hydrocele) or bowel (hernia).

Surgical Repair

Hydroceles that persist beyond 2 years of age require high ligation of the processus vaginalis. This surgery entails drainage of fluid from the scrotal sac and closure of the processus vaginalis (Nandivada et al., 2016).

Postoperative Assessment and Nursing Care

■ In the rare event that a hydrocele requires repair in the neonatal period, follow recommendations for postoperative care of the inguinal hernia.

Documentation

■ Vital signs
■ Assessment of surgical incision; include signs of infection and drainage

■ Pain scores

■ Parental teaching

INGUINAL HERNIA

TRICIA GRANDINETTI

Inguinal hernia is the escape of a bowel segment or other abdominal contents through the inguinal canal, which appears as a bulge in the groin.

Presentation

Inguinal hernias occur in both male and female infants. They usually present in the first 6 months of life and are six times more prevalent in male infants. The incidence of inguinal hernias is greater in preterm infants (Nandivada et al., 2016). In female infants, hernias can contain an ovary, with or without portions of the fallopian tube (15%–20% of the time; Goldstein & Potts, 1958). In females, when the ovary is present within the hernia, the risk of incarceration dramatically increases (Boley et al., 1991; Kapur et al., 1998). To prevent risks associated with incarceration such as impaired blood flow to vital structures and intestinal obstruction, hernias may be repaired prior to discharge home, especially if the infant was born premature and has other comorbidities (Nandivada et al., 2016).

Diagnosis

■ It is important to differentiate between a hydrocele, inguinal hernia, and incarcerated hernia because the first resolves on its own over time, the second requires surgical correction, and the third (respectively) requires emergent surgical intervention.

● Diagnostic studies to help differentiate between a hydrocele, inguinal hernia, and incarcerated hernia include x-ray and ultrasound (US).

■ The hernia presents as a firm, smooth mass in the scrotum or inguinal canal that may be exacerbated by increased abdominal pressure (Nandivada et al., 2016).

■ Symptoms of an incarcerated hernia include scrotal swelling or firmness, redness, tenderness or pain, emesis, and irritability.

● This condition can rapidly evolve into strangulation of the bowel and gangrenous hernia contents if not surgically corrected.

● Any hernia that cannot be reduced requires immediate surgical evaluation for incarceration.

■ Incarceration of the ovary occurs in approximately 43% of cases (Bronsther et al., 1972).

- As the ovary swells, it becomes incarcerated and less likely to reduce, unlike a bowel containing hernia.
- Any irreducible ovary should always be treated as an emergency, even if it is nontender (Boley et al., 1991).

Preoperative Assessment and Nursing Care

■ Perform daily reduction and assessment of the hernia by applying gentle pressure to determine if the intestines can be easily passed back through the processus vaginalis.

■ If the hernia is not reducible, this may indicate incarceration, which is a surgical emergency.

■ Symptoms of incarcerated hernia include a painful, nonreducible scrotal mass; emesis; and irritability (Nandivada et al., 2016).

■ These symptoms dictate the need for an emergency surgical consult.

■ All inguinal hernias are at risk for becoming incarcerated; therefore, surgical evaluation and correction are recommended as soon as possible, depending on the patient's age, weight, and condition.

■ Provide parental teaching that includes monitoring for signs of intestinal herniation and incarceration if discharged home prior to repair.

Surgical Repair

Surgical correction of the hernia is performed laparoscopically or via an open incision (Nandivada et al., 2016). The hernia is placed back into the abdominal cavity after being separated from the surrounding tissue and is followed by the closure of the processus vaginalis (Clarke, 2010).

Postoperative Assessment and Nursing Care

■ Place the infant in a supine or side-lying position. Ideally, keep the head turned to the side as this may minimize disruption to the suture line.

■ Monitor the incision site and/or suture line closely.

■ Report signs of infection.

■ Determine the timeline for removal if sutures are present.

- Often, dissolvable sutures are used.
- Check with the surgeon or the operative note to confirm suture material and plan.

■ Assess pain for a minimum of every 4 hours.

- Comfort may be achieved with acetaminophen alone but consider narcotics on a patient-specific basis.

■ Observation in an ICU for 24 hours is recommended for premature infants due to increased risk for apnea secondary to anesthesia exposure.

Documentation

■ Vital signs

■ Assessment of surgical incision, including signs of infection and drainage

■ Pain scores

■ Parental teaching

TESTICULAR TORSION

AVERY FORGET

Testicular torsion is a twisting of the spermatic cord; this structure is connected to the internal reproductive organs that contain blood vessels, nerves, muscles, and a tube for carrying semen. It is the result of incomplete attachment of the gubernaculum to the testis that allows for torsion and infarction.

Presentation

■ Of all testicular torsions diagnosed in the newborn period, it is reported that 70% develop prenatally (Ringer & Hansen, 2017).

■ The findings of testicular torsion include an enlarged swollen scrotum with a firm scrotal mass; the infant may experience varying levels of discomfort.

● Prenatal torsion is marked by minimal to no discomfort; the infant is generally asymptomatic, afebrile, and comfortable, but the skin overlying the torsion may be ecchymotic or edematous (Nandivada et al., 2016).

● Postnatal torsion presents with considerable tenderness and swelling of a previously normal testicle.

• Red or blue discoloration may be present.

Diagnosis

A diagnosis of testicular torsion is made by physical examination and can be confirmed by ultrasound (US). If the torsion is acute it will be extremely tender to palpation.

Preoperative Assessment and Nursing Care

Assess the scrotum daily to determine if the testicles have descended into the scrotal sac.

■ With torsion, the testicle is firm, nontender to painful, indurated, and swollen with a bluish or dusky cast of the affected side of the scrotum.

■ Without prompt identification and surgical treatment, the blood supply to the testicle is compromised and a testicle can die in as little as 4 to 6 hours (Nandivada et al., 2016).

■ Testicular torsion is a surgical emergency; thus, if detected on examination, the surgical team must be notified immediately.

Surgical Repair

■ If there is any suspicion of torsion, emergency exploration and detorsion should be performed within 4 to 6 hours of presentation in an attempt to preserve the testis (Ringer & Hansen, 2017).

■ If the testis is viable, it is detorsed and secured or pexed into the scrotum.

■ Due to the chance of contralateral torsion, the contralateral testis is prophylactically secured at the time of surgery.

Postoperative Assessment and Nursing Care

■ Admit premature infants to the ICU for 24 hours of observation with exposure to anesthesia and increased risk for apnea.

■ Monitor sutures and/or the incision line closely; observe the surgical site for signs of bleeding and infection.

■ Place the infant in a supine or side-lying position.

● Ideally, keep the head turned to the side as this may minimize the disruption of suture lines.

■ Assess pain for a minimum of every 4 hours.

● Comfort may be attainable with acetaminophen alone but consider narcotics on a patient-specific basis.

■ Remove dressings within 48 hours or as directed by the surgeon.

Documentation

■ Vital signs

■ Assessment of incision site

■ Pain scores

■ Dressing drainage amount

■ Parental teaching

UNDESCENDED TESTES

AVERY FORGET

Undescended testicle or cryptorchidism is a testicle that has not moved into the scrotal sac before birth.

Presentation

Usually just one testicle is undescended, although Nah et al., in 2014, observed both testicles were undescended in 24% of patients studied. An undescended testicle is uncommon in general but quite common among males born prematurely. In most cases, the undescended testicle moves into its proper position spontaneously; however, in some cases, it is necessary to correct surgically before 1 year of age.

Diagnosis

Diagnosis is by physical examination with the absence of testes in the scrotal sac.

Preoperative Assessment and Nursing Care

■ Assess for spontaneous resolution with the appearance of the testicles in the scrotal sac.

Surgical Repair

■ Surgical correction of the undescended testicle is called orchiopexy. It is the anchoring of the testes in the scrotum. This procedure is performed by laparoscope or open surgery.

Postoperative Assessment and Nursing Care

■ Admit premature infants to the ICU for 24 hours of observation due to exposure to anesthesia and increased risk for apnea.

■ Monitor incision and sutures (if present) closely for signs of bleeding and infection.

■ Place the infant in a supine or side-lying position.

  ● Ideally, position the head to the side as this may minimize disruption to the suture line.

■ Assess pain for a minimum of every 4 hours.

■ Achieve comfort with acetaminophen alone but consider narcotics on a patient-specific basis.

■ Remove dressing(s) within 48 hours or as directed by the provider.

Documentation

■ Vital signs

■ Assessment of incision site

■ Pain scores

■ Dressing drainage amount

■ Parental teaching

REFERENCES

Boley, S. J., Cahn, D., Lauer, L., Weinburg, G., & Kleinhaus, S. (1991). The irreducible ovary: A true emergency. *Journal of Pediatric Surgery, 26*(9), 1035–1038. https://doi.org/10.1016/0022-3468(91)90668-j

Bronsther, B., Abrams, M. W., & Elboim, C. (1972). Inguinal hernias in children: A study of 1,000 cases and a review of the literature. *Journal of the American Medical Women's Association, 10,* 522.

Clarke, S. (2010). Pediatric inguinal hernia and hydrocele: An evidence-based review in the era of minimal access surgery. [Review]. *Journal of Laparoendoscopic Advanced Surgical Techniques, 20*(3), 305–309. https://doi.org/10.1089/lap.2010.9997

Goldstein, R., & Potts, W. J. (1958). Inguinal hernias in female infants and children. *Annals of Surgery, 148*(5), 819–822. https://doi.org/10.1097/00000658-195811000-00013

Kapur, P., Caty, M. G., & Glick, P. L. (1998). Pediatric hernias and hydroceles. *Pediatric Clinics of North America, 45*(4), 773–789. https://doi.org/10.1016/s0031-3955(05)70044-4

Nah, S. A., Yeo, C. S., How, G. Y., Allen, J. C., Jr., Lakshmi, N. K., Yap, T. L., Jacobsen, A. S., Low, Y., & Ong, C. C. (2014). Undescended testis: 513 patients' characteristics, age at orchidopexy and patterns of referral. *Archives of Disease in Childhood, 99*(5), 401–406. https://doi.org/10.1136/archdischild-2013-305225

Nandivada, P., Fell, G. L., & Puder, M. (2016). Inguinal hernia. In A. R. Hansen & M. Puder (Eds.), *Manual of neonatal surgical intensive care* (3rd ed., pp. 333–341). People's Medical Publishing House.

Ringer, S. A., & Hansen, A. R. (2017). Surgical emergencies in the newborn. In E. C. Eichenwald, A. R. Hansen, C. R. Martin, & A. R. Stark (Eds.), *Cloherty and Stark's manual of neonatal care* (8th ed., pp. 825–826). Wolters Kluwer.

Skin Care

CAROLYN LUND

OVERVIEW

Neonatal skin care is an important clinical concern for neonatal nurses. Goals of skin care for newborn infants include protecting skin integrity, reducing exposure to potential toxicity from topical agents, and promoting healthy skin barrier function. An understanding of the unique anatomic and physiologic differences in premature, full-term newborn, and young infant skin is fundamental to providing effective care to these populations.

PHYSIOLOGIC AND ANATOMIC VARIATIONS IN NEWBORN, YOUNG INFANT, AND PREMATURE INFANT SKIN

Newborn skin undergoes an adaptation process during the transition from the aquatic environment of the uterus to the aerobic environment after birth. The skin assists in thermoregulation, serves as a barrier against toxins and microorganisms, is a reservoir for fat storage and insulation, and is a primary interface for tactile sensation and communication.

Stratum Corneum and Epidermis

The stratum corneum, which provides the important barrier function of the skin, contains 10 to 20 layers in the adult and in the full-term newborn. Although full-term newborns reportedly have skin barrier function comparable to that of adult skin, as indicated by a measurement called transepidermal water loss (TEWL), there is now some evidence that the stratum corneum does not function as well as adult skin during the first year of life. Infant skin is 30% thinner than adult skin, and the basal layer of the epidermis is 20% thinner than that of the adult, and the keratinocytes in this layer have a higher cell turnover rate, which may account for the faster wound healing that has been observed in neonates.

The premature infant has far fewer cell layers in the stratum corneum, with the specific number determined by gestational age. At less than 30 weeks' gestation, there may be as few as two or three layers, and the extremely premature infant of 23 to 24 weeks' gestation has almost no stratum corneum and negligible barrier function. The deficient stratum corneum results in excessive fluid and evaporative heat losses during the first weeks of life, leading to increased risk of dehydration and significant alterations in electrolyte levels, such as hypernatremia. Techniques used to reduce these losses include the use of polyethylene coverings immediately after delivery and use of high levels of relative humidity (>70% RH) in incubators for the first week of life. Maturation of the skin barrier, particularly for infants of 23 to 25 weeks' gestation, occurs over time, with evidence of mature barrier function delayed until about 30 to 32 weeks' postconceptional age.

Dermis

The dermis of the full-term newborn is thinner and not as well developed as the adult dermis. The collagen and elastin fibers are shorter and less dense, and the reticular layer of the dermis is absent, which makes the skin feel very soft.

Premature infant skin exhibits decreased cohesion between the epidermis and dermis, which places these babies at risk for skin injury from removal of medical adhesives. When extremely aggressive adhesives are used, the bond between adhesive and epidermis may be stronger than that between epidermis and dermis, resulting in stripping of the epidermal layer and loss of or significantly diminished skin barrier function.

Skin pH

Skin surface typically has an acidic pH, due to a number of chemical and biologic processes involving the stratum corneum. This "acid mantle" of the skin (pH<5) contributes to the immune function of the stratum corneum by inhibiting the growth of pathogenic microorganisms and supporting the proliferation of commensal, or "healthy," bacteria on the skin.

Full-term newborns are born with an alkaline skin surface (pH>6.0), but within the first 4 days after birth, the pH falls to less than 5.0. Skin surface pH in premature infants of varying gestational ages has·been reported to be greater than 6 on the first day of life; however, it decreases to 5.5 by the end of the first week, and 5.1 by the end of the first month. Bathing and other topical treatments transiently alter skin pH, and diapered skin has a higher pH due to the combined effects of urine contact and occlusion. The higher pH of diapered skin reduces the barrier function of the stratum corneum, rendering it more susceptible to mechanical damage from friction.

Risk of Toxicity From Topical Agents

Toxicity from topically applied substances has been discussed in numerous case reports due to the increased permeability of both preterm and full-term newborn skin. This is due to a number of factors including the fact that newborn skin is 20% to 40% thinner than adult skin, and the ratio of body surface to weight is nearly five times greater in newborns than in older children and adults, which places newborns at increased risk for percutaneous absorption and toxicity. Examples of toxicity from percutaneous absorption include encephalopathy and death among premature infants bathed with hexachlorophene and alterations in iodine levels and thyroid function related to routine use of povidone-iodine in NICUs.

SKIN CARE PRACTICES

Evidence-based skin care practices for neonates are provided in the third edition of the *Neonatal Skin Care: Evidence-Based Clinical Practice Guideline*, published by the Association of Women's Health, Obstetric and Neonatal Nurses (AWHONN; 2018). This guideline includes recommendations for 13 aspects of neonatal skin care, ranging from bathing to the use of disinfectants to diaper dermatitis. A brief summary of selected aspects is included in this handbook for neonatal nurses.

Bathing

The newborn's first bath should occur when temperature and vital signs are stable; the World Health Organization (WHO) recommends waiting at least 6 hours (WHO, 2015). Clear water or water and a mild baby wash product with a neutral or mildly acidic pH (5.5–7.0) may be used, but soap-based products are avoided as they can be drying or irritating to the skin. Leaving residual vernix caseosa intact has several benefits, including protecting from infection, moisturization, development of the acid mantle, and temperature regulation; it can be left in place to wear off with normal care and handling. Consider an "immersion" or tub bath even with the umbilical cord still in place, as this has been shown to be more soothing and has less temperature loss. For routine bathing, it is not necessary to bathe a newborn more than every other day (Lund, 2016).

Umbilical Cord Care

Cleanse the umbilical cord during bathing with clear water, and dry to remove excess water. Leave the umbilical cord stump clean, dry, and uncovered by keeping the diaper folded underneath the cord. Educate parents to use "natural drying" by keeping the cord area clean and dry, without the use of topical agents. This is also the recommendation of WHO (2015). In some developing countries, however, a single application of chlorhexidine gluconate has been shown to reduce infection.

Diaper Dermatitis

Maintaining a healthy skin environment in the diaper area is the primary goal. In the newborn period, changing the diaper when wet or soiled is beneficial, as often as every 1 to 3 hours. Avoid rubbing the perineal skin, and use soft cloths, water, or a gentle disposable diaper wipe that has been tested on newborn skin.

If diaper dermatitis occurs, determine the underlying cause. The most common type is irritant contact diaper dermatitis caused by fecal enzymes (Heimall et al., 2012). This type is seen in the peri-anal skin and can range from bright red to excoriated or denuded. Skin affected in this way can benefit from an immersion bath once daily and application of petrolatum-based ointment either as a preventive strategy or to protect reddened skin with each diaper change. For more severe skin excoriation, use a skin barrier product, such as those containing zinc oxide; the barrier should be applied in a very thick coating over the excoriated skin and reapplied with every diaper change. Other skin barrier products that provide even more effective barriers to fecal enzymes are also available for use in the most severe cases. Consider if there is an underlying cause, such as diarrhea that is infectious, opiate withdrawal, or significant malabsorption of nutrients due to a surgical condition; a change in diet or other medical interventions may be indicated.

Another type of diaper dermatitis involves *Candida albicans*; this may also be called a yeast or fungal diaper dermatitis. This type of diaper dermatitis is characterized by "beefy" red skin, with "satellite" lesions scattered at the edges; the skin may or may not be denuded. An antifungal ointment or cream is applied topically three or four times a day; if the rash does not respond in several days, it may be necessary to select another antifungal preparation.

Emollients

Emollients are topical substances composed of fat or oil, sometimes combined with water. The routine use of emollients in newborn skin care is not clear, although application of an emollient to skin that is dry or cracked is recommended. Large studies of very premature infants <1,000 g reported no differences in mortality when a petrolatum-based ointment was applied twice daily, compared to using this emollient only on an "as needed" basis for dry skin; they also reported an increase in bloodstream infections in the smallest infants <750 g with the routine use of this ointment. For this reason, the routine use of emollients in premature infants <1,000 g is not recommended.

In some cultures, the routine use of an emollient, usually in the form of an oil, is used during infant massage. Although some oils such as sunflower seed oil have been shown to be beneficial, others such as olive oil or grape seed oil may be more irritating according to some laboratory investigations. The role of these oils in the NICU is not well studied, and concerns about using them with infants who have central venous catheters, for example, have been raised.

Disinfectants

Disinfecting skin surfaces prior to invasive procedures such as insertion of central venous catheters, umbilical catheters, intravenous catheters, chest tubes, or venipuncture reduces the risk of infection. Current skin disinfectants used in this manner include 70% isopropyl alcohol, 10% povidone-iodine, and chlorhexidine gluconate, with concentrations ranging from 0.5% to 3.15%, some in aqueous solutions and many combined with 70% isopropyl alcohol. When evaluating different products used for skin disinfection, efficacy of skin sterilization, systemic toxicity, and skin irritation or chemical burns should be considered.

Chlorhexidine gluconate containing solutions have been shown to reduce the risk of bloodstream infection in adults with central venous catheters, but there is no study to date to demonstrate this in the NICU population. Povidone-iodine is next in terms of efficacy, with isopropyl alcohol the least effective for skin decontamination.

Systemic toxicity has been reported with povidone-iodine use in premature infants, affecting thyroid function transiently; if this solution is used, it is recommended to remove it completely using sterile water or saline to reduce skin exposure and absorption. Toxicity to chlorhexidine products has been seen with exposure to the eyes and ear structures. In adults, there have been reports of anaphylactic reactions when using chlorhexidine gluconate–impregnated urinary catheters or with large areas of exposure during repeated surgical procedures.

Chemical burns and skin irritation have been reported with alcohol-containing disinfectants. A number of reports involve the periumbilical skin that has been disinfected with chlorhexidine gluconate containing 70% isopropyl alcohol in extremely low-birth-weight premature infants, although there are even reports of skin injury with aqueous chlorhexidine gluconate. Disinfectants should be used with caution in this population.

Medical Adhesives

Medical adhesives such as tape, electrodes, and transparent adhesive dressings are applied and removed many times a day in the typical NICU. These secure both critical life support equipment, such as endotracheal tubes, intravenous and arterial catheters, and chest tubes, and numerous monitoring devices and probes. Skin injury from medical adhesives is a known problem in the NICU population (Lund, 2014). As mentioned previously, one reason is immature skin with decreased cohesion between the epidermis and dermis layers.

There are a number of different types of adhesive products, including cloth tape, plastic perforated tape, transparent adhesive dressings, hydrocolloid adhesives, hydrogel adhesives, and silicone adhesives. Depending on the critical need to adhere, different adhesives are selected for different indications. For example, hydrogel adhesives may work well for electrocardiogram electrodes but are not suitable to secure an endotracheal tube. Silicone adhesives work well as a border around dressings and to secure electroencephalogram electrodes to the scalp and hair and are very gentle when removed. However, silicone tapes do not adhere well to plastic tubes and cannulas.

Another strategy to reduce skin injury from adhesives is the use of silicone-based skin protectants that do not contain alcohol; these are commonly used on skin surrounding ostomy sites. They have been reported as beneficial in several small studies in premature infants. The use of bonding agents such as tincture of Benzoin to increase the stickiness of adhesives is not recommended, because the bond that these agents form between the adhesive and the epidermis may be stronger than the fragile cohesion between epidermis and dermis and can result in epidermal stripping when removed.

Silicone-based adhesive removal products are being seen in the literature and are described as very beneficial for infants with genetic skin disorders such as epidermolysis bullosa. It is possible that these, too, may benefit premature infants, but more research in this area is encouraged. Alcohol or organic-based skin removers contain hydrocarbon derivatives or petroleum distillates that have a potential for systemic toxicity and should not be used.

CONCLUSION

Newborn skin has unique properties that are important to understand when providing skin care. Both full-term and premature newborns require careful consideration during such daily care practices as bathing, skin disinfection, umbilical cord care, adhesive and emollient use, and management of diaper dermatitis. Optimal approaches for neonatal skin care that are evidence based have been shown to be practical in both the neonatal intensive care as well as "well baby" nursery settings, while improving the overall skin condition for newborns and young infants.

REFERENCES

Association of Women's Health, Obstetric and Neonatal Nurses. (2018). *Evidence-based clinical practice guideline: Neonatal skin care* (4th ed.). Author.

Heimall, L. M., Storey, B., Stellar, J. J., & Davis, K. F. (2012). Beginning at the bottom: Evidence-based care of diaper dermatitis. *American Journal of Maternal Child Nursing, 37*(1), 10–16. https://doi.org/10.1097/NMC.0b013e31823850ea

Lund, C. (2014). Medical adhesives in the NICU. *Newborn and Infant Nursing Reviews, 14*(4), 160–165. https://doi.org/10.1053/j.nainr.2014.10.001

Lund, C. (2016). Bathing and beyond: Current bathing controversies for newborn infants. *Advances in Neonatal Care, 16*(5S), S13–S20. https://doi.org/10.1097/ANC.00000000 00000336

World Health Organization. (2015). *Pregnancy, childbirth, postpartum and newborn care: A guide for essential practice.* World Health Organization. https://www.ncbi.nlm.nih.gov/books/NBK326678

Family-Centered Developmental Care

DOROTHY VITTNER AND JACQUELINE M. MCGRATH

OVERVIEW

Over 15 million premature infants are born annually around the world. One million children die from prematurity-related complications (Howson et al., 2012). Although survival rates of critically ill infants are steadily improving, the incidence of later developmental disabilities for these infants remains high (O'Reilly et al., 2020; Spittle & Treyvaud, 2016). The long-term implications for survivors of prematurity include differences in brain development, which include cognition, educational achievement, and behavioral differences, including social and emotional regulation (McAnulty et al., 2013; O'Reilly et al., 2020; Synnes & Hicks, 2018). It has been optimistically, yet incorrectly, proposed that healthy preterm infants without major complications eventually catch-up developmentally to term infants by school age (Duncan & Matthews, 2018; Hodel et al., 2017). However, evidence suggests that as premature infants move into school age and adolescence, the consequences of early birth continue to influence neurodevelopmental outcomes, and these influences cannot be ignored or minimized (Allotey et al., 2018; Chan et al., 2016; McAnulty et al., 2013). Despite advances in care for preterm infants and their families, it remains difficult to accurately predict adverse neurodevelopmental outcomes (Spittle et al., 2008; Spittle & Treyvaud, 2016). While some developmental differences and challenges seen in children born premature can be explained by the cumulative effect of medical complications associated with preterm birth and early-life experiences, many sequelae of prematurity are not as easily explained by medical complications alone (Als et al., 2005; Spittle & Treyvaud, 2016). Thus, the caregiving environment must also be considered; how medical care is delivered matters.

Individualized developmental care aims to support the infant's physiologic stability, neurobehavioral functioning, and the emotional and social well-being of the infant to facilitate the infant's growth and development. Based on each infant's maturity, competencies, vulnerabilities, and status of subsystem functioning, individualized developmental care integrates a supportive physical and social environment with individualized assessment and interventions for the hospitalized infant and their family. A collaborative partnership model for clinical practice provides personalized and consistent caregiving opportunities for infants and families to flourish and grow both individually and as a unit. Interventions include diffusing ambient light and sound levels in the nursery, providing supportive interactions with neutral postures, enhancing cue-based care, reducing the infant's pain and stress, and protecting and promoting restful sleep, along with implementation of family-centered care principles to support parent engagement.

INFANT DEVELOPMENT

The infant who is delivered early experiences a very different sensory environment in the task-driven, high-tech world of the NICU or other hospitalized settings than the womb where the foundation for their development should have occurred. It is imperative for infant development that their parents and caregivers understand the unique behavioral strategies the infant uses to cope during their early life experience in the hospital setting. At this point in development, the preterm infant neurobiologically expects a sensory experience that is quite different from those experienced in the NICU. This mismatch in neurobiological sensory expectations in the context of the developing brain is an important factor influencing long-term developmental outcomes (McAnulty et al., 2013).

INFANT BEHAVIORS, CUES, AND PATTERNS OF DEVELOPMENT

The infant's behavior is the window into understanding the functioning of the developing brain and provides a guide for the caregiver to estimate the infant's current strengths as well as their active efforts to cope with environmental experiences. Observation of the infant's behavior provides opportunities to infer from the patterns of behavior what the infant is trying to accomplish and their neurobehavioral goals and functioning. Observing and understanding the infant's behavioral patterns can be facilitated by utilizing the Synactive Theory of Development. This theoretical framework provides an approach to specifically document the complexity of the hospitalized infant by focusing on the interplay of behaviors within the systems of autonomic, motor, state organization, attention, and self-regulation as the infant's behavioral functioning interacts with the caregiver simultaneously with the environment (Als, 1982).

INFANT-DRIVEN CARE PRACTICES

Assessment and documentation of the infant's behavioral patterns offer the opportunity to identify competence and vulnerabilities, which provide an understanding of the infant's developing brain and nervous system. Using these assessments to make decisions about caregiving support and practices leads to the provision of developmentally appropriate experiences for the infant and their family in the hospital setting. Structuring a physical and social environment supportive and nurturant of the individual infant's successful coping along with the family's sense of competence becomes a critical component of care for infants in hospital settings (Als et al., 2004; Lisanti et al., 2019). Individualized developmental care ensures the infant's expectation for coregulatory care and for close, emotionally attuned and invested relationships, primarily with the infant's parents and then with other caregivers. It is pivotal to identify opportunities for increased effectiveness of hospital care delivery in supporting nonseparation and coregulation of the hospitalized infant and their family (D'Agata & McGrath, 2016; D'Agata et al., 2017). Implementation of such a framework requires knowledge and understanding of infant, parent, and family development, and of the interplay of the infant's medical issues with the developmental process to create an individualized plan of care specific to meet the needs and expectations for that infant and their family (D'Agata et al., 2016; Vittner et al., 2019).

WAKEFULNESS, STATE TRANSITIONS, RESTFUL SLEEP

The greater time spent sleeping in infancy and early childhood is thought to reflect the crucial role sleep (especially REM sleep) plays in fostering optimal brain development, cognition, and behavior. Sleep has important roles also in brain plasticity and the ability of the brain to change its structure and function in response to environmental changes and needs (Calciolari & Montirosso, 2011). The promotion and protection of sleep is essential and a cornerstone to implementing individualized developmental care for infants requiring intensive care settings (Griffiths et al., 2019). A lack of sleep in the neonatal period is associated with behavioral problems and reduced cerebral cortical size (Ednick et al., 2009). Strategies to promote sleep include modified sensory experiences creating a calm, quiet environment with dimmed lighting. Avoid sleep interruptions by postponing elective care activities while an infant is asleep.

The relationship between quantity and quality of sleep in preterm infants and neurocognitive and socioemotional outcomes has been established (Graven, 2006). Sleep and established sleep cycles are necessary for the normal neurosensory and cortex development. The interruption of normal sleep can lead to the modification of the expression of several genes that can reduce the brain plasticity (Calciolari & Montirosso, 2011).

The infant's wakefulness must be acknowledged and capitalized for interaction with the family whenever possible. Consider opportunities to awaken the infant gently by speaking softly prior to touching the infant; remember to pause as you begin your interaction to observe the infant's behavior to support the infant to actively participate in the interaction. Encourage the infant's family to actively participate in the caregiving activity. When the infant awakens, consider speaking softly to encourage the infant to open their eyes. After these interactions, it is important to speak with parents about the interaction and encourage them to better understand their infant's behaviors and how they can use supportive strategies to support these wakeful moments. In the beginning, these moments could seem fleeting and that could be discouraging to families. Helping them to understand these interactions with their infant will help parents to grow in better understanding their infant.

FACILITATING A NURTURING ENVIRONMENT

The physical, social, and emotional environments play a pivotal role in the developing infant and their family in hospital settings (Scatliffe et al., 2019). Parents are essential to support optimal infant development; high-risk birth with admission to the NICU only increases parents' vital role. Current evidence increasingly provides direction for how best to fully engage parents through increased opportunities for both physical and emotional closeness enhancing parent–infant interactions and participation in NICU caregiving activities (Lockridge, 2018; Smith, 2018). Parent engagement is defined as a dynamic process focused on enhancing and supporting the parent–infant experience; specifically, enhancing the acquisition of skills for problem-solving and provision of appropriate infant care based on the unique infant needs (Makris et al., 2019; Samra et al., 2015). Enhancing parent engagement is one means of decreasing what has been recently documented as posttraumatic stress disorder often experienced by parents who must traverse the chaotic hospital environment while supporting their high-risk infant (Feeg et al., 2016). Concurrently, the unique needs of the infant's developing brain demand that caregiving by parent and healthcare professionals be neuroprotective, matching the neurobiological expectations for experiences that nurture the infant's physical and emotional development (Feldman, 2015; Vittner et al., 2019).

STRATEGIES TO SUPPORT AND EMPOWER RELATIONSHIPS

The infant's developmental trajectory is influenced by evolving relationships. Parents are the infant's ideal nurturer and coregulator, enhancing the infant's competence and ability to build trust within the relationship (Als et al., 2004; Craig et al., 2015). Parents and infants benefit from the parent's awareness and responsiveness to the infant's behavioral capabilities and temperament. Parental ability to interpret the infant's behavioral cues has been shown to strengthen parent–infant interaction during the first year of life (Craig et al., 2015; Feldman, 2015). When parents have the skills to interpret their infant's cues and respond appropriately, the infant is better able to self-regulate and respond appropriately to the physical and social environment (Als et al., 2004). Providing infants with this foundation for trusting interactions increases their self-regulatory efforts and ability to respond to new situations.

SUPPORTING RECIPROCITY AND PARENTAL RESPONSIVENESS

In the early years of an infant's life, parent–infant contact is critical for establishing affectionate bonds that are formed through synchronous and responsive social interactions that lead to enduring attachment. Parental contact is fundamental to an infant's developmental trajectory, and these early-life experiences influence infant neurodevelopmental outcomes (Feeg et al., 2016; McAnulty et al., 2013). Synchronous interactions are not predetermined, yet emerge as self-organizing processes from the social inputs from those participating in the interaction (Feldman, 2015, 2017). This facilitates parents to provide coregulation which enables the integration of physiology while simultaneously utilizing behavior in a unique individualized repertoire of mutual support and self-regulation within the context of developing social skills (Feldman, 2015).

FACILITATING INFANT COPING AND COREGULATION WITH CAREGIVERS

Early social environments influence the neurobiology of the infant brain; thus, socialization through parent engagement is an important factor in the health of a premature infant (Vittner et al., 2019). Parent engagement is a dynamic process focused on enhancing and supporting the parent–infant experience, specifically targeting the acquisition of skills for parent problem-solving and provision of appropriate infant care based on the infant's strengths while supporting their weaknesses (Makris et al., 2019). Focusing on infant strengths is actualized by using the infant's cues to guide interactions such that the infant is in the most optimal state possible for interactions to occur. Providing environments that facilitate infant coping allows the infant to use their energies for interaction with parents and the environment as well as for enhancing cognitive development. If an infant's energy is entirely focused on surviving, such as breathing and eating, there is no energy left for interaction or growth. Providing a supportive environment increases the opportunities for growth in the infant's development and must be facilitated whenever possible. Stress, while inevitable, must be minimized and infant coping must be increased through interventions that provide support for interaction or restful sleep.

SKIN-TO-SKIN CARE IMPLEMENTATION

Skin-to-skin care (SSC) between the parent and infant is described as the upright prone positioning of the diaper-clad infant, skin to skin, on the parent's bare chest over the breast area. This approach was developed and initiated in Bogota, Colombia, in the late 1970s to help keep premature infants warm when incubators were not available (Whiteslaw & Sleath, 1985). There is a plethora of evidence to support kangaroo mother care (KMC) and SSC (Conde-Agudelo & Díaz-Rossello, 2016; Johnston et al., 2017; Mori et al., 2010). SSC is a vital component of individualized developmental care, especially for young infants hospitalized in intensive care or special care nurseries. SSC provides multisensory stimulation to the infant—including emotional, tactile, proprioceptive, vestibular, olfactory, auditory, visual, and thermal stimulation—in a unique interactive style. Fundamental to the infant's developmental trajectory is early parent–infant contact. Maternal touch, especially during SSC, has the potential to mitigate some of the adverse consequences of prematurity and hospitalized infants requiring intensive care. SSC is an evidence-based holding strategy that increases parental proximity and provides a continuous interactive environment known to enhance infant physiologic stability and affective closeness within the parent–infant dyad (Kostandy & Ludington-Hoe, 2019).

Continuous KMC, 24 hours per day, has been implemented as an ideally alternative measure for preterm infants in low-income settings and also in some high-income countries. Intermittent KMC has been recommended for hospitalized infants to consider the infant's adaptation as well as to promote sleep (Davanzo et al., 2013; Shattnawi & Al-Ali, 2019). KMC can be practiced by both mothers and fathers with their newborns immediately after birth and regularly throughout the first few months of life. It can also be used as an intervention to support parents who have difficulties with parent–infant bonding, breastfeeding, palliative care, or life-limiting conditions.

SUPPORTING SHORT- AND LONG-TERM DEVELOPMENT

While the focus in the NICU is often about *saving* the life of the preterm infant through procedures and treatments, the long-term effects of living in this environment must also be considered. Caregiving decision-making must be balanced not only with the immediate short-term benefits of this caregiving strategy but also with the long-term developmental sequelae of short-term interventions (McGrath et al., 2011; Papagreorgiou & Pelausa, 2014). Examples include the short-term use of steroids to support lung development and the long-term sequalae of poorer growth as well as other respiratory treatments like deep suctioning, vibration, and cupping. In the not-so-distant past, the long-term use of these respiratory strategies was routine care. Yet, we have learned that these practices, while beneficial, also have costs. Every caregiving practice in the NICU must be considered in the same way. Everything we do matters, as well as everything we do not do when potentially we should consider intervening. Weighing the cost and benefit of every intervention is important when considering both short- and long-term implications for development.

IMPLEMENTING STRATEGIES FOR MOTOR DEVELOPMENT

General principles for facilitating motor competence in the NICU (Marlow et al., 2007) begin with providing a supportive environment that enhances muscle development. Most commonly, this is done by providing supportive boundaries such as "nesting" an infant. However, the *nest* is not effective unless it encourages flexion of the extremities and the infant is able to stretch and extend to push against the nest or boundary (like the infant would experience in the womb) to increase muscle development and, in time, strength. Providing time for the infant to be both prone and supine with the proper supportive environment is also important to motor development as is providing time for the infant to look and see both to the right and to the left. For example, head tilts to the right or the left seen in preterm infants after discharge from the NICU are often the result of the infant being placed predominantly on the right or left side and not encouraging full range of motion. Focusing on both short- and long-term motor development while caring for the preterm infant may not always seem like the priority in the NICU, but these issues cannot be minimized, since they can cause long-term issues for the infant. It is well known that severe chronic lung disease is highly predictive of long-term development issues for preterm infants. These developmental issues are not just due to effects of oxygen deprivation on the brain; they are also related to poorer muscle development and lower levels of energy and inactivity in the NICU or even poorer reactive activity such as arching. While these concerns can have a cumulative effect on long-term development, there are focused strategies for caregiving that must also be considered that can help decrease the potential long-term effects from chronic lung disease.

IMPLEMENTING STRATEGIES FOR COGNITIVE DEVELOPMENT

Cognitive development is about attending to the visual and auditory stimuli surrounding the preterm infant. Generally speaking, the stimulation must be age appropriate (Synnes & Hicks, 2018). The appropriate strategies differ for a 24-week gestation infant as opposed to a 34-week gestation infant (Bader, 2014). Providing darkness for many hours of the day for a 24-week infant is often appropriate to facilitate sleep. However, the 34-week gestation infant will need a more routine cycle of both darkness at night and daylight during the day, which is important to neurologic development and helping the growing preterm infant transition to home after discharge. Auditory stimulation must be addressed in the same way. Observing the infant's behavior provides an opportunity to understand what they can tolerate and when the noise is overstimulation for the infant (Ohlsson & Jacobs, 2013).

In addition, to support cognitive development, the infant's behavioral cues must be acknowledged during every caregiving interaction and the caregiver's responsiveness to the infant's individualized cues. While a caregiver must have knowledge about infant cues to respond appropriately, the caregiver must also know this unique infant and their pattern of cues, as well as what these cues might mean or how this infant regularly uses those cues. An infant's behavioral repertoire is their language and it is unique. Providing a responsive environment that facilitates the infant to *actively participate* in the interaction is important to short- and long-term development. Responsiveness and synchrony in offering interaction are important in supporting the infant's short- and long-term development.

CONCLUSION

It is important for nurses to provide care in the context of knowing that every infant and family who must traverse the NICU environment with all of the competing demands did not choose to be there. It is our role to make sure their stay in this sometimes chaotic and medical environment is also mutually supportive and as positive as it can be. Weighing the cost/benefit of every strategy or intervention that is chosen to support the infant and the family must be a priority not only for supporting short-term outcomes but also for promoting long-term outcomes. The priority of caregiving must be individualized to acknowledge the core value that the hospitalized infant and family have an optimal start to not only these early-life experiences but also for their life together as a family.

REFERENCES

Allotey, J., Zamora, J., Cheong-See, F., Kalidindi, M., Arroyo-Manzano, D., Asztalos, E., Van der Post, J. A., Mol, B. W., Moore, D. G., Birtles, D., Khan, K. S., & Thangaratinam, S. (2018). Cognitive, motor, behavioural and academic performances of children born preterm: A metanalysis and systematic review involving 64,061 children. *International Journal of Obstetrics and Gynaecology, 125*, 16–25. https://doi.org/10.1111/1471-0528.14832

Als, H. (1982). Towards a synactive theory of development: Promise for infant individuality. *Infant Mental Health Journal, 3*(4), 229–243. https://doi.org/10.1002/1097-0355(198224) 3:4<229::AID-IMHJ2280030405>3.0.CO;2-H

Als, H., Butler, S., Kosta, S., & McAnulty, G. (2005). The assessment of preterm infant behavior (APIB): Furthering the understanding and measurement of neurodevelopmental competence in preterm and full-term infants. *Mental Retardation and Developmental Disabilities Research Reviews, 11*, 94–102. https://doi.org/10.1002/mrdd.20053

Als, H., Duffy, F., McAnulty, G. B., Rivkin, M., Vajapeyam, S., Mulkern, R., Warfield, S. K., Huppi, P. S., Butler, S. C., Conneman, N., Fischer, C., & Eichenwald, E. C. (2004). Early experience alters brain function and structure. *Pediatrics, 113*, 846–857. https://doi.org/ 10.1542/peds.113.4.846

Bader, L. (2014). Brain oriented care in the NICU: A case study. *Neonatal Network, 33*(5), 263–267. https://doi.org/10.1891/0730-0832.33.5.263

Calciolari, G., & Montirosso, R. (2011). The sleep protection in the preterm infants. *Journal of Maternal-Fetal Neonatal Medicine, 24*(S1), 12–14. https://doi.org/10.3109/14767058.2011 .607563

Chan, E., Leong, P., Malouf, R., & Quigley, M. (2016). Long-term cognitive and school outcomes of late preterm and early term births: A systematic review. *Child: Care, Health & Development, 42*(3), 297–312. https://doi.org/10.1111/cch.12320

Conde-Agudelo, A., & Díaz-Rossello, J. (2016). Kangaroo mother care to reduce morbidity and mortality in low birthweight infants. *Cochrane Database Systematic Reviews, 2016*(8), CD002771. https://doi.org/10.1002/14651858.CD002771.pub4

Craig, J., Glick, C., Phillip, R., Hall, S., Smith, J., & Browne, J. (2015). Recommendations for involving the family in developmental care of the NICU baby. *Journal of Perinatology, 35*, S5–S8. https://doi.org/10.1038/jp.2015.142

D'Agata, A., & McGrath, J. (2016). A framework of complex adaptive systems: Parents as partners in the Neonatal Intensive Care Unit. *Advances in Nursing Science, 39*(3), 244–256. https://doi.org/10.1097/ANS.0000000000000127

D'Agata, A., Walsh, S., Vittner, D., Cong, X., McGrath, J., & Young, E. (2017). FKBP5 genotype and early stress exposure predict neurobehavioral outcomes for preterm infants. *Developmental Psychobiology, 59*, 410–418. https://doi.org/10.1002/dev.21507

D'Agata, A., Young, E., Cong, X., Grosso, D., & McGrath, J. (2016). Infant medical trauma in the neonatal intensive care unit (IMTN): A proposed concept for science and practice. *Advances in Neonatal Care, 16*(4), 289–297. https://doi.org/10.1097/ANC.0000000000000309

Davanzo, R., Brovedani, P., Travan, L., Kennedy, J., Crocetta, A., Sanesi, C., Strajn, T., & De Cunto, A. (2013). Intermittent kangaroo mother care: A NICU protocol. *Journal of Human Lactation, 29*(3), 332–338. https://doi.org/10.1177/0890334413489375

Duncan, A., & Matthews, M. (2018). Neurodevelopmental outcomes in early childhood. *Clinics Perinatology, 45*, 377–392. https://doi.org/10.1016/j.clp.2018.05.001

Ednick, M., Cohen, A., McPhail, G., Beebe, D., Simaakajornboon, N., & Amin, R. (2009). A review of TGE effects of sleep during the first year of life on cognitive, psychomotor, and temperament development. *Sleep, 32*, 1449–1458. https://doi.org/10.1093/sleep/32.11.1449

Feeg, V., Paraszczuk, A., Cavusoglu, H., Sheilds, L., Pars, H., & Mamun, A. (2016). How is family centered care perceived by health care providers from different countries? An international comparison study. *Journal of Pediatric Nursing, 31*, 267–276. https://doi.org/10.1016/j.pedn.2015.11.007

Feldman, R. (2015). Sensitive periods in human social development: New insights from research on oxytocin, synchrony and high-risk parenting. *Development and Psychopathology, 27*, 369–395. https://doi.org/10.1017/S0954579415000048

Feldman, R. (2017). The neurobiology of human attachments. *Trends in Cognitive Sciences, 21*(2), 80–99. https://doi.org/10.1016/j.tics.2016.11.007

Graven, S. (2006). Sleep and brain development. *Journal of Perinatology, 33*, 693–706. https://doi.org/10.1016/j.clp.2006.06.009

Griffiths, N., Spence, K., Loughran-Fowlds, A., & Westrup, B. (2019). Individualised developmental care for babies and parents in the NICU: Evidence-based best practice guideline recommendations. *Early Human Development, 139*, E104840. https://doi.org/10.1016/j.earlhumdev.2019.104840

Hodel, A., Senich, K., Jokinen, C., Sasaon, O., Morris, A., & Thomas, K. (2017). Early executive function differences in infants born moderate to late preterm. *Early Human Development, 113*, 23–30. https://doi.org/10.1016/j.earlhumdev.2017.07.007

Howson, C. P., Kinney, M. V., & Lawn, J. E. (2012). *Born too soon: The global action report on preterm birth*. March of Dimes, PMNCH, Save the Children, WHO.

Johnston, C., Campell-Yeo, M., Disher, T., Benoit, B., Fernandes, A., Streiner, D., Inglis, D., & Zee, R. (2017). Skin-to-skin care for procedural pain in neonates. *Cochrane Database of Systematic Reviews, 2*, CD008435. https://doi.org/10.1002/14651858.CD008435.pub3

Kostandy, R., & Ludington-Hoe, S. (2019). The evolution of the science of kangaroo (mother) care (skin-to-skin contact). *Birth Defects Research, 111*(15), 1032–1043. https://doi.org/10.1002/bdr2.1565

Lisanti, A., Vittner, D., Medoff-Cooper, B., Fogl, J., & Butler, S. (2019). Individualized family-centered developmental care: An essential model to address the unique needs of infants with congential heart disease. *Journal of Cardiovascular Nursing, 34*(1), 85–93. https://doi.org/10.1097/JCN.0000000000000546

Lockridge, T. (2018). Neonatal neuroprotection: Bringing best practice to the bedside in the NICU. *Journal of Maternal Child Nursing, 43*(2), 66–76. https://doi.org/10.1097/NMC.0000000000000411

Makris, N., Vittner, D., Samra, H., & McGrath, J. (2019). The PREEMI as a measure of parent engagement in the NICU. *Applied Nursing Research, 47*, 24–28. https://doi.org/10.1016/j.apnr.2019.03.007

Marlow, N., Hennessy, E., Bracewell, M., Wolke, D., & Group, E. S. (2007). Motor and executive function at 6 years of age after extremely preterm birth. *Pediatrics, 120*, 793–804. https://doi.org/10.1542/peds.2007-0440

McAnulty, G., Duffy, F., Kosta, S., Weisenfeld, N., Warfield, S., Butler, S., Alidoost, M., Bernstein, J. H., Robertson, R., Zurakowski, D., & Als, H. (2013). School age effects of the newborn individualized developmental care and assessment program for preterm infants with intrauterine growth restriction: Preliminary findings. *BMC Pediatrics, 13*, 25. https://doi.org/10.1186/1471-2431-13-25

McGrath, J., Cone, S., & Hamra, H. (2011). Neuroprotection in preterm infant: Further understanding short- and long-term outcomes for brain development. *Newborn and Infant Nursing Reviews, 11*, 109–112. https://doi.org/10.1053/j.nainr.2011.007.002

Mori, R., Khanna, R., Pledge, D., & Nakayama, T. (2010). Meta analysis of physiologic effects of skin to skin contact for newborns and mothers. *Pediatrics International, 52*, 161–170. https://doi.org/10.1111/j.1442-200x.2009.02909.x

Ohlsson, A., & Jacobs, S. (2013). NIDCAP: A systematic and metanalysis of randomized controlled trials. *Pediatrics, 131*(3), e881–893. https://doi.org/10.1542/peds.2012.2121

O'Reilly, H., Johnson, S., Ni, Y., Wolke, D., & Marlow, N. (2020). Neuropsychological outcomes at 19 years of age following extreme preterm birth. *Pediatrics, 145*(2), e20192087. https://doi.org/10.1542/peds.2019-2087

Papagreorgiou, A., & Pelausa, E. (2014). Management and outcomes of extremely low birth weight infants. *Journal of Pediatric and Neonatal Individualized Medicine, 3*(3), 030209. https://doi.org/10.73631/030209

Samra, H., McGrath, J., Fischer, S., Schumacher, B., Dutcher, J., & Hansen, J. (2015). NICU Parent Risk Evaluation and Engagement Model Instrument (PREEMI) for neonates in intensive care units. *Journal of Obstetric Gynecologic and Neonatal Nursing, 44*, 114–126. https://doi.org/10.1111/1552-6909.12535

Scatliffe, N., Casavant, S., Vittner, D., & Cong, X. (2019). Oxytocin and early parent-infant interactions: A systematic review. *International Journal of Nursing Sciences, 6*, 445–453. https://doi.org/10.1016/j.ijnss.2019.09.009

Shattnawi, K. K., & Al-Ali, N. (2019). The effect of short duration skin to skin contact on premature infants' physiological and behavioral outcomes: A quasi-experimental study. *The Journal of Pediatric Nursing, 46*, e24–e28. https://doi.org/10.1016/j.pedn.2019.02.005

Smith, W. (2018). Concept analysis of family centered care of hospitalized pediatric patients. *Pediatric Nursing, 42*, 57–64. https://doi.org/10.1016/jpedn.2018.06.0147

Spittle, A., Doyle, L., & Boyd, R. (2008). A systematic review of clinimetric properties of neuromotor assessments for preterm infants during the first year of life. *Developmental Medicine and Child Neurology, 50*, 254–266. https://doi.org/10.1111/j.1469-8749.2008 .02025.x

Spittle, A., & Treyvaud, K. (2016). The role of early developmental intervention to influence neurobehavioral outcomes of children born preterm. *Seminars in Perinatology, 40*, 542–548. https://doi.org/10.1053/j.semperi.2016.09.006

Synnes, A., & Hicks, M. (2018). Neurodevelopmental outcomes of preterm children at school age and beyond. *Clinics Perinatology, 45*, 393–408. https://doi.org/10.1016/ j.clp.2018.05.002

Vittner, D., Butler, S., Smith, K., Makris, N., Brownell, E., Samra, H., & McGrath, J. (2019). Parent engagement correlates with parent and preterm infant oxytocin release during skin-to-skin contact. *Advances in Neonatal Care, 19*(1), 73–79. https://doi.org/10.1097/ ANC.0000000000000558

Whiteslaw, A., & Sleath, K. (1985). The myth of the marsupial mother. Homecare of very low birthweight babies in Bogota Columbia. *The Lancet, 1*(8439), 1206–1208. https://doi .org/10.1016/s0140-6736(85)92877-6

The Neonatal Intensive Care Unit Environment

LESLIE B. ALTIMIER AND RAYLENE M. PHILLIPS

OVERVIEW

Major advances in neonatal care have led to the increased survival of high-risk infants in recent decades, yet the long-term neurodevelopmental outcomes among such infants remain a concern. Infants born as early as 22 weeks' gestation now have a chance of survival, but this progress comes with great costs since these extremely premature infants must remain in the NICU for many weeks or months during a critical period of brain development and growth. Preterm birth is a leading cause of neurodevelopmental, neurocognitive, behavioral, language, motoric, neurosensory (visual or hearing), attentional, self-regulatory, social, and emotional impairments, all of which can significantly impact a child's social and academic functioning (Adams-Chapman et al., 2018; Ditzenberger et al., 2016; D. R. Moore et al., 2018; Neil & Inder, 2018; Symes, 2016).

More focus is now directed to preterm and low-birthweight infants who have mental health issues and long-term psychiatric diseases such as attention deficit and attention deficit hyperactivity disorders, anxiety disorders, and emotional disorders (Boardman & Counsell, 2020; Erdei et al., 2020; Fleiss & Gressens, 2019). Even moderate-to-late preterm infants are at risk of developing borderline intelligence functioning and attention problems at an early school age (Jin et al., 2020). Preterm infants born before 32 weeks' gestational age (GA) are at an increased risk to develop psychiatric disorders and are at higher risk for a wide range of sociocognitive and socioemotional impairments (Montagna & Nosarti, 2016; A. T. K. Spittle, 2016; Synnes & Hicks, 2018). Deficits in attention and executive functions, intelligence, poor growth, and physical problems later in life are frequently reported disabilities (Chiorean et al., 2020; Lundequist et al., 2015; Siahanidou & Spiliopoulou, 2020; A. J. Spittle et al., 2018; Tommiska et al., 2020; Twilhaar et al., 2018). Children born prematurely also have worse performance on achievement tests, lag behind in grade level, and receive more special education support compared to term-born peers (Dai et al., 2020; Grunewaldt et al., 2014; Jin et al., 2020; R. M. Joseph et al., 2016). Fortunately, some of these outcomes may be modifiable and responsive to programming and intervention (Church et al., 2020). Children born prematurely have been found to be at risk for autism spectrum disorder (ASD), which is defined by deficits in social communication and interaction as well as repetitive behaviors and restrictive interests and activities (Agrawal et al., 2018; Chen et al., 2020; Cogley et al., 2020; Xie et al., 2017). Visuospatial attention and processing at 1-year corrected age have been shown to be predictive for overall cognitive and motor development in preterm infants. A study using the nonverbal eye tracking–based test to assist in early detection of preterm children at risk of adverse neurodevelopment is the first of its kind to relate early visuospatial attention and processing with later neurodevelopmental outcomes in preterm children (Beunders et al., 2020). Earlier detection of preterm children at risk for adverse neurodevelopment will allow for more timely interventions and a decrease in adverse effects, not only for the child but also for the immediate and extended family, for health service and school education providers, and for society.

Although the cause of these findings remains unclear, it is thought that early environmental influences on the brain during "sensitive" or "critical" periods of development account for many of these adverse outcomes. Sensitive and/or critical periods in brain development are phases of enhanced susceptibility to experience. It is within such critical periods that highly active developmental processes are especially susceptible to positive and negative biological and environmental influences. This is particularly pertinent for preterm infants in the NICU. By necessity, these infants undergo a critical period of brain development while in the suboptimal ex-utero environment and are, therefore, vulnerable to brain injury and maldevelopment. Insults to brain development can include maternal/fetal infections or inflammation, intrauterine growth restriction, hypoxia–ischemia, and postnatal medical complications affecting multiple organ systems (Cheong et al., 2020).

In addition to medical conditions affecting physical and neurologic development and growth of preterm infants, the circumstances of early life in the NICU environment may have serious negative consequences on the emotional well-being and relationship quality of infants and parents (Givrad et al., 2020). These negative consequences have been ascribed to "toxic stress." Toxic stress is defined as profound or prolonged stress in the absence of the buffering protection of adult support. Parental absence and a lack of parental engagement and participation can lead to toxic stress (Bergman, 2019a; Shonkoff et al., 2012). Increasing parent engagement has the potential to enhance parent confidence, competence, and self-efficacy, which ultimately has potential to increase their ability to self-manage their child's care after discharge to optimize health and developmental outcomes for the child (Liyana Amin et al., 2018; Vance & Brandon, 2017; Wittkowski et al., 2017).

There is a paucity of research that has demonstrated the importance of environmental factors. It is critical to identify both positive and negative environmental influences, many of which are modifiable. The goal of improving long-term neurodevelopmental morbidity has led to an increased focus on improving neuroprotective, family-centered developmental care, not only in neonatal follow-up clinics but within the NICU itself to capture the period of earliest brain neuroplasticity. Neuroplasticity refers to the ability of the brain to make short-term or long-term modifications to the strength and number of its synaptic neuronal connections in response to incoming stimuli associated with activity and experience. Neuroplasticity is a lifelong property of the human brain, although it is most prominent from prenatal life until late childhood. It is thought that neuroplasticity peaks during early life because it is a period of rapid brain growth with the generation of excessive new synapses (synaptogenesis) and the activity-dependent and experience-dependent pruning of synapses. Therefore, identifying timely and effective strategies and interventions that can mitigate early adversity, increase resilience, improve outcomes, and support optimal development and mental health of both parents and infants is of significant importance.

The relationship between brain maturation, perinatal insult, and neurodevelopmental outcomes of the fragile infant is highly complex, multifactorial, and employs mechanisms and causal pathways that remain insufficiently understood. There are multiple mechanisms of insult which are recognized to disrupt or alter neonatal brain development, including preterm birth with its associated complications such as prenatal or postnatal brain injury, perinatal asphyxia, prenatal exposures to noxious substances, genetic conditions, bronchopulmonary dysplasia (BPD), infection and/or inflammation, and altered prenatal environment. Recent work has shed light on how the quality of the early postnatal neurosensory and social environment has a potentiating effect on newborn brain maturation and a long-lasting impact on child development (Bergman et al., 2019; Maitre et al., 2017). This is particularly pertinent for infants who spend weeks to months hospitalized in the NICU where they not only receive necessary medical care but also experience an atypical sensory (tactile, vestibular, olfactory, gustatory, auditory, visual) environment relative to healthy newborns (Altimier & White, 2020; Erdei et al., 2020). Long hospitalizations and inconsistent caregiving patterns in the NICU environment have been implicated in poor neurobehavioral and developmental outcomes (Pickler et al., 2020). Although much underlying brain damage can occur in utero or shortly after birth, neuroprotective interventions (NPIs) may stop progression of damage, particularly when these strategies are used during the most sensitive periods of neural plasticity 2 to 3 months before term age (Pickler et al., 2020).

NEUROPROTECTIVE CARE

Neuroprotection has been defined as strategies or interventions capable of preventing cell death. NPIs support the developing brain or facilitate the brain after a neuron injury in a way that allows it to heal through developing new connections and pathways for functionality and by decreasing neuronal death. Neuroprotective care (sometimes called neurosupportive care) is not only about protection from or prevention of harm but also a proactive and purposeful support for continuation of the normal fetal neurodevelopmental trajectory based on ecologically salient and expected sensory inputs that lead to physiological regulation and secure attachment, parallel processes that are based on the same limbic circuitry. As morbidity and mortality rates improve, we are challenged to enhance neuroprotective strategies for prematurely born infants that focus on the interpersonal experiences of the infant and their family while in the NICU (Bergman, 2015). Hospitalized infants of all ages, especially premature infants, have markedly improved outcomes when the stress of environmental overstimulation is reduced by incorporating neuroprotective strategies into the care of neonates as well as the design of a NICU (Altimier & Phillips, 2016).

Neuroprotective developmentally supportive care includes creating a healing environment that manages stress and pain while offering a calming and soothing approach to help involve the whole family in the infant's care and development (Altimier, 2015b; Altimier & Phillips, 2016; Altimier & White, 2020). Neuroprotective developmental care is grounded in research from a number of disciplines including nursing, medicine, neuroscience, and psychology (Altimier & Phillips, 2016; Browne et al., 2020; Cheong et al., 2020). Improvements in health outcomes and lengths of stay, as well as hospital costs and parental well-being, result when neuroprotective education and subsequent change of care practices were implemented (Altimier et al., 2005; Cong et al., 2017; Petteys & Adoumie, 2018; van Veenendaal et al., 2020).

The term "epigenetics" has evolved over time and today is generally accepted as any process that alters gene activity without changing the DNA sequence (Weinhold, 2006). Genes make proteins, and proteins make the brain and body tissues (Nelson & Panksepp, 1998). Some genes also make hormones, neurotransmitters, and their receptors, and these determine behaviors (Nestler, 2011). Each gene is responsive to many epigenes. The epigenes are sensitive to the environment, adaptation, and resultant neurobehavior in that environment. Some epigenes prevent or switch off gene expression, and even the proportion that is expressed can make different behaviors (Nestler, 2011). Other epigenes modify the expression of the gene in the way protein functions. Sensory experience and appraisal after behaviors give feedback to the brain, favoring neural connections (brain wiring) that are optimally suited to the environment, and unused connections are pruned away (Heck et al., 2008). The sum of all brain wiring is called the connectome (Turk et al., 2019). Genes, brains, and behavior are critical aspects of life (Nelson & Panksepp, 1998) and collectively form the genome, the connectome, and neurobehavior (Bergman, 2019b).

Incubator care is highly "abnormal" to the developing brain of an infant (Bergman, 2015). Skin-to-skin contact (SSC) provides the right environment (place) for the infant's epigenes, DNA, neural circuits, and physiologic regulation to function normally, making SSC the "optimal environment" for any newborn, especially premature infants (Bergman, 2019a).

Chi Luong et al. (2016) conducted a randomized controlled trial with low-birth-weight (LBW) infants (1,500–2,500 g) randomized at birth, 50 to routine care and 50 to skin-to-skin contact, with stabilization using the Stability of CardioRespiratory system in Preterms (SCRIP) score, measured repeatedly over the first 6 hours of life. Skin-to-skin contact was found to be an optimal environment for neonates without life-threatening conditions who weighed 1,500–2,500 g at birth. By preventing instability that requires subsequent medical treatment, it may also be a life-saving environment for neonates in low-income countries.

In fact, yet another randomized control trial was conducted in five countries by the World Health Organization (WHO) Immediate KMC Study Group. The group found that among infants with a birth weight between 1.0 and 1.799 kg, those who received immediate kangaroo mother care had lower mortality at 28 days than those who received conventional care with kangaroo mother care initiated after stabilization (Arya et al., 2021).

Creating the "optimal" or best sensory environment for preterm newborns is difficult given the conflicting data presented on the dangers of both overstimulation and sensory deprivation in this population. Just as the patent ductus serves an important purpose in utero but is a medical handicap after birth, incomplete attempts to mimic the sensory environment found in utero can be disadvantageous to neurodevelopment of the preterm infant ex utero (White, 2018). Circadian rhythm of the fetus, for example, is guided by multiple maternal zeitgebers, none of which is readily available to the newly born infant. Instead, new zeitgebers must be established, most notably lighting cycles (White, 2017). Accomplishing this is not as easy as turning a light on and off at the appropriate time of day. It is also not appropriate to simply leave the infant in a low-light environment continuously.

Sensory deprivation, as well as overstimulation of sound, touch, movement, taste, and smell, is also clearly undesirable. In addition to the challenge of getting the quantity of a particular stimulus right, the quality matters, and the target is continually moving, as the infant's medical condition, peripheral sensory apparatus, and brain maturity change almost daily (White, 2017). We may not even be aware of all of the sources of adverse stimuli; for example, there is evidence that preterm neonates are influenced by electromagnetic fields in their incubators (Bellieni et al., 2019). Not all sound is bad; stimulation provided by the auditory environment plays an important role in the auditory and emotional development of a baby. Because speech and other relevant sounds can be masked by noise, preterm infants may have difficulty making fine discriminations with respect to intonation of voice. Research performed so far confirms that the maternal voice makes an imprint, a memory trace in the immature cortical network during fetal life (Fellman, 2017; Filippa et al., 2019). However, enriching the NICU environment with more stimuli—for example, vocal recordings—is not always an improvement and there are risks to increased auditory exposure on preterm infants' sensory experiences (Filippa, 2019; Lejeune, Brand, et al., 2019). The goal is on individualizing care based on GA and creating an environment that seems most nurturing (White, 2017).

Additional studies on neuroprotective strategies indicate lighting should be circadian, without abrupt changes; noxious sounds should be minimized and replaced by parental conversation (Caskey et al., 2014) and probably music; and painful stimuli should be minimized but not to the point of continuous sedation (White, 2017). Effective NPIs are still missing and those that are known are inconsistently practiced. The Neonatal Integrative Developmental Care (IDC) Model highlights neuroprotective strategies and interventions to support the care of preterm and critically ill infants, along with their families in the NICU setting.

NEONATAL INTEGRATIVE DEVELOPMENTAL CARE MODEL

The Neonatal IDC Model (Philip's Healthcare, Cambridge, MA), which outlines seven core measures for neuroprotective family-centered developmental care of premature infants, is a framework that guides clinical practice in many NICUs around the globe. The seven neuroprotective core measures are: (1) the healing environment; (2) partnering with families; (3) positioning, handling, and caregiving; (4) safeguarding sleep; (5) minimizing stress and pain; (6) protecting skin; and (7) optimizing nutrition. They are depicted as overlapping petals of a lotus to illustrate

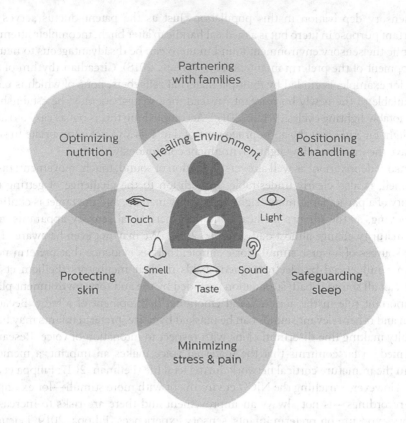

FIGURE 11.1 Neonatal Integrative Developmental Care (IDC) Model.
Source: Courtesy of Philips Healthcare, Cambridge, MA.

their distinct but overlapping contributions to neuroprotective family-centered developmental care (Altimier, 2015b; Altimier & Phillips, 2013, 2016; Altimier & White, 2020; see Figure 11.1).

The Neonatal IDC Model utilizes NPIs as strategies to support optimal synaptic neural connections; promote normal neurologic, physical, and emotional development; and help prevent disabilities (Altimier & Phillips, 2016). The mother–child dyad is the center of the lotus surrounded closely by symbols representing various aspects of the healing environment, highlighting the physical, extrauterine environment in which the infant now lives, the significance of the developing infant's sensory system, and the influence of people (patient, family, and staff) who help to create a healing environment for hospitalized infants and their families. Each of the seven neuroprotective core measures will be reviewed along with a thorough definition, standard/guideline/policy/procedure, idealized infant characteristics, identified goals to individualize for each infant to achieve, and evidence-based NPIs to incorporate into clinical practice (Altimier & Phillips, 2013, 2016; Altimier & White, 2020).

Numerous NICUs globally have utilized the Neonatal IDC Model for fully implementing neuroprotective family-centered developmental care into their unit design, practices, policies, and procedures (Bruton et al., 2018; Cardin et al., 2015; Lockridge, 2018; R. M. Phillips, 2015).

CORE MEASURE #1: HEALING ENVIRONMENT

The NICU is where an extraordinary period of growth and development will take place for premature infants. Because the infant is no longer protected in the uterus, their physiologic and neuroprotective needs have dramatically changed. The healing environment encompasses the physical environment, the people environment, and the sensory environment (Altimier, 2015b).

Given the disparate needs of infants, families, and caregivers—and even the differing needs of individual infants, each family, and individual caregivers—a strong case has been made for individualized NICU environments. To help meet this need, single-family rooms (SFRs) are a growing trend for NICUs around the world. Careful planning can avoid pitfalls in SFR design and workflow and bring benefit to babies, families, and caregivers alike (White, 2010).

Definition

The healing environment encompasses the physical environment of space, privacy, and safety; the people environment of the infant and family, as well as the healthcare staff; and the sensory environment which influences the infant's developing sensory system. The physical environment involves the space and characteristics, which affect maternal–infant attachment, parental engagement, and participation. The people environment highlights the infant and the family unit and equally all of the healthcare staff. The sensory system includes the tactile (touch), vestibular (movement, proprioception, and balance), gustatory (taste), olfactory (smell), auditory (noise), and visual (light) systems. (See Figure 11.2.)

There is considerable interaction between and within the physical, sensory, and social environments. They are differentiated for discussion purposes about opportunities for improvement in creating a holistic healing NICU environment. Adverse physical, sensory, or social environmental factors can significantly interfere with growth, health, and appropriate neurodevelopment and neuroprocessing, leading to lifelong alterations in function and well-being (Graven & Browne, 2008) while a carefully designed, healing environment provides support for optimal physical, mental, and emotional development (White, 2011).

Defining the optimal NICU sensory environment is elusive. Conflicting data exist regarding overstimulation and sensory deprivation in premature infants. Replicating the in-utero environment is not possible in the NICU environment nor most appropriate. Continuation of the in-utero sensory environment can be disadvantageous to neurodevelopment of the preterm infant ex utero (Altimier, 2015b).

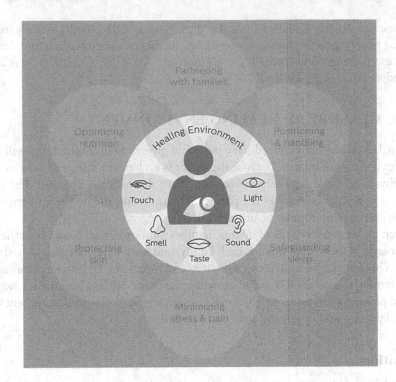

FIGURE 11.2 The healing environment.
Source: Courtesy of Philips Healthcare, Cambridge, MA.

Tactile (Touch)

Lower GA is associated with abnormal reactivity to deep pressure and vestibular stimulation. A potential explanation may relate to the altered sensory experiences inherent in the NICU hospitalization of preterm infants, such as procedural touch, supine immobilization, and unopposed gravitational forces during critical windows of neurologic development (Bock et al., 2005; Greenough et al., 1987). Firm rather than light touch is essential for premature infants. Light-touch stimulation elicits an abnormally defensive response in infants and is associated with poor adaptive motor function in infancy and worse motor and language scores (Wallace & Stein, 2007).

Vestibular/Proprioception (Balance & Motion)

Movement occurs in concert with tactile, vestibular, and proprioceptive input. The central and peripheral nervous systems must differentiate between vestibular signals imposed by the external world and those that result from spontaneous, self-directed actions. The critically ill and/or premature infant in the NICU receives vestibular input primarily through an external source (i.e., the parent or clinician) and is consequently vulnerable to sensory stimuli such as distress and excessive motor movements in an effort to stabilize and orient to a fixed surface during vestibular disturbances (Hunter et al., 2015).

Olfactory (Smell)

The olfactory system is functional by 28 weeks' gestation. Olfactory (smell) information is transmitted directly from the nose to the cerebral cortex. Maternal odor influences neonatal behavior. A mother's scent has been found to facilitate state regulation and optimal feeding experiences for both term and preterm infants. Since olfaction is functional in the second trimester, sensory stimuli from the NICU environment rather than the mother may interfere with its development, as well as other sensory development and attachment-bonding (Sarnat & Flores-Sarnat, 2019).

Absent or inefficient oral feeding performance is one of the major problems of premature newborns, sometimes requiring transient assistance with feeding tubes until oral performance improves (Bertoncelli et al., 2012; Lau & Smith, 2012). Improving newborns' oral feeding capacities is thus a key issue to better care and quicker hospital discharge. Many strategies have been tried and shown to be helpful, such as non-nutritive sucking, sensory–motor–oral stimulation, and/or the smell of milk applied to the nipple (Bertoncelli et al., 2012; Lau & Smith, 2012). However, in premature infants before 33 weeks GA, other strategies are needed since coordination of sucking–swallowing–breathing is not fully mature. Several studies suggest that early training accelerates maturation of oro-pharyngeal coordination mechanisms, including kinesthetic (massage), auditory, and possibly olfactory stimulation (Bertoncelli et al., 2012; Simpson et al., 2002), all of which seem to have an impact on energy expenditure in growing preterm infants (Lubetzky et al., 2010). Results from a randomized controlled investigation conducted by Cao Van et al. (2018) suggest that olfactory stimulation may promote a faster switch from feeding tube to satisfactory oral feeding in premature newborns. The odor-stimulated newborns (experimental group) in their study could be discharged on average more than 3.4 days earlier than the non-odor stimulated (control group) of newborns. Although their results were not statistically significant, their observed effect was a trend, and in light of the vulnerability of these newborns, and regarding the fact that in early phases of their life, 3 days may be crucial, the study emphasizes that olfaction may have its place in early feeding stimulation (Cao Van et al., 2018). In yet another study, premature infants born at less than 31 weeks GA exposed to olfactory stimulation with their mother's own milk learned to feed sooner than infants exposed to water (Davidson et al., 2019).

Gustatory (Taste)

In utero, fetuses begin swallowing amniotic fluid between 10 and 14 weeks' gestation (Delaney & Arvedson, 2008). Amniotic fluid provides gustatory stimulation (i.e., taste) and exposes the lymphoid tissue in the oropharynx to immune modulating and growth-stimulating factors that are important for the development of the immune system and gastrointestinal tract (Garofalo & Caplan, 2019). After birth, the mother's own milk provides similar gustatory stimulation, immune support, and growth-stimulating factors (Garofalo & Caplan, 2019). Infants who are fed by feeding tube directly into the stomach miss opportunities for oral exposure to gustatory and immune stimulation. The taste of a mother's milk has been shown to facilitate the infant's mouthing, sucking, arousal, and calming from irritability, especially in preparation for oral feeding (Davidson et al., 2019). Provision of oro-pharyngeal mother's own milk during gavage feeding may stimulate the gastroin-testinal tract to release digestive hormones and help infants associate the taste of milk with feelings of satiety to support later oral feeding. Placement of small amounts of the mother's own milk into the oral cavity of infants who are not yet able to feed by mouth has been found to improve breastfeeding rates (Snyder et al., 2017), improve growth (Seigel et al., 2013), reduce sepsis, and increase immune-protective factors. Giving infants a pacifier with the mother's milk has been shown to increase nonnutritive sucking (NNS), intake, and growth, and to shorten the length of hospitalization (Harding et al., 2018) and multisensory environment (Altimier, 2015b; Beker et al., 2019; Cao Van et al., 2018).

Much of brain development in the first 24 weeks of gestation is dependent on strong genetic factors, but brain development in the last trimester of fetal develop-ment (24–40 weeks GA) through 3 years of corrected age is greatly dependent on environmental factors (Altimier, 2015a; Pletikos et al., 2014; Vasung et al., 2019). The period of time in which infants are hospitalized in the NICU is a very vulner-able time for brain development. Strategies to protect infants from noxious stimuli and promote positive sensory experiences support neonatal brain development during this critical time and support an infant's ability to manage the complexity of future oral feeding. Providing multisensory experiences such as combining odor and taste can potentiate sensory organization during feeding. Providing supports for mothers and infants to be together early in the NICU stay is essential in sup-porting both the olfactory and gustatory sensory development. Holding the baby close to the caregiver's body, especially in skin-to-skin contact, serves to provide an organized multisensory environment (Altimier, 2015b; Beker et al., 2019; Cao Van et al., 2018).

Auditory (Sound/Noise)

The auditory function in prematurely born children tends to be unstable, especially at a very early age. In very preterm infants, it may either deteriorate or improve. Fetal auditory pathways to the central nervous system (CNS) appear to be complete by 24 weeks' gestation. The hearing threshold (the intensity at which one perceives sound) is approximately 40 dB at 27 to 29 weeks. Noise can cause abrupt physio-logic changes in behavioral state, blood pressure, heart rate, blood flow, respiratory effort, alternations in oxygen saturation, and increased oxygen consumption sec-ondary to elevated heart and respiratory rates and may, therefore, decrease the number of calories available for growth; in a vulnerable premature infant, all of this can have serious neurologic sequelae. Exposure to 10 to 15 dB sound peaks during active sleep resulted in a significantly increased mean heart rate and decreased mean respiratory rate and mean systemic and cerebral oxygen saturations relative to baseline (Kuhn et al., 2012). These changes also can affect sleep either by awak-ening infants or by changing sleep state, which causes infants to experience unnec-essary stress. Elevated levels of speech are needed to overcome the noisy environment in the NICU, thereby increasing the negative impacts on staff, newborns, and their families. High noise levels are associated with an increased rate of errors and accidents, leading to decreased performance among staff.

Habituation is the simplest form of nonassociative learning. It is defined as a behavioral decrement that results from repeated stimulation and does not involve sensory or motor fatigue (Aldrete-Cortez et al., 2021). This implies a physiological process of adaptation to the environment and is related to the speed at which a novel stimulus is no longer perceived as novel and therefore should no longer be eliciting distress. This phenomenon, called habituation, is characterized in the newborn by the capacity to diminish their behavioral responses when exposed to frequent and repeated stimuli (Aldrete-Cortez et al., 2021; Castillo et al., 2014; Weber et al., 2016). Castillo et al. (2014) identified that preterm infants had higher habituation response scores for sound stimuli than for light and tactile stimuli (Castillo et al., 2014). Habituation responses can account for the system that regulates behavioral states, since both habituation and behavioral states are resources required for newborns to avoid or approach stimuli in the environment (Brazelton & Nugent, 2014; Kiblawi et al., 2014). Habituation has also been used as a paradigm for the early, quick, and easy identification of cognitive injury.

Visual (Light)

The visual system is the last sense to develop functionally. Protecting the development of the visual system remains important because visual problems continue to be common among NICU graduates who were preterm births. Infants at or before 32 weeks' gestation have thin eyelids and little or no pupillary constriction. This allows little ability to limit light reaching the retina (LeVay et al., 1980). By 34 to 36 weeks' gestation, the pupillary constriction is more consistent and the eyelids are thicker, allowing some ability to limit light exposure to the retina. The pathways from the retina to the visual cortex that transmit visual images become functional at 39 to 40 weeks' gestation. All processes involved in the development of the structure and function of the human visual system have a critical period between 20 and 40 weeks' gestation during which epigenetic events, toxic exposures, and inappropriate exogenous stimulation can produce significant alterations in the structure and function of the infant's visual system. Proper visual system development requires appropriate endogenous stimuli generated by the spontaneous activity of neuronal cells and the preservation of active sleep, especially rapid eye movements (REMs; Graven, 2011).

All sensory stimuli carry social and emotional connections and characteristics. Adverse environmental sensory insults can significantly interfere with health, appropriate neurodevelopment, and neuroprocessing, resulting in lifelong alterations in brain development and function (Aldrete-Cortez et al., 2021; Dumont et al., 2017; Lejeune et al., 2016; Lejeune, Lordier, et al., 2019; Maitre et al., 2017). Since the NICU is a replacement for the intrauterine environment during the third trimester and early "fourth trimester" and a home away from home for many newly expanded families, it is important to prioritize creating and maintaining a healing environment for babies and their families (White, 2020a).

Standard

A policy/procedure/guideline on creating a healing environment, which includes the physical environment (space, privacy, and safety), the people environment (infant, family, and healthcare staff), and sensory environment, exists and is followed throughout the infant's NICU stay.

Infant Characteristics

Characteristics include stability of the infant's autonomic, sensory, motor, and state regulatory systems.

Goals

An environment will be maintained that promotes healing by minimizing the negative impacts of the artificial, extrauterine NICU environment on the developing infant's brain, behavior, and its impact on the entire family unit in support of bonding and attachments, and family well-being.

Neuroprotective Interventions

Physical Environment

■ Provide appropriate environmental modifications or construction/renovation of new NICU facilities.

● The latest recommended standards for NICU design should always be utilized. While many of these standards are minimums, the intent is to optimize design within the constraints of available resources and to facilitate excellent healthcare for the infant in a setting that supports the central role of the family and the needs of the staff (White, 2020b).

■ Provide a physical design that meets the neurodevelopmental needs of the infant and provides adequate private space and facilities to support a family-integrated care approach, while at the same time meeting the needs of the multidisciplinary staff that participate in that infant and family's care.

● Increasing family integration into the care has progressed from almost total exclusion during the early days of modern neonatal intensive care to full participation as members of the care team in many NICUs. These changes have been evidence based with steadily improving outcomes attributable not only to better treatments but also to better environments of care.

■ Provide a sufficient number of SFRs to meet the needs of parents who wish to stay with their babies.

● There is now good evidence that SFRs lead to improved outcomes, reduced costs, and improved parent and staff satisfaction. There is also evidence that parents are the "active ingredient" for this improvement, and that placing a baby in a private room when the family is rarely present may be detrimental.

These babies, as well as multiples, may be better cared for in multibed pods or rooms (van Veenendaal et al., 2020; White, 2020b).

People Environment

■ Provide opportunities for all staff, as well as parents, to participate in multidisciplinary rounds.

  ● Despite the interplay between all healthcare staff, it has been shown that the neonatologist has the most essential role in impeding or supporting parental participation in the communication and decision-making process that occurs during multidisciplinary rounds.

■ Promote bonding and attachment opportunities between parents and infants.

  ● More attention is needed on the parents' psychosocial needs. Supporting maternal mental health both improves maternal well-being and enables mothers to be emotionally available and responsive to their extremely preterm infant.

■ Respect family members that have an integral role to play in optimizing their baby's outcomes.

Sensory Environment

Tactile

■ Facilitate early, frequent, and prolonged SSC to provide positive tactile experiences through gentle, safe contact with parent's bare chest.

■ Provide gentle, yet firm touch in all positioning, handling, and caregiving interactions.

■ Maintain midline, flexion, containment, and comfort when positioning the infant.

■ Provide a neutral thermal environment (NTE) for the infant utilizing SSC or incubator humidity for very low-birthweight (VLBW) infants during the first 2 weeks after birth.

■ Incorporate noninvasive monitoring and testing whenever possible.

■ Minimize routine labs and procedures that provide noxious touch.

■ Encourage vocal interactions between parents and infant(s).

Vestibular

■ Facilitate early, frequent, and prolonged SSC to provide opportunities to experience the gentle movement of parent's breathing while positioned on parent's chest.

■ Change infant's position slowly and gradually with no sudden movements using two-person/four-handed support.

■ Provide supportive circumferential boundaries when moving or positioning infant.

■ Utilize facilitative tucking and containment principles during cares.

■ Provide balanced clustering of care.

■ Coordinate assessments, treatments, examinations, and care between multidisciplinary healthcare staff.

Olfactory

■ Facilitate early, frequent, and prolonged SSC to provide opportunities to smell mother's familiar scent.

■ Maintain a scent-free and fragrance-free unit; evaluate all cleaners utilized in the unit.

■ Provide mother's scent when possible via breast pad or soft cloth.

■ Open alcohol/chloraprep/mastisol pads away from the infant (outside incubator/ away from infant and mother).

■ Provide NNS with mother's own milk (when possible) during tube feedings.

Gustatory

■ Facilitate early, frequent, and prolonged SSC to provide proximity to the breast and opportunities for positive oral experiences of nuzzling at the mother's breast as a precursor to breastfeeding.

■ Position infant with hands near the face/mouth.

■ Provide colostrum or expressed breast milk (EBM) oral care per protocol.

■ Provide NNS opportunities, especially during tube feedings.

■ Provide positive oral feeding experiences, promoting nuzzling and breastfeeding when appropriate.

■ Minimize adhesives around the mouth, nose, and face.

Auditory

■ Facilitate early, frequent, and prolonged SSC promoting opportunities to hear mother's and father's voices.

■ Monitor noise levels in patient rooms.

● Infant rooms (including airborne infection isolation rooms) and adult sleep rooms, as well as the hallways or other areas in open communication with them, shall be designed to mitigate a combination of continuous background sound and operational sound of at least L50 of 45 dB A-weighted, slow response, and an L10 of 65 dB A-weighted, slow response, as measured 3 feet from any infant bed or other relevant listener position (White, 2020b).

■ Set alarms at minimal effective level, and silence alarms as quickly as possible.

■ Implement NICU-wide "Quiet Times."

■ Facilitate "approach behavior" through a calm, quiet voice prior to and during interactions while closely monitoring baby's behavioral cues.

■ Cover incubator (when appropriate) and protect the incubator/bed by eliminating items placed on top of the incubator.

■ Minimize or eliminate extraneous sounds.

■ Consider ceiling tiles with high noise reduction coefficients (NRCs).

■ Evaluate noisy equipment/carts/cabinets/doors in the unit and fix or eliminate when possible.

Visual

■ Facilitate early, frequent, and prolonged SSC to provide opportunities to visualize the parents' faces when baby is ready to do so.

■ Provide adjustable light levels at the infant's bedspace through a range of at least 10 to no more than 600 lux (approximately 1 to 60 foot-candles [ftc]).

■ Avoid purposeful visual stimulation prior to 38 weeks' GA.

■ Promote enface visual opportunities with parents.

■ Cover infant's eyes during assessments, examinations, procedures, and treatments with procedure lights.

■ Utilize eye patches when exposed to phototherapy lights or direct lighting.

■ Cover and protect the incubator/bed (when appropriate) to protect from excessive light.

■ Cycle lighting at 28 weeks (or sooner if stable).

CORE MEASURE #2: PARTNERING WITH FAMILIES

Family-centered care (FCC) feels safe and familiar to families when they find themselves in the unfamiliar hospital environment. The infant is first and foremost a family member and care is individualized to the family and infant (Hill et al., 2018). FCC is the foundation for caregiving; the family is visible, available, and supportive of their infant's needs because they are an integral aspect of every decision that affects their child even if not present at the bedside 24 hours a day, just like any other member of the health professional team (Craig et al., 2015; Miyagishima et al., 2017). Thus, their presence is noted in all aspects of care.

Parents are essential caregivers for their infants. While admission to the NICU may temporarily shift some of the caregiving responsibilities, it does not negate the importance of a parent's lifelong role in their child's overall health and development (French & Altimier, 2020; French & French, 2016; Niela-Vilén et al., 2017). Actively fostering family involvement is a fundamental component of collaborative caregiving that supports the full integration of neuroprotective, family-centered partnerships (Altimier & Holditch-Davis, 2020; Altimier & White, 2020; Boyle & Altimier, 2019; Bruton et al., 2018; Namprom et al., 2020; Phillips, 2020b).

There is strong evidence that NICU family-centered developmental care, which includes an effective partnership between professionals and families, results in improved neonatal and neurodevelopmental outcomes and promotes cerebral cortical development, decreased length of stay, increased family satisfaction, and even enhanced employee satisfaction once a culture change has been adopted (Als et al., 1994, 2004; Altimier & White, 2020; Bergman, 2019a, 2019b; Bergman et al., 2019; Bruton et al.,

2018; Darcy Mahoney et al., 2020; Dittman & Hughes, 2018; Franck et al., 2020; Klawetter et al., 2019; Lee & O'Brien, 2014; Pineda et al., 2018; Pisoni et al., 2021).

The care environment also plays a critical role in the emotional and cognitive development of infants. The most important aspect of the care environment is the quality of relationships infants develop with their primary caregivers and their experience in these relationships (Zeanah, 2019). The parent–infant relationship is the basis of infant mental health. These early relationships set an internal working model or template for the individual about who they are, what world they live in, and how they experience their relationships (Altimier & Boyle, 2021).

Because of the high rates of negative developmental consequences among prematurely born children, attention is shifting to modifiable aspects of the NICU environment, with a priority of enhancing parental partnerships in order to optimize developmental outcomes (R. J. Ludwig & Welch, 2019, 2020; Porges et al., 2019; Welch, Barone, et al., 2020). In spite of ample evidence of benefits to infants and families, implementing the known principles of family-centered developmental care into the NICU and creating the needed culture changes have often been fraught with internal and external challenges (Cardin et al., 2015; Malik et al., 2015; Mörelius et al., 2020; R. M. Phillips, 2015). True collaboration and shared decision-making with families in the care of their baby has not yet become a fully embraced standard of care. The overwhelming and often traumatic experience of being the parent of a critically ill infant can preclude such collaboration (Coughlin, 2021; D'Agata et al., 2018; Hall et al., 2016).

FCC begins wherever and whenever a family enters the healthcare system and continues throughout the hospitalization to discharge. Families should encounter this philosophy of care before birth in antenatal care, then continue it into the delivery room and beyond into the postpartum period. Families are not replaceable at any level in the overall development of the child. Within FCC implementation, their impact always supersedes that of the healthcare system (Whitehead et al., 2018).

Minimize the separation of parents and infant and provide expertise in bonding and attachment that can support parents directly or indirectly. Nonseparation of infant and parents also has ethical and legal support from the United Nations Convention on the Rights of the Child (UNCRC; UNICEF, 1989).

One way to encourage nonseparation of infant and parents is through the implementation of SFRs which encourage 24/7 family access. Couplet care is another emerging concept within the neonatal intensive care environment that provides facilities for parents to live in the neonatal intensive care nursery along with their infants throughout the entire hospitalization by coupling the care of the infant with the care of the newly delivered mother (Westrup, 2015; White, 2016, 2020b). This model has been practiced in several European countries (Sweden, the Netherlands, etc.) for over 20 years, and the first NICU in the United States to adopt this practice was Beacon Children's Hospital in South Bend, IN (USA) under the direction of Dr. Robert White. It includes postpartum care after a normal delivery and care of mothers with more advanced needs. After the immediate postpartum period, approximately half of all mothers with infants born prematurely have a prolonged need for medical care and would otherwise be separated from their infants during the very important first days of bonding and attachment (White, 2016, 2020b).

When introducing couplet care, appropriately adjust the design and structure of the nursery. The NICU design should include accommodations and considerations for the comfort and support of families. Parents must be viewed as partners in the care of their infant. Consideration should be given to attractive and clear signage in the primary languages spoken by the populations served by the hospital. Adequate and convenient storage of personal family belongings should be made available. Comfortable chairs should be present at every bedside to facilitate prolonged SSC. Providing parents computer and internet access, educational materials, and space to socialize supports the emotional and psychosocial needs. It is ideal to have spaces with equipment for parents to make meals, wash clothes, shower, and sleep in close proximity to their NICU baby (White, 2020b). Private spaces for therapeutic inter-actions with NICU mental health providers will facilitate psychosocial support for NICU parents who are at significantly increased risk for postpartum depression, anxiety disorders, and posttraumatic stress disorder (Altimier & White, 2020; Barton & White, 2016; Shepley et al., 2014; Vohr et al., 2017; White, 2020a, 2020b).

Premature and medically vulnerable infants who experience early and some-times prolonged separation from their parents, intrusive and unnatural environments, painful and distressing procedures, difficulties with physiological regulation, and increased biological and neurologic vulnerabilities often grow up to have higher rates of neurocognitive and psychosocial difficulties (Erdei et al., 2020; Givrad et al., 2020; R. M. Joseph et al., 2016). Parents of these infants born prematurely or with medical vulnerabilities, in turn, experience significant distress and are a psychiatrically vulnerable population, with very high rates of depression, anxiety, and post-traumatic stress disorder (Bonacquisti et al., 2020; Carson et al., 2015; Givrad et al., 2020; Greene et al., 2015; Hynan et al., 2015; Kim et al., 2015; Lean et al., 2018; Petersen & Quinlivan, 2020; Soghier et al., 2020). Depressive symptoms in parents of preterm and full-term infants at NICU discharge are high, with 45% of parents reporting depressive symptoms and 43% reporting elevated perceived stress. Older GA, greater parental stress, and lower levels of social support are strong correlates of depressive symptoms (Soghier et al., 2020). Maternal anxiety and depression negatively impact maternal–infant attachment (Bonacquisti et al., 2020).

NICU admission is stressful for both parents. Nurses often focus on maternal well-being and fail to acknowledge the stress of fathers. Fathers are increasingly recognized as playing a critical role in the family unit and the emotional development of their children (Provenzi & Santoro, 2015; Saliba et al., 2020; Shorey et al., 2016). Following birth of a preterm baby, persisting anxiety may affect the quality of life of fathers (Petersen & Quinlivan, 2020). Parental role alteration, infant appearance, NICU environment, and staff communication have been identified as stressors by fathers (Prouhet et al., 2018). By recognizing the extent and types of psychological stress in fathers, nurses can provide better support for fathers in their new role. Younger fathers and those with very low-birthweight premature infants may need additional support and resources (Busse et al., 2013; Carson et al., 2015; Hall et al., 2015; Petersen & Quinlivan, 2020; Prouhet et al., 2018). Strategies to support all parents, including depression screening, stress reduction strategies, and mental health referrals, are greatly needed (Hall et al., 2016).

Given the critical importance of early relationships with primary caregivers for infant mental health and long-term developmental outcomes, NPIs promoting healthy infant and parent mental health, bonding, and attachment should be targeted to facilitate an optimal infant–parent relationship in the NICU population (Ash & Williams, 2016; Browne, 2021; Chiorean et al., 2020; Del Fabbro & Cain, 2016; Erdei et al., 2020; Givrad et al., 2020; Gordon et al., 2021; Hynan et al., 2015; Tomlin et al., 2016). Supporting maternal mental health improves maternal well-being and, thus, enables mothers to be emotionally available and responsive to their extremely preterm or critically ill infant.

Early NPIs have long been considered crucial for reducing the severity of neuro-developmental disorders (Fontana et al., 2020; Pisoni et al., 2021) and improving infant and family outcomes after the NICU experience (Ågren, 2020; Asztalos et al., 2017; Bergman et al., 2019; DeMaster et al., 2019; Detmer et al., 2020; Fleiss & Gressens, 2019; Gaffari & Jindal, 2019; Painter et al., 2019; Petteys & Adoumie, 2018; Pineda et al., 2018; Pisoni et al., 2021; A. T. K. Spittle, 2016; Standley & Gutierrez, 2020). Many NICU interventions and programs exist with the aim to improve family-centered neurodevelopmental outcomes of premature infants. Developmental care programs such as the Newborn Developmental Care and Assessment Program (NIDCAP; Als, 2009; Als et al., 2012; Ohlsson & Jacobs, 2013) and the Wee Care Program® (Philips, Cambridge, MA; Altimier et al., 2005, 2015; Bruton et al., 2018; Cardin et al., 2015; R. M. Phillips, 2015) provide detailed education for staff on how to interact and promote intentional relationships with infants by individualizing the neuroprotective developmental care provided to each infant and family unit. The Family Integrated Care (FICare) and the Family Nurture Intervention (FNI) programs help achieve valuable family–professional partnerships and relationships in the NICU. The FICare program uses a strengths-based approach based on FCC principles to promote parental empowerment, learning, shared decision-making, and positive parent–infant caregiving experiences (Lee & O'Brien, 2014). FiCare outcomes include increased self-efficacy upon discharge and improved parent–infant relationships and infant developmental outcomes (Franck et al., 2020). FICare in the NICU has a sustained effect on child behavior and improving self-regulation at 18 to 21 months corrected age (Church et al., 2020).

The FNI is an intervention designed to overcome the maladaptive conditioning effects of maternal separation and the NICU environment on the premature infant. It is hypothesized to do so by facilitating an emotional connection and by establishing an adaptive classical homeostatic conditioning routine between mother and infant, referred to as the Calming Cycle (Welch & Ludwig, 2017a).

Skin-to-Skin Contact (Kangaroo Care)

SSC is called out separately to emphasize its critical importance to the health of infants and well-being of parents. Besides the intrauterine environment, the optimal environment for any newborn, particularly for the premature infant, is SSC with the mother (or father), which has also been called kangaroo care (KC). The defining feature is direct contact between maternal/paternal skin and infant skin.

SSC is much more than an intervention. Essentially, it is a "place of care" and is the normal, developmentally expected, and most optimal environment for all infants after birth, but preterm infants are the most dependent on SSC for physiologic stability and normal neurodevelopment (Bergman, 2015, 2019a, 2019b).

Continuous SSC is the developmental expectation of all newborns and where they are usually the most stable (R. Phillips, 2020b). Although continuous SSC is necessary for optimal normal development, even intermittent SSC provides well-documented short- and long-term benefits for babies and parents (Angelhoff et al., 2018; Bergman, 2015; Casper et al., 2018; Feldman et al., 2014; E. R. Moore et al., 2016). The need for SSC to support physiologic stability and neuroprotection is inversely proportional to GA. Babies born prematurely require the close proximity to their mother/parent that SSC provides to maintain maximum stability and continue normal gestational maturation (R. Phillips, 2020b). SSC increases survival and supports numerous vital quality measures of neonatal care, such as improved thermal control, cardiorespiratory stability, parent–infant bonding, attachment, and interaction, breastfeeding, growth, and longer-term development (Ågren, 2020; Boundy et al., 2016; Conde-Agudelo & Díaz-Rossello, 2016; Sahlén Helmer et al., 2020). Early and prolonged daily SSC promotes breastfeeding; is associated with a reduced risk of developing BPD and cholestasis; and leads to a lower incidence of hospital-acquired infections (HAIs; Casper et al., 2018; Oras et al., 2016). SSC is indisputably one of the most powerful measures to improve the care of newborn infants and is a fundamental component of neuroprotective and family-integrated care for hospitalized preterm and critically ill infants (Bergman et al., 2019).

There is overwhelming evidence for the benefits of SSC/KC in various settings and for at-risk infants, including premature and low-birthweight infants, infants with congenital heart disease (CHD), and infants with neonatal abstinence syndrome (NAS). In the past two decades, the number of infants born with NAS has quadrupled, causing a strain on NICUs. Although there are recommended pharmacological and nonpharmacological approaches for the management of NAS, recently, more emphasis has been placed on taking a holistic approach to NAS management (Kondili & Duryea, 2019). SSC/KC is effective in managing NAS symptoms and helps the mother–infant dyad bond and attach. In infants with NAS, SSC/KC was associated with improved autonomic nervous system (ANS) function, reduction in withdrawal symptoms, and increased length of quiet sleep (Arora, 2017).

SSC plays a role in establishing an infant's microbiome (R. Phillips & Smith, 2020). The infant microbiome describes the population of microorganisms that inhabit our body inside and out including our skin and gastrointestinal tract that colonizes the baby at birth. A mature human microbiome is a complex ecosystem essential to normal physiological, metabolic, and immune function for our health, and an abnormal microbiome can lead to disease (Kelsey et al., 2021). Infancy represents a sensitive period in gut microbiome formation as the gut microbiome changes from a relatively sterile environment to a diverse ecosystem with over 3×10^{13} species of microorganisms (Borre et al., 2014; Cryan & Dinan, 2012; Sender et al., 2016). Importantly, the gut microbiome is thought to impact psychological functioning and mental health through the microbiota–gut–brain axis (Borre et al., 2014).

Yet, little is known about how the gut microbiome impacts developing brain function and psychological health during this sensitive period of early human development (Cowan et al., 2020; Kelsey et al., 2019).

Kelsey and colleagues (2021) found that gut microbiota composition is linked to individual variability in brain network connectivity, which, in turn mediates individual differences in behavioral temperament among infants. Results demonstrated that gut microbiota taxa diversity was positively associated with functional connectivity in two resting-state brain networks in newborn infants and increased taxa diversity was linked to frontoparietal connectivity, a brain network previously associated with positive mental health outcomes in adults and positive behavioral traits in infants. Specifically, greater connectivity in the frontoparietal network has been linked to decreased incidence of internalizing disorder in adulthood and increased regulation and orienting behaviors in infancy (Kaiser et al., 2015). Their findings corroborated data from previous infant studies, showing a positive association between taxa diversity and parietal cortex structure and function, pointing to a consistent pattern of association between gut microbiome diversity and the developing brain (Carlson et al., 2018; W. Gao et al., 2019; Rosin et al., 2020).

Hendricks-Muñoz et al. (2015) explored the development of oral microbial colonization repertoires and health characteristics in preterm infants with or without SSC. Neisseria and Acinetobacter, important oral bacteria, were more prevalent in the SSC infants, demonstrating that SSC during the earlier postnatal period was associated with a distinct microbial pattern and an accelerated pace of oral microbial repertoire maturity. SSC was associated with shorter hospitalizations (Hendricks-Muñoz et al., 2015).

SSC decreases procedural pain in term and preterm infants (Johnston et al., 2017). EEG studies on KC in stable term infants have shown a different activity in the prefrontal regions of the brain, known to be responsible for attachment (Welch, Grieve, et al., 2020). Stable preterm infants cared for in SSC also have better temperature control (Ågren, 2020) and significant improvements in both cerebral blood flow and cardiovascular performance when preterm infants were placed skin to skin with their mother/father (Sehgal et al., 2020). These findings complement previous conclusions of the beneficial effects on heart rate variability (HRV) and oxygenation. They show a better physiologic regulation and sleep–wake cyclicity in the neonatal period (Bastani et al., 2017), a sleep pattern more similar to infants born at term (Dereymaeker et al., 2017), better neurodevelopment at 6 months, and behavioral organization throughout childhood (El-Farrash et al., 2020).

Cortisol is a glucocorticoid that has properties that are beneficial when released in response to short-term stress but become detrimental when the body is exposed to elevated levels over a prolonged period of time. Prolonged elevation of cortisol levels results in increased levels of glutamate, which contributes to overstimulation of neurons, neuronal cell death (Mooney-Leber & Brummelte, 2017, 2020; Mooney-Leber et al., 2018), and ultimately poor brain growth and structural changes to the brain (Fumagalli et al., 2018). Additional consequences of prolonged cortisol levels contribute to lipolysis in the extremities (i.e., poor somatic growth), inhibition of bone formation (i.e., increased risk of metabolic bone disease), increased gastric acid secretion, and suppression of the immune system through atrophy of lymphoid tissue and reduction in T lymphocyte and natural killer cell activity (McCance & Huether, 2019). These changes in response to prolonged stress likely contribute to some of the long-term neurodevelopmental abnormalities in infants who survive being critically ill (Bergman, 2019a, 2019b; Casavant et al., 2019; Cong et al., 2017; D'Agata et al., 2019; Fumagalli et al., 2018; Montirosso & Provenzi, 2015; Nist et al., 2020). Stress, as measured by cortisol levels, decreases in response to SSC in the stable preterm infant (Angelhoff et al., 2018). Since prolonged stress is harmful to neurodevelopment, the decreased stress found with infants in SSC supports this important NPI provided by parents in the NICU.

Research with moderately preterm infants has demonstrated the safety of SSC during the first hours of life, with more normal blood glucose levels and body temperature (Kristoffersen et al., 2016; Linnér et al., 2020). Positive maternal outcomes of SSC include higher rates of exclusive breastfeeding (Lefmann, 2020; E. R. Moore et al., 2016), better maternal mental health (Dongre et al., 2020; Mehler et al., 2020; Scime et al., 2019), enhanced mother–infant bonding, and strengthened maternal–infant interactions (Casper et al., 2018; Hucklenbruch-Rother et al., 2020; Mehler et al., 2020).

Social relationships throughout the life span are critical for health and well-being. It has been suggested that oxytocin, often called the "hormone of attachment," plays an important role in early-life nurturing and resulting social bonding (Angelhoff et al., 2018; Bergman et al., 2019; Cong et al., 2015; Filippa et al., 2019; Norholt, 2020; Scatliffe et al., 2019; Vittner et al., 2018, 2019; Welch & Ludwig, 2017a). The complexities of oxytocinergic mechanisms are rooted in neurobiological, genetic, and social factors. A positive correlation between parent–infant contact and oxytocin levels in the infancy period has been demonstrated, with increased maternal oxytocin levels significantly relating to more affectionate contact behaviors in mothers following mother–infant contact, synchrony, and engagement (Bigelow et al., 2018; Vittner et al., 2019), while increased paternal oxytocin levels were found to be significantly related to more stimulatory contact behaviors in fathers following father–infant contact (Cong et al., 2015; Dongre et al., 2020; Olsson et al., 2017; Prouhet et al., 2018; Provenzi & Santoro, 2015; Shorey et al., 2016).

Oxytocin levels have been found to significantly increase in infants, mothers, and fathers during SSC, and parents with higher oxytocin levels exhibit more synchrony and responsiveness in their infant interactions (Filippa et al., 2019; Welch & Ludwig, 2017a). The release of oxytocin during SSC also makes the mother and infant relax, fall asleep, and feel safe, all of which are necessary for quality sleep (Bergman et al., 2019; Cong et al., 2015; Norholt, 2020; Vittner et al., 2018, 2019).

Mother–infant SSC is a bonding and attachment promoting NPI. Current evidence supports the original bonding and attachment research that early maternal touch influences infant socioemotional development and attachment quality, with positive implications for mother–child relationship functioning (Norholt, 2020). Parent–infant bonding and attachment quality has also gained prominence as a trauma-resilience factor and a predictor of adult physical health.

Early bonding with both physical and psychological components leads to secure attachment, which includes parental relationships and parenting behaviors, as well as the unfolding ability of the infant, child, and adult to form and maintain meaningful and enduring relationships (Norholt, 2020). Studies of extended mother–infant physical contact have demonstrated positive effects in multiple domains. For infants, these include sleep organization, temperature and heart rate regulation, behavioral response, crying/colic, socioemotional development, attachment quality, speech development opportunities, and mother–child interactions (Ågren, 2020; Bergman, 2019b; Carvalho et al., 2019; Conde-Agudelo & Díaz-Rossello, 2016; El-Farrash et al., 2020; Evereklian & Posmontier, 2017; Feldman et al., 2014; Hucklenbruch-Rother et al., 2020; Johnston et al., 2017; Kostandy & Ludington-Hoe, 2019; Kristoffersen et al., 2016; Mehler et al., 2020; Oras et al., 2016; R. M. Phillips, 2013; Sehgal et al., 2020). For mothers, studies demonstrate improved depressive symptomatology, physiological stress regulation, contingent responsivity, breastfeeding, and mother–child interactions (Angelhoff et al., 2018; Bergman, 2019a; Bergman et al., 2019; Bonacquisti et al., 2020; Browne et al., 2020; Buil et al., 2020; Montirosso et al., 2014; Oras et al., 2016; Petersen & Quinlivan, 2020; Scime et al., 2019; Welch & Ludwig, 2017b).

Based on five decades of evidence, these SSC/KC recommendations and areas of research were identified for future implementation (Bergman, 2014; Kostandy & Ludington-Hoe, 2019):

■ Separating infants from their mothers and families is harmful and toxic to the infant development and well-being. Separation needs to be eliminated or at least minimized. Mothers need to be with their infants at least for the first 6 weeks of life and especially during the sensitive period immediately after birth.

■ Infants need to be held in SSC/KC as early and as long as possible as it is their "natural habitat" and their expected environment. Being in SSC/KC is therapeutic for all neonates (minimal exceptions).

■ Strategies and policies to support mothers and families to be in the hospital during the infants' hospital stay should be developed and implemented.

Education and support should be provided to all healthcare professionals to increase the implementation and compliance of SSC/KC for all infants. One comprehensive simulation-based KC education program improved nurses' perception of SSC/KC value, their competency and comfort in infant transfer for SSC/KC, and successfully promoted SSC/KC parent utilization for the preterm infant in the NICU (Hendricks-Munoz & Mayers, 2014).

Partnering With Families

Establishing family–professional partnerships in the NICU environment can be challenging; yet, because families are the constant in the infant's life, helping families achieve a positive outcome from their NICU experience should be a priority while providing care (Altimier, 2015b; Altimier & Phillips, 2020; Altimier & White, 2020). The Parent Risk Evaluation and Engagement Model and Instrument is an assessment tool that has been successful in initiating strategies designed to increase empowerment for parents who are propelled into a sudden and stressful position of learning how to care for a premature infant. Using this instrument to help increase communication and clinician understanding has the potential to break down parental barriers of uncertainties and allow them to find comfort in the chaotic environment of the NICU (Makris et al., 2019).

Effective communication among healthcare team members is a mainstay of patient safety, especially in a NICU, given small errors can have serious and life-threatening consequences. Ineffective communication with families of hospitalized children can lead to decreased satisfaction and trust in the healthcare team. To improve communication, education of the nursing staff and other team members, as well as the development of a rounding script, enhances the roles they play in multidisciplinary patient rounds (Dittman & Hughes, 2018). Family presence and participation in bedside rounds is a key component of a family-centered partnership and knowledge exchange between healthcare providers and families. Participation on medical rounds helps parents be less worried and anxious (Grzyb et al., 2014). Despite the interplay between all healthcare staff, the neonatologist has the most essential role in impeding or supporting parental participation in the communication and decision-making process that occurs during multidisciplinary rounds (Axelin et al., 2018).

An international survey conducted in high-income countries investigated if there was a link between the availability of NICU family rooms and neonatal outcomes. Of 331 units studied, 13.3% (44/331) provided infant–parent rooms, and of the infants studied, 28% of them were cared for in units with infant–parent rooms. The availability versus absence of infant–parent rooms was associated with lower odds of composite outcome of mortality or major morbidity, including lower odds of sepsis and BPD, than those from units without infant–parent rooms. The adjusted mean length of stay was 3.4 days shorter in the units with infant–parent rooms (Axelin et al., 2010). These results demonstrate that parental presence positively contributes to the health and well-being of their infants and supports parents.

The NICU staff's well-being is equally important. NICU staff often suffer from caregiving fatigue and secondary posttraumatic stress. Prioritizing equipment and workspace in the NICU design that optimizes staff workflows will support NICU staff in providing the best care with the greatest efficiency. NICU design that includes spaces for rest and relaxation in a pleasant environment during work breaks will give NICU staff tangible evidence of the value placed on their well-being (Hogan et al., 2018; Huerkamp et al., 2018; Kuhn et al., 2018; Lehtonen et al., 2020; Mann, 2016; Meredith et al., 2017; White, 2020a, 2020b).

Compassion Rounds are spiritual care interventions that focus solely on emotional and spiritual well-being, rather than physical diagnoses. The correlation between spiritual wellness and clinical outcomes is also widely established in the literature. Compassion Rounds have positive effects on spiritual wellness for NICU parents and their healthcare providers, while also allowing chaplains to model and provide spiritual care for physicians. Compassion Rounds have a restorative effect on caregivers and have the potential to prevent or overcome burnout, return meaning to the work of clinicians, and create trust within multidisciplinary care teams (McManus & Robinson, 2020).

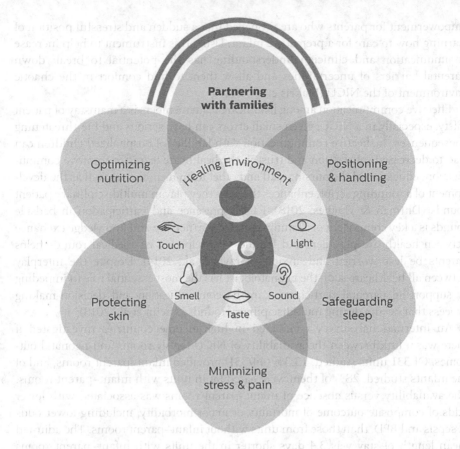

FIGURE 11.3 Partnering with families.
Source: Courtesy of Philips Healthcare, Cambridge, MA.

Focusing on the health and well-being of families and staff does not detract from focusing on infant care. FCC improves infant outcomes, family well-being, and staff satisfaction. Advances in medical technology cannot compensate for lack of parent–infant contact and interaction, especially in the critical weeks after birth. With this knowledge, efforts must be made to expand and improve family partnerships and increase active parent involvement with their NICU infant (see Figure 11.3).

The social and practical constructs that will enable parents to practice zero separation are a nonnegotiable condition for neurosupportive care (Bergman, 2014, 2019a, 2019b; Csaszar-Nagy & Bókkon, 2018). Zero separation from parents will ensure neurodevelopment is supported to normal standards (as in optimal development assumed for term infants), not merely protected from the effects of toxic stress (Bergman, 2019a, 2019b; Shonkoff et al., 2012). Reciprocal tactile stimulation between mother and infant may contribute to increased maternal responsiveness and infant attachment (Álvarez-Álvarez et al., 2019; André et al., 2020; Dumont et al., 2017; Gaffari & Jindal, 2019; Lejeune et al., 2020; Molina et al., 2015; Norholt, 2020). When the quality and/or quantity of parental care toward infants is limited, these adverse experiences can lead to changes in brain architecture and function (Keunen et al., 2017; Maitre et al., 2017; Matas et al., 2016; McAdams & Traudt, 2018; Montirosso & Provenzi, 2017; Mooney-Leber & Brummelte, 2020; Mörelius, Örtenstrand, et al., 2016; Pisoni et al., 2021; Tataranno & Benders, 2019).

Promoting a healing social environment requires a NICU design that prioritizes the need to support all members of the multidisciplinary team involved in caring for preterm and sick infants in the NICU including medical, nursing, and therapy staff, as well as parents. Equilateral respect and support among all members involved in this partnership will promote optimal patient care, enhance family satisfaction, and engage the healthcare team (Altimier & White, 2020).

Definition

The concept of partnering with families in the NICU includes a philosophy of care, which acknowledges that over time the family has the greatest influence over an infant's health and well-being. Compassionately delivered FCC, with zero separation, where SSC is the norm is currently seen as the ideal model of care to encourage parental involvement, attachment, and bonding, as well as create partnerships with the healthcare team (Altimier, 2015a, 2015b; Altimier & White, 2020; Bergman, 2019a; Bergman et al., 2019).

Standard 1

A policy/procedure/guideline on partnering with families exists and is followed throughout the infant's stay.

Standard 2

There is a specific mission statement addressing partnering with families.

Infant Characteristics

Characteristics include the infant's response to parental relationships and interactions.

Goals

■ Parents will be viewed not as "visitors" but as vital members of the caregiving team with zero separation encouraged (24-hr/d access).
■ Parents will be supported as the primary and most important caregivers for their infant.
■ Infants will develop secure attachment with parents.

Neuroprotective Interventions

■ Facilitate early, frequent, and prolonged SSC to promote emotional connections that support parent–infant bonding and attachment.

■ Encourage zero separation of infants from their mothers/fathers.

■ Promote active participation via medical rounds, shift-to-shift report, parent conferences, and phone updates.

■ Acknowledge where the family is in regard to stages of grief and loss and provide individualized and appropriate resources as needed.

■ Actively observe and listen to families' feelings and concerns (both verbal and nonverbal).

■ Communicate the infant's medical and developmental needs in a culturally appropriate and understandable way.

■ Encourage and support breastfeeding and breast milk expression.

■ Assist parents in becoming competent in caring for their baby.

■ Encourage parents as they develop confidence in their own abilities to continue providing SSC for their baby after going home.

■ Educate parents on infant attachment, development, and safety issues.

■ Provide parents with information about language development and strategies to promote communication with their babies.

■ Provide social networking opportunities for parents of premature infants in the NICU.

CORE MEASURE #3: POSITIONING, HANDLING, AND CAREGIVING

Developmentally appropriate neuroprotective care must include developmentally supportive positioning, handling, and caregiving activities. In utero, the infant is contained in a circumferential enclosed space with 360° of well-defined boundaries. Conversely, the spontaneous resting posture of a third-trimester NICU infant often is flat, extended, asymmetrical with the head to one side (usually the right), and with the extremities abducted and externally rotated (Danner-Bowman & Cardin, 2015; de Bijl-Marcus et al., 2017; Hunter et al., 2015; Romantsik et al., 2017; Santos et al., 2017). Over time, neuronal connections can be reinforced that favor this flattened, externally rotated, and asymmetrical resting posture as baseline for these infants.

Improper positioning may cause muscle contractures that interfere with the infant's neurologic and psychomotor development. Positioning is one of the important aspects of developmental care to keep the baby flexed, aligned, contained, and comfortable; to decrease days on ventilation; to shorten hospital stay; to promote self-regulation and sleep; and to reduce pain responses (Charafeddine et al., 2018; Eskandari et al., 2020; Pölkki et al., 2018; Santos et al., 2017; Wiley et al., 2020). (See Figure 11.4.)

Common musculoskeletal consequences of inadequate NICU positioning include abnormal spinal curvatures; excessive abduction and external rotation in the hips (called a "frog leg" posture); "W" arm positioning in which the shoulders

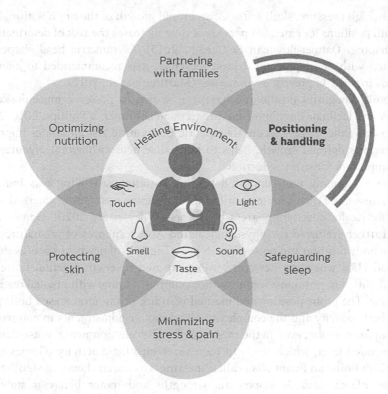

FIGURE 11.4 Positioning, handling, and caregiving.
Source: Courtesy of Philips Healthcare, Cambridge, MA.

are elevated, abducted, and externally rotated; and skull deformities (Hunter et al., 2015). These body misalignments can lead to motor delays and functional limitations that may follow an infant from the NICU into childhood and subsequently extend across the life span. Parents are essential care partners who should be encouraged to participate in their infant's positioning. Preterm infants whose parents were involved in their positioning have improved motor development at term-equivalent age compared to preterm infants whose positioning had been done only by healthcare professionals (Fjørtoft et al., 2017; Øberg et al., 2019, 2020). Parents need to be supported in positioning their infant through education and training. Direct face-to-face and video training has been shown to improve parents' handling activities better than written or pictorial instructions (Byrne & Garber, 2013).

Inappropriate positioning support in the NICU can affect the infant's early muscle and bone formation. Prolonged medical positioning and necessary medical intervention can lead to deformational infant head shapes and tightness of neck musculature. The pliability of a newborn's head is the antecedent of changes in head shape, particularly in premature infants whose cranial bones are even softer and thinner than those of term infants (Danner-Bowman & Cardin, 2015; Hunter et al., 2015). In premature infants, the head is the body part that takes the greatest amount of pressure whether in supine, prone, or side-lying positions. In addition to relatively high pressure, skull softness, and rapid growth of the brain within, lying in certain positions for extended periods of time increases the risk of deformational head shaping (Danner-Bowman & Cardin, 2015). Asymmetric head shapes are associated with developmental delays; therefore, it is recommended to alternate positions in order to prevent asymmetries (Martiniuk et al., 2017).

Careful, thoughtful positioning has been shown to preserve musculoskeletal integrity and facilitate developmental progression (Altimier & Phillips, 2016, 2020; Altimier & White, 2020). Secure therapeutic positioning also promotes improved rest, supports optimal growth, helps to normalize neurobehavioral organization, and is important for stress reduction.

Prone positioning was supported by three studies, side-lying was found to reduce stress more than supine positioning, and supine positioning emerged as the least effective for controlling stress behaviors (Wiley et al., 2020). Gomes et al. (2019) further evaluated the physiological and ANS responses of premature newborns to body position and noise in the NICU. The ANS of newborns was evaluated based on HRV when the newborns were exposed to environmental noise and placed in different positions: supine without support, supine with manual restraint, and prone. The prone position and manual restraint position increased both parasympathetic activity and the complexity of autonomic adjustments in comparison to the supine position, even in the presence of higher environmental noise than the recommended level, which tends to increase sympathetic activity (Gomes et al., 2019). Containing an infant (also called "nesting") has been shown to significantly enhance infants' neurodevelopmental strengths and motor behavior stabilities (Eskandari et al., 2020).

Positioning infants in the NICU is a neuromotor developmental intervention used to minimize positional deformities and to improve muscle tone, postural alignment, movement patterns, and ultimately developmental milestones (Hunter et al., 2015). Developmentally supportive positioning positively influences physiologic function and stability, sensory development, neurobehavioral organization, skin integrity, thermoregulation, bone density, sleep facilitation, optimal growth, brain development, and neonatal developmental outcomes (Aldana Acosta et al., 2019; Altimier & Phillips, 2016, 2018; Chen et al., 2020; Danner-Bowman & Cardin, 2015; Eskandari et al., 2020; Francisco et al., 2020; Hunter et al., 2015; Santos et al., 2017).

The core measure "Positioning and Handling" incorporates the Infant Positioning Assessment Tool (IPAT; Philips, 2018), which was developed with three goals for use as:

1. A reference and educational tool for teaching
2. An evaluation instrument
3. A method of standardizing best positioning practices of premature infants in the NICU

The IPAT is a validated and reliable easy-to-use pictorial tool used to evaluate posture of premature infants in six areas of the body (head, neck, shoulders, hands, hips/pelvis, and knees/ankles/feet), with cumulative scores ranging from 0 to 12. (See Exhibit 11.1.)

Infant Positioning Assessment Tool (IPAT)

Patient's name: _____   Birth gestational age/corrected gestational age: _____

Clinician's name: _____   Date/time of assessment: _____

Infant position: ☐ Supine   ☐ Side-lying   ☐ Prone

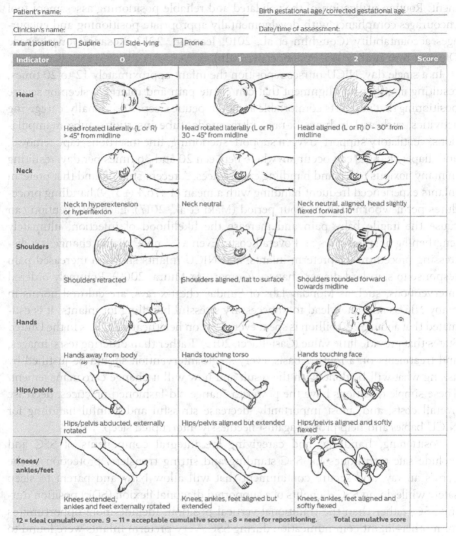

Indicator	0	1	2	Score
Head	Head rotated laterally (L or R) > 45° from midline	Head rotated laterally (L or R) 30 – 45° from midline	Head aligned (L or R) 0 – 30° from midline	
Neck	Neck in hyperextension or hyperflexion	Neck neutral	Neck neutral, aligned, head slightly flexed forward 10°	
Shoulders	Shoulders retracted	Shoulders aligned, flat to surface	Shoulders rounded forward towards midline	
Hands	Hands away from body	Hands touching torso	Hands touching face	
Hips/pelvis	Hips/pelvis abducted, externally rotated	Hips/pelvis aligned but extended	Hips/pelvis aligned and softly flexed	
Knees/ankles/feet	Knees extended, ankles and feet externally rotated	Knees, ankles, feet aligned but extended	Knees, ankles, feet aligned and softly flexed	

12 = Ideal cumulative score. 9 – 11 = acceptable cumulative score. ≤8 = need for repositioning.   Total cumulative score ____

EXHIBIT 11.1 Infant Positioning Assessment Tool.
Source: Courtesy of Philips Healthcare, Cambridge, MA.

A two-point scoring system is used on each area of the body with a score of 2 for ideal therapeutic positioning, 1 for acceptable positioning, and 0 for unacceptable positioning. Any asymmetrical positioning of the arms or legs is scored a 1 (a full score of 2 is never granted for asymmetrical positioning). According to the IPAT, a full score of 12 is indicative of ideal positioning, scores of 9 to 11 are acceptable as it accommodates for asymmetry of positioning often needed when technology interfaces are present (i.e., infants with various venous or arterial access needs, drains, surgical sites), and scores of 8 or lower indicate a need for positioning support that offers containment, promotes flexion, and ensures proper body alignment. Routine utilization of the validated and reliable positioning assessment tool encourages compliance with developmentally appropriate positioning and encourages accountability (Coughlin et al., 2010; Jeanson, 2013; Rosana Gonçalves de Oliveira Toso et al., 2015; Spilker et al., 2016).

In a single day, NICU nurses reposition the infant approximately 12 to 20 times, resulting in either misalignment that can create pain and interrupt sleep or secure positioning that supports comfortable and therapeutic sleep. Additionally, caregiving activities, such as lab draws, x-rays, ultrasounds, tube insertions, tube manipulations, ventilatory support, oxygen support, suctioning, line insertions, tape removal, and diaper changes can occur anywhere between 20 and 36 times per day, resulting in many noxious touch and handling experiences. A recent study found that preterm infants experienced frequent handling with a mean of 176.4 ($\pm$37.9) handling procedures per newborn each 24-hour period (Maki et al., 2017). Each intervention can cause the fragile baby pain and increase the likelihood of infection, ultimately lengthening hospital stays and overall costs. Even a "simple" diaper change is a distressing procedure for preterm infants, and NICU infants show an increased pain response to standard diaper changes (Comaru & Miura, 2009). Routinely ordered interventions, such as Monday labs or Sunday chest-x-rays, are cultural norms in many NICUs and often lead to unnecessary stressful handling for infants. It is estimated that about $200 billion is spent every year on healthcare services in the United States that provide little value (Castellucci, 2019). Rather than ordering tests, images, and treatments on a routine basis, every single intervention should be justified by asking what will be done with the result and how will it change care management. These simple questions have the power to change old-fashioned practices, decrease overall costs, and, most importantly, decrease stressful and painful handling for NICU babies and help protect against needlessly interrupted sleep.

Positioning, handling, and caregiving are integral components of SSC and include safe techniques for SSC standing and sitting transfers, protection of the baby's airway, and secure containment that will allow baby and parent to sleep safely while doing SSC. Benefits of a supported diagonal flexion (SDF) position during SSC, rather than the traditional vertical position, include more opportunities for mother–infant communication during SSC. Very preterm infants were found to vocalize three times more and mothers vocalized, gazed at their baby's face, and smiled more in the SDF than in the vertical control group. The SDF position in SSC, thus, fosters a greater multimodal temporal proximity and supports a more qualitative mother–infant communication (Buil et al., 2016, 2020).

Definition

NICU positioning has traditionally been a neuromotor developmental intervention to minimize positional deformities and improve muscle tone, postural alignment, movement patterns, and ultimately developmental milestones. Each body position that is experienced while in the NICU affects alignment and shaping of the musculoskeletal system. Therapeutic positioning as a fundamental NPI can influence not only neuromotor and musculoskeletal development but also physiologic function and stability, skin integrity, thermal regulation, bone density, head shaping, sleep facilitation, and brain development. Adapting positioning to the preterm infant's GA as well as their individual and developmental needs is essential.

Handling and caregiving in the NICU should include gentle, slow movements of the baby when handled and an overarching goal to justify each caregiving activity and every test and procedure being ordered to ask why it is needed and what might be changed with each result (Castellucci, 2019; Godarzi et al., 2018; Murthy et al., 2020; Orsi et al., 2017).

Standard

A policy/procedure/guideline on positioning, handling, and caregiving exists and is followed throughout the infant's stay.

Infant Characteristics

■ Autonomic stability during positioning, handling, and caregiving activities

■ Ability to maintain tone and flexed postures with and without supports

Goals

■ Autonomic stability will be maintained throughout positioning changes, handling, and caregiving activities, as well as during periods of rest and sleep.

■ Preventable positional deformities will be eliminated or minimized by maintaining infants in a midline, flexed, contained, and comfortable position throughout their NICU stay.

■ The caregiver sees their role as in partnership with the baby so that caregiving procedures are performed "with" the infant rather than "to" the infant.

■ Infants will be provided age-appropriate, developmentally supportive stimulation/play only as they mature (i.e., mobiles, swings).

Neuroprotective Interventions

■ Facilitate early, frequent, and prolonged SSC with appropriate handling during standing and sitting transfers and adequate positioning support throughout the duration of SSC.

■ Utilize a validated and reliable positioning assessment tool (i.e., IPAT) routinely to ensure appropriate positioning and encourage accountability.

■ Anticipate, prioritize, and support the infant's individualized needs during each caregiving interaction to minimize stressors known to interfere with normal development.

■ Maintain a midline, flexed, contained, and comfortable position at all times utilizing appropriate positioning aids and boundaries.

■ Provide appropriate ventral support when positioning prone to ensure flexed shoulders/hips.

■ Provide appropriate gel-filled positioning supports to protect fragile skin and support musculoskeletal development.

■ Assess the infant sleep–wake cycle to evaluate appropriate timing of positioning, handling, and caregiving.

■ Reposition the infant with care and minimally every 4 hours.

■ Gently change the extremely preterm infant's diaper by turning baby side to side.

■ Implement minimal handling protocols when warranted.

■ Provide two-person/four-handed support during positioning and caring activities.

■ Provide swaddled bathing and weighing.

■ Promote hand to mouth/face contact.

■ Educate parents about the principles of positioning, containment, and handling, as well as how to recognize their baby's behavioral signs of stress or relaxation in response to positioning, containment, and handling. Encourage parents to provide positive touch whenever appropriate to help balance the overabundance of negative touch and handling in the NICU.

CORE MEASURE #4: SAFEGUARDING SLEEP

Sleep is the main behavioral state of a preterm infant and is a crucial human physiologic need playing a significant role in the maturation of the CNS, memory consolidation, learning, energy maintenance, thermoregulation, promotion of protein synthesis, and the production of certain hormones, such as growth, thyroid stimulation, melatonin, prolactin, renin, and cortisol (Bennet et al., 2018; Calciolari & Montirosso, 2011; Fraiwan & Alkhodari, 2020). Newborns spend most of their time in the sleep state and their brain grows and functions following an endogenous activity. This has been found to be of high importance to brain maturity and neuronal survival at an early stage of life (Ansari et al., 2018; Dereymaeker et al., 2017). In addition, the pattern of sleep provides an indication about any brain growth risks that could lead to developing behavioral, psychomotor, and cognitive disorders (Dereymaeker et al., 2017; Fraiwan & Alkhodari, 2020). Therefore, qualitative assessment of neonatal sleep patterns, through daily monitoring tools, provides the necessary support to clinicians in the NICU for optimal feeding and neonatal care periods (Dereymaeker et al., 2017).

Sleep organization begins during fetal life, at which time it is influenced by multiple maternal zeitgebers. A zeitgeber (German: literally "time-givers") is any external or environmental cue that entrains or synchronizes an organism's biological rhythms to the earth's 24-hour light/dark cycle. Circadian rhythm of the fetus, for example, is guided by multiple maternal zeitgebers, none of which is readily available to the newborn. Instead, new zeitgebers must be established, most notably lighting cycles and breast milk (White, 2018). Preterm infants are further deprived of these maternal factors, so they develop a sleep structure based on the environment of the NICU, typically sleep less, and have seriously disrupted and fragmented patterns of sleep (Bonan et al., 2015; Fink et al., 2018; Godarzi et al., 2018; Graven & Browne, 2008; Levy et al., 2017; Maki et al., 2017; Modesto et al., 2016; Mony et al., 2018; Orsi et al., 2017; Pugliesi et al., 2018; Ryan et al., 2020; Saré et al., 2016; Tarullo et al., 2011; Venkataraman et al., 2018; White, 2015; Zores et al., 2018).

Fetal circadian rhythms can be observed in utero from 30 weeks' gestation and are coupled to the maternal rhythm. The fetus receives multiple circadian cues from the mother, including transplacental hormones (e.g., melatonin and cortisol) as well as her body temperature and activity, and after birth, circadian cues come from the external environment (McKenna & Reiss, 2018; White, 2015, 2017; Whitehead et al., 2018). Important external cues for circadian synchronization include the light/dark cycle, the timing of feeding, and exposure to melatonin in breast milk. Disruption to these cues occurs during admission to the NICU and can impair the development of circadian rhythms and influence survival and function in the neonatal period with a potential to impact health and well-being throughout adult life.

Dismissing the importance of the circadian system because it is immature in premature infants makes no more sense than disregarding the immune system or the brain because they too are immature. Circadian biology is far more complex than simply the effects of light on the pineal gland; nearly all tissues have biological clocks, at least some of which develop in utero under maternal influence and then continue to develop ex utero with whatever circadian stimuli we provide (Bartman et al., 2020; Guyer et al., 2015; D. Joseph et al., 2015; Lan et al., 2019; Morag & Ohlsson, 2016; White, 2020c; Zores-Koenig et al., 2020). Even ex utero, the mother has a potential role through her breast milk (Bueno & Menna-Barreto, 2016; Italianer et al., 2020; White, 2017) and likely through other signals (i.e., body temperature and activity) transmitted during SSC.

Melatonin is a natural sleep-inducing hormone secreted by the pineal gland, and its rhythmic secretion is induced by the light/dark cycle and inhibited by artificial light (Colella et al., 2016). Melatonin has antioxidant, anti-inflammatory, and anti-excitotoxic effects in neonates and plays a neuroprotective role in perinatal brain injury, preventing brain insults associated with prematurity or birth asphyxia (Biran et al., 2014, 2019; Bruni et al., 2015). The fetus is exposed to a circadian rhythm of melatonin from the mother; after delivery, this same circadian rhythm is delivered via the breast milk (Italianer et al., 2020; White, 2017). Most preterm infants, however, receive little melatonin and rarely get it in a circadian pattern unless breast milk is fed at a similar time of day as when it was expressed. The preterm infant, then, exists in a chronic state of melatonin deficiency (White, 2015).

Chronopharmacology, the study of how the response to and toxicity of drugs may be affected by the body's circadian rhythm, may have relevance to other drugs used in newborns, especially those that affect hormones that exhibit a circadian rhythm in the mother and fetus, such as steroids (White, 2015). In addition, high doses of sedative and depressing drugs can depress the endogenous firing of cells, thus interfering with visual development, REM (active sleep), and nonrapid eye movement (NREM; quiet sleep) sleep cycles and decreasing REM time. In the developing brain, sedatives such as barbiturates and benzodiazepines can cause neuronal and oligodendroglia apoptosis, impair synaptogenesis, inhibit neurogenesis, and trigger long-term neurocognitive sequelae, reducing the ability for learning and memory (Grigg-Damberger, 2016; Noguchi et al., 2020).

Sleep disturbance at the onset of life, besides causing newborns discomfort, can also result in future changes related to cognition, attention, increased risk of asthmatic diseases, obesity, anxiety, depression, and behavioral and social impairments/disorders (Aldrete-Cortez et al., 2021; Bennet et al., 2018; Bonan et al., 2015; Fink et al., 2018; Graven & Browne, 2008; Krause et al., 2017; Levy et al., 2017; Maki et al., 2017; Orsi et al., 2017; Pugliesi et al., 2018; Saré et al., 2016). The disruption of sleep can also negatively affect growth, development, and clinical status; delay hospital discharge; and trigger behavioral disorders in adulthood (Rioualen et al., 2017; Wachman & Lahav, 2011). According to the American Academy of Sleep Medicine (AASM), about 10% of U.S. newborns require intensive care at the NICU, which is a noisy environment that leaves an impact on neonate sleep patterns (AASM, 2018). Neonates with unorganized sleep have a higher risk of sudden infant death syndrome (SIDS) and sleep apnea and suffer from poor emotional and cognitive development by the age of 5 years (Levy et al., 2017).

Sleep is essential for brain development and synaptic plasticity during early life (Bennet et al., 2018; Callaghan & Fifer, 2019; Dang-Vu et al., 2006; Fraiwan & Alkhodari, 2020; Park, 2020; Pisch et al., 2019; Wolfe & Ralls, 2019). Brain plasticity refers to the ability of the brain to change its structure and function according to environmental changes and needs, thereby affecting an infant's ability to interact with the environment and accomplish necessary developmental milestones (Dang-Vu et al., 2006). Quiet sleep is associated with neural activities that potentially induce synaptic plasticity (Dang-Vu et al., 2006). The quality of sleep in early life predicts developmental outcomes in several areas, including physical, cognitive, motor, neurologic, and psychosocial (Franco et al., 2019; Shellhaas et al., 2019; Smithson et al., 2018; Winkler et al., 2017).

Quiet sleep, active sleep, and indeterminate sleep are well-defined sleep states that can be identified as early as 25 weeks of GA (Altimier & Holditch-Davis, 2020). Because infants spend most of their time sleeping in the neonatal period, extrinsic sensory stimulation is very limited. High levels of endogenous neural activation are required for the development of appropriate neural connections in the growing brain. Active sleep plays an important role in providing endogenous stimulation to the sensory processing areas in the brain, which positively affect early neural development. Active sleep is equivalent to REM and is characterized by the presence of REM, sporadic motor movements, irregular respiration, and a continuous EEG pattern. Quiet sleep is equivalent to NREM sleep and is characterized by the absence of REM, no motor movements, respiration with regular patterns, and a discontinuous EEG pattern. Quiet sleep is characterized by the increased secretion of essential hormones, such as melatonin, growth hormones, dehydroepiandrosterone, and sex hormones. During quiet sleep the information acquired during waking is further processed and consolidated, contributing to learning and memory consolidation. Protein production increases and protein breakdown decreases during quiet sleep, which improves regeneration and healing of body functions. Indeterminate sleep is a state in which the characteristics of sleep cannot be clearly classified as active or quiet sleep. The period of the indeterminate sleep that occurs at the beginning of sleep and between quiet sleep and active sleep is called transitional sleep or sleep–wake transition (Altimier & Holditch-Davis, 2020; Bennet et al., 2018; Dang-Vu et al., 2006; Fink et al., 2018; Graven, 2006; Pugliesi et al., 2018; White, 2015; Whitehead et al., 2018).

Each sleep state is responsible for different developmental tasks. Recent findings have demonstrated that REM sleep selectively prunes newly formed dendritic spines and strengthens new synapses in the developing brain. This process is critical for normal neuronal circuit development and behavioral improvement after learning. Developmental neuroplasticity refers to the continuous change of the developing brain during fetal development. Lack of plasticity may result in reduced intellectual ability, reduced learning and memory consolidation, and mental illness (Wolfe & Ralls, 2019).

A lack of active (REM) sleep is associated with reduced size of the cerebral cortex and brainstem (Calciolari & Montirosso, 2011), and it also delays the development of the neural connection in the visual system (Graven, 2011). Long-term behavioral changes result from deprivation of active sleep in early life, including anxiety, hyperactivity, attention and learning difficulties, increased alcohol consumption, and reduced sexual activity (Krause et al., 2017; Saré et al., 2016).

The presence of distinct sleep states is a marker of brain maturation and is essential for the homeostasis of infants. During the early stages of brain development, active sleep takes up a large proportion of sleep time and is the major sleep state up to 40 weeks of GA. Afterward, the proportion of active sleep gradually decreases in favor of quiet sleep, which then becomes the predominant sleep state. Each sleep cycle includes one complete active sleep and quiet sleep, in which infants tend to fall asleep in active sleep, followed by a short period of indeterminate sleep, and then they move into quiet sleep. If an infant experiences frequent disruptions, quiet sleep cannot be achieved.

Although sleep cycle length can vary depending on individual and environmental factors, the mean duration of a sleep cycle is 40 minutes at 27 to 30 weeks of GA, 45 minutes at 31 to 34 weeks of GA, and 50 to 70 minutes at 35 to 41 weeks of GA (Rioualen et al., 2017). Preterm infants demonstrate a significant amount of variation in sleep patterns depending on a multitude of infant and environmental factors, including birthweight, GA, sex, illness severity, light, noise, caregiving, and feeding methods (Altimier & Holditch-Davis, 2020; Altimier & White, 2020; Orsi et al., 2017; Thomas, 2000). Infants with younger GA or those with medical complications, such as intraventricular hemorrhage, demonstrate more active sleep, less alertness, and a narrower range of states than infants without these conditions (Del Rio-Bermudez & Blumberg, 2018; dos Santos et al., 2014). Boys show less active sleep, more drowsiness, and more waking state than girls (Geva et al., 2016).

Sleep and wake states are clusters of behaviors that represent the level of arousal of the infant, which affects the infant's ability to respond to external stimulations. Therefore, an infant's responsiveness to nursing interventions and to parental interactions heavily relies on the infant's state when the stimulation begins. Careful assessment of sleep and wake states enables nurses to understand an infant's physiologic needs and adjust the timing of their care in response to the infant's present state in a way that maximizes their responsiveness to nursing interventions and minimizes sleep disruption. The goal of caregivers in the NICU environment should focus on the development of interventions that promote preterm infants' sleep periods while mitigating the negative influences of sleep disruption on their health and development. Because sleep and wake states are closely related to an infant's neurologic function, sleep and wake state patterns can be used to identify infants at risk for neurologic complications or poor developmental outcomes and who may benefit more from NPIs (Park, 2020). Several sleep- and wake-state scoring systems exist; however, direct behavioral observation has shown a high degree of agreement with other objective measures, such as EEG and actigraphy scoring (Altimier & Holditch-Davis, 2020); therefore, direct behavioral observation can enable nurses to reliably score sleep and wake states (Park, 2020).

Preterm infants are frequently exposed to painful procedures in the NICU that disturb their sleep cycle and affect their growth and neurodevelopment. Supportive care bundles (modulation of the infants' states, NNS, facilitated tucking, and oral sucrose feeding) significantly increase preterm infants' sleep efficiency and total sleep time and also significantly decrease duration of sleep latency and frequency of wake bouts (Lan et al., 2018, 2019). Since peak sound levels during sleep can compromise the development of hospitalized infants, quiet time is recommended. Quiet time during a dedicated time each day is a strategy implemented in neonatal units to promote the sleeping of neonates by reducing noise levels, luminosity, and handling during particular periods of the day (Pugliesi et al., 2018; Zauche et al., 2021).

Researchers classify light as the environmental factor that most influences the establishment of circadian rhythm synchronization of the infant (E. Brooks & Canal, 2013; Guyer et al., 2015; D. Joseph et al., 2015; Lan et al., 2019; Morag & Ohlsson, 2016; White, 2020c). Short-term effects on infants have been observed with minor changes in light levels (Zores et al., 2018), and a Cochrane review on cycled lighting demonstrated improved outcomes for infants in a cycled lighting environment compared with either continuous dim or continuous bright light (Morag & Ohlsson, 2016). However, there are conflicting data in the literature regarding the presence of a circadian rhythm in preterm infants. Some researchers showed that the fetus is already sensitive to light by the 24th gestational week and that the exposure to low-intensity light can help regulate the circadian rhythm (Guyer et al., 2015; D. Joseph et al., 2015; Lan et al., 2019; Morag & Ohlsson, 2016; White, 2011).

Autonomic indices demonstrate the presence of anxious arousal while infants are alone in a crib, with greatly prolonged time to sleep onset. In cribs, quiet sleep is greatly reduced by more than 85% and sleep cycles are eliminated. Infants who received SSC showed better organization of sleep and wake states, namely, less time in active sleep and indeterminate sleep, with an increase in quiet sleep percentage, increased alertness, decreased crying, and increased sleep–wake cycle. During SSC, preterm infants using frontal EEGs demonstrate regular patterns of sleep and normal cycling, compared to infants separated from their parents. Maternal scent stimulates the infant's olfactory system, promoting sleep cycling, which further emphasizes the necessity of SSC. Studies have found that excessive handling and sleep deprivation in preterm infants may impair neuromotor development, induce hyperexcitability, trigger or exacerbate psychiatric diseases, and cause excessive daytime sleepiness (Bennet et al., 2018; Calciolari & Montirosso, 2011). (See Figure 11.5.)

The premature infant has challenges in safeguarding sleep because of the NICU environment, care procedures, and interventions required to support life. Continuous bright lights in the NICU can disrupt sleep–wake states. Any event,

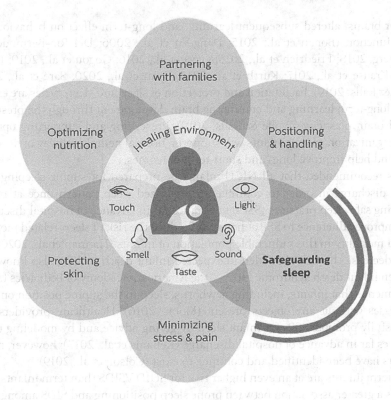

FIGURE 11.5 Safeguarding sleep.
Source: Courtesy of Philips Healthcare, Cambridge, MA.

process, or drug that disrupts REM sleep will disrupt the organization of the eye cells, structures, and connections. Patients of any age who are trying to sleep find direct light unpleasant. Premature infants are photophobic; however, they will open their eyes with dim lights. If the light levels never change, infants never experience the diurnal rhythm necessary for development. Reducing light levels may facilitate rest and subsequent energy conservation, as well as promote organization and growth (Altimier, 2015b; Altimier & White, 2020; White, 2015). Most clinical interventions, tasks, and procedures are scheduled at the convenience of staff. To be most neuroprotective and developmentally appropriate, they should be performed at the most optimal time for the baby, which is in a manner that does not disrupt their age-appropriate sleep–wake cycle.

Definition

Sleep is one of the primary activities of the brain during early development and plays an important role in healthy cognitive and psychosocial development in early life. REM and NREM sleep cycling are essential for early neurosensory development, learning and memory, and preservation of brain plasticity for the life of the individual (Graven, 2006; Graven & Browne, 2008; Jiang, 2020). Sleep deprivation (both REM and NREM) results in a loss of brain plasticity, which is manifested by smaller brains, altered subsequent learning, and long-term effect on behavior and brain function (Bonan et al., 2015; Dang-Vu et al., 2006; Del Rio-Bermudez & Blumberg, 2018; Friedrich et al., 2020; Geva et al., 2016; Gogou et al., 2019; Jiang, 2020; Krause et al., 2017; Kurth et al., 2015; Ryan et al., 2020; Saré et al., 2016; Wolfe & Ralls, 2019). Facilitation and protection of sleep and sleep cycles are essential to long-term learning and continuing brain development through the preservation of brain plasticity (Wolfe & Ralls, 2019). Preserving and supporting optimal sleep organization among infants will support a normal neural pathway of development and help improve long- and short-term outcomes.

It is recommended that all NICU infants be prepared for supine sleeping well before discharge in order to continue an organized sleep pattern once at home. Modeling safe sleep practices (SSPs) to families far in advance of hospital discharge may improve adherence to SSP at home and reduce the risk of sleep-related morbidity and mortality in this vulnerable population of infants (Hannan et al., 2020).

To decrease the risk of sudden unexpected infant death (SUID), also known as "sudden infant death syndrome (SIDS)," the American Academy of Pediatrics (AAP) recommends that infants, including newborns, sleep in the supine position on firm mattresses without any objects present (Moon, 2016). Healthcare providers can successfully promote SSPs for infant sleep by giving advice and by modeling these practices far in advance of hospital discharge (Kellams et al., 2017); however, many barriers have been identified and continue to exist (Colson et al., 2019).

Preterm infants are at an even higher risk for SUIDS/SIDS than term infants, and there is a greater association between prone sleep positioning and SIDS among low-birthweight infants, yet SSPs are rarely integrated into the routine clinical care of these infants in the NICU (Hwang et al., 2015). Many NICU staff do not consistently model recommended SSPs, which contributes to the lack of adherence to SSP by parents and others who care for infants at home (Bergman et al., 2019; Kellams et al., 2017; Naugler & DiCarlo, 2018).

The AAP Task Force on SIDS recommends that preterm infants be placed in supine sleep position by 32 weeks' postmenstrual age if they are clinically stable (Moon, 2011). Despite these recommendations, preterm infants are less likely than term infants to be placed supine in the hospital, as well as after discharge to home (Kellams et al., 2017). However, mothers of late preterm infants admitted to a NICU were more likely to initiate breastfeeding (which independently protects against SIDS) and practice supine sleep position than mothers of late preterm infants not admitted to a NICU (Hannan et al., 2020; Thompson et al., 2017).

Although 24 years have passed since the AAP's first recommended nonprone sleeping and nurses are aware of the AAP safe sleep recommendations, many hospital staff still believe this practice is not feasible or credible for themselves or for infant caregivers because of concerns about choking, the infant's respiratory status, and infant comfort (Geyer et al., 2016; Kellams et al., 2017; Kuhlmann et al., 2016; Naugler & DiCarlo, 2018; Rholdon, 2017; Rholdon & Dailey, 2016). If healthcare professionals are concerned about or disagree with aspects of the safe sleep recommendations, or if they do not know how to explain the recommendations to families, change is unlikely to occur. When hospital staff model SSPs and integrated SSPs into routine clinical care, parents are more likely to do the same at home

(Colson et al., 2019; Hwang et al., 2018; Kuhlmann et al., 2016; Raines et al., 2016). Supervised wakeful prone promotes motor milestones; however, many infants do not receive adequate prone with poor tolerance as a contributing factor. Increasing positional support helps to facilitate tolerance for the prone position for infants of all sizes (Guidetti et al., 2017).

Standard

A policy/procedure/guideline on safeguarding sleep in the NICU and back-to-sleep practices exist and are followed throughout the infant's stay as medically appropriate and role modeled prior to discharge.

Infant Characteristics

■ Infant demonstrates sleep–wake states, cycles, and transitions
■ Infant's maturity and readiness for back-to-sleep protocol

Goals

■ Infant sleep–wake states will be assessed before initiating all caregiving activities.
■ Prolonged periods of uninterrupted sleep will be protected.
■ Infants will be transitioned to the back-to-sleep protocol when developmentally appropriate, or according to the NICU guidelines. Parents will be included in timing and implementation of SSPs.

Neuroprotective Interventions

■ Facilitate early, frequent, and prolonged SSC to support restful sleep with improved sleep cycles and increased quiet sleep.
■ Utilize a valid and reliable sleep-state scale or direct observation methods.
■ Provide nonpharmacologic age-appropriate developmentally supportive care practices.
  ● Approach the infant using a soft voice followed by gentle firm touch.
  ● Facilitate gentle touch and touch via early and prolonged SSC.
  ● Promote noise control in a quiet environment to ensure uninterrupted sleep.
  ● When possible, utilize SFRs to encourage family presence to enhance sleep.
  ● In multibay/pod NICUs, when the census is lower, provide more space between infant beds to encourage decreased disturbances, increased sleep, and more privacy between parents and their infant(s).
  ● Provide soothing auditory stimuli, such as maternal voice, heartbeat, and music, when appropriate.

■ Protect sleep and sleep cycles, especially REM sleep

● Promote early and prolonged SSC.

● Protect the infant's eyes from direct light exposure and maintain low levels of ambient light (utilize incubator covers) for light control.

● Provide some daily exposure to light, preferably including shorter wavelengths, for entrainment of the circadian rhythm.

● Educate parents on how to read their infant's behavioral cues related to sleep–wake states and how to promote sleep cycling.

● Cluster or group care and individualize caregiving activities around sleep–wake states to keep the longest periods free of manipulations and enabling infant sleep.

● Provide NICU-wide "Quiet-Time."

■ Provide developmentally supportive therapeutic positioning.

■ Avoid high doses of sedative and depressing drugs which can depress the endogenous firing of cells, thus interfering with visual development, as well as REM and NREM sleep cycles.

■ Assure the infant is able to maintain a normal sleep pattern in a supine position (back-to-sleep) well before discharge and role model this behavior.

● Provide tummy time/prone-to-play time routinely for infants who are medically and developmentally ready for sleeping in the back-to-sleep position.

● Educate NICU staff and parents about the importance and rationale for SSPs and the need for supervised tummy time (inform parents to communicate this importance to other family members and anyone who will be caring for the infant at home; Altimier & Phillips, 2016).

CORE MEASURE #5: MINIMIZING STRESS AND PAIN

The development of the brain depends on an individual's nature (genes) and nurture (environments). This interaction between genetic predispositions and environmental events during brain development drives the maturation of functional brain circuits such as sensory, motor, emotional, and complex cognitive pathways. Pain has many dimensions and is processed at multiple different levels of the nervous system (Fitzgerald, 2005, 2015). When tissue is injured, nociceptive pathways in the peripheral and CNS trigger essential behaviors, mediated by reflex motor circuits in the spinal cord and brainstem, to ensure that the body is protected from further harm (Verriotis et al., 2016).

Noxious information is not processed in the brain in the same way as other sensory modalities. There is no dedicated primary "pain" cortex analogous to the primary somatosensory or visual cortices; rather, noxious stimulation evokes a diffuse pattern of activity in many brain areas; therefore, it is not known when and how the brain develops the ability to encode noxious stimuli and create the experience of pain (Verriotis et al., 2016). Nociceptive systems become functional at 24 to 28 weeks' gestation with the development of thalamocortical connections: however, brainstem-mediated endogenous pain modulation only develops closer to term-equivalent age (Fitzgerald, 2005; Verriotis et al., 2016). Exposure to pain at earlier GAs may have differential effects on the developing brain. How and when this complex brain network develops to encode noxious stimuli and create the experience of pain has clear clinical implications for devising analgesic strategies in hospitalized newborn infants, tailored and individualized to the developmental stage of the individual.

Early-life exposure to abnormal sensory stimulation is a major determinant for future pain susceptibility. Neonates admitted to NICUs typically receive 10 to 14 painful procedures and considerable handling each day, often without adequate preemptive analgesic (Roofthooft et al., 2014). Negative sensory interventions in the neonatal period can lead to alterations in behavioral and neurophysiological measures of pain processing (Brummelte et al., 2012; Grunau et al., 2009). For example, the analgesic requirement for surgery is higher in infants who have undergone previous surgical procedures during the neonatal period (Peters et al., 2005).

In adults, physiological stress causes hyperalgesia and increased background stress increases pain, but these data have not been extrapolated to infants (Jennings et al., 2014; Jones et al., 2017; Reinhardt et al., 2013). One infant study simultaneously measured nociceptive behavior, brain activity, and levels of physiological stress in a sample of newborn human infants. Salivary cortisol (hypothalamic pituitary axis), HRV (sympathetic adrenal medullary system), EEG event-related potentials (nociceptive cortical activity), and facial expression (behavior) were acquired in individual infants following a clinically required heel lance. Infants with higher levels of stress exhibited larger amplitude cortical nociceptive responses, but this was not reflected in their behavior. Furthermore, while nociceptive behavior and cortical activity are normally correlated, this relationship was disrupted in infants with high levels of physiological stress. This study demonstrated that brain activity evoked by noxious stimulation is enhanced by stress, but this cannot be deduced from observation of pain behavior. These results may be important in the prevention of adverse effects of early repetitive pain on brain development (Jones et al., 2017).

Infants born preterm are confronted with stressful sensory experiences such as exposure to pain, light, and sound. In particular, infants in the NICU are exposed to essential life saving but often painful and stressful interventions ranging from heel lancing for blood tests and oral interventions including nasogastric tube and endotracheal tube insertions, to long-term ventilation and major surgery. Factors relevant to neurodevelopment here include the effects of pain experienced by the infant, the medical condition giving rise to the painful experience or intervention, and anesthetic or analgesic treatments (Cheong et al., 2020). Because adverse environmental conditions such as early-life stress and painful events can interfere with the functional development of emotional and cognitive brain systems, an increased risk of developing psychiatric disorders later in life has been identified (Matas et al., 2016).

Preterm infants experienced a high degree of pain/stressors in the NICU, both in numbers of daily acute events and cumulative times of chronic/stressful exposure. Both acute and chronic pain/stress experienced during early life significantly contribute to impaired neurobehavioral outcomes (Cong et al., 2017). Greater numbers of painful and stressful procedures in very preterm infants (GA ≤29 weeks) are related to altered brain development and cortisol (stress hormone) regulation which affects neurodevelopment and behavior in this vulnerable population (Grunau, 2020; Valeri et al., 2015).

Neonatal pain and/or stress is also predictive of white matter maturity (Vinall et al., 2014), cortical thickness (Ranger et al., 2013; Valeri et al., 2015), regional cerebellar volumes (Ranger et al., 2015), lower IQ in toddlers born very preterm (GA ≤32 weeks; Dai et al., 2020; Valeri et al., 2015), and neuronal activity at school age, and, in turn, cognitive function, behavior, and motor development at 1 year of age (Grunau, 2020; Valeri et al., 2015). Experiencing a higher number of painful procedures has been associated with alterations in brain development across the preterm to term-equivalent periods. Early exposure (but not later exposure to pain) is associated with reduced white matter maturation at term age and reduced subcortical gray matter maturation with pain exposure throughout the neonatal period (Brummelte et al., 2012), including the thalamus in very preterm infants (Duerden et al., 2020). Greater exposure to neonatal invasive procedures is also associated with lower volumes in the amygdala, thalamus, and hippocampal subregions (Chau et al., 2019). Surgery early in life significantly contributes to poorer brain maturation in the neonatal period (Brummelte et al., 2012) and at school age (Chau et al., 2019) over and above pain in the NICU and other clinical factors related to prematurity. More surgeries, days of ventilation, and lower GA are also related to smaller volumes in various subcortical regions. These reduced volumes are differentially related to poorer cognitive, visual motor, and behavioral outcomes (Chau et al., 2019).

The unnatural NICU environment and stressful stimuli have not only been associated with epigenetic alterations but, by their very nature, they lead to altered parent–infant bonding (Casavant et al., 2019; Feldman et al., 2014). Infants born preterm have the neuronal connections required to perceive pain; however, the functional response is immature, meaning they are often unable to distinguish between noxious and nonnoxious stimuli (Green et al., 2019; Harrison et al., 2015; Orovec et al., 2019; Ranger & Grunau, 2014; Tataranno & Benders, 2019; Verriotis et al., 2016). The accumulation of painful stressors in preterm infants is especially detrimental to the rapidly developing central nervous and neuroendocrine systems and has been associated with increased risk of neurodevelopmental and behavioral disorders (Agut et al., 2020; Aroke et al., 2019; Cheong et al., 2020; Cong et al., 2017; Ganguly et al., 2020; Grunau, 2020; Harrison et al., 2015; Mooney-Leber & Brummelte, 2017; Mooney-Leber et al., 2018; Orovec et al., 2019; Ranger et al., 2014; Valeri et al., 2015, 2016).

The most commonly selected biomarker to measure stress is cortisol. The skin is the barrier between the external environment and communicates with our neurologic, endocrine, and immune regulatory networks. Stress level and cortisol reactivity vary by gestation age. Higher stress results in higher cortisol for infants >28 weeks; lower stress scores are associated with higher stress for infants <28 weeks. Skin cortisol has been shown to be a preterm biomarker of chronic stress exposure (Brummelte et al., 2015; D'Agata et al., 2019). Seemingly typical handling and caregiving by the NICU staff, such as bathing, weighing, and diaper changes, can be perceived as stressful to the infant (Comaru & Miura, 2009). NICU stressors and painful interventions may raise cortisol levels, limiting neuroplastic reorganization, and, therefore, the learning and memory of motor skills (Brummelte et al., 2015). Measurement of stress exposure is challenging with multiple measures of stress exposure in use, including counts of skin breaking or invasive procedures or counts of noxious sensory exposures. Even a single adverse sensation or situation is enough to increase cortisol; high-cortisol levels signal stress, even when the infant appears to be resting and calm. NICU-related pain-related stress events affect the developmental trajectories of preterm infants and children via epigenetic alterations of imprinted and stress-related genes (Provenzi et al., 2018).

The birth of a preterm infant and witnessing one's infant in pain is remembered by parents as being among the most stressful aspects of the NICU. Elevated post-traumatic stress symptoms (PTSSs) are highly prevalent among mothers of preterm infants, and it has been shown that mothers of infants exposed to greater numbers of invasive procedures have more elevated PTSSs at discharge (Vinall et al., 2018).

Morphine is widely used in NICU care to treat ongoing pain/stress and the distress of mechanical ventilation (Ancora et al., 2019; Tataranno et al., 2020; Zwicker et al., 2016). There are long-standing concerns that exposure to opiates may have adverse effects on the immature brain (Ancora et al., 2019; H. Gao et al., 2021; Orovec et al., 2019; Siahanidou & Spiliopoulou, 2020). On the whole, studies have been reassuring that morphine treatment is not related to severe brain injury or major impairments; however, greater internalizing (anxiety/depressive) symptoms have been associated with higher morphine exposure (Chau et al., 2019; Ranger et al., 2014). Oral morphine administration for painful clinical procedures was explored in the psychological outcomes, preventative psychological intervention (POPPI) randomized control trial (RCT). The objective was to investigate whether or not a single 100 mcg/kg morphine sulphate dose administered orally prior to acute painful clinical procedures would provide effective analgesia. Results demonstrated that the administration of 100 mcg/kg of oral morphine to nonventilated premature infants had the potential for harm without analgesic benefit. Oral morphine is not recommended for retinopathy of prematurity screening, and caution is strongly advised if this is being considered for other acute painful procedures in nonventilated premature infants (Monk et al., 2019).

Prevention and management of stress and pain is an important NPI in the NICU. It is essential that appropriate and adequate support be given prior to every potentially stressful intervention. Likewise, appropriate and adequate analgesia must be given prior to every potentially painful procedure. SSC with parents, containment, sucrose, and pacifiers are appropriate foundational nonpharmacological supports with appropriate analgesia added as needed. (See Figure 11.6.)

Routine procedures can cause pain and stress and can be harmful to the rapidly growing brain of preterm infants. Minimizing stress and pain in preterm infants has many neurologic benefits and can help preserve existing neuroplastic capacity. Mitigating pain and stress can be accomplished by pharmacologic and nonpharmacologic means; yet many pharmacologic therapies have negative side effects and negative impacts long term. Therefore, exploring nonpharmacologic alternatives to be used first, and when stronger medications are not necessary, can benefit both the infant and parents. Many nonpharmacologic NPIs that, either individually or in combination, have been explored have been found to be efficacious. These include, but are not limited to, parent partnerships with increased participation; parental odors consisting of odor cloth exchange; olfaction stimulation; SSC; breastfeeding;

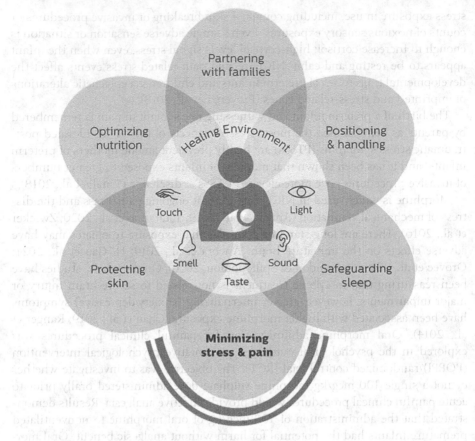

FIGURE 11.6 Minimizing stress and pain.
Source: Courtesy of Philips Healthcare, Cambridge, MA.

breast milk; NNS; pacifier; sucrose; decreased noise and light levels; gentle, yet firm and sustained, human touch; massage; therapeutic positioning; facilitative tuck; containment; swaddling; gentle handling and caregiving; and swaddled bathing, as well as music therapy (Aita et al., 2020; Akbari et al., 2021; Altimier & Holditch-Davis, 2020; Altimier & Phillips, 2016, 2020; Altimier & White, 2020; Apaydin Cirik & Efe, 2020; De Clifford-Faugère et al., 2017; Melançon et al., 2021).

An integrated approach to training and supporting parents in the NICU on how to recognize and reduce their infant's stress and pain, including components of parent contact, resulted in more mature brain connectivity as seen on MRI (Welch & Ludwig, 2017a). Higher-quality parent–infant interaction mediates the relationship between perinatal risk and neurodevelopment (Lean et al., 2018). Very early SSC may play a role in the later infant emotion regulation process and can also act as a protective factor in chronically stressed mothers of NICU infants (Selman et al., 2020). Early SSC and infant massage have both shown a decrease in cortisol levels (Angelhoff et al., 2018; Asmarani et al., 2020). Maternal and neonatal stress levels synchronously decrease during SSC. Just 20 minutes of SSC reduces cortisol levels by 60% in infants greater than 25 weeks' GA (Angelhoff et al., 2018; Mörelius,

He, et al., 2016). Breastfeeding and SSC in tandem may be the most profound analgesic available, with no side effects. A simple gentle nurturing touch from parents to their infants can influence pain sensitivity, affect, and growth in neonates.

Preterm infants exposed to music interventions have demonstrated significantly improved white matter maturation as well as larger amygdala volumes. These results suggest a structural maturational effect of a music intervention on premature infants' auditory and emotional processing neural pathways during a key period of brain development (Sa de Almeida et al., 2020). NICU music therapists (NICU-MTs) often provide services to parents and involve them in developmental care of their child (Standley & Gutierrez, 2020). NICU-MT is highly effective in reducing parental stress, enhancing parent/infant attachment, and training parents to reduce overstimulation of their infant (Browne, 2017; Coombes & Muzaffar, 2021; Detmer, 2017, 2019; Detmer & Whelan, 2017; Lejeune, Lordier, et al., 2019). Music is carefully selected for each intervention depending on the GA of the infant and on their developmental progress (Detmer, 2017). When premature infants are smallest and at their most fragile, the selected music should be quiet lullabies sung in their native language in a style meant to soothe that removes alerting stimuli, such as changes in key, accompaniment, dynamics, and rhythm. Infants learn language concepts by overhearing their mother's voice during the final trimester of gestation. Because lullabies from every culture contain a preponderance of the beginning language sounds for that culture, they meet dual criteria for infant development: soothing aural stimulation and language stimulation (Standley & Gutierrez, 2020). Combined pharmacological, behavioral, and physical interventions (sucrose, massage, music, NNS, and gentle human touch) may remain efficacious and safe for reducing repeated procedural pain, decrease basal cortisol levels at discharge from the NICU, and promote early neurobehavioral development in preterm infants.

Definition

Sources of stress and pain for infants include the physical environment, caregiver interventions, medical and surgical procedures, distress, pathologic processes, temperature changes, handling and multiple modes of stimulation, and, most importantly, the separation from parents. Consequences of neonatal stress and pain include increased energy expenditure, decreased healing and recovery, altered growth, impaired physiologic stability, and altered brain development and organization.

Standard

A policy/procedure/guideline on the assessment and management of stress and pain exists and is followed throughout the infant's stay.

Infant Characteristics

Characteristics include behavioral cues indicating stress or regulation.

Goal

■ The goal is to promote physiologic regulation and neurodevelopmental organization.

Neuroprotective Interventions

■ Facilitate early and prolonged SSC to decrease stress and during minor painful procedures when possible to decrease pain.

■ Utilize a validated and reliable pain assessment tool.

■ Develop a stepwise algorithm to assess, prevent, and manage stress and pain.

■ Provide individualized care in a manner that anticipates, prioritizes, and supports the needs of infants to minimize stress and pain.

■ Provide nonpharmacologic support with all minor invasive interventions.

■ Involve parents in supporting their infant during stressful and painful procedures if they choose by providing SSC, as well as by assisting with sucrose, positioning, and containment strategies.

■ Educate parents on how to read their infant's behavioral cues related to stress and pain and how to provide comforting interventions.

■ Provide psychosocial support (with a dedicated mental health professional) to NICU parents to reduce and manage the stress of having a baby in the NICU as well as coping with anxiety, depression, and grief.

CORE MEASURE #6: PROTECTING SKIN

Protecting skin becomes of particular importance when dealing with neonates at the limits of viability (22–24 weeks), when the skin is especially fragile. NICU infants are at risk for skin injury due to immature skin, compromised perfusion, fluid retention, compromised immune system, medical diagnosis, and procedural skin breaks, as well as the presence of dressings, tapes, adhesives, and various medical devices that are essential to their care. At the moment of birth, the skin is sterile; within 24 hours, it has been colonized with its own bacteria. An acid mantle with a pH of less than 5 is created by the skin to protect it from microorganisms (Kusari et al., 2019; Narendran, 2015; Visscher & Narendran, 2014; Visscher et al., 2015). Maintaining skin integrity is an important healthcare goal because of the essential role of the skin in protecting the infant and providing innate immunity. Achievement of this goal requires constant vigilance and awareness of factors that can negatively impact the skin.

SSC minimizes transepidermal water loss (TEWL), which improves the skin barrier function. The kangaroo position reduces infant heat loss by minimizing the skin surface area exposed to the cooler environment and allows conductive heat gain through SSC between the infant and parent (Conde-Agudelo & Díaz-Rossello, 2016); therefore, SSC can be safely used in extremely preterm infants. SSC can be initiated during the first week of life and is feasible in infants requiring neonatal intensive care, including ventilator treatment. During SSC, the conduction of heat from parent to infant is sufficiently high to compensate for the increase in

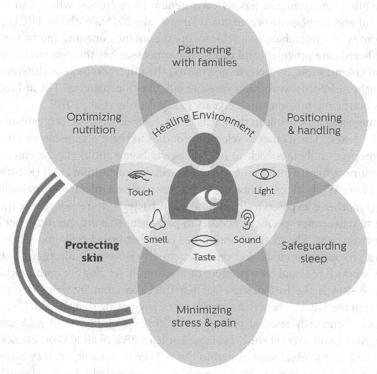

FIGURE 11.7 Protecting skin.
Source: Courtesy of Philips Healthcare, Cambridge, MA.

evaporative and convective heat loss. The increased water loss through the skin during SSC is small and should not affect the infant's fluid balance. Maternal breasts, as well as fathers' chests, warm up and conduct heat to the infant, as well as regulate the infant's temperature. (See Figure 11.7.)

HAIs remain a major problem in the United States. One out of every 31 patients will experience an HAI, costing the United States approximately billions of dollars per year (Centers for Disease Control and Prevention [CDC], 2020). Infants hospitalized in NICUs are particularly susceptible to infection due to their underdeveloped immune and skin systems (Arrieta et al., 2015). To protect against infection, infants are often prescribed antibiotics during the first week of life. In fact, antibiotics are three of the six most commonly administered medications in the NICU (Gasparrini et al., 2016). This treatment likely kills microbes acquired during the birthing process (Raveh-Sadka et al., 2015) and promotes a categorically different colonization pattern in preterm infants relative to full-term infants (Groer et al., 2014). Preterm infants are often colonized by ESKAPE organisms (*Enterococcus* spp-species pluralis, *Staphylococcus aureus*, *Klebsiella* spp., *Acinetobacter* spp., *Pseudomonas aeruginosa*, and other *Enterobacteriaceae*), which are also the most frequent cause of HAIs (Hu et al., 2015). The relatively sterile preterm infant gut microbiome and the high frequency at which infants are colonized by hospital-associated microbes create a valuable study setting to better understand how the room microbiome is shaped by its occupants.

Every NICU environment has its own genera of microbes, which can include commensal and pathogenic organisms (Hartz et al., 2015). With the NICU genera as the context for microbiome development, the infant's ongoing interaction with multiple healthcare providers and caregiving processes has the potential to impact microbial colonization. In preterm newborns, the gut microbiota is different from that of term newborns, with high variable colonization patterns. GA at birth still imprints on the microbiome up to 4 years of age (Fouhy et al., 2019).

Both mom and baby, while in the NICU, are colonized with NICU organisms (bacteria and viruses). The mother develops antibodies to these organisms and transfers these protective antibodies back to her infant via breast milk, via the enteromammary immune system, which in turn helps protect the infant from HAIs (Kleinman & Walker, 1979). While in SSC contact with her hospitalized infant, a breastfeeding (or pumping) mother is exposed to the infant's skin bacteria. In response, the mother's immune system creates specific antibodies to pathogens that are specific to her baby's NICU environment. The mother's antibodies enter her breast milk and when fed to the infant provide immune protection to potential nosocomial infections. This process only works if SSC and breastfeeding or breast milk feeding are both practiced.

Because skin is the first defense against infection, skin integrity is especially important in the NICU. There is strong evidence suggesting that the NICU serves as a reservoir of clinically relevant pathogens. Outbreaks of disease in ICUs are relatively common, and a recent study estimated at least 38% of all ICU outbreaks could be attributed to microbial sources within the ICU environment, such as equipment or personnel (Gastmeier et al., 2007). In addition, upward of 63% of extremely preterm infants develop life-threatening infections (Stoll et al., 2010). Epidemiologic investigations indicate environmental sources of infective agents in air or heating, ventilation, and air-conditioning (HVAC) systems (Adler et al., 2005), mobile phones (Dorost et al., 2018; Kirkby & Biggs, 2016; Simmonds et al., 2020), infant incubators (Cadot et al., 2019; Fattorini et al., 2018), NICU surfaces (Brons et al., 2020; B. Brooks et al., 2018; Hartz et al., 2015; Heisel et al., 2019), sink drains (Qiao et al., 2020; Tracy et al., 2020; Weng et al., 2019), soap dispensers (Buffet-Bataillon et al., 2009), thermometers (Pestourie et al., 2014), and baby toys (Naesens et al., 2009).

Although many touched surfaces were associated with skin-associated bacteria, a gut-associated *Klebsiella* also dominated environments such as the surface monitors, countertops, and scanners. Surprisingly, the floor in front of the infant's incubator had the highest density of microbes relative to any other environment within the NICU (B. Brooks et al., 2018). Samples from the HVAC system had the highest biomass of all organism types, and bioaerosol samples had the lowest. Sinks had the highest biomass of the swabbed samples and hands had the lowest average count. Resuspension or deposits of particles from occupants are the largest contributors of aerosolized particles in the NICU and human-associated taxa dominate most surfaces. Human-associated taxa are likely sourced and trafficked throughout the NICU by healthcare providers (Kembel et al., 2014). Despite regular cleaning of hospital surfaces, bacterial biomasses of organisms were detectable at varying densities. A room-specific microbiome signature was detected, suggesting microbes seeding NICU surfaces are sourced from reservoirs within the room and that these reservoirs contain actively dividing cells. Data suggests that hospitalized infants, in combination with their caregivers, can actually shape the microbiome of NICU rooms (B. Brooks et al., 2014, 2018).

The mobile phone has become an extension of its owner and shares some of their microbiome (Meadow et al., 2014). The personal microbiome, here defined as the collection of microbes associated with an individual's personal effects (i.e., possessions regularly worn or carried on one's person), likely varies uniquely from person to person (Meadow et al., 2014). Research has shown there can be significant interpersonal variation in human microbiota, including for those microbes found on the skin (Flowers & Grice, 2020). Moving constantly with their user into new surroundings, phones come into contact with bacteria from different environments and may feasibly be responsible for the transmission of bacteria from place to place, or person to person. The average person touches their mobile phone anywhere from 200 up to 2,617 times a day—or one million times a year (Cha & Seo, 2018; Nelson, 2016), providing colonizing bacteria with constant nutrition in the form of amino acids and minerals from shed skin cells and sweat (Leyden et al., 1987). Combined with the heat generated by the device and the crevices of cracked screens and phone covers, smartphones (staff and families) provide an excellent habitat for bacteria to colonize (Simmonds et al., 2020). *Enterococci* are normally found in the intestines; therefore, their presence on mobile phones might suggest poor hand hygiene (Wu et al., 2020). It is estimated that 75% of the population use their mobile devices while in the bathroom (Lindsley et al., 2020), which may explain the presence of *enterococci* on participant's mobile phones. Additionally, *enterococci* are known to survive for several weeks on dry surfaces (Wendt et al., 1998).

Clearly there is a growing need for comprehensive ecological surveys of the hospital bacterial environment to better understand the overall process of microbe migration and establishment on and in the body of occupants. While daily cleaning substantially lowers the bioburden (Bokulich et al., 2013), the harshest cleaning methods cannot sterilize hospital surfaces (Hu et al., 2015).

Definition

Functions of the skin include thermoregulation; fat storage and insulation; fluid and electrolyte balance; barrier and immune protection against penetration and absorption of bacteria and toxins; sensation of touch, pressure, and pain; and conduit of sensory information to the brain. Skin care practices outlining humidity practices, cleaning practices, bathing practices, emollient usage, and use of adhesives for babies in each stage of development should be incorporated into unit practices and policies. Additionally, premature infant microbiomes are especially susceptible to environmental influences.

Standard

A policy/procedure/guideline on skin care exists and is followed throughout the infant's stay.

Infant Characteristics

Characteristics include maturity and integrity of the infant's skin.

Goals

Maintain skin integrity of the infant from birth to discharge.

■ Reduce transepidural water loss of extremely low-birthweight (ELBW) infants.

■ Provide developmentally appropriate gentle touch and infant massage.

Neuroprotective Interventions

■ Facilitate early and prolonged SSC to promote development of the infant's microbiome and support the enteromammary immune system with breastfeeding mothers.

■ Utilize a validated and reliable skin assessment tool (i.e., Braden Q) on admission and routinely according to hospital protocol.

■ Provide appropriate humidity via SSC with the mother or incubator to facilitate *stratum corneum* maturation during the first 2 weeks of life.

■ Implement evidence-based catheter insertion practices.

■ Minimize use of adhesives and use caution when removing adhesives to prevent epidermal stripping.

■ Utilize products that protect the skin from adhesive damage.

■ Provide appropriate positioning aids to protect skin and prevent skin breakdown.

■ Avoid soaps and routine use of emollients.

■ Provide full-body swaddled bathing no more than every 96 hours.

■ Use water only for bathing infants who are less than 1,000 g.

■ Use pH-neutral cleansers for bathing infants who are greater than 1,000 g.

■ Educate parents on protecting skin, swaddled bathing, SSC, and delivery of developmentally appropriate infant massage.

CORE MEASURE #7: OPTIMIZING NUTRITION

Breast milk is the optimal nutrition for NICU infants; any breast milk the infant receives is valuable. SSC provides a safe habitat for the infant, thus promoting breast milk production and breastfeeding. Breastfeeding or breast milk feeding supports the early anchoring of the healthy microbiome and ensures direct immune protection. Breastfeeding is a regulator of cardiorespiratory stability. SSC promotes initiation of prefeeding behaviors, exclusivity of breastfeeding, longer duration of breastfeeding, better recognition of mother's milk, and higher milk production (Klaus & Klaus, 2010; Oras et al., 2016). Early, regular, and prolonged SSC also has a positive impact on premature infants' health. In particular, early SSC is associated with a reduced risk of BPD development, cholestasis, and HAI. Prolonged daily SSC is associated with a lower incidence of HAI and promotes breastfeeding (Casper et al., 2018). Breastfeeding is the primary outcome of SSC; infants who have been provided with SSC are discharged earlier and are breastfeeding more successfully than infants who have not been provided SSC (Conde-Agudelo & Díaz-Rossello, 2016). A longer daily duration of SSC in the NICU was associated with earlier attainment of exclusive breastfeeding (Oras et al., 2016). The semirecumbent position of SSC helps to release primitive neonatal reflexes that stimulate breastfeeding. Additionally, preterm neonates who receive SSC for long durations reach full enteral feeds faster and have better breastfeeding success, neurobehavioral performance, thermal control, and tissue oxygenation (El-Farrash et al., 2020). (See Figure 11.8.)

NNS or "dry" sucking without fluid, such as on a fist or pacifier, is present but usually disorganized in infants younger than 30 weeks. Sucking rhythm generally improves by 30 to 32 weeks' postconception, and sucking strength and stamina are usually mature enough for adequate feeding by 36 to 37 weeks' GA. Because NNS does not interrupt breathing, it is usually (but not always) established before an infant has the neurologic maturation to coordinate sucking with swallows and breathing. Benefits of NNS have been summarized as increased oxygenation, faster transition to nipple feeding, and better bottle-feeding performance (Hunter et al., 2015).

Neurosupportive feeding focuses on the infant. Neurologic maturation, medical issues, ongoing physiologic status, current stage of feeding readiness and skills, and psychosocial and interactive skills have redefined feeding success in the NICU. In infant-led feeding, quantity becomes secondary to the safety and quality of the feed.

Definition

Breastfeeding is considered the most optimal mode of feeding for neonates and mothers. Human milk changes over the course of lactation in order to perfectly suit the infant's nutritional and immunological needs. Its composition also varies throughout the day. Circadian fluctuations in some bioactive components are suggested to transfer chronobiological information from mother to child to assist the development of the biological clock, which may play a role in the child's growth and development (Italianer et al., 2020; White, 2017).

Breastfeeding is the single most powerful and well-documented preventive modality available to healthcare providers to reduce the risk of common causes of infant morbidity. Even when adequate breast milk is available, most premature neonates learn to eat via nipple feeding. Nipple feeding is a complex task for premature infants and requires a skilled caregiver in assisting the infant in achieving a safe, functional, and nurturing feeding experience. Infant-led feeding scales that address feeding readiness and quality of nippling, as well as developmentally supportive caregiver interventions, are beneficial when initiating oral feedings in the premature neonate (Holloway, 2014; S. Ludwig & Waitzman, 2007; Thoyre et al., 2018; Waitzman et al., 2014).

Studies have demonstrated that preterm infants can safely breastfeed before learning to bottle-feed. Mothers who wish to breastfeed their preterm babies should be supported in breastfeeding directly from the breast well before infant discharge.

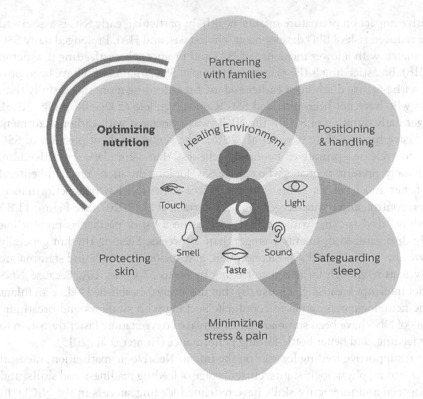

FIGURE 11.8. Optimizing nutrition.
Source: Courtesy of Philips Healthcare, Cambridge, MA.

Preterm infants who alternate between breastfeeding and bottle-feeding while learning to nipple feed can become competent at both by the time of discharge without increasing the length of hospital stay (Phillips, 2020a).

Standard 1

A policy/procedure/guideline on optimizing nutrition (cue-based/infant-driven breastfeeding or bottle-feeding), which includes infant readiness; quality of nippling and caregiver techniques is followed throughout the infant's stay.

Standard 2

A policy/procedure/guideline on SSC exists and is followed throughout the infant's stay.

Infant Characteristics

■ Physiologic stability with handling and feeding
■ Feeding readiness cues

■ Coordinated suck/swallow/breathing (SSB) throughout breastfeeding or bottle-feeding

■ Endurance to maintain nutritional intake and support growth

Goals

■ Feeding will be safe, functional, nurturing, and neurosupportive.

■ Optimized nutrition will be enhanced by individualizing all feeding care practices.

■ Oral aversions will be prevented by assuring it is a positive experience for the infant.

■ Infants of breastfeeding mothers will be competent at breastfeeding prior to discharge.

Neuroprotective Interventions

■ Facilitate early, frequent, and prolonged SSC to promote early opportunities to practice breastfeeding.

■ Utilize validated and reliable infant-driven feeding scale.

■ Support mothers in initiation and maintenance of an adequate breast milk supply.

■ Provide the taste and smell of mother's breast milk with gavage feedings.

■ Minimize negative perioral stimulation (adhesives, suctioning, etc.).

■ Utilize indwelling gavage tubes rather than intermittent tubes.

■ Promote NNS at the mother's breast during gavage feeds.

■ Hold the infant and use NNS with an appropriate-sized pacifier during gavage feeds when the mother is not available.

■ Individualize care by incorporating cue-based/infant-led feeding practices.

■ Once orally feeding, focus on the quality of feeding experience versus quantity of feeds.

■ Utilize caregiver techniques when nippling infant to avoid twisting, jiggling, excessive chin and neck support, and so on.

■ Promote the side-lying position close to the parent/caregiver when bottle-feeding.

■ Educate parents about infant feeding cues.

■ Support breastfeeding mothers in feeding infants at the breast.

CONCLUSIONS

Premature and medically vulnerable infants experience early and sometimes prolonged separation from their parents, intrusive and unnatural environments, painful and distressing procedures, difficulties with physiological regulation, increased biological and neurologic vulnerabilities, grow up to have higher rates of neurocognitive and intellectual impairments, and are also at increased risk of psychosocial and psychiatric illnesses later in life. Parents of infants born prematurely or with medical vulnerabilities, in turn, experience significant distress and are a psychiatrically vulnerable population, with very high rates of depression, anxiety, and posttraumatic stress disorder. The combination of these factors causes significant challenges for many NICU infants and parents in developing an early optimal relationship and emotional connections.

The current challenge is to develop neuroprotective approaches to improve adverse outcomes in preterm and critically ill NICU survivors. Learning the principles of neurodevelopment and understanding the meaning of preterm behavior make it possible for NICU caregivers to provide individualized, developmentally appropriate, neuroprotective, FCC to each infant and family in the NICU environment.

The seven core measures of the Neonatal IDC Model provide specific and structured guidance in optimizing care for infants and families in the NICU. Acknowledging challenges and potentially negative impacts the NICU environment can have on the infant's developing sensory system is critical in order to mitigate risks to the NICU infant and to provide optimal support for who that child will become. Partnering with families, eliminating separation, and encouraging SSC promotes parent–infant bonding and attachment and sets the stage for emotional stability throughout the life span. Providing gentle containment, supportive boundaries, and midline flexed positions helps to simulate the womb positioning that was lost prematurely. By safeguarding sleep, minimizing stress and pain, protecting skin, and optimizing nutrition, NICU caregivers can enhance the experience of infants and families in their care, increasing the likelihood of achieving optimal physical and neurodevelopmental outcomes.

Organizational change is a continual process and occurs for better or worse depending on the change management priorities of organizational leaders. To create effective changes, specific, focused efforts must be made to align an organization's culture (i.e., beliefs and ways of behaving) with goals for improvement. By making new practices and changes, such as incorporating evidence-based NPIs, NICUs can achieve improved neonatal outcomes for babies and families and also increase staff fulfilment and satisfaction in their chosen profession of neonatal nursing.

REFERENCES

Adams-Chapman, I., Heyne, R., DeMauro, S., Duncan, A., Hintz, S., Pappas, A., Vohr, B. R., McDonald, S. A., Das, A., Newman, J. E., Higgins, R. D., & Follow-Up Study of the Eunice Kennedy Shriver National Institute of Child Health and Human Development Neonatal Research Network. (2018). Neurodevelopmental impairment among extremely preterm infants in the neonatal research network. *Pediatrics, 141*(5), e20173091. https://doi .org/10.1542/peds.2017-3091

Adler, A., Gottesman, G., Dolfin, T., Arnon, S., Regev, R., Bauer, S., & Litmanovitz, I. (2005). *Bacillus* species sepsis in the neonatal intensive care unit. *Journal of Infection, 51*(5), 390–395. https://doi.org/10.1016/j.jinf.2004.12.006

Agrawal, S., Rao, S., Bulsara, M., & Patole, S. (2018). Prevalence of autism spectrum disorder in preterm infants: A meta-analysis. *Pediatrics, 142*(3), E20180134. https://doi.org/10.1542/peds.2018-0134

Ågren, J. (2020). Using skin-to-skin contact for thermal control in very and extremely preterm infants must optimise heat exchange in order to maintain body temperature. *Acta Paediatrica, 109*(4), 647–648. https://doi.org/10.1111/apa.15117

Agut, T., Alarcon, A., Cabañas, F., Bartocci, M., Martinez-Biarge, M., Horsch, S., & eurUS. brain group. (2020). Preterm white matter injury: Ultrasound diagnosis and classification. *Pediatric Research, 87*, 37–49. https://doi.org/10.1038/s41390-020-0781-1

Aita, M., Héon, M., Savanh, P., De Clifford-Faugère, G., & Charbonneau, L. (2020). Promoting family and siblings' adaptation following a preterm birth: A quality improvement project of a family-centered care nursing educational intervention. *Journal of Pediatric Nursing, 58*, 21–27. https://doi.org/10.1016/j.pedn.2020.11.006

Akbari, N., Moradi, Z., Sabzi, Z., Mehravar, F., Fouladinejad, M., & Asadi, L. (2021). The effect of narrative writing on fathers' stress in neonatal intensive care settings. *Journal of Maternal-Fetal and Neonatal Medicine, 34*(3), 403–408. https://doi.org/10.1080/14767058.2019.1609926

Aldana Acosta, A. C., Tessier, R., Charpak, N., & Tarabulsy, G. (2019). Randomised controlled trial on the impact of kinesthetic stimulation on early somatic growth of preterm infants in kangaroo position. *Acta Paediatrica, 108*(7), 1230–1236. https://doi.org/10.1111/apa.14675

Aldrete-Cortez, V., Tafoya, S. A., Ramírez-García, L. A., & Poblano, A. (2021). Habituation alteration in infants with periventricular echogenicity as an indicator of neurocognitive impairment. *Developmental Neuropsychology, 46*(1), 82–92. https://doi.org/10.1080/87565641.2020.1871482

Als, H. (2009). NIDCAP: Testing the effectiveness of a relationship-based comprehensive intervention. *Pediatrics, 124*(4), 1208–1210. https://doi.org/10.1542/peds.2009-1646

Als, H., Duffy, F. H., McAnulty, G., Butler, S. C., Lightbody, L., Kosta, S., Warfield, S. K., Huppi, P. S., Butler, S. C., Conneman, N., Fischer, C., & Warfield, S. K. (2012). NIDCAP improves brain function and structure in preterm infants with severe intrauterine growth restriction. *Journal of Perinatology, 32*(10), 797–803. https://doi.org/10.1038/jp.2011.201

Als, H., Duffy, F. H., McAnulty, G. B., Rivkin, M. J., Vajapeyam, S., Mulkern, R. V., Weisenfeld, N. I., Robertson, R., Parad, R. B., Ringer, S. A., Blickman, J. G., Zurakowski, D., & Eichenwald, E. C. (2004). Early experience alters brain function and structure. *Pediatrics, 113*(4), 846–857. https://doi.org/10.1542/peds.113.4.846

Als, H., Lawhon, G., Duffy, F. H., McAnulty, G. B., Gibes-Grossman, R., & Blickman, J. G. (1994). Individualized developmental care for the very low-birth-weight preterm infant. Medical and neurofunctional effects. *JAMA, 272*(11), 853–858. https://doi.org/10.1001/jama.1994.03520110033025

Altimier, L. (2015a). Compassionate family care framework: A new collaborative compassionate care model for NICU families and caregivers. *Newborn and Infant Nursing Reviews, 15*(1), 33–41. https://doi.org/10.1053/j.nainr.2015.01.005

Altimier, L. (2015b). Neuroprotective core measure 1: The healing NICU environment. *Newborn and Infant Nursing Reviews, 15*(3), 89–94. http://doi.org/10.1053/j.nainr.2015.06.014

Altimier, L., & Boyle, B. (2021). Unprecedented opportunities for a transformational change. *Journal of Neonatal Nursing, 27*(3), 157–164. https://doi.org/10.1016/j.jnn.2021.04.001

Altimier, L., Eichel, M., Warner, B., Tedeschi, L., & Brown, B. (2005). Developmental care: Changing the NICU physically and behaviorally to promote patient outcomes and contain costs. *Neonatal Intensive Care, 18*(4), 12–16.

Altimier, L., & Holditch-Davis, D. (2020). Neurobehavioral system. In A. Kenner, L. Altimier, & M. V. Boykova (Eds.), *Comprehensive neonatal nursing care* (6th ed., pp. 675–712). Springer Publishing Company.

Altimier, L., Kenner, C., & Damus, K. (2015). The effect of a comprehensive developmental care training program: Wee Care neuroprotective program (Wee Care) on seven neuroprotective core measures for family-centered developmental care of premature neonates. *Newborn and Infant Nursing Reviews, 15*(1), 6–16. https://doi.org/10.1053/j.nainr.2015.01.006

Altimier, L., & Phillips, R. (2016). The neonatal integrative developmental care model: Advanced clinical applications of the seven core measures for neuroprotective family-centered developmental care. *Newborn and Infant Nursing Reviews, 16*(4), 230–244. https://doi.org/10.1053/j.nainr.2016.09.030

Altimier, L., & Phillips, R. (2018). Neuroprotective care of extremely preterm infants in the first 72 hours after birth. *Critical Care Nursing Clinics of North America, 30*, 563–583. https://doi.org/10.1016/j.cnc.2018.07.010

Altimier, L., & Phillips, R. (2020). Neonatal diagnostic and care protocols. Neuroprotective interventions. In C. Kenner, L. Altimier, & M. V. Boykova (Eds.), *Comprehensive neonatal nursing care* (6th ed., pp. 963–977). Springer Publishing Company.

Altimier, L., & Phillips, R. M. (2013). The neonatal integrative developmental care model: Seven neuroprotective core measures for family-centered developmental care. *Newborn and Infant Nursing Reviews, 13*(1), 9–22. https://doi.org/10.1053/j.nainr.2012.12.002

Altimier, L., & White, R. (2020). The NICU environment. In A. Kenner, L. Altimier, & M. V. Boykova (Eds.), *Comprehensive neonatal nursing care* (6th ed., pp. 713–726). Springer Publishing Company.

Álvarez-Álvarez, M. J., Fernández-García, D., Gómez-Salgado, J., Ordás, B., Rodríguez-González, M. D., & Martínez-Isasi, S. (2019). Effectiveness of the application of massage therapy and kinesitherapy by parents on premature neonates: A research protocol. *Journal of Advanced Nursing, 75*(11), 3097–3104. https://doi.org/10.1111/jan.14135

American Academy of Sleep Medicine. (2018). *Preterm newborns sleep better in NICU while hearing their mother's voice.* American Academy of Sleep Medicine. https://aasm.org/preterm-newborns-sleep-better-in-nicu-while-hearing-their-mothers-voice/

Ancora, G., Lago, P., Garetti, E., Merazzi, D., Savant Levet, P., Bellieni, C. V., Pieragostini, L., & Pirelli, A. (2019). Evidence-based clinical guidelines on analgesia and sedation in newborn infants undergoing assisted ventilation and endotracheal intubation. *Acta Paediatrica, 108*(2), 208–217. https://doi.org/10.1111/apa.14606

André, V., Durier, V., Beuchée, A., Roué, J.-M., Lemasson, A., Hausberger, M., Sizun, J., & Henry, S. (2020). Higher tactile sensitivity in preterm infants at term-equivalent age: A pilot study. *PLoS One, 15*(3), e0229270. https://doi.org/10.1371/journal.pone.0229270

Angelhoff, C., Blomqvist, Y. T., Sahlén Helmer, C., Olsson, E., Shorey, S., Frostell, A., & Mörelius, E. (2018). Effect of skin-to-skin contact on parents' sleep quality, mood, parent-infant interaction and cortisol concentrations in neonatal care units: Study protocol of a randomised controlled trial. *BMJ Open, 8*(7), e021606. https://doi.org/10.1136/bmjopen-2018-021606

Ansari, A. H., De Wel, O., Lavanga, M., Caicedo, A., Dereymaeker, A., Jansen, K., Vervisch, J., De Vos, M., Naulaers, G., & Van Huffel, S. (2018). Quiet sleep detection in preterm infants using deep convolutional neural networks. *Journal of Neural Engineering, 15*(6), 066006. https://doi.org/10.1088/1741-2552/aadc1f

Apaydin Cirik, V., & Efe, E. (2020). The effect of expressed breast milk, swaddling and facilitated tucking methods in reducing the pain caused by orogastric tube insertion in preterm infants: A randomized controlled trial. *International Journal of Nursing Studies, 104*, 103532. https://doi.org/10.1016/j.ijnurstu.2020.103532

Aroke, E. N., Joseph, P. V., Roy, A., Overstreet, D. S., Tollefsbol, T. O., Vance, D. E., & Goodin, B. R. (2019). Could epigenetics help explain racial disparities in chronic pain? *Journal of Pain Research, 12*, 701–710. https://doi.org/10.2147/JPR.S191848

Arora, G. (2017). *Skin-to-skin interventions in infants with neonatal abstinence syndrome* (Order No. 10615768). Department of Medicine. https://open.bu.edu/handle/2144/26606

Arrieta, M.-C., Stiemsma, L. T., Dimitriu, P. A., Thorson, L., Russell, S., Yurist-Doutsch, S., Kuzeljevic, B., Gold, M. J., Britton, H. M., Lefebvre, D. L., Subbarao, P., Mandhane, P., Becker, A., McNagny, K. M., Sears, M. R., Kollmann, T., CHILD Study Investigators, Mohn, W. W., Turvey, S. E., & Finlay, B. B. (2015). Early infancy microbial and metabolic alterations affect risk of childhood asthma. *Science Translational Medicine, 7*(307), 307ra152. https://doi.org/10.1126/scitranslmed.aab2271

Arya, S., Naburi, H., Kawaza, K., Newton, S., Anyabolu, C. H., Bergman, N., Rao, S. P. N., Mittal, P., Assenga, E., Gadama, L., Larsen-Reindorf, R., Kuti, O., Linnér, A., Yoshida, S., Chopra, N., Ngarina, M., Msusa, A. T., Boakye-Yiadom, A., Kuti, B. P., & Morgan, B. (2021). Immediate "Kangaroo Mother Care" and survival of infants with low birth weight. *New England Journal of Medicine, 384*(21), 2028–2038. https://doi.org/10.1056/NEJMoa2026486

Ash, J., & Williams, M. E. (2016). Policies and systems support for infant mental health in the care of fragile infants and their families. *Newborn and Infant Nursing Reviews, 16*(4), 316–321. https://doi.org/10.1053/j.nainr.2016.09.015

Asmarani, R. I., Irwanto, I., Suryawan, A., Irmawati, M., & Utomo, M. T. (2020). Effect of massage on salivary cortisol level in preterm neonates. *Iranian Journal of Neonatology, 11*(1), 12–16. https://doi.org/10.22038/ijn.2019.40771.1664

Asztalos, E. V., Church, P. T., Riley, P., Fajardo, C., & Shah, P. S. (2017). Neonatal factors associated with a good neurodevelopmental outcome in very preterm infants. *American Journal of Perinatology, 34*(4), 388–396. https://doi.org/10.1055/s-0036-1592129

Axelin, A., Kirjavainen, J., Salanterä, S., & Lehtonen, L. (2010). Effects of pain management on sleep in preterm infants. *European Journal of Pain, 14*(7), 752–758. https://doi.org/10.1016/j.ejpain.2009.11.007

Axelin, A., Outinen, J., Lainema, K., Lehtonen, L., & Franck, L. (2018). Neonatologists can impede or support parents' participation in decision-making during medical rounds in neonatal intensive care units. *Acta Paediatrica, 107*(12), 2100–2108. https://doi.org/10.1111/apa.14386

Bartman, C. M., Matveyenko, A., & Prakash, Y. S. (2020). It's about time: Clocks in the developing lung. *Journal of Clinical Investigation, 130*(1), 39–50. https://doi.org/10.1172/JCI130143

Barton, S., & White, R. (2016). Advancing NICU care with a new multi-purpose room concept. *Newborn and Infant Nursing Reviews, 16*(4), 222–224. https://doi.org/10.1053/j.nainr.2016.09.010

Bastani, F., Rajai, N., Farsi, Z., & Als, H. (2017). The effects of kangaroo care on the sleep and wake states of preterm infants. *Journal of Nursing Research, 25*(3), 231–239. https://doi.org/10.1097/JNR.0000000000000194

Beker, F., Macey, J., Liley, H., Hughes, I., Davis, P. G., Twitchell, E., & Jacobs, S. (2019). The effect of smell and taste of milk during tube feeding of preterm infants (the Taste trial): A protocol for a randomised controlled trial. *BMJ Open, 9*(7), e027805. https://doi.org/10.1136/bmjopen-2018-027805

Bellieni, C. V., Nardi, V., Buonocore, G., Di Fabio, S., Pinto, I., & Verrotti, A. (2019). Electromagnetic fields in neonatal incubators: The reasons for an alert. *Journal of Maternal-Fetal and Neonatal Medicine, 32*(4), 695–699. https://doi.org/10.1080/14767058.2017.1390559

Bennet, L., Walker, D. W., & Horne, R. S. C. (2018). Waking up too early—The consequences of preterm birth on sleep development. *Journal of Physiology, 596*(23), 5687–5708. https://doi.org/10.1113/JP274950

Bergman, N. J. (2014). The neuroscience of birth—And the case for zero separation. *Curationis, 37*(2), 1–4. https://doi.org/10.4102/curationis.v37i2.1440

Bergman, N. J. (2015). Neuroprotective core measures 1–7: Neuroprotection of skin-to-skin contact (SSC). *Newborn and Infant Nursing Reviews, 15*(3), 142–146. https://doi .org/10.1053/j.nainr.2015.06.006

Bergman, N. J. (2019a). Birth practices: Maternal-neonate separation as a source of toxic stress. *Birth Defects Research, 111*(15), 1087–1109. https://doi.org/10.1002/bdr2.1530

Bergman, N. J. (2019b). Historical background to maternal-neonate separation and neonatal care. *Birth Defects Research, 111*(15), 1081–1086. https://doi.org/10.1002/bdr2.1528

Bergman, N. J., Ludwig, R. J., Westrup, B., & Welch, M. G. (2019). Nurturescience versus neuroscience: A case for rethinking perinatal mother-infant behaviors and relationship. *Birth Defects Research, 111*(15), 1110–1127. https://doi.org/10.1002/bdr2.1529

Bertoncelli, N., Cuomo, G., Cattani, S., Mazzi, Pugliese, M., Coccolini, E., Zagni, P., Mordini, B., & Ferrari, F. (2012). Oral feeding competences of healthy preterm infants: A review. *International Journal of Pediatrics, 2012*, 896257. https://doi.org/10.1155/2012/896257

Beunders, V. A. A., Vermeulen, M. J., Roelants, J. A., Rietema, N., Swarte, R. M. C., Reiss, I. K. M., Pel, J. J. M., Joosten, K. F. M., & Kooiker, M. J. G. (2020). Early visuospatial attention and processing and related neurodevelopmental outcome at 2 years in children born very preterm. *Pediatric Research.* https://doi.org/10.1038/s41390-020-01206-7

Bigelow, A. E., Power, M., MacLean, K., Gillis, D., Ward, M., Taylor, C., Berrigan, L., & Wang, X. (2018). Mother–infant skin-to-skin contact and mother–child interaction 9 years later. *Social Development, 27*(4), 937–951. https://doi.org/10.1111/sode.12307

Biran, V., Decobert, F., Bednarek, N., Boizeau, P., Benoist, J.-F., Claustrat, B., Barré, J., Colella, M., Frérot, A., Garnotel, R., Graesslin, O., Haddad, B., Launay, J. M., Schmitz, T., Schroedt, J., Virlouvet, A. L., Guilmin-Crépon, S., Yacoubi, A., Jacqz-Aigrain, E., . . . Baud, O. (2019). Melatonin levels in preterm and term infants and their mothers. *International Journal of Molecular Sciences, 20*(9), 2077. https://doi.org/10.3390/ijms20092077

Biran, V., Phan Duy, A., Decobert, F., Bednarek, N., Alberti, C., & Baud, O. (2014). Is melatonin ready to be used in preterm infants as a neuroprotectant? *Developmental Medicine and Child Neurology, 56*(8), 717–723. https://doi.org/10.1111/dmcn.12415

Boardman, J. P., & Counsell, S. J. (2020). Invited review: Factors associated with atypical brain development in preterm infants: Insights from magnetic resonance imaging. *Neuropathology and Applied Neurobiology, 46*(5), 413–421. https://doi.org/10.1111/nan .12589

Bock, J., Gruss, M., Becker, S., & Braun, K. (2005). Experience-induced changes of dendritic spine densities in the prefrontal and sensory cortex: Correlation with developmental time windows. *Cerebral Cortex, 15*(6), 802–808. https://doi.org/10.1093/cercor/bhh181

Bokulich, N. A., Mills, D. A., & Underwood, M. A. (2013). Surface microbes in the neonatal intensive care unit: Changes with routine cleaning and over time. *Journal of Clinical Microbiology, 51*(8), 2617–2624. https://doi.org/10.1128/JCM.00898-13

Bonacquisti, A., Geller, P. A., & Patterson, C. A. (2020). Maternal depression, anxiety, stress, and maternal-infant attachment in the neonatal intensive care unit. *Journal of Reproductive and Infant Psychology, 38*(3), 297–310. https://doi.org/10.1080/02646838.2019.1695041

Bonan, K. C. S. C., Pimentel Filho, J. C., Tristão, R. M., Jesus, J. A. L., & Campos Junior, D. (2015). Sleep deprivation, pain and prematurity: A review study. *Arquivos De Neuro-Psiquiatria, 73*(2), 147–154. https://doi.org/10.1590/0004-282X20140214

Borre, Y. E., O'Keeffe, G. W., Clarke, G., Stanton, C., Dinan, T. G., & Cryan, J. F. (2014). Microbiota and neurodevelopmental windows: Implications for brain disorders. *Trends in Molecular Medicine, 20*(9), 509–518. https://doi.org/10.1016/j.molmed.2014.05.002

Boundy, E. O., Dastjerdi, R., Spiegelman, D., Fawzi, W. W., Missmer, S. A., Lieberman, E., Kajeepeta, S., Wall, S., & Chan, G. J. (2016). Kangaroo mother care and neonatal outcomes: A meta-analysis. *Pediatrics, 137*(1), e20152238. https://doi.org/10.1542/ peds.2015-2238

Boyle, B., & Altimier, L. (2019). The role of families in providing neuroprotection for infants in the NICU. *Journal of Neonatal Nursing, 25*(4), 155–159. https://doi.org/10.1016/j.jnn.2019.05.004

Brazelton, T. B., & Nugent, J. K. (2011). *The neonatal behavioral assessment scale* (4th ed.). Mac Keith Press.

Brons, J. A., Bierman, A., White, R., Benner, K., Deng, L., & Rea, M. S. (2020). An assessment of a hybrid lighting system that employs ultraviolet-A for mitigating healthcare-associated infections in a newborn intensive care unit. *Lighting Research and Technology, 52*(6), 704–721. https://doi.org/10.1177/1477153520904107

Brooks, B., Firek, B. A., Miller, C. S., Sharon, I., Thomas, B. C., Baker, R., Morowitz, M. J., & Banfield, J. F. (2014). Microbes in the neonatal intensive care unit resemble those found in the gut of premature infants. *Microbiome, 2*(1), 1. https://doi.org/10.1186/2049-2618-2-1

Brooks, B., Olm, M. R., Firek, B. A., Baker, R., Geller-McGrath, D., Reimer, S. R., Soenjoyo, K. R., Yip, J. S., Dahan, D., Thomas, B. C., Morowitz, M. J., & Banfield, J. F. (2018). The developing premature infant gut microbiome is a major factor shaping the microbiome of neonatal intensive care unit rooms. *Microbiome, 6*(1), 112. https://doi.org/10.1186/s40168 -018-0493-5

Brooks, E., & Canal, M. M. (2013). Development of circadian rhythms: Role of postnatal light environment. *Neuroscience and Biobehavioral Reviews, 37*(4), 551–560. https://doi .org/10.1016/j.neubiorev.2013.02.012

Browne, J. V. (2017). Recorded maternal voice, recorded music, or live intervention: A bio-ecological perspective. In M. Filippa, P. Kuhn, & B. Westrup (Eds.), *Early vocal contact and preterm infant brain development: Bridging the gaps between research and practice* (pp. 183–204). Springer Publishing Company.

Browne, J. V. (2021). Infant mental health in intensive care: Laying a foundation for social, emotional and mental health outcomes through regulation, relationships and reflection. *Journal of Neonatal Nursing, 27*(1), 33–39. https://doi.org/10.1016/j.jnn.2020.11.011

Browne, J. V., Jaeger, C. B., & Kenner, C. (2020). Executive summary: Standards, competencies, and recommended best practices for infant- and family-centered developmental care in the intensive care unit. *Journal of Perinatology, 40*, 5–10. https://doi.org/10.1038/s41372-020-0767-1

Brummelte, S., Chau, C. M. Y., Cepeda, I. L., Degenhardt, A., Weinberg, J., Synnes, A. R., & Grunau, R. E. (2015). Cortisol levels in former preterm children at school age are predicted by neonatal procedural pain-related stress. *Psychoneuroendocrinology, 51*, 151–163. https://doi.org/10.1016/j.psyneuen.2014.09.018

Brummelte, S., Grunau, R., Chau, V., Poskitt, K., Brant, R., Vinall, J., Gover, A., Synnes, A. R., & Miller, S. P. (2012). Procedural pain and brain development in premature newborns. *Annals of Neurology, 71*(3), 385–396. https://doi.org/10.1002/ana.22267

Bruni, O., Alonso-Alconada, D., Besag, F., Biran, V., Braam, W., Cortese, S., Moavero, R., Parisi, P., Smits, M., Van der Heijden, K., & Curatolo, P. (2015). Current role of melatonin in pediatric neurology: Clinical recommendations. *European Journal of Paediatric Neurology, 19*(2), 122–133. https://doi.org/10.1016/j.ejpn.2014.12.007

Bruton, C., Meckley, J., & Nelson, L. (2018). NICU nurses and families partnering to provide neuroprotective, family-centered, developmental care. *Neonatal Network, 37*(6), 351–357. https://doi.org/10.1891/0730-0832.37.6.351

Bueno, C., & Menna-Barreto, L. (2016). Development of sleep/wake, activity and temperature rhythms in newborns maintained in a neonatal intensive care unit and the impact of feeding schedules. *Infant Behavior and Development, 44*, 21–28. https://doi.org/10.1016/j.infbeh.2016.05.004

Buffet-Bataillon, S., Rabier, V., Bétrémieux, P., Beuchée, A., Bauer, M., Pladys, P., Le Gall, E., Cormier, M., & Jolivet-Gougeon, A. (2009). Outbreak of *Serratia marcescens* in a neonatal intensive care unit: Contaminated unmedicated liquid soap and risk factors. *Journal of Hospital Infection, 72*(1), 17–22. https://doi.org/10.1016/j.jhin.2009.01.010

Buil, A., Carchon, I., Apter, G., Laborne, F., Granier, M., & Devouche, E. (2016). Kangaroo supported diagonal flexion positioning: New insights into skin-to-skin contact for communication between mothers and very preterm infants. *Archives De Pédiatrie, 23*(9), 913–920. https://doi.org/10.1016/j.arcped.2016.04.023

Buil, A., Sankey, C., Caeymaex, L., Apter, G., Gratier, M., & Devouche, E. (2020). Fostering mother-very preterm infant communication during skin-to-skin contact through a modified positioning. *Early Human Development, 141,* 104939. https://doi.org/10.1016/j.earlhumdev.2019.104939

Busse, M., Stromgren, K., Thorngate, L., & Thomas, K. (2013). Parents' responses to stress in the neonatal intensive care unit. *Critical Care Nurse, 33*(4), 52–60. https://doi.org/10.4037/ccn2013715

Byrne, E., & Garber, J. (2013). Physical therapy intervention in the neonatal intensive care unit. *Physical and Occupational Therapy in Pediatrics, 33*(1), 75–110. https://doi.org/10.3109/01942638.2012.750870

Cadot, L., Bruguière, H., Jumas-Bilak, E., Didelot, M.-N., Masnou, A., de Barry, G., Cambonie, G., Parer, S., & Romano-Bertrand, S. (2019). Extended spectrum beta-lactamase-producing *Klebsiella pneumoniae* outbreak reveals incubators as pathogen reservoir in neonatal care center. *European Journal of Pediatrics, 178*(4), 505–513. https://doi.org/10.1007/s00431-019-03323-w

Calciolari, G., & Montirosso, R. (2011). The sleep protection in the preterm infants. *Journal of Maternal-Fetal and Neonatal Medicine, 24,* 12–14. https://doi.org/10.3109/14767058.2011.607563

Callaghan, B., & Fifer, W. P. (2019). Perinatal attention, memory and learning during sleep. *Enfance, 2019*(3), 349–361. https://doi.org/10.4074/S0013754517003056

Cao Van, H., Guinand, N., Damis, E., Mansbach, A., Poncet, A., Hummel, T., & Landis, B. (2018). Olfactory stimulation may promote oral feeding in immature newborn: A randomized controlled trial. *European Archives of Oto-Rhino-Laryngology, 275*(1), 125–129. https://doi.org/10.1007/s00405-017-4796-0

Cardin, A., Rens, L., Stewart, S., Danner-Bowman, K., McCarley, R., & Kopsas, R. (2015). Neuroprotective core measures 1–7: A developmental care journey: Transformations in NICU design and caregiving attitudes. *Newborn and Infant Nursing Reviews, 15*(3), 132–141. http://doi.org/10.1053/j.nainr.2015.06.007

Carlson, A. L., Xia, K., Azcarate-Peril, M. A., Goldman, B. D., Ahn, M., Styner, M. A., Thompson, A. L., Geng, X., Gilmore, J. H., & Knickmeyer, R. C. (2018). Infant gut microbiome associated with cognitive development. *Biological Psychiatry, 83*(2), 148–159. https://doi.org/10.1016/j.biopsych.2017.06.021

Carson, C., Redshaw, M. E., Gray, R., & Quigley, M. A. (2015). Risk of psychological distress in parents of preterm children in the first year: Evidence from the UK Millennium Cohort Study. *BMJ Open, 5*(12), e007942. https://doi.org/10.1136/bmjopen-2015-007942

Carvalho, M. E. S., Justo, J. M. R. M., Gratier, M., Tomé, T., Pereira, E., & Rodrigues, H. (2019). Vocal responsiveness of preterm infants to maternal infant-directed speaking and singing during skin-to-skin contact (kangaroo care) in the NICU. *Infant Behavior and Development, 57,* 101332. https://doi.org/10.1016/j.infbeh.2019.101332

Casavant, S. G., Cong, X., Moore, J., & Starkweather, A. (2019). Associations between preterm infant stress, epigenetic alteration, telomere length and neurodevelopmental outcomes: A systematic review. *Early Human Development, 131,* 63–74. https://doi.org/10.1016/j.earlhumdev.2019.03.003

Caskey, M., Stephens, B., Tucker, R., & Vohr, B. (2014). Adult talk in the NICU with preterm infants and developmental outcomes. *Pediatrics, 133*(3), e578–e584. https://doi.org/10.1542/peds.2013-0104

Casper, C., Sarapuk, I., & Pavlyshyn, H. (2018). Regular and prolonged skin-to-skin contact improves short-term outcomes for very preterm infants: A dose-dependent intervention. *Archives De Pédiatrie, 25*(8), 469–475. https://doi.org/10.1016/j.arcped.2018.09.008

Castellucci, M. (2019). Fewer tests, treatments for NICU babies reduces infections, cuts costs. *Modern Healthcare, 49*(15), 30. https://www.modernhealthcare.com/care-delivery/fewer-tests-treatments-nicu-babies-reduces-infections-cuts-costs

Castillo, M. U., Barros, M. C. M., & Guinsburg, R. (2014). Habituation responses to external stimuli: Is the habituation of preterm infants at a postconceptual age of 40 weeks equal to that of term infants? *Archives of Disease in Childhood. Fetal and Neonatal Edition, 99*(5), F402–F407. https://doi.org/10.1136/archdischild-2013-305626

Centers for Disease Control and Prevention. (2020). *HAI data and statistics.* https://www.cdc.gov/hai/data/index.html

Cha, S.-S., & Seo, B.-K. (2018). Smartphone use and smartphone addiction in middle school students in Korea: Prevalence, social networking service, and game use. *Health Psychology Open, 5*(1), 2055102918755046. https://doi.org/10.1177/2055102918755046

Charafeddine, L., Masri, S., Ibrahim, P., Badin, D., Cheayto, S., & Tamim, H. (2018). Targeted educational program improves infant positioning practice in the NICU. *International Journal for Quality in Health Care, 30*(9), 642–648. https://doi.org/10.1093/intqhc/mzy123

Chau, C. M. Y., Ranger, M., Bichin, M., Park, M. T. M., Amaral, R. S. C., Chakravarty, M., Poskitt, K., Synnes, A. R., Miller, S. P., & Grunau, R. E. (2019). Hippocampus, amygdala, and thalamus volumes in very preterm children at 8 years: Neonatal pain and genetic variation. *Frontiers in Behavioral Neuroscience, 13*, 51. https://doi.org/10.3389/fnbeh.2019.00051

Chen, L. W., Wang, S. T., Wang, L. W., Kao, Y. C., Chu, C. L., Wu, C. C., Chiang, C. H., & Huang, C. C. (2020). Early neurodevelopmental trajectories for autism spectrum disorder in children born very preterm. *Pediatrics, 146*(4), 1–9. https://doi.org/10.1542/peds.2020-0297

Cheong, J. L. Y., Burnett, A. C., Treyvaud, K., & Spittle, A. J. (2020). Early environment and long-term outcomes of preterm infants. *Journal of Neural Transmission, 127*(1), 1–8. https://doi.org/10.1007/s00702-019-02121-w

Chi Luong, K., Long Nguyen, T., Huynh Thi, D. H., Carrara, H. P. O., & Bergman, N. J. (2016). Newly born low birthweight infants stabilise better in skin-to-skin contact than when separated from their mothers: A randomised controlled trial. *Acta Paediatrica, 105*(4), 381–390. https://doi.org/10.1111/apa.13164

Chiorean, A., Savoy, C., Beattie, K., El Helou, S., Silmi, M., & Van Lieshout, R. J. (2020). Childhood and adolescent mental health of NICU graduates: An observational study. *Archives of Disease in Childhood, 105*(7), 684–689. https://doi.org/10.1136/archdischild-2019-318284

Church, P. T., Banihani, R., Luther, M., Maddalena, P., & Asztalos E. (2018) Premature infants: The behavioral phenotype of the preterm survivor. In H. Needelman & B. Jackson (Eds.), *Follow-up for NICU graduates* (pp. 111–126). Springer Publishing Company. https://doi.org/10.1007/978-3-319-73275-6_6

Church, P. T., Cavanagh, A., Lee, S. K., & Shah, V. (2019). Academic challenges for the preterm infant: Parent and educators' perspectives. *Early Human Development, 128*, 1–5. https://doi.org/10.1016/j.earlhumdev.2018.09.016

Church, P. T., Grunau, R. E., Mirea, L., Petrie, J., Soraisham, A. S., Synnes, A., Ye, X. Y., & O'Brien, K. (2020). Family Integrated Care (FICare): Positive impact on behavioural outcomes at 18 months. *Early Human Development, 151*, 105196. https://doi.org/10.1016/j.earlhumdev.2020.105196

Cogley, C., O'Reilly, H., Bramham, J., & Downes, M. (2020). A systematic review of the risk factors for autism spectrum disorder in children born preterm. *Child Psychiatry and Human Development.* https://doi.org/10.1007/s10578-020-01071-9

Colella, M., Biran, V., & Baud, O. (2016). Melatonin and the newborn brain. *Early Human Development, 102*, 1–3. https://doi.org/10.1016/j.earlhumdev.2016.09.001

Colson, E. R., Schaeffer, P., Hauck, F. R., Provini, L., McClain, M., Corwin, M. J., Drake, E. E., Kellams, A. L., Geller, N. L., Tanabe, K., & Moon, R. Y. (2019). Facilitators and barriers to implementation of safe infant sleep recommendations in the hospital setting. *Journal of Obstetric, Gynecologic, and Neonatal Nursing, 48*(3), 332–340. https://doi.org/10.1016/j.jogn.2019.02.005

Comaru, T., & Miura, E. (2009). Postural support improves distress and pain during diaper change in preterm infants. *Journal of Perinatology, 29*(7), 504–507. https://doi.org/10.1038/jp.2009.13

Conde-Agudelo, A., & Díaz-Rossello, J. L. (2016). Kangaroo mother care to reduce morbidity and mortality in low birthweight infants. *Cochrane Database of Systematic Reviews, 2016*(8), CD002771. https://doi.org/10.1002/14651858.CD002771.pub4

Cong, X., Ludington-Hoe, S. M., Hussain, N., Cusson, R. M., Walsh, S., Vazquez, V., Briere, C. E., & Vittner, D. (2015). Parental oxytocin responses during skin-to-skin contact in pre-term infants. *Early Human Development, 91*(7), 401–406. https://doi.org/10.1016/j.earlhumdev.2015.04.012

Cong, X., Wu, J., Vittner, D., Xu, W., Hussain, N., Galvin, S., Fitzsimons, M., McGrath, J. M., & Henderson, W. A. (2017). The impact of cumulative pain/stress on neurobehavioral development of preterm infants in the NICU. *Early Human Development, 108*, 9–16. https://doi.org/10.1016/j.earlhumdev.2017.03.003

Coombes, E., & Muzaffar, I.-A. (2021). The singing unit—A pilot study investigating the efficacy of a music therapy singing intervention in a local neonatal unit to support parent/infant bonding and reduce parental anxiety. *Journal of Neonatal Nursing, 27*(1), 47–51. https://doi.org/10.1016/j.jnn.2020.07.002

Coughlin, M. (2021). *Transformative nursing in the NICU: Trauma-informed age-approriate care* (2nd ed.). Springer Publishing Company.

Coughlin, M., Lohman M. B., & Gibbins, S. (2010). Reliability and effectiveness of an infant positioning assessment tool to standardize developmentally supportive positioning practices in the neonatal intensive care unit. *Newborn and Infant Nursing Reviews, 10*(2), 104–106. https://doi.org/10.1053/j.nainr.2010.03.003

Cowan, C. S. M., Dinan, T. G., & Cryan, J. F. (2020). Annual research review: Critical windows—The microbiota–gut–brain axis in neurocognitive development. *Journal of Child Psychology and Psychiatry, 61*(3), 353–371. https://doi.org/10.1111/jcpp.13156

Craig, J. W., Glick, C., Phillips, R., Hall, S. L., Smith, J., & Browne, J. (2015). Recommendations for involving the family in developmental care of the NICU baby. *Journal of Perinatology, 35*, S5–S8. https://doi.org/10.1038/jp.2015.142

Cryan, J. F., & Dinan, T. G. (2012). Mind-altering microorganisms: The impact of the gut microbiota on brain and behavior. *Nature Reviews Neuroscience, 13*(10), 701–712. https://doi.org/10.1038/nrn3346

Csaszar-Nagy, N., & Bókkon, I. (2018). Mother-newborn separation at birth in hospitals: A possible risk for neurodevelopmental disorders? *Neuroscience and Biobehavioral Reviews, 84*, 337–351. https://doi.org/10.1016/j.neubiorev.2017.08.013

D'Agata, A. L., Coughlin, M., & Sanders, M. R. (2018). Clinician perceptions of the NICU infant experience: Is the NICU hospitalization traumatic? *American Journal of Perinatology, 35*(12), 1159–1167. https://doi.org/10.1055/s-0038-1641747

D'Agata, A. L., Roberts, M. B., Ashmeade, T., Dutra, S. V. O., Kane, B., & Groer, M. W. (2019). Novel method of measuring chronic stress for preterm infants: Skin cortisol. *Psychoneuroendocrinology, 102*, 204–211. https://doi.org/10.1016/j.psyneuen.2018.12.223

Dai, D. W. T., Wouldes, T. A., Brown, G. T. L., Tottman, A. C., Alsweiler, J. M., Gamble, G. D., & Harding, J. E. (2020). Relationships between intelligence, executive function and academic achievement in children born very preterm. *Early Human Development, 148*, 105122. https://doi.org/10.1016/j.earlhumdev.2020.105122

Dang-Vu, T. T., Desseilles, M., Peigneux, P., & Maquet, P. (2006). A role for sleep in brain plasticity. *Pediatric Rehabilitation, 9*(2), 98–118. https://doi.org/10.1080/13638490500138702

Danner-Bowman, K., & Cardin, A. (2015). Neuroprotective core measure 3: Positioning & handling—A look at preventing positional plagiocephaly. *Newborn and Infant Nursing Reviews, 15*(3), 111–113. https://doi.org/10.1053/j.nainr.2015.06.009

Darcy Mahoney, A., White, R. D., Velasquez, A., Barrett, T. S., Clark, R. H., & Ahmad, K. A. (2020). Impact of restrictions on parental presence in neonatal intensive care units related to coronavirus disease 2019. *Journal of Perinatology, 40*, 36–46. https://doi.org/10.1038/s41372-020-0753-7

Davidson, J., Ruthazer, R., & Maron, J. L. (2019). Optimal timing to utilize olfactory stimulation with maternal breast milk to improve oral feeding skills in the premature newborn. *Breastfeeding Medicine, 14*(4), 230–235. https://doi.org/10.1089/bfm.2018.0180

de Bijl-Marcus, K. A., Brouwer, A. J., de Vries, L. S., & van Wezel-Meijler, G. (2017). The effect of head positioning and head tilting on the incidence of intraventricular hemorrhage in very preterm infants: A systematic review. *Neonatology, 111*, 267–279. https://doi.org/10.1159/000449240

De Clifford-Faugère, G., Lavallée, A., & Aita, M. (2017). Olfactive stimulation interventions for managing procedural pain in preterm and full-term neonates: A systematic review protocol. *Systematic Reviews, 6*(1), 203. https://doi.org/10.1186/s13643-017-0589-1

Delaney, A. L., & Arvedson, J. C. (2008). Development of swallowing and feeding: Prenatal through first year of life. *Developmental Disabilities Research Reviews, 14*(2), 105–117. https://doi.org/10.1002/ddrr.16

Del Fabbro, A., & Cain, K. (2016). Infant mental health and family mental health issues. *Newborn and Infant Nursing Reviews, 16*(4), 281–284. https://doi.org/10.1053/j.nainr.2016.09.020

Del Rio-Bermudez, C., & Blumberg, M. S. (2018). Active sleep promotes functional connectivity in developing sensorimotor networks. *BioEssays, 40*(4), e1700234. https://doi.org/10.1002/bies.201700234

DeMaster, D., Bick, J., Johnson, U., Montroy, J. J., Landry, S., & Duncan, A. F. (2019). Nurturing the preterm infant brain: Leveraging neuroplasticity to improve neurobehavioral outcomes. *Pediatric Research, 85*(2), 166–175. https://doi.org/10.1038/s41390-018-0203-9

Dereymaeker, A., Pillay, K., Vervisch, J., De Vos, M., Van Huffel, S., Jansen, K., & Naulaers, G. (2017). Review of sleep-EEG in preterm and term neonates. *Early Human Development, 113*, 87–103. https://doi.org/10.1016/j.earlhumdev.2017.07.003

Detmer, M. R. (2017). Extending the therapeutic impact of music in the NICU through developmentally appropriate recorded music. *Imagine, 8*(1), 79–83.

Detmer, M. R. (2019). Music in the NICU: An evidence-based healthcare practice with proven benefits. *Neonatal Intensive Care, 32*(1), 20–23. https://www.nicmag.ca/pdf/NIC-32-1-Winter-2019-R14.pdf

Detmer, M. R., Evans, K., Shina, E., Walker, K., DeLoach, D., & Malowitz, J. R. (2020). Multimodal neurologic enhancement improves preterm infants' developmental outcomes: A longitudinal pilot study. *Neonatal Network, 39*(1), 16–23. https://doi.org/10.1891/0730-0832.39.1.16

Detmer, M. R., & Whelan, M. L. (2017). Music in the NICU: The role of nurses in neuroprotection. *Neonatal Network, 36*(4), 213–217. https://doi.org/10.1891/0730-0832.36.4.213

Dittman, K., & Hughes, S. (2018). Increased nursing participation in multidisciplinary rounds to enhance communication, patient safety, and parent satisfaction. *Critical Care Nursing Clinics of North America, 30*(4), 445. https://doi.org/10.1016/j.cnc.2018.07.002

Ditzenberger, G., Blackburn, S., Brown, B., & Altimier, L. (2016). Neurologic system. In C. Kenner & J. W. Lott (Eds.), *Neonatal nursing care handbook: An evidence-based approach to conditions and procedures* (2nd ed., pp. 83–172). Springer Publishing Company.

Dongre, S., Desai, S., & Nanavati, R. (2020). Kangaroo father care to reduce paternal stress levels: A prospective observational before-after study. *Journal of Neonatal-Perinatal Medicine, 13*(3), 403–411. https://doi.org/10.3233/NPM-180190

Dorost, A., Safari, Y., Akhlaghi, M., Soleimani, M., & Yoosefpour, N. (2018). Microbial contamination data of keypad and touch screen of cell phones among hospital and non-hospital staffs—A case study: Iran. *Data in Brief, 20*, 80–84. https://doi.org/10.1016/j.dib.2018.07.041

dos Santos, A. Á., Khan, R. L., Rocha, G., & Nunes, M. L. (2014). Behavior and EEG concordance of active and quiet sleep in preterm very low birth weight and full-term neonates at matched conceptional age. *Early Human Development, 90*(9), 507–510. https://doi.org/10.1016/j.earlhumdev.2014.06.014

Duerden, E. G., Grunau, R. E., Chau, V., Groenendaal, F., Guo, T., Chakravarty, M. M., Benders, M., Wagenaar, N., Eijsermans, R., Koopman, C., Synnes, A., Vries, L., & Miller, S. P. (2020). Association of early skin breaks and neonatal thalamic maturation: A modifiable risk? *Neurology, 95*(24), e3420–e3427. https://doi.org/10.1212/WNL.0000000000010953

Dumont, V., Bulla, J., Bessot, N., Gonidec, J., Zabalia, M., Guillois, B., & Roche-Labarbe, N. (2017). The manual orienting response habituation to repeated tactile stimuli in preterm neonates: Discrimination of stimulus locations and interstimulus intervals. *Developmental Psychobiology, 59*(5), 590–602. https://doi.org/10.1002/dev.21526

El-Farrash, R. A., Shinkar, D. M., Ragab, D. A., Salem, R. M., Saad, W. E., Farag, A. S., Salama, D. H., & Sakr, M. F. (2020). Longer duration of kangaroo care improves neurobehavioral performance and feeding in preterm infants: A randomized controlled trial. *Pediatric Research, 87*(4), 683–688. https://doi.org/10.1038/s41390-019-0558-6

Erdei, C., Liu, C. H., Machie, M., Church, P. T., & Heyne, R. (2020). Parent mental health and neurodevelopmental outcomes of children hospitalized in the neonatal intensive care unit. *Early Human Development, 154*, 105278. https://doi.org/10.1016/j.earlhumdev.2020.105278

Eskandari, Z., Seyedfatemi, N., Haghani, H., Almasi-Hashiani, A., & Mohagheghi, P. (2020). Effect of nesting on extensor motor behaviors in preterm infants: A randomized clinical trial. *Iranian Journal of Neonatology, 11*(3), 64–70. https://doi.org/10.22038/ijn.2020.42355.1703

Evereklian, M., & Posmontier, B. (2017). The impact of kangaroo care on premature infant weight gain. *Journal of Pediatric Nursing, 34*, e10–e16. https://doi.org/10.1016/j.pedn.2017.02.006

Fattorini, M., Buonocore, G., Lenzi, D., Burgassi, S., Cardaci, R. M. R., Biermann, K. P., Cevenini, G., & Messina, G. (2018). Public health since the beginning: Neonatal incubators safety in a clinical setting. *Journal of Infection and Public Health, 11*(6), 788–792. https://doi.org/10.1016/j.jiph.2018.03.001

Feldman, R., Rosenthal, Z., & Eidelman, A. I. (2014). Maternal-preterm skin-to-skin contact enhances child physiologic organization and cognitive control across the first 10 years of life. *Biological Psychiatry, 75*(1), 56–64. https://doi.org/10.1016/j.biopsych.2013.08.012

Fellman, V. (2017). More voice, less noise in NICUs. *Acta Paediatrica, 106*(8), 1210–1211. https://doi.org/10.1111/apa.13927

Filippa, M. (2019). Auditory stimulations in the NICU: The more is it always the best? *Acta Paediatrica, 108*(3), 392–393. https://doi.org/10.1111/apa.14667

Filippa, M., Poisbeau, P., Mairesse, J., Monaci, M. G., Baud, O., Hüppi, P., Grandjean, D., & Kuhn, P. (2019). Pain, parental involvement, and oxytocin in the neonatal intensive care unit. *Frontiers in Psychology, 10*, 715. https://doi.org/10.3389/fpsyg.2019.00715

Fink, A., Bronas, U., & Calik, M. (2018). Autonomic regulation during sleep and wakefulness: A review with implications for defining the pathophysiology of neurological disorders. *Clinical Autonomic Research, 28*(6), 509–518. https://doi.org/10.1007/s10286-018-0560-9

Fitzgerald, M. (2005). The development of nociceptive circuits. *Nature Reviews Neuroscience, 6*(7), 507–520. https://doi.org/10.1038/nrn1701

Fitzgerald, M. (2015). What do we really know about newborn infant pain? *Experimental Physiology, 100*(12), 1451–1457. https://doi.org/10.1113/EP085134

Fjørtoft, T., Ustad, T., Follestad, T., Kaaresen, P. I., & Øberg, G. K. (2017). Does a parent-administered early motor intervention influence general movements and movement character at 3 months of age in infants born preterm? *Early Human Development, 112,* 20–24. https://doi.org/10.1016/j.earlhumdev.2017.06.008

Fleiss, B., & Gressens, P. (2019). Neuroprotection of the preterm brain. *Handbook of Clinical Neurology, 162,* 315–328. https://doi.org/10.1016/B978-0-444-64029-1.00015-1

Flowers, L., & Grice, E. A. (2020). The skin microbiota: Balancing risk and reward. *Cell Host and Microbe, 28*(2), 190–200. https://doi.org/10.1016/j.chom.2020.06.017

Fontana, C., De Carli, A., Ricci, D., Dessimone, F., Passera, S., Pesenti, N., Bonzini, M., Bassi, L., Squarcina, L., Cinnante, C., Mosca, F., & Fumagalli, M. (2020). Effects of early intervention on visual function in preterm infants: A randomized controlled trial. *Frontiers in Pediatrics, 8,* 291. https://doi.org/10.3389/fped.2020.00291

Fouhy, F., Watkins, C., Hill, C. J., O'Shea, C.-A., Nagle, B., Dempsey, E. M., O'Toole, P. W., Ross, R. P., Ryan, C. A., & Stanton, C. (2019). Perinatal factors affect the gut microbiota up to four years after birth. *Nature Communications, 10*(1), 1517. https://doi.org/10.1038/s41467-019-09252-4

Fraiwan, L., & Alkhodari, M. (2020). Neonatal sleep stage identification using long short-term memory learning system. *Medical and Biological Engineering and Computing, 58*(6), 1383–1391. https://doi.org/10.1007/s11517-020-02169-x

Francisco, A. S. P. G., Montemezzo, D., Ribeiro, S. N. D. S., Frata, B., Menegol, N. A., Okubo, R., Sonza, A., & Sanada, L. S. (2020). Positioning effects for procedural pain relief in NICU: Systematic review. *Pain Management Nursing, 22*(2), 121–132. https://doi.org/10.1016/j.pmn.2020.07.006

Franck, L. S., Waddington, C., & O'Brien, K. (2020). Family integrated care for preterm infants. *Critical Care Nursing Clinics of North America, 32*(2), 149–165. https://doi.org/10.1016/j.cnc.2020.01.001

Franco, P., Guyon, A., Stagnara, C., Flori, S., Bat-Pitault, F., Lin, J.-S., Patural, H., & Plancoulaine, S. (2019). Early polysomnographic characteristics associated with neuro-cognitive development at 36 months of age. *Sleep Medicine, 60,* 13–19. https://doi.org/10.1016/j.sleep.2018.11.026

French, K. B., & Altimier, L. B. (2020). Through a mother's eyes. In A. Kenner, L. Altimier, & M. V. Boykova (Eds.), *Comprehensive neonatal nursing care* (6th ed., pp. 727–731). Springer Publishing Company.

French, K. B., & French, T. (2016). *Juniper: The girl who was born too soon.* Little, Brown and Company.

Friedrich, M., Mölle, M., Friederici, A. D., & Born, J. (2020). Sleep-dependent memory con-solidation in infants protects new episodic memories from existing semantic memories. *Nature Communications, 11*(1), 1298. https://doi.org/10.1038/s41467-020-14850-8

Fumagalli, M., Provenzi, L., De Carli, P., Dessimone, F., Sirgiovanni, I., Giorda, R., Cinnante, C., Squarcina, L., Pozzoli, U., Triulzi, F., Brambilla, P., Borgatti, R., Mosca, F., & Montirosso, R. (2018). From early stress to 12-month development in very preterm infants: Preliminary findings on epigenetic mechanisms and brain growth. *PLoS One, 13*(1), e0190602. https://doi.org/10.1371/journal.pone.0190602

Gaffari, M., & Jindal, P. (2019). Concept of neuroprotective NICU. *Qatar Medical Journal, 2019*(2), 1–2. https://doi.org/10.5339/qmj.2019.qccc.29

Ganguly, A., Bhadesia, P. J., Phatak, A. G., Nimbalkar, A. S., & Nimbalkar, S. M. (2020). Pain profile of premature infants during routine procedures in neonatal intensive care: An observational study. *Journal of Family Medicine and Primary Care, 9*(3), 1517–1521. https://doi.org/10.4103/jfmpc.jfmpc_1033_19

Gao, H., Xu, G., Li, F., Lv, H., Rong, H., Mi, Y., & Li, M. (2021). Effect of combined pharmacological, behavioral, and physical interventions for procedural pain on salivary cortisol and neurobehavioral development in preterm infants: A randomized controlled trial. *Pain, 162*(1), 253–262. https://doi.org/10.1097/j.pain.0000000000002015

Gao, W., Salzwedel, A. P., Carlson, A. L., Xia, K., Azcarate-Peril, M. A., Styner, M. A., Thompson, A. L., Geng, X., Goldman, B. D., Gilmore, J. H., & Knickmeyer, R. C. (2019). Gut microbiome and brain functional connectivity in infants—a preliminary study focusing on the amygdala. *Psychopharmacology, 236*(5), 1641–1651. https://doi.org/10.1007/s00213-018-5161-8

Garofalo, N. A., & Caplan, M. S. (2019). Oropharyngeal Mother's milk: State of the science and influence on necrotizing enterocolitis. *Clinics in Perinatology, 46*(1), 77–88. https://doi.org/10.1016/j.clp.2018.09.005

Gasparrini, A. J., Crofts, T. S., Gibson, M. K., Tarr, P. I., Warner, B. B., & Dantas, G. (2016). Antibiotic perturbation of the preterm infant gut microbiome and resistome. *Gut Microbes, 7*(5), 443–449. https://doi.org/10.1080/19490976.2016.1218584

Gastmeier, P., Loui, A., Stamm-Balderjahn, S., Hansen, S., Zuschneid, I., Sohr, D., Behnke, M., Obladen, M., Vonberg, R. P., & Rüden, H. (2007). Outbreaks in neonatal intensive care units—They are not like others. *American Journal of Infection Control, 35*(3), 172–176. https://doi.org/10.1016/j.ajic.2006.07.007

Geva, R., Yaron, H., & Kuint, J. (2016). Neonatal sleep predicts attention orienting and distractibility. *Journal of Attention Disorders, 20*(2), 138–150. https://doi.org/10.1177/1087054713491493

Geyer, J. E., Smith, P. K., & Kair, L. R. (2016). Safe sleep for pediatric inpatients. *Journal for Specialists in Pediatric Nursing, 21*(3), 119–130. https://doi.org/10.1111/jspn.12146

Givrad, S., Hartzell, G., & Scala, M. (2020). Promoting infant mental health in the neonatal intensive care unit (NICU): A review of nurturing factors and interventions for NICU infant-parent relationships. *Early Human Development, 154*, 105281. https://doi.org/10.1016/j.earlhumdev.2020.105281

Godarzi, Z., Zarei, K., Shariat, M., Sadeghniat, K., Nikafs, N., & Sepaseh, H. (2018). Correlations of handling procedures and sleep patterns of the infants admitted to the neonatal intensive care unit. *Iranian Journal of Neonatology, 9*(3), 35–41. https://doi.org/10.22038/ijn.2018.23783.1299

Gogou, M., Haidopoulou, K., & Pavlou, E. (2019). Sleep and prematurity: Sleep outcomes in preterm children and influencing factors. *World Journal of Pediatrics, 15*(3), 209–218. https://doi.org/10.1007/s12519-019-00240-8

Gomes, E. L. F. D., Santos, C. M. D., Santos, A. C. S., Silva, A. G., França, M. A. M., Romanini, D. S., Mattos, M. C. V., Leal, A. F., & Costa, D. (2019). Autonomic responses of premature newborns to body position and environmental noise in the neonatal intensive care unit. *Revista Brasileira de Terapia Intensiva, 31*(3), 296–302. https://doi.org/10.5935/0103-507X.20190054

Gordon, J. M., Robidoux, H., Gaffney, K., Cirrito, B. L., & Lauerer, J. A. (2021). Conceptualizing the early detection and intervention of infant mental health disorders in neonatal nursing. *Journal of Neonatal Nursing, 27*(1), 6–13. https://doi.org/10.1016/j.jnn.2020.10.002

Graven, S. N. (2006). Sleep and brain development. *Clinics in Perinatology, 33*(3), 693–706. https://doi.org/10.1016/j.clp.2006.06.009

Graven, S. N. (2011). Early visual development: Implications for the neonatal intensive care unit and care. *Clinics in Perinatology, 38*(4), 671–683. https://doi.org/10.1016/j.clp.2011.08.006

Graven, S. N., & Browne, J. V. (2008). Sleep and brain development: The critical role of sleep in fetal and early neonatal brain development. *Newborn and Infant Nursing Reviews, 8*(4), 173–179. https://doi.org/10.1053/j.nainr.2008.10.008

Green, G., Hartley, C., Hoskin, A., Duff, E., Shriver, A., Wilkinson, D., Adams, E., Rogers, R., Moultrie, F., & Slater, R. (2019). Behavioural discrimination of noxious stimuli in infants is dependent on brain maturation. *Pain, 160*(2), 493–500. https://doi.org/10.1097/j.pain.0000000000001425

Greene, M. R. B., Patra, K., Kratovil, A., Janes, J., & Meier, P. (2015). Depression, anxiety, and perinatal-specific posttraumatic distress in mothers of very low birth weight infants in the neonatal intensive care unit. *Journal of Developmental and Behavioral Pediatrics, 36*(5), 362–370. https://doi.org/10.1097/DBP.0000000000000174

Greenough, W. T., Black, J. E., & Wallace, C. S. (1987). Experience and brain development. *Child Development, 58*(3), 539–559.

Grigg-Damberger, M. M. (2016). The visual scoring of sleep in infants 0 to 2 months of age. *Journal of Clinical Sleep Medicine, 12*(3), 429–445. https://doi.org/10.5664/jcsm.5600

Groer, M. W., Luciano, A. A., Dishaw, L. J., Ashmeade, T. L., Miller, E., & Gilbert, J. A. (2014). Development of the preterm infant gut microbiome: A research priority. *Microbiome, 2*, 38. https://doi.org/10.1186/2049-2618-2-38

Grunau, R., Whitfield, M., & Petrie-Thomas, J. (2009). Neonatal pain, parenting stress and interaction, in relation to cognitive and motor development at 8 and 18 months in preterm infants. *Pain, 143*, 138–146. https://doi.org/10.1016/j.pain.2009.02.014

Grunau, R. E. (2020). Personal perspectives: Infant pain—A multidisciplinary journey. *Paediatric and Neonatal Pain, 2*(2), 50–57. https://doi.org/10.1002/pne2.12017

Grunewaldt, K. H., Fjørtoft, T., Bjuland, K. J., Brubakk, A.-M., Eikenes, L., Håberg, A. K., Løhaugen, G. C., & Skranes, J. (2014). Follow-up at age 10 years in ELBW children—Functional outcome, brain morphology and results from motor assessments in infancy. *Early Human Development, 90*(10), 571–578. https://doi.org/10.1016/j.earlhumdev.2014.07.005

Grzyb, M. J., Coo, H., Rühland, L., & Dow, K. (2014). Views of parents and health-care providers regarding parental presence at bedside rounds in a neonatal intensive care unit. *Journal of Perinatology, 34*(2), 143–148. https://doi.org/10.1038/jp.2013.144

Guidetti, J., Wells, J., Worsdall, A., & Metz, A. E. (2017). The effect of positional support on tolerance of wakeful prone in infants. *Physical and Occupational Therapy in Pediatrics, 37*(3), 308–321. https://doi.org/10.1080/01942638.2016.1185506

Guyer, C., Huber, R., Fontijn, J., Bucher, H. U., Nicolai, H., Werner, H., Molinari, L., Latal, B., & Jenni, O. G. (2015). Very preterm infants show earlier emergence of 24-hour sleep–wake rhythms compared to term infants. *Early Human Development, 91*(1), 37–42. https://doi.org/10.1016/j.earlhumdev.2014.11.002

Hall, S., Phillips, R. M., & Hynan, M. (2016). Transforming NICU care to provide comprehensive family support. *Newborn and Infant Newborn Reviews, 16*(2), 5. https://doi.org/10.1053/j.nainr.2016.03.008

Hall, S. L., Hynan, M. T., Phillips, R., Press, J., Kenner, C., & Ryan, D. J. (2015). Development of program standards for psychosocial support of parents of infants admitted to a neonatal intensive care unit: A national interdisciplinary consensus model. *Newborn and Infant Nursing Reviews, 15*(1), 24–27. https://doi.org/10.1053/j.nainr.2015.01.007

Hannan, K. E., Smith, R. A., Barfield, W. D., & Hwang, S. S. (2020). Association between neonatal intensive care unit admission and supine sleep positioning, breastfeeding, and postnatal smoking among mothers of late preterm infants. *Journal of Pediatrics, 227*, 114. https://doi.org/10.1016/j.jpeds.2020.07.053

Harding, C., Cockerill, H., Cane, C., & Law, J. (2018). Using non-nutritive sucking to support feeding development for premature infants: A commentary on approaches and current practice. *Journal of Pediatric Rehabilitation Medicine, 11*(3), 147–152. https://doi.org/10.3233/PRM-170442

Harrison, D., Reszel, J., Wilding, J., Abdulla, K., Bueno, M., Campbell-Yeo, M., Dunn, S., Harrold, J., Nicholls, S., Squires, J., & Stevens, B. (2015). Neuroprotective core measure 5: Minimizing stress and pain—Neonatal pain management practices during heel lance and venipuncture in Ontario, Canada. *Newborn and Infant Nursing Reviews, 15*(3), 116–123. https://doi.org/10.1053/j.nainr.2015.06.010

Hartz, L. E., Bradshaw, W., & Brandon, D. H. (2015). Potential NICU environmental influences on the neonate's microbiome: A systematic review. *Advances in Neonatal Care, 15*(5), 324–335. https://doi.org/10.1097/ANC.0000000000000220

Heck, N., Golbs, A., Riedemann, T., Sun, J.-J., Lessmann, V., & Luhmann, H. J. (2008). Activity-dependent regulation of neuronal apoptosis in neonatal mouse cerebral cortex. *Cerebral Cortex, 18*(6), 1335–1349. https://doi.org/10.1093/cercor/bhm165

Heisel, T., Nyaribo, L., Sadowsky, M. J., & Gale, C. A. (2019). Breastmilk and NICU surfaces are potential sources of fungi for infant mycobiomes. *Fungal Genetics and Biology, 128*, 29–35. https://doi.org/10.1016/j.fgb.2019.03.008

Hendricks-Munoz, K. D., & Mayers, R. M. (2014). A neonatal nurse training program in kangaroo mother care (KMC) decreases barriers to KMC utilization in the NICU. *American Journal of Perinatology, 31*(11), 987–991. https://doi.org/10.1055/s-0034-1371359

Hendricks-Munoz, K. D., Xu, J., Parikh, H. I., Xu, P., Fettweis, J. M., Kim, Y., Louie, M., Buck, G. A., Thacker, L. R., & Sheth, N. U. (2015). Skin-to-skin care and the development of the preterm infant oral microbiome. *American Journal of Perinatology, 32*(13), 1205–1216. https://doi.org/10.1055/s-0035-1552941

Hill, C., Knafl, K. A., & Santacroce, S. J. (2018). Family-centered care from the perspective of parents of children cared for in a pediatric intensive care unit: An integrative review. *Journal of Pediatric Nursing, 41*, 22–33. https://doi.org/10.1016/j.pedn.2017.11.007

Hogan, M. C., Norton, J. N., & Reynolds, R. P. (2018). Environmental factors: Macroenvironment versus microenvironment. In R. H. Weichbrod, G. A. H. Thompson, & J. N. Norton (Eds.), *Management of animal care and use programs in research, education, and testing* (pp. 461–478). CRC Press.

Holloway, E. (2014). The dynamic process of assessing infant feeding readiness. *Newborn and Infant Nursing Reviews, 14*(3), 119–123. https://doi.org/10.1053/j.nainr.2014.06.006

Hu, H., Johani, K., Gosbell, I. B., Jacombs, A. S. W., Almatroudi, A., Whiteley, G. S., Deva, A. K., Jensen, S., & Vickery, K. (2015). Intensive care unit environmental surfaces are contaminated by multidrug-resistant bacteria in biofilms: Combined results of conventional culture, pyrosequencing, scanning electron microscopy, and confocal laser microscopy. *Journal of Hospital Infection, 91*(1), 35–44. https://doi.org/10.1016/j.jhin.2015.05.016

Hucklenbruch-Rother, E., Vohlen, C., Mehdiani, N., Keller, T., Roth, B., Kribs, A., & Mehler, K. (2020). Delivery room skin-to-skin contact in preterm infants affects long-term expression of stress response genes. *Psychoneuroendocrinology, 122*, 104883. https://doi.org/10.1016/j.psyneuen.2020.104883

Huerkamp, M. J., Mallon, D., & Percifield, G. (2018). Facility design, planning, and renovation. In R. H. Weichbrod, G. A. H. Thompson, & J. N. Norton (Eds.), *Management of animal care and use programs in research, education, and testing* (pp. 377–430). CRC Press.

Hunter, J., Lee, A., & Altimier, L. (2015). Neonatal intensive care unit. In J. Case-Smith & J. C. O'Brien (Eds.), *Occupational therapy for children and adolescents* (7th ed., pp. 595–635). Elsevier.

Hwang, S. S., Melvin, P., Diop, H., Settle, M., Mourad, J., & Gupta, M. (2018). Implementation of safe sleep practices in Massachusetts NICUs: A state-wide QI collaborative. *Journal of Perinatology, 38*(5), 593–599. https://doi.org/10.1038/s41372-018-0046-6

Hwang, S. S., O'Sullivan, A., Fitzgerald, E., Melvin, P., Gorman, T., & Fiascone, J. M. (2015). Implementation of safe sleep practices in the neonatal intensive care unit. *Journal of Perinatology, 35*(10), 862–866. https://doi.org/10.1038/jp.2015.79

Hynan, M. T., Steinberg, Z., Baker, L., Cicco, R., Geller, P. A., Lassen, S., Milford, C., Mounts, K. O., Patterson, C., Saxton, S., Segre, L., & Stuebe, A. (2015). Recommendations for mental health professionals in the NICU. *Journal of Perinatology, 35*(Suppl. 1), S14–S18. https://doi.org/10.1038/jp.2015.144

Italianer, M. F., Naninck, E. F. G., Roelants, J. A., van der Horst, G. T. J., Reiss, I. K. M., Goudoever, J. B. V., Joosten, K. F. M., Chaves, I., & Vermeulen, M. J. (2020). Circadian variation in human milk composition, a systematic review. *Nutrients, 12*(8), 2328. https://doi.org/10.3390/nu12082328

Jeanson, E. (2013). One-to-one bedside nurse education as a means to improve positioning consistency. *Newborn and Infant Nursing Reviews, 13*(1), 27–30. https://doi.org/10.1053/j.nainr.2012.12.004

Jennings, E. M., Okine, B. N., Roche, M., & Finn, D. P. (2014). Stress-induced hyperalgesia. *Progress in Neurobiology, 121*, 1–18. https://doi.org/10.1016/j.pneurobio.2014.06.003

Jiang, F. (2020). Sleep and early brain development. *Annals of Nutrition and Metabolism, 75*(Suppl. 1), 44–54. https://doi.org/10.1159/000508055

Jin, J. H., Yoon, S. W., Song, J., Kim, S. W., & Chung, H. J. (2020). Long-term cognitive, executive, and behavioral outcomes of moderate and late preterm at school age. *Clinical and Experimental Pediatrics, 63*(6), 219–225. https://doi.org/10.3345/kjp.2019.00647

Johnston, C., Campbell-Yeo, M., Disher, T., Benoit, B., Fernandes, A., Streiner, D., Inglis, D., & Zee, R. (2017). Skin-to-skin care for procedural pain in neonates. *Cochrane Database of Systematic Reviews, 2*, CD008435. https://doi.org/10.1002/14651858.CD008435.pub3

Jones, L., Fabrizi, L., Laudiano-Dray, M., Whitehead, K., Meek, J., Verriotis, M., & Fitzgerald, M. (2017). Nociceptive cortical activity is dissociated from nociceptive behavior in newborn human infants under stress. *Current Biology, 27*(24), 3846. https://doi.org/10.1016/j.cub.2017.10.063

Joseph, D., Chong, N. W., Shanks, M. E., Rosato, E., Taub, N. A., Petersen, S. A., Symonds, M. E., Whitehouse, W. P., & Wailoo, M. (2015). Getting rhythm: How do babies do it? *Archives of Disease in Childhood. Fetal and Neonatal Edition, 100*(1), F50–F54. https://doi.org/10.1136/archdischild-2014-306104

Joseph, R. M., O'Shea, T. M., Allred, E. N., Heeren, T., Hirtz, D., Jara, H., Leviton, A., & Kuban, K. C. K. (2016). Neurocognitive and academic outcomes at age 10 years of extremely preterm newborns. *Obstetrical and Gynecological Survey, 71*(8), 457–458. https://doi.org/10.1097/OGX.0000000000000354

Kaiser, R. H., Andrews-Hanna, J. R., Wager, T. D., & Pizzagalli, D. A. (2015). Large-scale network dysfunction in major depressive disorder: A meta-analysis of resting-state functional connectivity. *JAMA Psychiatry, 72*(6), 603–611. https://doi.org/10.1001/jamapsychiatry.2015.0071

Kellams, A., Parker, M. G., Geller, N. L., Moon, R. Y., Colson, E. R., Drake, E., Corwin, M. J., McClain, M., Golden, W. C., & Hauck, F. R. (2017). TodaysBaby quality improvement: Safe sleep teaching and role modeling in 8 US maternity units. *Pediatrics, 140*(5), e20171816. https://doi.org/10.1542/peds.2017-1816

Kelsey, C., Dreisbach, C., Alhusen, J., & Grossmann, T. (2019). A primer on investigating the role of the microbiome in brain and cognitive development. *Developmental Psychobiology, 61*(3), 341–349. https://doi.org/10.1002/dev.21778

Kelsey, C. M., Prescott, S., McCulloch, J. A., Trinchieri, G., Valladares, T. L., Dreisbach, C., Alhusen, J., & Grossmann, T. (2021). Gut microbiota composition is associated with newborn functional brain connectivity and behavioral temperament. *Brain, Behavior, and Immunity, 91*, 472–486. https://doi.org/10.1016/j.bbi.2020.11.003

Kembel, S. W., Meadow, J. F., O'Connor, T. K., Mhuireach, G., Northcutt, D., Kline, J., Moriyama, M., Brown, G. Z., Bohannan, B. J., & Green, J. L. (2014). Architectural design drives the biogeography of indoor bacterial communities. *PLoS One, 9*(1), e87093. https://doi.org/10.1128/mBio.00602-12

Keunen, K., Counsell, S., & Benders, M. (2017). The emergence of functional architecture during early brain development. *Neuroimage, 160,* 2–14. https://doi.org/10.1016/j.neuroimage.2017.01.047

Kiblawi, Z. N., Smith, L. M., Diaz, S. D., LaGasse, L. I , Derauf, C., Newman, E., Shah, R., Arria, A., Huestis, M., Haning, W., Strauss, A., DellaGrotta, S., Dansereau, L. M., Neal, C., & Lester, B. (2014). Prenatal methamphetamine exposure and neonatal and infant neurobehavioral outcome: Results from the IDEAL study. *Substance Abuse, 35*(1), 68–73. https://doi.org/10.1080/08897077.2013.814614

Kim, W. J., Lee, E., Kim, K. R., Namkoong, K., Park, E. S., & Rha, D. W. (2015). Progress of PTSD symptoms following birth: A prospective study in mothers of high-risk infants. *Journal of Perinatology, 35*(8), 575–579. https://doi.org/10.1038/jp.2015.9

Kirkby, S., & Biggs, C. (2016). Cell phones in the neonatal intensive care unit: How to eliminate unwanted germs. *Advances in Neonatal Care, 16*(6), 404–409. https://doi.org/10.1097/ANC.0000000000000328

Klaus, M. H., & Klaus, P. (2010). Academy of breastfeeding medicine founder's lecture 2009: Maternity care re-evaluated. *Breastfeeding Medicine, 5*(1), 3–8. https://doi.org/10.1089/bfm.2009.0086

Klawetter, S., Greenfield, J. C., Speer, S. R., Brown, K., & Hwang, S. S. (2019). An integrative review: Maternal engagement in the neonatal intensive care unit and health outcomes for U.S.-born preterm infants and their parents. *AIMS Public Health, 6*(2), 160–183. https://doi.org/10.3934/publichealth.2019.2.160

Kleinman, R. E., & Walker, W. A. (1979). The enteromammary immune system: An important new concept in breast milk host defense. *Digestive Diseases and Sciences, 24*(11), 876–882. https://doi.org/10.1007/BF01324906

Kondili, E., & Duryea, D. G. (2019). The role of mother-infant bond in neonatal abstinence syndrome (NAS) management. *Archives of Psychiatric Nursing, 33*(3), 267–274. https://doi.org/10.1016/j.apnu.2019.02.003

Kostandy, R. R., & Ludington-Hoe, S. M. (2019). The evolution of the science of kangaroo (mother) care (skin-to-skin contact). *Birth Defects Research, 111*(15), 1032–1043. https://doi.org/10.1002/bdr2.1565

Krause, A. J., Simon, E. B., Mander, B. A., Greer, S. M., Saletin, J. M., Goldstein-Piekarski, A. N., & Walker, M. P. (2017). The sleep-deprived human brain. *Nature Reviews Neuroscience, 18*(7), 404–418. https://doi.org/10.1038/nrn.2017.55

Kristoffersen, L., Støen, R., Rygh, H., Sognnæs, M., Follestad, T., Mohn, H. S., Nissen, I., & Bergseng, H. (2016). Early skin-to-skin contact or incubator for very preterm infants: Study protocol for a randomized controlled trial. *Trials, 17*(1), 593. https://doi.org/10.1186/s13063-016-1730-5

Kuhlmann, S., Ahlers-Schmidt, C. R., Lukasiewicz, G., & Truong, T. M. (2016). Interventions to improve safe sleep among hospitalized infants at eight children's hospitals. *Hospital Pediatrics, 6*(2), 88–94. https://doi.org/10.1542/hpeds.2015-0121

Kuhn, P., Sizun, J., & Casper, C. (2018). Recommendations on the environment for hospitalised newborn infants from the French Neonatal Society: Rationale, methods and first recommendation on neonatal intensive care unit design. *Acta Paediatrica, 107*(11), 1860–1866. https://doi.org/10.1111/apa.14501

Kuhn, P., Zores, C., Pebayle, T., Hoeft, A., Langlet, C., Escande, B., Astruc, D., & Dufour, A. (2012). Infants born very preterm react to variations of the acoustic environment in their incubator from a minimum signal-to-noise ratio threshold of 5 to 10 dBA. *Pediatric Research, 71*(4 Pt 1), 386–392. https://doi.org/10.1038/pr.2011.76

Kurth, S., Olini, N., Huber, R., & LeBourgeois, M. (2015). Sleep and early cortical development. *Current Sleep Medicine Reports, 1*(1), 64–73. https://doi.org/10.1007/s40675-014-0002-8

Kusari, A., Han, A. M., Virgen, C. A., Matiz, C., Rasmussen, M., Friedlander, S. F., & Eichenfield, D. Z. (2019). Evidence-based skin care in preterm infants. *Pediatric Dermatology, 36*(1), 16–23. https://doi.org/10.1111/pde.13725

Lan, H., Yang, L., Hsieh, K., Yin, T., Chang, Y., & Liaw, J. (2018). Effects of a supportive care bundle on sleep variables of preterm infants during hospitalization. *Research in Nursing & Health, 41*(3), 281–291. https://doi.org/10.1002/nur.21865

Lan, H.-Y., Yin, T., Chen, J.-L., Chang, Y.-C., & Liaw, J.-J. (2019). Factors associated with preterm infants' circadian sleep/wake patterns at the hospital. *Clinical Nursing Research, 28*(4), 456–472. https://doi.org/10.1177/1054773817724960

Lau, C., & Smith, E. O. (2012). Interventions to improve the oral feeding performance of preterm infants. *Acta Paediatrica, 101*(7), e269–e274. https://doi.org/10.1111/j.1651-2227.2012.02662.x

Lean, R. E., Rogers, C. E., Paul, R. A., & Gerstein, E. D. (2018). NICU hospitalization: Long-term implications on parenting and child behaviors. *Current Treatment Options in Pediatrics, 4*(1), 49–69. https://doi.org/10.1007/s40746-018-0112-5

Lee, S. K., & O'Brien, K. (2014). Parents as primary caregivers in the neonatal intensive care unit. *Canadian Medical Association Journal, 186*(11), 845–847. https://doi.org/10.1503/cmaj.130818

Lefmann, T. (2020). Breastfeeding as a best practice for mitigating the negative effects of stress. *Best Practice in Mental Health, 16*(1), 32–45.

Lehtonen, L., Lee, S. K., Kusuda, S., Lui, K., Norman, M., Bassler, D., Håkansson, S., Vento, M., Darlow, B. A., Adams, M., Puglia, M., Isayama, T., Noguchi, A., Morisaki, N., Helenius, K., Reichman, B., Shah, P. S., & International Network for Evaluating Outcomes of Neonates. (2020). Family rooms in neonatal intensive care units and neonatal outcomes: An international survey and linked cohort study. *Journal of Pediatrics, 226*, 112–117.E4. https://doi.org/10.1016/j.jpeds.2020.06.009

Lejeune, F., Brand, L. A., Palama, A., Parra, J., Marcus, L., Barisnikov, K., Debillon, T., Gentaz, E., & Berne-Audéoud, F. (2019). Preterm infant showed better object handling skills in a neonatal intensive care unit during silence than with a recorded female voice. *Acta Paediatrica, 108*(3), 460–467. https://doi.org/10.1111/apa.14552

Lejeune, F., Delacroix, E., Gentaz, E., Berne-Audéoud, F., Marcus, L., & Debillon, T. (2020). Influence of swaddling on tactile manual learning in preterm infants. *Early Human Development, 153*, 105288. https://doi.org/10.1016/j.earlhumdev.2020.105288

Lejeune, F., Lordier, L., Pittet, M. P., Schoenhals, L., Grandjean, D., Hüppi, P. S., Filippa, M., & Borradori Tolsa, C. (2019). Effects of an early postnatal music intervention on cognitive and emotional development in preterm children at 12 and 24 months: Preliminary findings. *Frontiers in Psychology, 10*, 494. https://doi.org/10.3389/fpsyg.2019.00494

Lejeune, F., Parra, J., Berne-Audéoud, F., Marcus, L., Barisnikov, K., Gentaz, E., & Debillon, T. (2016). Sound interferes with the early tactile manual abilities of preterm infants. *Scientific Reports, 6*, 23329. https://doi.org/10.1038/srep23329

LeVay, S., Wiesel, T. N., & Hubel, D. H. (1980). The development of ocular dominance columns in normal and visually deprived monkeys. *Journal of Complex Neurology, 191*(1), 1–51. https://doi.org/10.1002/cne.901910102

Levy, J., Hassan, F., Plegue, M., Sokoloff, M., Kushwaha, J., Chervin, R., Barks, J. D., & Shellhaas, R. (2017). Impact of hands-on care on infant sleep in the neonatal intensive care unit. *Pediatric Pulmonology, 52*(1), 84–90. https://doi.org/10.1002/ppul.23513

Leyden, J. J., McGinley, K. J., Nordstrom, K. M., & Webster, G. F. (1987). Skin microflora. *Journal of Investigative Dermatology, 88*, 65s–72s. https://doi.org/10.1038/jid.1987.13

Lindsley, J. A., Reynolds, C. D., Williams, T., Underwood, J., Ingram, A. N., Jowitt, J., & Gelinas, L. S. (2020). How dirty is your phone? Evaluating restroom behavior and cell phone surface contamination. *Joint Commission Journal on Quality and Patient Safety, 46*(10), 588–590. https://doi.org/10.1016/j.jcjq.2020.06.008

Linnér, A., Westrup, B., Lode-Kolz, K., Klemming, S., Lillieskold, S., Markhus Pike, H., Morgan, B., Bergman, N. J., Rettedal, S., & Jonas, W. (2020). Immediate parent-infant skin-to-skin study (IPISTOSS): Study protocol of a randomised controlled trial on very preterm infants cared for in skin-to-skin contact immediately after birth and potential physiological, epigenetic, psychological and neurodevelopmental consequences. *BMJ Open, 10*(7), e038938. https://doi.org/10.1136/bmjopen-2020-038938

Liyana Amin, N. A., Tam, W. W. S., & Shorey, S. (2018). Enhancing first-time parents' self-efficacy: A systematic review and meta-analysis of universal parent education interventions' efficacy. *International Journal of Nursing Studies, 82*, 149–162. https://doi.org/10.1016/j.ijnurstu.2018.03.021

Lockridge, T. (2018). Neonatal neuroprotection: Bringing best practice to the bedside in the NICU. MCN. *American Journal of Maternal Child Nursing, 43*(2), 66–76. https://doi.org/10.1097/NMC.0000000000000411

Lubetzky, R., Mimouni, F. B., Dollberg, S., Reifen, R., Ashbel, G., & Mandel, D. (2010). Effect of musclly Mozart on energy expenditure in growing preterm infants. *Pediatrics, 125*(1), e24–e28. https://doi.org/10.1542/peds.2009-0990

Ludwig, R. J., & Welch, M. G. (2019). Darwin's other dilemmas and the theoretical roots of emotional connection. *Frontiers in Psychology, 10*, 683. https://doi.org/10.3389/fpsyg.2019.00683

Ludwig, R. J., & Welch, M. G. (2020). How babies learn: The autonomic socioemotional reflex. *Early Human Development, 151*, 105183. https://doi.org/10.1016/j.earlhumdev.2020.105183

Ludwig, S., & Waitzman, K. (2007). Changing feeding documentation to reflect infant-driven feeding practice. *Newborn and Infant Nursing Reviews, 7*(3), 155–160. https://doi.org/10.1053/j.nainr.2007.06.007

Lundequist, A., Böhm, B., Lagercrantz, H., Forssberg, H., & Smedler, A. C. (2015). Cognitive outcome varies in adolescents born preterm, depending on gestational age, intrauterine growth and neonatal complications. *Acta Paediatrica, 104*(3), 292–299. https://doi.org/10.1111/apa.12864

Maitre, N. L., Key, A. P., Chorna, O. D., Slaughter, J. C., Matusz, P. J., Wallace, M. T., & Murray, M. M. (2017). The dual nature of early-life experience on somatosensory processing in the human infant brain. *Current Biology, 27*(7), 1048–1054. https://doi.org/10.1016/j.cub.2017.02.036

Maki, M. T., Sbampato Calado Orsi, K. C., Tsunemi, M. H., Hallinan, M. P., Pinheiro, E. M., & Machado Avelar, A. F. (2017). The effects of handling on the sleep of preterm infants. *Acta Paulista de Enfermagem, 30*(5), 489–496. https://doi.org/10.1590/1982-0194201700071

Makris, N. M., Vittner, D., Samra, H. A., & McGrath, J. M. (2019). The PREEMI as a measure of parent engagement in the NICU. *Applied Nursing Research, 47*, 24–28. https://doi.org/10.1016/j.apnr.2019.03.007

Malik, G., McKenna, L., & Plummer, V. (2015). Perceived knowledge, skills, attitude and contextual factors affecting evidence-based practice among nurse educators, clinical coaches and nurse specialists. *International Journal of Nursing Practice, 21*, 46–57. https://doi.org/10.1111/ijn.12366

Mann, D. (2016). Design, implementation, and early outcome indicators of a new family-integrated neonatal unit. *Nursing for Women's Health, 20*(2), 158–166. https://doi.org/10.1016/j.nwh.2016.01.007

Martiniuk, A. L. C., Vujovich-Dunn, C., Park, M., Yu, W., & Lucas, B. R. (2017). Plagiocephaly and developmental delay: A systematic review. *Journal of Developmental and Behavioral Pediatrics, 38*(1), 67–78. https://doi.org/10.1097/DBP.0000000000000376

Matas, E., Bock, J., & Braun, K. (2016). The impact of parent-infant interaction on epigenetic plasticity mediating synaptic adaptations in the infant brain. *Psychopathology, 49*(4), 201–210. https://doi.org/10.1159/000448055

McAdams, R. M., & Traudt, C. M. (2018). Brain injury in the term infant. In C. A. Gleason & S. E. Juul (Eds.), *Avery's diseases of the newborn* (10th ed., pp. 897–910). Elsevier.

McCance, K. L., & Huether, S. E. (2019). *Pathophysiology: The biologic basis for disease in adults and children* (8th ed.). Mosby.

McKenna, H., & Reiss, I. (2018). The case for a chronobiological approach to neonatal care. *Early Human Development, 126,* 1–5. https://doi.org/10.1016/j.earlhumdev.2018.08.012

McManus, K., & Robinson, P. S. (2020). A thematic analysis of the effects of compassion rounds on clinicians and the families of NICU patients. *Journal of Health Care Chaplaincy,* 1–12. https://doi.org/10.1080/08854726.2020.1745489

Meadow, J. F., Altrichter, A. E., & Green, J. L. (2014). Mobile phones carry the personal microbiome of their owners. *PeerJ, 2,* e447. https://doi.org/10.7717/peerj.447

Mehler, K., Hucklenbruch-Rother, E., Trautmann-Villalba, P., Becker, I., Roth, B., & Kribs, A. (2020). Delivery room skin-to-skin contact for preterm infants: A randomized clinical trial. *Acta Paediatrica, 109*(3), 518–526. https://doi.org/10.1111/apa.14975

Melançon, J., Aita, M., Belzile, S., & Lavallée, A. (2021). Clinical intervention involving parents in their preterm infant's care to promote parental sensitivity: A case study. *Journal of Neonatal Nursing, 27*(1), 58–62. https://doi.org/10.1016/j.jnn.2020.05.003

Meredith, J. L., Jnah, A., & Newberry, D. (2017). The NICU environment: Infusing single-family room benefits into the open-bay setting. *Neonatal Network, 36*(2), 69–76. https://doi.org/10.1891/0730-0832.36.2.69

Miyagishima, S., Himuro, N., Kozuka, N., Mori, M., & Tsutsumi, H. (2017). Family-centered care for preterm infants: Parent and physical therapist perceptions. *Pediatrics International, 59*(6), 698–703. https://doi.org/10.1111/ped.13266

Modesto, I., Avelar, A., Pedreira, M., Pradella-Hallinan, M., Avena, M., & Pinheiro, E. M. (2016). Effect of sleeping position on arousals from sleep in preterm infants. *Journal for Specialists in Pediatric Nursing, 21*(3), 131–138. https://doi.org/10.1111/jspn.12147

Molina, M., Sann, C., David, M., Touré, Y., Guillois, B., & Jouen, F. (2015). Active touch in late-preterm and early-term neonates. *Developmental Psychobiology, 57*(3), 322–335. https://doi.org/10.1002/dev.21295

Monk, V., Moultrie, F., Hartley, C., Hoskin, A., Green, G., Bell, J. L., Stokes, C., Juszczak, E., Norman, J., Rogers, R., Patel, C., Adams, E., & Slater, R. (2019). *Oral morphine analgesia for preventing pain during invasive procedures in non-ventilated premature infants in hospital: The Poppi RCT.* NIHR Journals Library. https://doi.org/10.3310/eme06090

Montagna, A., & Nosarti, C. (2016). Socio-emotional development following very preterm birth: Pathways to psychopathology. *Frontiers in Psychology, 7,* 80. https://doi.org/10.3389/fpsyg.2016.00080

Montirosso, R., Fedeli, C., Del Prete, A., Calciolari, G., Borgatti, R., & Group, N.-A. S. (2014). Maternal stress and depressive symptoms associated with quality of developmental care in 25 Italian Neonatal Intensive Care Units: A cross sectional observational study. *International Journal of Nursing Studies, 51*(7), 994–1002. https://doi.org/10.1016/j.ijnurstu.2013.11.001

Montirosso, R., & Provenzi, L. (2015). Implications of epigenetics and stress regulation on research and developmental care of preterm infants. *Journal of Obstetric, Gynecologic, and Neonatal Nursing, 44*(2), 174–182. https://doi.org/10.1111/1552-6909.12559

Montirosso, R., & Provenzi, L. (2017). Implications of epigenetics in developmental care of preterm infants in the NICU: Preterm behavioral epigenetics. In M. Filippa, P. Kuhn, & B.

Westrup (Eds.), *Early vocal contact and preterm infant brain development: Bridging the gaps between research and practice* (pp. 295–310). Springer Publishing Company.

Mony, K., Selvam, V., Diwakar, K., & Vijaya, R. R. (2018). Effect of nesting on sleep pattern among preterm infants admitted in NICU. *Biomedical Research, 29*(10), 1994–1997. http://doi.org/10.4066/biomedicalresearch.29-18-326

Moon, R. Y. (2011). SIDS and other sleep-related infant deaths: Expansion of recommendations for a safe infant sleeping environment. *Pediatrics, 128*(5), 1030–1039. https://doi.org/10.1542/peds.2011-2284

Moon, R. Y. (2016). SIDS and other sleep-related infant deaths: Evidence base for 2016 updated recommendations for a safe infant sleeping environment. *Pediatrics, 138*(5), e20162940. https://doi.org/10.1542/peds.2016-2940

Mooney-Leber, S. M., & Brummelte, S. (2017). Neonatal pain and reduced maternal care: Early-life stressors interacting to impact brain and behavioral development. *Neuroscience, 342,* 21–36. https://doi.org/10.1016/j.neuroscience.2016.05.001

Mooney-Leber, S. M., & Brummelte, S. (2020). Neonatal pain and reduced maternal care alter adult behavior and hypothalamic–pituitary–adrenal axis reactivity in a sex-specific manner. *Developmental Psychobiology, 62*(5), 631–643. https://doi.org/10.1002/dev.21941

Mooney-Leber, S. M., Spielmann, S. S., & Brummelte, S. (2018). Repetitive neonatal pain and reduced maternal care alter brain neurochemistry. *Developmental Psychobiology, 60*(8), 963–974. https://doi.org/10.1002/dev.21777

Moore, D. R., Sieswerda, S. L., Grainger, M. M., Bowling, A., Smith, N., Perdew, A., Eichert, S., Alston, S., Hilbert, L. W., Summers, L., Lin, L., & Hunter, L. L. (2018). Referral and diagnosis of developmental auditory processing disorder in a large, United States hospital-based audiology service. *Journal of the American Academy of Audiology, 29*(5), 364–377. https://doi.org/10.3766/jaaa.16130

Moore, E. R., Bergman, N., Anderson, G. C., & Medley, N. (2016). Early skin-to-skin contact for mothers and their healthy newborn infants. *Cochrane Database of Systematic Reviews, 11,* CD003519. https://doi.org/10.1002/14651858.CD003519.pub4

Morag, I., & Ohlsson, A. (2016). Cycled light in the intensive care unit for preterm and low birth weight infants. *Cochrane Database of Systematic Reviews, 8,* CD006982. https://doi.org/10.1002/14651858.CD006982.pub4

Mörelius, E., He, H., & Shorey, S. (2016). Salivary cortisol reactivity in preterm infants in neonatal intensive care: An integrative review. *International Journal of Environmental Research and Public Health, 13*(3), 337. https://doi.org/10.3390/ijerph13030337

Mörelius, E., Olsson, E., Sahlén Helmer, C., Thernström Blomqvist, Y., & Angelhoff, C. (2020). External barriers for including parents of preterm infants in a randomised clinical trial in the neonatal intensive care unit in Sweden: A descriptive study. *BMJ Open, 10*(12), e040991. https://doi.org/10.1136/bmjopen-2020-040991

Mörelius, E., Örtenstrand, A., Theodorsson, E., & Frostell, A. (2016). OC09—Early maternal contact has an impact on preterm infants' brain systems that manage stress. *Nursing Children and Young People, 28*(4), 62–63. https://doi.org/10.7748/ncyp.28.4.62.s40

Murthy, P., Zein, H., Thomas, S., Scott, J. N., Abou Mehrem, A., Esser, M. J., Lodha, A., Metcalfe, C., Kowal, D., Irvine, L., Scotland, J., Leijser, L., & Mohammad, K. (2020). Neuroprotection care bundle implementation to decrease acute brain injury in preterm infants. *Pediatric Neurology, 110,* 42–48. https://doi.org/10.1016/j.pediatrneurol.2020.04.016

Naesens, R., Jeurissen, A., Vandeputte, C., Cossey, V., & Schuermans, A. (2009). Washing toys in a neonatal intensive care unit decreases bacterial load of potential pathogens. *Journal of Hospital Infection, 71*(2), 197–198. https://doi.org/10.1016/j.jhin.2008.10.018

Namprom, N., Woragidpoonpol, P., Altimier, L., Jintrawet, U., Chotibang, J., & Klunklin, P. (2020). Maternal participation on preterm infants care reduces the cost of delivery of preterm neonatal healthcare services. *Journal of Neonatal Nursing, 26*(5), 291–296. https://doi.org/10.1016/j.jnn.2020.03.005

Narendran, V. (2015). Neuroprotective core measure 6: Protecting skin—Neuroprotective care in the newborn: Does skin protect the immature brain from hyperbilirubinemia? *Newborn and Infant Nursing Reviews, 15*, 124–127. https://doi.org/10.1053/j.nainr.2015.06.013

Naugler, M. R., & DiCarlo, K. (2018). Barriers to and interventions that increase nurses' and parents' compliance with safe sleep recommendations for preterm infants. *Nursing for Women's Health, 22*(1), 24–39. https://doi.org/10.1016/j.nwh.2017.12.009

Neil, J. J., & Inder, T. E. (2018). Neonatal neuroimaging. In C. A. Gleason & S. E. Juul (Eds.), *Avery's diseases of the newborn* (10th ed., pp. 923–951). Elsevier.

Nelson, E. E., & Panksepp, J. (1998). Brain substrates of infant–mother attachment: Contributions of opioids, oxytocin, and norepinephrine. *Neuroscience and Biobehavioral Reviews, 22*(3), 437–452. https://doi.org/10.1016/S0149-7634(97)00052-3

Nelson, P. (2016, July 7). We touch our phones 2,617 times a day, says study. *NetworkWorld.* https://www.networkworld.com/article/3092446/we-touch-our-phones-2617-times-a-day-says-study.html

Nestler, E. J. (2011). Hidden switches in the mind. *Scientific American, 305*(6), 76–83. https://doi.org/10.1038/scientificamerican1211-76

Niela-Vilén, H., Feeley, N., & Axelin, A. (2017). Hospital routines promote parent-infant closeness and cause separation in the birthing unit in the first 2 hours after birth: A pilot study. *Birth, 44*(2), 167–172. https://doi.org/10.1111/birt.12279

Nist, M. D., Harrison, T. M., Pickler, R. H., & Shoben, A. B. (2020). Measures of stress exposure for hospitalized preterm infants. *Nursing Research, 69*, S3–S10. https://doi.org/10.1097/NNR.0000000000000444

Noguchi, K. K., Fuhler, N. A., Wang, S. H., Capuano, S., 3rd, Brunner, K. R., Larson, S., Crosno, K., Simmons, H. A., Mejia, A. F., Martin, L. D., Dissen, G. A., Brambrink, A., & Ikonomidou, C. (2020). Brain pathology caused in the neonatal macaque by short and prolonged exposures to anticonvulsant drugs. *Neurobiology of Disease, 149*, 105245. https://doi.org/10.1016/j.nbd.2020.105245

Norholt, H. (2020). Revisiting the roots of attachment: A review of the biological and psychological effects of maternal skin-to-skin contact and carrying of full-term infants. *Infant Behavior and Development, 60*, 101441. https://doi.org/10.1016/j.infbeh.2020.101441

Øberg, G. K., Girolami, G. L., Campbell, S. K., Ustad, T., Heuch, I., Jacobsen, B. K., Kaaresen, P. I., Aulie, V. S., & Jørgensen, L. (2020). Effects of a parent-administered exercise program in the neonatal intensive care unit: Dose does matter—a randomized controlled trial. *Physical Therapy, 100*(5), 860–869. https://doi.org/10.1093/ptj/pzaa014

Øberg, G. K., Ustad, T., Jørgensen, L., Kaaresen, P. I., Labori, C., & Girolami, G. L. (2019). Parents' perceptions of administering a motor intervention with their preterm infant in the NICU. *European Journal of Physiotherapy, 21*(3), 134–141. https://doi.org/10.1080/21679169.2018.1503718

Ohlsson, A., & Jacobs, S. (2013). NIDCAP: A systematic review and meta-analyses of randomized controlled trials. *Pediatrics, 131*(3), e881–e893. https://doi.org/10.1542/peds.2012-2121

Olsson, E., Eriksson, M., & Anderzén-Carlsson, A. (2017). Skin-to-skin contact facilitates more equal parenthood—A qualitative study from fathers' perspective. *Journal of Pediatric Nursing, 34*, e2–e9. https://doi.org/10.1016/j.pedn.2017.03.004

Oras, P., Blomqvist, Y. T., Nyqvist, K. H., Gradin, M., Rubertsson, C., Hellström-Westas, L., & Funkquist, E. L. (2016). Skin-to-skin contact is associated with earlier breastfeeding attainment in preterm infants. *Acta Paediatrica, 105*(7), 783–789. https://doi.org/10.1111/apa.13431

Orovec, A., Disher, T., Caddell, K., & Campbell-Yeo, M. (2019). Assessment and management of procedural pain during the entire neonatal intensive care unit hospitalization. *Pain Management Nursing, 20*(5), 503–511. https://doi.org/10.1016/j.pmn.2018.11.061

Orsi, K. C. S. C., Avena, M. J., Lurdes de Cacia Pradella-Hallinan, M., da Luz Gonçalves Pedreira, M., Tsunemi, M. H., Machado Avelar, A. F., & Pinheiro, E. M. (2017). Effects of handling and environment on preterm newborns sleeping in incubators. *Journal of Obstetric, Gynecologic, and Neonatal Nursing, 46*(2), 238–247. https://doi.org/10.1016/j.jogn.2016.09.005

Painter, L., Lewis, S., & Hamilton, B. K. (2019). Improving neurodevelopmental outcomes in NICU patients. *Advances in Neonatal Care, 19*(3), 236–243. https://doi.org/10.1097/ANC.0000000000000583

Park, J. (2020). Sleep promotion for preterm infants in the NICU. *Nursing for Women's Health, 24*(1), 24–35. https://doi.org/10.1016/j.nwh.2019.11.004

Pestourie, N., Garnier, F., Barraud, O., Bedu, A., Ploy, M.-C., & Mounier, M. (2014). Outbreak of AmpC □-lactamase-hyper-producing *Enterobacter cloacae* in a neonatal intensive care unit in a French teaching hospital. *American Journal of Infection Control, 42*(4), 456–458. https://doi.org/10.1016/j.ajic.2013.11.005

Peters, J. W. B., Schouw, R., Anand, K. J. S., van Dijk, M., Duivenvoorden, H. J., & Tibboel, D. (2005). Does neonatal surgery lead to increased pain sensitivity in later childhood? *Pain, 114*(3), 444–454. https://doi.org/10.1016/j.pain.2005.01.014

Petersen, I. B., & Quinlivan, J. A. (2020). Fatherhood too soon. Anxiety, depression and quality of life in fathers of preterm and term babies: A longitudinal study. *Journal of Psychosomatic Obstetrics and Gynaecology, 42*(2), 162–167. https://doi.org/10.1080/01674 82X.2020.1808620

Petteys, A. R., & Adoumie, D. (2018). Mindfulness-based neurodevelopmental care: Impact on NICU parent stress and infant length of stay; a randomized controlled pilot study. *Advances in Neonatal Care, 18*(2), E12–E22. https://doi.org/10.1097/ANC.0000000000000474

Philips, H. (2018). *Infant Positioning and Assessment Tool* (Version 4522 991 40131) [Mobile application software].

Phillips, R. (2020a). *Breastfeeding practice before bottle feeding increases breastfeeding rates for preterm infants at time of NICU discharge* [Paper presentation]. Academy of Breastfeeding Medicine Annual Meeting, Virtual.

Phillips, R. (2020b). Guidelines for supporting skin-to-skin contact in the NICU. In A. Kenner, L. Altimier, & M. V. Boykova (Eds.), *Comprehensive neonatal nursing care* (6th ed., pp. 936–938). Springer Publishing Company.

Phillips, R., & Smith, K. (2020). First consensus conference on standards, competencies and recommended best practices for infant and family centered developmental care in the intensive care unit: Infant and family-centered developmental care recommendations for skin-to-skin contact with intimate family members. *Journal of Perinatology, 40*, 2–4. https://doi.org/10.1038/s41372-020-0766-2

Phillips, R. M. (2013). The sacred hour: Uninterrupted skin-to-skin contact immediately after birth. *Newborn and Infant Nursing Reviews, 13*(2), 67–72. https://doi.org/10.1053/j.nainr.2013.04.001

Phillips, R. M. (2015). Seven core measures of neuroprotective family-centered developmental care: Creating an infrastructure for implementation. *Newborn and Infant Nursing Reviews, 15*, 87–90. https://doi.org/10.1053/j.nainr.2015.06.004

Pickler, R. H., Meinzen-Derr, J., Moore, M., Sealschott, S., & Tepe, K. (2020). Effect of tactile experience during preterm infant feeding on clinical outcomes. *Nursing Research, 69*, S21–S28. https://doi.org/10.1097/NNR.0000000000000453

Pineda, R., Bender, J., Hall, B., Shabosky, L., Annecca, A., & Smith, J. (2018). Parent participation in the neonatal intensive care unit: Predictors and relationships to neurobehavior and developmental outcomes. *Early Human Development, 117*, 32–38. https://doi.org/10.1016/j.earlhumdev.2017.12.008

Pisch, M., Wiesemann, F., & Karmiloff-Smith, A. (2019). Infant wake after sleep onset serves as a marker for different trajectories in cognitive development. *Journal of Child Psychology and Psychiatry, 60*(2), 189–198. https://doi.org/10.1111/jcpp.12948

Pisoni, C., Provenzi, L., Moncecchi, M., Caporali, C., Naboni, C., Stronati, M., Montirosso, R., Borgatti, R., & Orcesi, S. (2021). Early parenting intervention promotes 24-month psychomotor development in preterm children. *Acta Paediatrica, 110*(1), 101–108. https://doi.org/10.1111/apa.15345

Pletikos, M., Sousa, A. M., Sedmak, G., Meyer, K. A., Zhu, Y., Cheng, F., Li, M., Kawasawa, Y. I., & Sestan, N. (2014). Temporal specification and bilaterality of human neocortical topographic gene expression. *Neuron, 81*(2), 321–332. https://doi.org/10.1016/j.neuron.2013.11.018

Pölkki, T., Korhonen, A., & Laukkala, H. (2018). Parents' use of nonpharmacologic methods to manage procedural pain in infants. *Journal of Obstetric, Gynecologic, and Neonatal Nursing, 47*(1), 43–51. https://doi.org/10.1016/j.jogn.2017.10.005

Porges, S. W., Davila, M. I., Lewis, G. F., Kolacz, J., Okonmah-Obazee, S., Hane, A. A., Kwon, K. Y., Ludwig, R. J., Myers, M. M., & Welch, M. G. (2019). Autonomic regulation of preterm infants is enhanced by family nurture intervention. *Developmental Psychobiology, 61*(6), 942–952. https://doi.org/10.1002/dev.21841

Prouhet, P. M., Gregory, M. R., Russell, C. L., & Yaeger, L. H. (2018). Fathers' stress in the neonatal intensive care unit: A systematic review. *Advances in Neonatal Care, 18*(2), 105–120. https://doi.org/10.1097/ANC.0000000000000472

Provenzi, L., Guida, E., & Montirosso, R. (2018). Preterm behavioral epigenetics: A systematic review. *Neuroscience and Biobehavioral Reviews, 84*, 262–271. https://doi.org/10.1016/j.neubiorev.2017.08.020

Provenzi, L., & Santoro, E. (2015). The lived experience of fathers of preterm infants in the neonatal intensive care unit: A systematic review of qualitative studies. *Journal of Clinical Nursing, 24*(13–14), 1784–1794. https://doi.org/10.1111/jocn.12828

Pugliesi, R. R., Campillos, M. S., Calado Orsi, K. C. S., Avena, M. J., Pradella-Hallinan, M. L. C., Tsunemi, M. H., Avelar, A. F. M., & Pinheiro, E. M. (2018). Correlation of premature infant sleep/wakefulness and noise levels in the presence or absence of "quiet time." *Advances in Neonatal Care, 18*(5), 393–399. https://doi.org/10.1097/ANC.0000000000000549

Qiao, F., Wei, L., Feng, Y., Ran, S., Zheng, L., Zhang, Y., Xiang, Q., Liu, Y., Wu, X., Duan, X., Zhang, W., Li, Q., Guo, H., Huang, W., Zhu, S., Wen, H., & Zong, Z. (2020). Handwashing sink contamination and carbapenem-resistant *klebsiella* infection in the intensive care unit: A prospective multicenter study. *Clinical Infectious Diseases, 71*(Suppl. 4), S379–S385. https://doi.org/10.1093/cid/ciaa1515

Raines, D. A., Barlow, K., Manquen, D., Povmelli, T., & Wagner, A. (2016). Teaching evaluation of an evidence-based program for newborn safe sleep. *Neonatal Network, 35*(6), 397–400. https://doi.org/10.1891/0730-0832.35.6.397

Ranger, M., Chau, C. M. Y., Garg, A., Woodward, T. S., Beg, M. F., Bjornson, B., Poskitt, K., Fitzpatrick, K., Synnes, A. R., Miller, S. P., & Grunau, R. E. (2013). Neonatal pain-related stress predicts cortical thickness at age 7 years in children born very preterm. *PLoS One, 8*(10), e76702. https://doi.org/10.1371/journal.pone.0076702

Ranger, M., & Grunau, R. E. (2014). Early repetitive pain in preterm infants in relation to the developing brain. *Pain Management, 4*(1), 57–67. https://doi.org/10.2217/pmt.13.61

Ranger, M., Synnes, A. R., Vinall, J., & Grunau, R. E. (2014). Internalizing behaviours in school-age children born very preterm are predicted by neonatal pain and morphine exposure. *European Journal of Pain, 18*(6), 844–852. https://doi.org/10.1002/j.1532-2149.2013.00431.x

Ranger, M., Zwicker, J. G., Chau, C. M. Y., Park, M. T. M., Chakravarthy, M. M., Poskitt, K., Miller, S. P., Bjornson, B. H., Tam, E. W., Chau, V., Synnes, A. R., & Grunau, R. E. (2015). Neonatal pain and infection relate to smaller cerebellum in very preterm children at school age. *Journal of Pediatrics, 167*(2), 292–298. https://doi.org/10.1016/j.jpeds.2015.04.055

Raveh-Sadka, T., Thomas, B. C., Singh, A., Firek, B., Brooks, B., Castelle, C. J., Sharon, I., Baker, R., Good, M., Morowitz, M. J., & Banfield, J. F. (2015). Gut bacteria are rarely shared by co-hospitalized premature infants, regardless of necrotizing enterocolitis development. *ELife, 4*, e05477. https://doi.org/10.7554/eLife.05477

Reinhardt, T., Kleindienst, N., Treede, R. D., Bohus, M., & Schmahl, C. (2013). Individual modulation of pain sensitivity under stress. *Pain Medicine, 14*(5), 676–685. https://doi.org/10.1111/pme.12090

Rholdon, R. D. (2017). Outcomes of a quality improvement project: An implementation of inpatient infant safe sleep practices. *Pediatric Nursing, 43*(5), 229–232.

Rholdon, R. D., & Dailey, L. (2016). Implementation of inpatient infant safe sleep practices. *Journal of Obstetric, Gynecologic and Neonatal Nursing, 45*, S40–S41. https://doi.org/10.1016/j.jogn.2016.03.104

Rioualen, S., Bertelle, V., Roué, J. M., & Sizun, J. (2017). How to improve sleep in a neonatal intensive care unit: A systematic review. *Early Human Development, 115*, 1. https://doi.org/10.1016/j.earlhumdev.2017.08.001

Romantsik, O., Calevo, M. G., & Bruschettini, M. (2017). Head midline position for preventing the occurrence or extension of germinal matrix-intraventricular hemorrhage in preterm infants. *Cochrane Database of Systematic Reviews, 7*(7), CD012362. https://doi.org/10.1002/14651858.CD012362.pub3

Roofthooft, D. W. E., Simons, S. H. P., Anand, K. J. S., Tibboel, D., & van Dijk, M. (2014). Eight years later, are we still hurting newborn infants? *Neonatology, 105*(3), 218–226. https://doi.org/10.1159/000357207

Rosana Gonçalves de Oliveira Toso, B., Silveira Viera, C., Martins Valter, J., Delatore, S., & Mazoti Scalabrin Barreto, G. (2015). Validation of newborn positioning protocol in intensive care unit. *Revista Brasileira de Enfermagem, 68*(6), 835–841. https://doi.org/10.1590/0034-7167.2015680621i

Rosin, S., Xia, K., Azcarate-Peril, M. A., Carlson, A. L., Propper, C. B., Thompson, A. L., Grewen, K., & Knickmeyer, R. C. (2020). A preliminary study of gut microbiome variation and HPA axis reactivity in healthy infants. *Psychoneuroendocrinology, 124*, 105046. https://doi.org/10.1016/j.psyneuen.2020.105046

Ryan, M. A., Mathieson, S., Livingstone, V., O'Sullivan, M. P., Dempsey, E., & Boylan, G. B. (2020). Nocturnal sleep architecture of preterm infants in the NICU. *Infant, 16*(5), 209–214. https://www.infantjournal.co.uk/journal_article.html?id=7177

Sa de Almeida, J., Lordier, L., Zollinger, B., Kunz, N., Bastiani, M., Gui, L., Adam-Darque, A., Borradori-Tolsa, C., Lazeyras, F., & Hüppi, P. S. (2020). Music enhances structural maturation of emotional processing neural pathways in very preterm infants. *Neuroimage, 207*, 116391. https://doi.org/10.1016/j.neuroimage.2019.116391

Sahlén Helmer, C., Birberg Thornberg, U., Frostell, A., Örtenstrand, A., & Mörelius, E. (2020). A randomized trial of continuous versus intermittent skin-to-skin contact after premature birth and the effects on mother-infant interaction. *Advances in Neonatal Care, 20*(3), E48–E56. https://doi.org/10.1097/ANC.0000000000000675

Saliba, S., Gratier, M., Filippa, M., Devouche, E., & Esseily, R. (2020). Fathers' and mothers' infant directed speech influences preterm infant behavioral state in the NICU. *Journal of Nonverbal Behavior, 44*(4), 437–451. https://doi.org/10.1007/s10919-020-00335-1

Santos, A. M. G., Viera, C. S., Bertolini, G. R. F., Osaku, E. F., Costa, C. R. L. M., & Grebinski, A. T. K. G. (2017). Physiological and behavioural effects of preterm infant positioning in a neonatal intensive care unit. *British Journal of Midwifery, 25*(10), 647–654. https://doi.org/10.12968/bjom.2017.25.10.647

Saré, R. M., Levine, M., Hildreth, C., Picchioni, D., & Smith, C. B. (2016). Chronic sleep restriction during development can lead to long-lasting behavioral effects. *Physiology and Behavior, 155*, 208–217. https://doi.org/10.1016/j.physbeh.2015.12.019

Sarnat, H. B., & Flores-Sarnat, L. (2019). Development of the human olfactory system. *Handbook of Clinical Neurology, 164*, 29–45. https://doi.org/10.1016/B978-0-444-63855-7.00003-4

Scatliffe, N., Casavant, S., Vittner, D., & Cong, X. (2019). Oxytocin and early parent-infant interactions: A systematic review. *International Journal of Nursing Sciences, 6*(4), 445–453. https://doi.org/10.1016/j.ijnss.2019.09.009

Scime, N. V., Gavarkovs, A. G., & Chaput, K. H. (2019). The effect of skin-to-skin care on postpartum depression among mothers of preterm or low birthweight infants: A systematic review and meta-analysis. *Journal of Affective Disorders, 253*, 376–384. https://doi.org/10.1016/j.jad.2019.04.101

Sehgal, A., Nitzan, I., Jayawickreme, N., & Menahem, S. (2020). Impact of skin-to-skin parent-infant care on preterm circulatory physiology. *Journal of Pediatrics, 222*, 91. https://doi.org/10.1016/j.jpeds.2020.03.041

Seigel, J. K., Smith, P. B., Ashley, P. L., Cotten, C. M., Herbert, C. C., King, B. A., Maynor, A. R., Neill, S., Wynn, J., & Bidegain, M. (2013). Early administration of oropharyngeal colostrum to extremely low birth weight infants. *Breastfeeding Medicine, 8*(6), 491–495. https://doi.org/10.1089/bfm.2013.0025

Selman, S. B., Dilworth-Bart, J., Selman, H., Cook, J. G., & Duncan, L. G. (2020). Skin-to-skin contact and infant emotional and cognitive development in chronic perinatal distress. *Early Human Development, 151*, 105182. https://doi.org/10.1016/j.earlhumdev.2020.105182

Sender, R., Fuchs, S., & Milo, R. (2016). Revised estimates for the number of human and bacteria cells in the body. *PLoS Biology, 14*(8), e1002533. https://doi.org/10.1371/journal.pbio.1002533

Shellhaas, R. A., Burns, J. W., Barks, J. D. E., Hassan, F., & Chervin, R. D. (2019). Maternal voice and infant sleep in the neonatal intensive care unit. *Pediatrics, 144*(3), e20190288. https://doi.org/10.1542/peds.2019-0288

Shepley, M. M., Smith, J. A., Sadler, B. L., & White, R. D. (2014). The business case for building better neonatal intensive care units. *Journal of Perinatology, 34*(11), 811–815. https://doi.org/10.1038/jp.2014.174

Shonkoff, J. P., Garner, A. S., Committee on Psychosocial Aspects of Child and Family Health; Committee on Early Childhood, Adoption, and Dependent Care; Section on Developmental and Behavioral Pediatrics. (2012). The lifelong effects of early childhood adversity and toxic stress. *Pediatrics, 129*(1), e232–e246. https://doi.org/10.1542/peds.2011-2663

Shorey, S., He, H.-G., & Morelius, E. (2016). Skin-to-skin contact by fathers and the impact on infant and paternal outcomes: An integrative review. *Midwifery, 40*, 207–217. https://doi.org/10.1016/j.midw.2016.07.007

Siahanidou, T., & Spiliopoulou, C. (2020). Pharmacological neuroprotection of the preterm brain: Current evidence and perspectives. *American Journal of Perinatology.* https://doi.org/10.1055/s-0040-1716710

Simmonds, R., Lee, D., & Hayhurst, E. (2020). Mobile phones as fomites for potential pathogens in hospitals: Microbiome analysis reveals hidden contaminants. *Journal of Hospital Infection, 104*(2), 207–213. https://doi.org/10.1016/j.jhin.2019.09.010

Simpson, C., Schanler, R. J., & Lau, C. (2002). Early introduction of oral feeding in preterm infants. *Pediatrics, 110*(3), 517–522. https://doi.org/10.1542/peds.110.3.517

Smithson, L., Baird, T., Tamana, S. K., Lau, A., Mariasine, J., Chikuma, J., Lefebvre, D. L., Subbarao, P., Becker, A. B., Turvey, S. E., Sears, M. R., CHILD Study Investigators, Beal, D. S., Pei, J., & Mandhane, P. J. (2018). Shorter sleep duration is associated with reduced cognitive development at two years of age. *Sleep Medicine, 48*, 131–139. https://doi.org/10.1016/j.sleep.2018.04.005

Snyder, R., Herdt, A., Mejias-Cepeda, N., Ladino, J., Crowley, K., & Levy, P. (2017). Early provision of oropharyngeal colostrum leads to sustained breast milk feedings in preterm infants. *Pediatrics and Neonatology, 58*(6), 534–540. https://doi.org/10.1016/j.pedneo.2017.04.003

Soghier, L. M., Kritikos, K. I., Carty, C. L., Glass, P., Tuchman, L. K., Streisand, R., & Fratantoni, K. R. (2020). Parental depression symptoms at neonatal intensive care unit discharge and associated risk factors. *Journal of Pediatrics, 227*, 163. https://doi.org/ 10.1016/j.jpeds.2020.07.040

Spilker, A., Hill, C., & Rosenblum, R. (2016). The effectiveness of a standardised position-ing tool and bedside education on the developmental positioning proficiency of NICU nurses. *Intensive and Critical Care Nursing, 35*, 10–15. https://doi.org/10.1016/j .iccn.2016.01.004

Spittle, A. J., Cameron, K., Doyle, L. W., & Cheong, J. L. (2018). Motor impairment trends in extremely preterm children: 1991–2005. *Pediatrics, 141*(4), 1–8. https://doi.org/10.1542/ peds.2017-3410

Spittle, A. T. K. (2016). The role of early developmental intervention to influence neurobe-havioral outcomes of children born preterm. *Seminars in Perinatology, 40*(8), 542–548. https://doi.org/10.1053/j.semperi.2016.09.006

Standley, J. M., & Gutierrez, C. (2020). Benefits of a comprehensive evidence-based NICU-MT program: Family-centered, neurodevelopmental music therapy for premature infants. *Pediatric Nursing, 46*(1), 40–46.

Stoll, B. J., Hansen, N. I., Bell, E. F., Shankaran, S., Laptook, A. R., Walsh, M. C., Hale, E. C., Newman, N. S., Schibler, K., Carlo, W. A., Kennedy, K. A., Poindexter, B. B., Finer, N. N., Ehrenkranz, R. A., Duara, S., Sánchez, P. J., O'Shea, T. M., Goldberg, R. N., Van Meurs, K. P., . . . Eunice Kennedy Shriver National Institute of Chi. (2010). Neonatal outcomes of extremely preterm infants from the NICHD neonatal research network. *Pediatrics, 126*, 443–456. https://doi.org/10.1542/peds.2009-2959

Symes, A. (2016). Developmental outcomes. In M. G. MacDonald & M. M. Seshia (Eds.), *Avery's neonatology: Pathophysiology & management of the newborn* (7th ed., pp. 1157–1168). Wolters Kluwer.

Synnes, A., & Hicks, M. (2018). Neurodevelopmental outcomes of preterm children at school age and beyond. *Clinics in Perinatology, 45*(3), 393–408. https://doi.org/10.1016/ j.clp.2018.05.002

Tarullo, A., Balsam, P., & Fifer, W. (2011). Sleep and infant learning. *Infant and Child Development, 20*, 35–46. https://doi.org/10.1002/icd.685

Tataranno, M. L., & Benders, M. M. J. N. L. (2019). The effects of early stress and pain on brain development in extremely preterm infants. *Psychoneuroendocrinology, 107*, 69–70. https://doi.org/10.1016/j.psyneuen.2019.07.200

Tataranno, M. L., Gui, L., Hellström-Westas, L., Toet, M., Groenendaal, F., Claessens, N. H. P., Schuurmans, J., Fellman, V., Sävman, K., de Vries, L. S., Huppi, P., & Benders, M. J. N. L. (2020). Morphine affects brain activity and volumes in preterms: An observational multi-center study. *Early Human Development, 144*, 104970. https://doi.org/10.1016/ j.earlhumdev.2020.104970

Thomas, K. A. (2000). Differential effects of breast- and formula-feeding on preterm infants' sleep-wake patterns. *Journal of Obstetric, Gynecologic, and Neonatal Nursing, 29*(2), 145–152. https://doi.org/10.1111/j.1552-6909.2000.tb02034.x

Thompson, J. M. D., Tanabe, K., Moon, R. Y., Mitchell, E. A., McGarvey, C., Tappin, D., Blair, P. S., & Hauck, F. R. (2017). Duration of breastfeeding and risk of SIDS: An individual participant data meta-analysis. *Pediatrics, 140*(5), e20171324. https://doi.org/10.1542/peds.2017-1324

Thoyre, S. M., Pados, B. F., Shaker, C. S., Fuller, K., & Park, J. (2018). Psychometric proper-ties of the early feeding skills assessment tool. *Advances in Neonatal Care, 18*(5), E13–E23. https://doi.org/10.1097/ANC.0000000000000537

Tomlin, A., Deloian, B., & Wollesen, L. (2016). Infant/early childhood mental health and collaborative partnerships: Beyond the NICU. *Newborn and Infant Nursing Reviews, 16*(4), 309–315. https://doi.org/10.1053/j.nainr.2016.09.025

Tommiska, V., Lano, A., Kleemola, P., Klenberg, L., Lehtonen, L., Löppönen, T., Olsen, P., Tammela, O., Fellman, V., & Finnish ELBW Cohort Study Group. (2020). Analysis of neurodevelopmental outcomes of preadolescents born with extremely low weight revealed impairments in multiple developmental domains despite absence of cognitive impairment. *Health Science Reports, 3*(3), e180. https://doi.org/10.1002/hsr2.180

Tracy, M., Ryan, L., Samarasekara, H., Leroi, M., Polkinghorne, A., & Branley, J. (2020). Removal of sinks and bathing changes to control multidrug-resistant Gram-negative bacteria in a neonatal intensive care unit: A retrospective investigation. *Journal of Hospital Infection, 104*(4), 508–510. https://doi.org/10.1016/j.jhin.2020.01.014

Turk, E., van den Heuvel, M. I., Benders, M. J., de Heus, R., Franx, A., Manning, J. H., Hect, J. L., Hernandez-Andrade, E., Hassan, S. S., Romero, R., Kahn, R. S., Thomason, M. E., & van den Heuvel, M. P. (2019). Functional connectome of the fetal brain. *Journal of Neuroscience, 39*(49), 9716–9724. https://doi.org/10.1523/JNEUROSCI.2891-18.2019

Twilhaar, E. S., Wade, R. M., de Kieviet, J. F., van Goudoever, J. B., van Elburg, R. M., & Oosterlaan, J. (2018). Cognitive outcomes of children born extremely or very preterm since the 1990s and associated risk factors: A meta-analysis and meta-regression. *Obstetrical and Gynecological Survey, 73*(10), 562–563. https://doi.org/10.1097/01.ogx .0000547169.91377.70

UNICEF. (1989). *What is the Convention on the Rights of the Child.* https://www.unicef.org/ child-rights-convention/what-is-the-convention

Valeri, B., Holsti, L., & Linhares, M. (2015). Neonatal pain and developmental outcomes in children born preterm. *Clinical Journal of Pain, 31*(4), 355–362. https://doi.org/10.1097/ AJP.0000000000000114

Valeri, B. O., Ranger, M., Chau, C. M. Y., Cepeda, I. L., Synnes, A., Linhares, M. B. M., & Grunau, R. E. (2016). Neonatal invasive procedures predict pain intensity at school age in children born very preterm. *Clinical Journal of Pain, 32*(12), 1086–1093. https://doi .org/10.1097/AJP.0000000000000353

van Veenendaal, N. R., van der Schoor, S. R. D., Heideman, W. H., Rijnhart, J. J. M., Heymans, M. W., Twisk, J. W. R., van Goudoever, J. B., & van Kempen, A. A. M. W. (2020). Family integrated care in single family rooms for preterm infants and late-onset sepsis: A retrospective study and mediation analysis. *Pediatric Research, 88*(4), 593–600. https://doi.org/10.1038/s41390-020-0875-9

Vance, A. J., & Brandon, D. H. (2017). Delineating among parenting confidence, parenting self-efficacy, and competence. *Advances in Nursing Science, 40*(4), E18–E37. https://doi .org/10.1097/ANS.0000000000000179

Vasung, L., Abaci Turk, E., Ferradal, S. L., Sutin, J., Stout, J. N., Ahtam, B., Lin, P. Y., & Grant, P. E. (2019). Exploring early human brain development with structural and physiological neuroimaging. *NeuroImage, 187*, 226–254. https://doi.org/10.1016/j.neuroimage.2018.07.041

Venkataraman, R., Kamaluddeen, M., Amin, H., & Lodha, A. (2018). Is less noise, light and parental/caregiver stress in the neonatal intensive care unit better for neonates? *Indian Pediatrics, 55*(1), 17–21. https://doi.org/10.1007/s13312-018-1220-9

Verriotis, M., Chang, P., Fitzgerald, M., & Fabrizi, L. (2016). The development of the nociceptive brain. *Neuroscience, 338*, 207–219. https://doi.org/10.1016/j.neuroscience.2016.07.026

Vinall, J., Miller, S. P., Bjornson, B. H., Fitzpatrick, K. P., Poskitt, K. J., Brant, R., Synnes, A. R., Cepeda, I. L., & Grunau, R. E. (2014). Invasive procedures in preterm children: Brain and cognitive development at school age. *Pediatrics, 133*, 412–421. https://doi.org/10.1542/ peds.2013-1863

Vinall, J., Noel, M., Disher, T., Caddell, K., & Campbell-Yeo, M. (2018). Memories of infant pain in the neonatal intensive care unit influence posttraumatic stress symptoms in mothers of infants born preterm. *Clinical Journal of Pain, 34*(10), 936–943. https://doi .org/10.1097/AJP.0000000000000620

Visscher, M., Adam, R., Brink, S., & Odio, M. (2015). Newborn infant skin: Physiology, development, and care. *Clinics in Dermatology, 33*(3), 271–280. https://doi.org/10.1016/j.clindermatol.2014.12.003

Visscher, M., & Narendran, V. (2014). Neonatal infant skin: Development, structure and function. *Newborn and Infant Nursing Reviews, 14*(4), 135–141. https://doi.org/10.1053/j.nainr.2014.10.004

Vittner, D., Butler, S., Smith, K., Makris, N., Brownell, E., Samra, H., & McGrath, J. (2019). Parent engagement correlates with parent and preterm infant oxytocin release during skin-to-skin contact. *Advances in Neonatal Care, 19*(1), 73–79. https://doi.org/10.1097/ANC.0000000000000558

Vittner, D., McGrath, J., Robinson, J., Lawhon, G., Cusson, R., Eisenfeld, L., Walsh, S., Young, E., & Cong, X. (2018). Increase in oxytocin from skin-to-skin contact enhances development of parent-infant relationship. *Biological Research for Nursing, 20*(1), 54–62. https://doi.org/10.1177/1099800417735633

Vohr, B., McGowan, E., McKinley, L., Tucker, R., Keszler, L., & Alksninis, B. (2017). Differential effects of the single-family room neonatal intensive care unit on 18- to 24-month Bayley scores of preterm infants. *Journal of Pediatrics, 185*, 42–48 e41. https://doi.org/10.1016/j.jpeds.2017.01.056

Wachman, E. M., & Lahav, A. (2011). The effects of noise on preterm infants in the NICU. *Archives of Disease in Childhood. Fetal and Neonatal Edition, 96*(4), F305–309. https://doi.org/10.1136/adc.2009.182014

Waitzman, K., Ludwig, S., & Nelson, C. (2014). Contributing to content validity of the Infant-Driven Feeding Scales© through Delphi surveys. *Newborn and Infant Nursing Reviews, 14*(3), 88–91. https://doi.org/10.1053/j.nainr.2014.06.010

Wallace, M. T., & Stein, B. E. (2007). Early experience determines how the senses will inter-act. *Journal of Neurophysiology, 97*(1), 921–926. https://doi.org/10.1152/jn.00497.2006

Weber, P., Depoorter, A., Hetzel, P., & Lemola, S. (2016). Habituation as parameter for prediction of mental development in healthy preterm infants: An electrophysiological pilot study. *Journal of Child Neurology, 31*(14), 1591–1597. https://doi.org/10.1177/0883073816665312

Weinhold, B. (2006). Epigenetics: The science of change. *Environmental Health Perspectives, 114*(3), A160–A167. https://doi.org/10.1289/ehp.114-a160

Welch, M. G., Barone, J. L., Porges, S. W., Hane, A. A., Kwon, K. Y., Ludwig, R. J., Stark, R. I., Surman, A. L., Kolacz, J., & Myers, M. M. (2020). Family nurture intervention in the NICU increases autonomic regulation in mothers and children at 4–5 years of age: Follow-up results from a randomized controlled trial. *PLoS One, 15*(8), e0236930. https://doi.org/10.1371/journal.pone.0236930

Welch, M. G., Grieve, P. G., Barone, J. L., Ludwig, R. J., Stark, R. I., Isler, J. R., & Myers, M. M. (2020). Family nurture intervention alters relationships between preterm infant EEG delta brush characteristics and term age EEG power. *Clinical Neurophysiology, 131*(8), 1909–1916. https://doi.org/10.1016/j.clinph.2020.05.020

Welch, M. G., & Ludwig, R. J. (2017a). Calming cycle theory and the co-regulation of oxytocin. *Psychodynamic Psychiatry, 45*(4), 519–541. https://doi.org/10.1521/pdps.2017.45.4.519

Welch, M. G., & Ludwig, R. J. (2017b). Mother/infant emotional communication through the lens of visceral/autonomic learning. In M. Filippa, P. Kuhn, & B. Westrup (Eds.), *Early vocal contact and preterm infant brain development: Bridging the gaps between research and practice* (pp. 271–294). Springer Publishing Company.

Wendt, C., Wiesenthal, B., Dietz, E., & Rüden, H. (1998). Survival of vancomycin-resistant and vancomycin-susceptible enterococci on dry surfaces. *Journal of Clinical Microbiology, 36*(12), 3734–3736. https://doi.org/10.1128/JCM.36.12.3734-3736.1998

Weng, M. K., Brooks, R. B., Glowicz, J., Keckler, M. S., Christensen, B. E., Tsai, V., Mitchell, C. S., Wilson, L. E., Laxton, R., Moulton-Meissner, H., & Fagan, R. (2019). Outbreak investigation of *Pseudomonas aeruginosa* infections in a neonatal intensive care unit. *American Journal of Infection Control, 47*(9), 1148–1150. https://doi.org/10.1016/j.ajic.2019.03.009

Westrup, B. (2015). Family-centered developmentally supportive care: The Swedish example. *Archives De Pédiatrie, 22*(10), 1086–1091. https://doi.org/10.1016/j.arcped.2015.07.005

White, R. D. (2010). Single-family room design in the neonatal intensive care unit—challenges and opportunities. *Newborn and Infant Nursing Reviews, 10*(2), 83–86. https://doi.org/10.1053/j.nainr.2010.03.011

White, R. D. (2011). The newborn intensive care unit environment of care: How we got here, where we're headed, and why. *Seminars in Perinatology, 35*(1), 2–7. https://doi.org/10.1053/j.semperi.2010.10.002

White, R. D. (2015). Neuroprotective core measure 4: Safeguarding sleep—Its value in neuroprotection of the newborn. *Newborn and Infant Nursing Reviews, 15*, 114–115. https://doi.org/10.1053/j.nainr.2015.06.012

White, R. D. (2016). The next big ideas in NICU design. *Journal of Perinatology, 36*(4), 259–262. https://doi.org/10.1038/jp.2016.6

White, R. D. (2017). Circadian variation of breast milk components and implications for care. *Breastfeeding Medicine, 12*(7), 398–400. https://doi.org/10.1089/bfm.2017.0070

White, R. D. (2018). Defining the optimal sensory environment in the NICU: An elusive task. *Acta Paediatrica, 107*(7), 1. https://doi.org/10.1111/apa.14296

White, R. D. (2020a). Next steps in newborn intensive care unit design and developmental care. *Journal of Perinatology, 40*, 1–1. https://doi.org/10.1038/s41372-020-0748-4

White, R. D. (2020b). Recommended standards for newborn ICU design, 9th edition. *Journal of Perinatology, 40*, 2–4. https://doi.org/10.1038/s41372-020-0766-2

White, R. D. (2020c). Right lighting the NICU. *Acta Paediatrica, 109*(7), 1288–1289. https://doi.org/10.1111/apa.15193

Whitehead, K., Laudiano-Dray, M., Meek, J., & Fabrizi, L. (2018). Emergence of mature cortical activity in wakefulness and sleep in healthy preterm and full-term infants. *Sleep, 41*(8). https://doi.org/10.1093/sleep/zsy096

Wiley, F., Raphael, R., & Ghanouni, P. (2020). NICU positioning strategies to reduce stress in preterm infants: A scoping review. *Early Child Development and Care.* https://doi.org/10.1080/03004430.2019.1707815

Winkler, M. R., Park, J., Pan, W., Brandon, D. H., Scher, M., & Holditch-Davis, D. (2017). Does preterm period sleep development predict early childhood growth trajectories? *Journal of Perinatology, 37*(9), 1047–1052. https://doi.org/10.1038/jp.2017.91

Wittkowski, A., Garrett, C., Calam, R., & Weisberg, D. (2017). Self-report measures of parental self-efficacy: A systematic review of the current literature. *Journal of Child and Family Studies, 26*(11), 2960–2978. https://doi.org/10.1007/s10826-017-0830-5

Wolfe, K., & Ralls, F. M. (2019). Rapid eye movement sleep and neuronal development. *Current Opinion in Pulmonary Medicine, 25*(6), 555–560. https://doi.org/10.1097/MCP.0000000000000622

Wu, Y.-H., Chen, C.-J., Wu, H.-Y., Chen, I., Chang, Y.-H., Yang, P.-H., Wang, T. Y., Chen, L. C., Liu, K. T., Yeh, I. J., Wu, D. C., Hou, M. F., Liu, H. L., & Su, W.-H. (2020). Plastic wrap combined with alcohol wiping is an effective method of preventing bacterial colonization on mobile phones. *Medicine, 99*(44), e22910. https://doi.org/10.1097/MD.00000000000022910

Xie, S., Heuvelman, H., Magnusson, C., Rai, D., Lyall, K., Newschaffer, C. J., Dalman, C., Lee, B. K., & Abel, K. (2017). Prevalence of autism spectrum disorders with and without intellectual disability by gestational age at birth in the Stockholm Youth Cohort: A Register Linkage Study. *Paediatric and Perinatal Epidemiology, 31*(6), 586–594. https://doi.org/10.1111/ppe.12413

Zauche, L. H., Zauche, M. S., & Williams, B. L. (2021). Influence of quiet time on the auditory environment of infants in the NICU. *Journal of Obstetric, Gynecologic and Neonatal Nursing, 50*(1), 68–77. https://doi.org/10.1016/j.jogn.2020.09.159

Zeanah, C. H. (2019). *Handbook of infant mental health* (4th ed.). Guilford.

Zores, C., Dufour, A., Pebayle, T., Dahan, I., Astruc, D., & Kuhn, P. (2018). Observational study found that even small variations in light can wake up very preterm infants in a neonatal intensive care unit. *Acta Paediatrica, 107*(7), 1191–1197. https://doi.org/10.1111/apa.14261

Zores-Koenig, C., Kuhn, P., & Caeymaex, L. (2020). Recommendations on neonatal light environment from the French Neonatal Society. *Acta Paediatrica, 109*(7), 1292–1301. https://doi.org/10.1111/apa.15173

Zwicker, J. G., Miller, S. P., Grunau, R. E., Chau, V., Brant, R., Studholme, C., Liu, M., Synnes, A., Poskitt, K. J., Stiver, M. L., & Tam, E. W. Y. (2016). Smaller cerebellar growth and poorer neurodevelopmental outcomes in very preterm infants exposed to neonatal morphine. *The Journal of Pediatrics, 172*, 81–87e82. https://doi.org/10.1016/j.jpeds.2015.12.024

Trauma-Informed Developmental Care

MARY COUGHLIN, TARA DEWOLFE, AND KRISTY FULLER

OVERVIEW

The adverse childhood experience (ACE) study was the largest investigation into the relationship between childhood adversity and adult morbidity and mortality (Felitti et al., 1998). Replicated across a multitude of demographic populations, the results stand firm. Adversity in childhood negatively impacts health and wellness across the life span. Infants across all gestational ages requiring newborn intensive care are exposed to a myriad of traumatic experiences ranging from painful and stressful procedures, sleep fragmentation, and social isolation, to maternal separation (Montirosso et al., 2017). For the family, NICU hospitalization has been described as a traumatic event that shatters hopes, dreams, and expectations for parenthood. Finally, research has shown that clinicians repeatedly exposed to the suffering of others become vulnerable to compassion fatigue, secondary trauma, burnout, and posttraumatic stress disorder. Acknowledging the nature of traumatic experiences endured by infants, families, and clinicians within the setting of intensive critical care assists in identifying and developing strategies aimed at reducing traumatization and retraumatization while creating effective compassionate caring encounters. Trauma-informed developmental care invites us to move past procedure-driven practices and create a culture of care that focuses on the human experience of critical care for the infant, the family, and the clinician. This requires a shift in mindset, intention, and language. As language shapes the way we think, act, and perceive the world around us, the words we choose to describe the experiences we create and the individuals we serve frame how we engage with others.

DEFINITIONS

What is trauma? Trauma results from an event, a series of events, or a set of circumstances that is experienced by an individual as physically and/or emotionally harmful or life-threatening and has lasting adverse effects on the individual's functioning and mental, physical, social, emotional, or spiritual well-being (Substance Abuse and Mental Health Services Administration [SAMHSA], 2014). Within the context of the infant in the NICU, trauma experiences can be big or small and may include

TABLE 12.1 Examples of Trauma for the Infant, the Family, and the Clinician

INFANT	FAMILY	CLINICIAN
■ Maternal separation/ deprivation ■ Social isolation ■ Unsafe eating experiences ■ Unmanaged/undermanaged pain and stress ■ Fragmented/disrupted sleep	■ Separation ■ Fear of the unknown ■ Loss of control ■ Role confusion ■ Uncertainty of survival/ outcome	■ Bearing witness ■ Understaffing ■ Professional practice ■ Environment

anything from life-threatening illness to the day-to-day experiences of parental separation, fragmented sleep, a disruptive environment, painful experiences, stressful eating encounters, limited mobility, prolonged time in bed, and more. Table 12.1 presents examples of traumatic experiences in the NICU for the infant, family, and clinician.

What is a trauma-informed approach to care? A trauma-informed approach realizes the widespread impact of trauma; recognizes the signs and symptoms of trauma in patients, families, colleagues, and self; responds by fully integrating knowledge about trauma into policies, procedures, and practices; and seeks to actively resist re-traumatization.

What is trauma-informed language? Trauma-informed language acknowledges the personhood of the individual and reflects an awareness of our shared human experiences, our shared humanity.

Examples of trauma-informed language include

■ referring to an individual by their name and *not* their diagnosis and

■ using language that reflects "being with" another person and *not* "doing to" another person (e.g., supporting a pleasant eating experience vs. feeding the infant and supporting postural alignment vs. positioning the infant).

PHYSIOLOGY OF TOXIC STRESS AND TRAUMA

Adverse early-life experiences lead to disruptions, dysregulation, and perturbations of the developing human during critical and sensitive periods of development mediated by the hypothalamic–pituitary–adrenal (HPA) axis and the stress response system. Individual vulnerabilities such as genetic background, fetal programming, timing, duration, and intensity of the stressor, coupled with varied coping strategies and social supports, all have implications for the long-term biopsychological effects of early-life adversity to include medical and childhood trauma on infants and families (Agorastos et al., 2019). Fragmented, unpredictable patterns of maternal care, aberrant rhythms of early sensory input, and other social determinants of health influence the developmental trajectory and maturation of cognitive and emotional brain circuits (Blaze et al., 2015; Chen & Baram, 2016; Glynn & Baram, 2019; Weber & Harrison, 2018).

Research indicates that early-life adversity amplifies bidirectional communication between peripheral inflammation and neural circuitry responsible for the threat and reward system, as well as executive control (Nusslock & Miller, 2016). These adverse experiences sensitize the corticoamygdala region of the brain responsible for threat detection and response, as well as systemic immune cells responsible for the propagation of inflammation. Chronic perceived threat sets up a low-grade inflammatory reaction, both peripherally and centrally, which undermines and eventually degrades homeostatic integrity, leading to HPA axis dysregulation, oxidative stress, cytotoxicity, and epigenetic modifications. These epigenetic modifications have been linked to reduced brain volumes at hospital discharge and alterations in socioemotional development (Fumagalli et al., 2018).

As depicted in the ecobiodevelopmental framework put forth by the American Academy of Pediatrics, environmental experiences, both physical and social, are appraised by the individual as stressful or not. These experiences prompt a biological adaptation, which may become maladaptive over time, leading to derailed life-long health and development (Shonkoff et al., 2012). Experiences elicit an emotional response that is detected at the subcortical level of the central nervous system, which then activates an appropriate physiologic response (Sanders & Hall, 2018). In the case of experiences appraised as stressful, a negative emotional response prompts activation of the sympathetic adrenal medullary (SAM) pathway and the HPA axis, which drive physiologic changes in response to the stressor (Godoy et al., 2018). As an individual appraises a situation as stressful and experiences negative emotions, the stress response transitions from acute to chronic stress, producing an allostatic load. This phenomenon can become a self-perpetuating cycle unraveling biologic integrity when the stress experience is not buffered and the affected individual is not able to experience a felt sense of safety, security, and connectedness (Sanders & Hall, 2018).

NEUROSCIENTIFIC AND SOCIOEMOTIONAL CONSEQUENCES OF TOXIC STRESS IN THE NEONATAL INTENSIVE CARE UNIT

Prolonged activation of the stress response system during early life, in the absence of the buffering effect of maternal care, results in an allostatic load that induces:

- Immunosuppression
- Oxidative damage
- Aberrant metabolic modulation

- Stimulation of bacterial growth
- Increased oxygen consumption
- Compromised cardiac function (Casavant, Cong, Fitch, et al., 2019; Weber & Harrison, 2018)

Prematurity has been referred to as a traumatic beginning requiring intensive critical care management confounded by toxic stress and reduced exposure to the buffering effects of maternal care (Karr-Morse, 2012; Montirosso & Provenzi, 2015).

Research has found connections between highly stressful experiences in children and an increased risk for later mental illnesses including:

- Generalized anxiety disorder
- Major depressive disorders
- Poorer emotion regulation
- Increased risk for suicide (Blasco-Fontcella et al., 2013; Lammertink et al., 2020; Montagna & Nosarti, 2016; Nosarti et al., 2012)

Atypical stress responses over a lifetime can also result in increased risk for physical ailments to include:

- Cardiovascular disease
- Metabolic syndromes
- Obesity
- Fibromyalgia
- Migraines
- Central sensitizing syndromes (Basch et al., 2015; Lewandowski et al., 2013; Low & Schweinhardt, 2012; Posod et al., 2016; Tinnion et al., 2014)

Implications of Toxic Stress

Infants

- Early adverse experiences affect gene expression through epigenetic mechanisms, which alter developmental trajectories in preterm infants (Casavant, Cong, Moore, et al., 2019; Provenzi et al., 2015).
- Greater pain-related stress was related to increased DNA methylation from birth to discharge, and at 3 months, the methylation level was associated with temperamental difficulties and increased negativity in response to social stress (Casavant, Cong, Moore, et al., 2019; Provenzi et al., 2015).
- Adverse experiences associated with NICU practices increase demands for energy, which further deplete preterm infants' limited resources (Casavant, Cong, Moore, et al., 2019; Provenzi et al., 2015).

Family

- Mothers of preterm newborns scored significantly greater on measures of distress (27.3% vs. 3.7%) and depression (15.1% vs. 3.7%) than mothers of full term, healthy newborns (Roque et al., 2017).
- Twenty percent of fathers and 24% of mothers reported symptoms of anxiety, and almost a third (30.8%) of fathers and 35% of mothers reported depression symptoms (Roque et al., 2017).
- Studies showed a greater incidence (52%) of posttraumatic stress symptoms 2 weeks after birth, as well as clinically significant depression (28%) and anxiety (17%; Roque et al., 2017).

Clinicians

- Compassion fatigue, burnout (Lipsky, 2009; Reith, 2018)
- Absenteeism and/or presenteeism (Gillet et al., 2020)

■ Trauma exposure responses (see the following "Clinical Manifestations" section; Lipsky, 2009)

Certain types of stress-induced epigenetic modifications can be reversed and function restored when infants are supported during stressful experiences facilitating the development of resilience.

NURSING INTENTION AND ASSESSMENT

Intention

When approaching caregiving and assessment, the clinician must consider the intention for the caring moment. When one is able to come from a place of alignment and conscious awareness, they are able to be more present within that moment. Infants make meaning out of the world based on how the world makes them feel (Korl et al., 2019; Tronick & Beeghly, 2011). Questions to consider during a caring encounter include the following:

■ Does the baby feel safe, secure, and/or connected?

■ Do they feel unsafe, insecure, and/or isolated?

One effective strategy that supports presence and intention in a caring encounter is practicing G.R.A.C.E. (Halifax, 2014). This mnemonic was developed by Joan Halifax, a Buddhist nun, when working with palliative care, end-of-life nurses. Disengaging from the human experience of those we serve denies us the joy that is inherent in intentionally easing the suffering of another human being. The practice of nursing is deeply embedded in relationships and the cultivation and expression of compassion (Halifax, 2014). Grounded in Dr. Halifax's model of compassion, the G.R.A.C.E. intervention suggests as follows:

■ Gathering attention

■ Recalling intention

■ Attuning to self and others

■ Considering what will serve in the moment

■ Engaging and ending

These elements allow nurses to pause and become aware and present for the caring encounter, priming them to cultivate more compassion in life and with those they enagage with.

Assessment

Assessment begins with observation. Given the highly technical and task-based nature of NICU care, one can easily overlook the language of the baby. All behavior is communication, and behavior is the primary mode of communication of babies, informing their foundational relationship with the world around them, answering the question, Is the world a safe and secure place, or is the world a scary and insecure place? The socioemotional foundation for infants begins with a felt sense of safety, sense of security, and sense of connectedness (Sanders & Hall, 2018).

The Developmental Participation Skills (DPS) Assessment tool is an observational tool designed to guide the clinician in assessing:

1. An infant's readiness for a caring encounter
2. The quality of the infant's participation in the encounter
3. If an opportunity exists for the clinician to reflect on the cost of the caring encounter determined by the infant's autonomic and systemic stability

The DPS *Readiness for Caregiving* section of the tool offers a trauma-informed way to interpret and respect infant communication and readiness for a care encounter (Fuller et al., 2021). See Box 12.1.

BOX 12.1   Developmental Participation Skills Assessment Tool Readiness Portion

Readiness for Caregiving Interaction	
Baby does not wake or show signs of readiness for care. Minimal fluctuations in autonomic system (heart rate, breathing, and oxygen saturations).	1
Baby is beginning to stir but remains drowsy or returns to sleep. Limited rooting and/or minimal active hands to face and mouth. May show fluctuations in heart rate or have fast breathing.	2
Baby is awake prior to caregiving. Beginning to show signs of readiness for care. May show fluctuations in heart rate and have variable breathing. Baby may require more than 2L breathing support.	3
Baby is beginning to stir but initially drowsy. Begins to wake, showing signs of readiness for care and eating through rooting/mouthing/sucking. Steady breathing less than 60 breaths per minute. Baby on 2L or less oxygen.	4
Baby is awake prior to caregiving. Showing more eager signs of readiness for care and eating through rooting/mouthing/sucking. Steady breathing less than 60 breaths per minute. Baby on 2L or less oxygen. *(If baby meets all of the previous criteria, but on greater than 2L of oxygen, score = 3)*	5

Readiness Indications for Care (Skin-to-Skin Holding Is Always Encouraged Regardless of Readiness Score)

1—Protect sleep. Provide only medically necessary care for urgent needs or adjustments to promote stability and comfort.
2 and 3—Greet baby. Initiate supportive, caring interaction. Offer pleasurable, nurturing experience and/or opportunity at breast.
4 and 5—Greet baby. Initiate supportive, caring interaction. Offer pleasurable, nurturing prefeeding or eating experience (breast OR bottle).

Source: Fuller, K., DeWolfe, T., & Coughlin, M. (2021). *The Developmental Participation Skills assessment: development and content validation.* Manuscript submitted for publication. Reprinted with Permission from Caring Essentials Collaborative, LLC.

CLINICAL MANIFESTATIONS: WHAT DOES TRAUMA EXPOSURE LOOK LIKE?

Within the Caregiving Experience

Throughout each caregiver interaction, the trauma-informed clinician is attuned to the physiological and behavioral communication of the infant. Clinical manifestations of stress and pain include changes within the subsystems of autonomic, motor, state, attention/interaction, and self-regulation as defined by the synactive theory (Als, 1982). The absence of clinical manifestations does not exclude the presence of stress or pain, and the sensitively attuned trauma-informed clinician is able to adjust caregiving in order to provide the most nurturing, supportive experience.

Examples of Distress Indicators in Babies

Early Signs of Stress

It is key to recognize the early signs of stress in order to respond, pause, make adjustments in care, and/or offer additional support to prevent further stress and dysregulation.

- Eyebrows raised (one or both)
- Eyelid flutter or blinking
- Furrowed brow
- Worried look
- Looking away
- Finger splay
- Clenched toes/fists
- Hiccups or yawning

Late Signs of Stress

An infant who is not adequately supported or is unable to competently use the support provided may have more serious and lasting consequences.

- Facial grimace
- Gape face
- Pulling or turning away
- Flailing or stop sign
- Tense body or limp body
- Fussing/crying
- Decrease in oxygen saturation
- Shutdown
- Rapid state transitions
- Increased work of breathing
- Breath holding
- Fast or slow heart rate
- Blood pressure changes
- Color changes

Examples of Distress Indicators in Families

- Anger
- Cynicism
- Withdrawal
- Abruptness
- Emotional lability
- Anxiety

Examples of Trauma Exposure Responses in Clinicians

■ Feeling helpless and hopeless
■ A sense that one can never do enough
■ Hypervigilance
■ Diminished creativity
■ Inability to embrace complexity
■ Minimizing
■ Chronic exhaustion/physical ailments
■ Inability to listen/deliberate avoidance

■ Dissociative moments
■ Sense of persecution
■ Guilt
■ Fear
■ Anger/cynicism
■ Inability to empathize/numbing
■ Addictions
■ Grandiosity: an inflated sense of importance related to one's work

(Lipsky, 2009)

Throughout the Neonatal Intensive Care Unit Experience

Signs and symptoms of trauma manifest within the infant, the family, and the clinician. The daily stress of the NICU experience is cumulative. Examples of signs and symptoms of trauma are listed in the following:

Infant signs and symptoms of trauma

■ Exaggerated responses to acute stress; intense fight-or-flight responses

■ Hyporeactivity and/or immobilization to increasing stress; fright-and-freeze responses

■ Feeding intolerance

■ Sympathetic nervous system arousal

■ Autonomic dysregulation

■ Poor weight gain

Family signs and symptoms of trauma

■ Feelings of guilt and inadequacy in parental role

■ Less affectionate and less responsive to their infant; withdrawn, flat affect; and/or hostility or intrusiveness with their infant

■ Fatigue and sleep disruptions

■ Protracted sadness and worry

■ Hypervigilance and avoidance behaviors

■ Physical and emotional withdrawal

Clinician signs and symptoms of trauma

■ Hypervigilance, diminished creativity, an inability to embrace complexity, minimizing, chronic exhaustion and physical ailments, inability to listen/deliberate avoidance, dissociative moments, sense of persecution, guilt, fear, anger and cynicism, inability to empathize/numbing, addictions, grandiosity: an inflated sense of importance related to one's work, feeling helpless and hopeless, a sense that one can never do enough

■ Medical errors, patient mortality, hospital-transmitted infections, dishonest behavior, reduced altruism, substance abuse

TREATMENT: BUFFERING THE TRAUMA EXPERIENCE

Figure 12.1 provides a framework of trauma-informed care:

■ The five guiding principles of trauma-informed care

■ The five core measures of trauma-informed care

■ The eight attributes of the Trauma Informed Professional (TIP)

This evidence-based framework embraces all ways of providing trauma-informed developmentally supportive care to ensure consistently reliable, compassionate evidence-based care.

The Five Guiding Principles of a Trauma-Informed Paradigm

Providing trauma-informed care begins with the adoption of the five principles of a trauma-informed paradigm to guide human-to-human interactions.

■ Safety

■ Choice

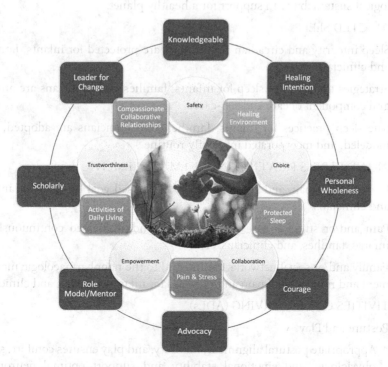

FIGURE 12.1 Framework of the Trauma Informed Professional.
Source: Reprinted with Permission from Caring Essentials Collaborative, LLC

■ Collaboration

■ Empowerment

■ Trustworthiness

The Core Measures of Trauma-Informed Developmental Care

Coughlin (2021) has updated the original disease-independent five core measures for developmentally supportive care (Coughlin et al., 2009) endorsed by the National Association of Neonatal Nurses (Coughlin, 2011, 2016). The current five core measures have implications and relevance for the infant, the family, and the clinician and are listed with their corresponding attributes in the text that follows:

1. HEALING ENVIRONMENT

   ● The physical environment is a soothing, spacious, and aesthetically pleasing healing space conducive to rest, growth, and establishing connectedness.

   ● The human environment emanates compassion, authenticity, and healing intention while preserving the natural world and practicing environmental stewardship.

   ● The organizational environment reflects a commitment to healing spaces and experiences that align with a trauma-informed approach while fostering ecological sustainability in support for a healthy planet.

2. PROTECTED SLEEP

   ● Sleep integrity and circadian rhythmicity are protected for infants, families, and clinicians.

   ● Strategies that support sleep for infants, families, and clinicians are an integral component of care and self-care.

   ● Safe sleep practices for infants, families, and clinicians are adopted, role-modeled, and incorporated into daily routine.

3. PAIN AND STRESS PREVENTION AND MANAGEMENT

   ● Prevention of pain and stress is a daily expressed goal for infants, families, and clinicians.

   ● Pain and/or stress is assessed, managed, and reassessed continuously for infants, families, and clinicians.

   ● Family and/or social networks are integral to the nonpharmacologic management and mitigation of pain and/or stress for infants, families, and clinicians.

4. ACTIVITIES OF DAILY LIVING (ADLs)

   ● Posture and Play

     • Appropriate postural alignment, mobility, and play ensures comfort, safety, physiologic, and emotional stability and support optimal neuromotor integrity for infants, families, and clinicians.

- Eating and Nourishment
    - Eating experiences are positive, pleasant, nurturing, and nourishing for infants, families, and clinicians.
- Skin care and hygiene
    - Appropriate hygiene and skin care routines preserve barrier function and tissue integrity while ensuring a calming and nurturing experience for infants, families, and clinicians.
5. Compassionate Collaborative Relationships
    - Assessing and supporting emotional well-being is a priority.
    - Strategies to cultivate and maintain self-efficacy are mentored, supported, and validated.
    - Communication is consistent, compassionate, and reciprocated with respectful active listening.

The Attributes of the Trauma Informed Professional

Eight attributes of the TIP have been identified by an international, interdisciplinary faculty board of neonatal experts. Meeting the whole-person needs of the baby and family in crisis hinges on the wholeness of the clinician. One cannot give what one does not have; what one does not give to oneself.

Eight Attributes and Competencies of a Trauma Informed Professional

- Knowledgeable
- Healing intention
- Personal wholeness
- Courage
- Advocacy
- Role model and mentor
- Scholarship
- Leader for change

Becoming a TIP begins with unbundling one's passion, mission, and noble purpose from the myriad of tasks, rituals, and routines that often overshadow and overpower one's presence in the caring moment. The attributes provide a road map for personal and professional growth and development that is the cornerstone for cultural transformation within the NICU and beyond.

CONCLUSION

Awareness of the experience of trauma in the NICU for babies, families, and clinicians is a first step to transform and humanize this fragile, yet critical care environment. Trauma-informed care is an effective, compassionate, and evidence-based strategy. Through this paradigm, clinicians are invited to actively buffer the trauma experienced by the babies and families they serve in the NICU and beyond. In mitigating the needless suffering of babies and families, NICU nurses are empowered to transform the experience of intensive care for vulnerable infants, families in crisis, and themselves.

REFERENCES

Agorastos, A., Pervanidou, P., Chrousos, G. P., & Baker, D. G. (2019). Developmental trajectories of early life stress and trauma: A narrative review on neurobiological aspects beyond stress system dysregulation. *Frontiers in Psychiatry, 10,* 118. https://doi.org/10.3389/fpsyt.2019.00118

Als, H. (1982). Toward a synactive theory of development: Promise for the assessment and support of infant individuality. *Infant Mental Health Journal, 3*(4), 229–243. https://doi.org/10.1002/1097-0355(198224)3:4<229::AID-IMHJ2280030405>3.0.CO;2-H

Blasco-Fontecilla, H., Jaussent, I., Olie, E., Garcia, E. B., Beziat, S., Malafosse, A., Guillaume, S., & Courtet, P. (2013). Additive effects between prematurity and postnatal risk factors of suicidal behavior. *Journal of Psychiatric Research, 47*(7), 937–943. https://doi.org/10.1016/j.jpsychires.2013.02.017

Blaze, J., Asok, A., & Roth, T. L. (2015). The long-term impact of adverse caregiving environments on epigenetic modifications and telomeres. *Frontiers in Behavioral Neuroscience, 9*(79), 1–12. https://doi.org/10.3389/fnbeh.2015.00079

Casavant, S. G., Cong, X., Fitch, R. H., Moore, J., Rosenkrantz, T., & Starkweather, A. (2019). Allostatic load and biomarkers of stress in the preterm infant: An integrative review. *Biological Research in Nursing, 21*(2), 210–223. https://doi.org/10.1177/1099800418824415

Casavant, S. G., Cong, X., Moore, J., & Starkweather, A. (2019). Associations between preterm infant stress, epigenetic alterations, telomere length and neurodevelopmental outcome: A systematic review. *Early Human Development, 131,* 63–74. https://doi.org/10.1016/j.earlhumdev.2019.03.003

Chen, Y., & Baram, T. Z. (2016). Toward understanding how early-life stress reprograms cognitive and emotional brain networks. *Neuropsychopharmacology, 41*(1), 197–206. https://doi.org/10.1038/npp.2015.181

Coughlin, M. (2011). *Age-appropriate care of the premature and critically ill hospitalized infant: Guideline for practice.* National Association of Neonatal Nurses.

Coughlin, M. (2016). *Trauma-informed care in the NICU: Evidence-based practice guidelines for neonatal clinicians.* Springer Publishing Company.

Coughlin, M. (2021). *Transformative nursing in the NICU: Trauma-informed, age-appropriate care* (2nd ed.). Springer Publishing Company.

Coughlin, M., Gibbins, S., & Hoath, S. (2009). Core measures for developmentally supportive care in neonatal intensive care: Theory, precedence and practice. *Journal of Advanced Nursing, 65* (10), 2239–2248. https://doi.org/10.1111/j.1365-2648.2009.05052.x

Felitti, V. J., Anda, R. F., Nordenberg, D., Williamson, D. F., Spitz, A. M., Edwards. V., Koss, M. P., & Marks, J. S. (1998). Relationship of childhood abuse and household dysfunction to many leading causes of death in adults. The adverse childhood experience (ACE) study. *American Journal of Preventive Medicine, 14*(4), 245–258. https://doi.org/10.1016/s0749-3797(98)00017-8

Fuller, K., DeWolfe, T., & Coughlin, M. (2021). *The Developmental Participation Skills assessment: Development and content validation.* Manuscript submitted for publication.

Fumagalli, M., Provenzi, L., De Carli, P., Dessimone, F., Sirgiovanni, I., Giorda, R., Cinnante, C., Squarcina, L., Pozzoli, U., Triulzi, F., Brambilla, P., Borgatti, R., Mosca, F., & Montirosso, R. (2018). From early stress to 12-month development in very preterm infants: Preliminary findings on epigenetic mechanisms and brain growth. *PLoS One, 13,* e0190602. https://doi.org/10.1371/journal.pone.0190602

Gillet, N., Huyghebaert-Zouaghi, T., Reveillere, C., Colombat, P., & Fouquereau, E. (2020). The effects of job demands on nurses' burnout and presenteeism through sleep quality and relaxation. *Journal of Clinical Nursing, 29*(3–4), 583–592. https://doi.org/10.1111/jocn.15116

Glynn, L. M., & Baram, T. Z. (2019). The influence of unpredictable, fragmented parental signals on the developing brain. *Frontiers in Neuroendocrinology, 53,* 100736. https://doi .org/10.1016/j.yfrne.2019.01.002.

Godoy, L. D., Rossignoli, M. T., Delfino-Pereira, P., Garcia-Cairasco, N., & de Lima Umeoka, E. H. (2018). A comprehensive overview on stress neurobiology: basic concepts and clinical implications. *Frontiers in Behavioral Neuroscience, 2018*(12), 127. https://doi.org/10.3389/ fnbeh.2018.00127

Halifax, J. (2014). G.R.A.C.E. for nurses: Cultivating compassion in nurse/patient interactions. *Journal of Nursing Education and Practice, 4*(1), 121–128. https://doi.org/10.5430/ jnep.v4n1p121

Karr-Morse, R. (2012). *Scared sick. The role of childhood trauma in adult disease.* Basic Books.

Krol, K. M., Moulder, R. G., Lillard, T. S., Grossmann, T., & Connelly, J. J. (2019). Epigenetic dynamics in infancy and the impact of maternal engagement. *Science Advances, 5*(10), eaay0680. https://doi.org/10.1126/sciadv.aay0680.

Lewandowski, A. J., Augustine, D., Lamata, P., Davis, E. F., Lazdam, M., Francis, J., McCormick, K., Wilkinson, A. R., Singhal, A., Lucas, A., Smith, N. P., Neubauer, S., & Leeson, P. (2013). Preterm heart in adult life: Cardiovascular magnetic resonance reveals distinct differences in left ventricular mass, geometry, and function. *Circulation, 127*(2), 197–206. https://doi.org/10.1161/CIRCULATIONAHA.112.126920

Lipsky, L. D. (2009). *Trauma stewardship: An everyday guide to caring for self while caring for others.* Berrett-Koehler.

Low, L. A., & Schweinhardt, P. (2012). Early life adversity as a risk factor for fibromyalgia in later life. *Pain Research and Treatment, 2012,* 140832. https://doi.org/10.1155/2012/140832

Montagna, A., & Nosarti, C. (2016). Socio-emotional development following very preterm birth: Pathways to psychopathology. *Frontiers in Psychology, 7,* 80. https://doi.org/10.3389/ fpsyg.2016.00080

Montirosso, R., & Provenzi, L. (2015). Implications of epigenetics and stress regulation on research and developmental care of preterm infants. *Journal of Obstetric, Gynecologic, & Neonatal Nursing, 44*(2), 174–182. https://doi.org/10.1111/1552-6909.12559

Montirosso, R., Tronick, E., & Borgatti, R. (2017). Promoting neuroprotective care in neonatal intensive care units and preterm infant development: Insights from the Neonatal Adequate Care for Quality of Life study. *Child Development Perspectives, 11*(1), 9–15. https:// doi.org/10.1111/cdep.12208

Nosarti, C., Reichenberg, A., Murray, R. M., Cnattingius, S., Lambe, M. P., Yin, L., MacCabe, J., Rifkin, L., & Hultman, C. M. (2012). Preterm birth and psychiatric disorders in young adult life. *Archives in General Psychiatry, 69*(6), e1–e8. https://doi.org/10.1001/archgen psychiatry.2011.1374

Nusslock, R., & Miller, G. E. (2016). Early-life adversity and physical and emotional health across the lifespan: A neuro-immune network hypothesis. *Biological Psychiatry, 80*(1), 23–32. https://doi.org/10.1016/j.biopsych.2015.05.017

Posod, A., Odri Komazec, I., Kager, K., Pupp Peglow, U., Griesmaier, E., Schermer, E., Wurtinger, P., Baumgartner, D., & Kiechl-Kohlendorfer, U. (2016). Former very preterm infants show an unfavorable cardiovascular risk profile at a preschool age. *PLoS One, 11*(12), e0168162. https://doi.org/10.1371/journal.pone.0168162

Provenzi, L., Fumagalli, M., Sirigiovanni, I., Giorda, R., Pozzoli, U., Morandi, F., Beri, S., Menozzi, G., Mosca, F., Borgatti, R., & Montirosso, R. (2015). Pain-related stress during the neonatal intensive care unit stay and SLC6A4 methylation in very preterm infants. *Frontiers in Behavioral Neuroscience, 9,* 99. https://doi.org/10.3389/fnbeh.2015.00099

Reith, T. P. (2018). Burnout in United States healthcare professionals: A narrative review. *Cureus, 10*(12), e3681. https://doi.org/10.7759/cureus.3681

Roque, A. T. F., Lasiuk, G. C., Radunz, V., & Hegadoren, K. (2017). Scoping review of the mental health of parents of infants in the NICU. *Journal of Obstetric, Gynecologic, & Neonatal Nursing, 46*, 576–587. https://doi.org/10.1016/j.jogn.2017.02.005

Sanders, M. R., & Hall, S. L. (2018). Trauma-informed care in the newborn intensive care unit: Promoting safety, security and connectedness. *Journal of Perinatology, 38*(1), 3–10. https://doi.org/10.1038/jp.2017.124

Shonkoff, J. P., Garner, A. S., & The Committee on Psychosocial Aspects of Child and Family Health, Committee on Early Childhood, Adoption, and Dependent Care and Section on Developmental and Behavioral Pediatrics. (2012). The lifelong effects of early childhood adversity and toxic stress. *Pediatrics, 129*(1), e232. https://doi.org/10.1542/peds.2011-2663

Substance Abuse and Mental Health Services Administration. (2014). *SAMHSA's concept of trauma and guidance for a trauma-informed approach.* HHS Publication No. (SMA) 14-4884. Substance Abuse and Mental Health Services Administration.

Tronick, E., & Beeghly, M. (2011). Infants' meaning-making and the development of mental health problems. *American Psychologist, 66*(2), 107–119. https://doi.org/10.1037/a0021631

Weber, A., & Harrison, T. M. (2018). Reducing toxic stress in the NICU to improve infant outcomes. *Nursing Outlook, 67*(2), 169–189. https://doi.org/10.1016/j.outlook.2018.11.002

Neonatal Abstinence Syndrome/ Neonatal Opioid Withdrawal

GAIL A. BAGWELL

OVERVIEW

■ *Opioid Use Disorder:* This chronic lifelong disorder affects 3.2 million people in the United States (Substance Abuse and Mental Health Services Administration [SAMHSA], 2019). The disorder can lead to disability, relapses, and even death. Opioid use disorder is similar to a substance use disorder but has two unique features in that physical dependence can occur in as short of time as 4 to 8 weeks and the abrupt cessation will lead to severe physical symptoms such as nausea, vomiting, diarrhea, generalized pain, chills, muscle cramps, dilated pupils, restlessness, anxiety, insomnia, and intense craving (American Psychiatric Association [APA], n.d.). There are multiple factors that increase the chance of developing an opioid use disorder such as genetics, environmental issues, and past traumas. The fifth edition of the *Diagnostic and Statistical Manual of Mental Disorders* (*DSM-5*; APA, 2013) describes it as a pattern of opioid use that leads to problems or distress with at least two of several features over a 12-month period. These features are as follows:

- Using more of a medication or using it for a longer duration than originally intended
- A desire to continue use or being unable to discontinue use
- Focusing on obtaining and using the medication, or recovering from the medication and its effects
- Having a craving for the opioid
- Having trouble fulfilling obligations at work, home, or school
- Continuing the use of the opioid despite the negative consequences associated with the use
- Using the opioids in an unsafe method or place
- Continuing to use the opioid in spite of the negative effects on physical and mental health
- Developing a tolerance to the opioid requiring increased usage or experiencing withdrawal when abruptly stopping the opioid or using the opioid to prevent withdrawal

459

▮ *Substance Use Disorder:* This is similar to the opioid use disorder but includes substances besides opioids. These include legal substances, such as alcohol, tobacco, and prescription medications such as benzodiazepines, amphetamines, and barbiturates, as well as illegal substances such as marijuana, although this substance is becoming legal in many states for both recreational and medical purposes. As with opioid use disorder, there are risk factors that lead to this disorder and the diagnosis follows similar criteria (APA, 2013).

▮ *Neonatal Abstinence Syndrome (NAS):* This term, coined by Dr. Loretta Finnegan, describes neonates exposed to opioids and other substances, such as benzodiazepines, in utero (Finnegan & MacNew, 1974). Common signs of the disorder are central nervous system irritability, as well as respiratory, autonomic, and gastrointestinal system distress (Hudak et al., 2012).

▮ *Neonatal Opioid Withdrawal Syndrome (NOWS):* This is a more recent term used to describe neonates exposed to opioids only in utero (U.S. Food and Drug Administration [FDA], 2016). Many use the terms "NAS" and "NOWS" interchangeably.

EPIDEMIOLOGY

▮ The opioid epidemic in the United States for the past 20 years has not spared the pregnant woman or her unborn child.

▮ SAMHSA of the U.S. Department of Health and Human Services (USDHHS) does a yearly National Survey on Drug Use and Health (NSDUH). The survey, which is voluntary and self-reporting, asks about illicit substance use in the past month, which can affect survey results. The most recent survey done in 2019 and released in 2020 showed that:

   ● The number of pregnant women who admitted to using an illicit substance was 5.8%, a decrease from a high of 8.5% in 2017.

   ● Of the illicit substances, the number of people who admitted to abusing opioids decreased, while those using marijuana and cocaine increased.

▮ A complication of in utero exposure of opioids and other substances is NAS/NOWS. Since 2000, the number of neonates diagnosed with NAS/NOWs has skyrocketed from 1.2/1,000 live births to 7.3/1,000 live births in 2017 (Hirai et al., 2021; Patrick et al., 2012, 2015). This equals approximately one baby born every 15 minutes.

▮ There is great variability in the incidence of NAS/NOWS based on geographical location. Rural areas of the United States have been hit the hardest with a rate of 7.5/1,000 live births compared to neonates born in urban areas having a rate of 4.8/1,000 live births (Villapiano et al., 2017). There is also variation by state with rates ranging from 0.7/1,000 live births in Hawaii to 53.5/1,000 live births in West Virginia (Hirai et al., 2021; Ko et al., 2016).

▮ In addition to geographical location, ethnic groups are affected differently by the current epidemic. The Native American/Alaskan Native has been the most affected with 15.8/1,000 live births having a diagnosis of NAS/NOWS followed by non-Hispanic Whites at 10.5/1,000 live births and Blacks at 3.4/1,000 live births, and then Hispanic neonates at 2.5/1,000 live births (Strahan et al., 2019).

■ NICUs where the majority of these infants have been cared for saw an increase in admissions from 7/1,000 admissions in 2004 to 27/1,000 admissions in 2013, an almost four-fold increase (Tolia et al., 2015).

PATHOPHYSIOLOGY

■ Currently, mechanisms of withdrawal from opioids and other substances in the newborn are not well understood, but in animal models it appears that it is distinctively different from adult withdrawal. This occurs because of the neonate's immature neural development, decreased neuroprocessing, and variable levels of the opioid receptors (Mu, Kappa, and Delta) and neurotransmitters, as well as the pharmacokinetics between the mother, fetus, and placenta (Grossman & Berkwitt, 2019; Kocherlakota, 2014).

■ Neonatal withdrawal from opiates and other substances is influenced by a dysregulation of the hormonal system in the body. The hormone and their corresponding signs are noted in the list that follows (Grossman & Berkwitt, 2019; Kocherlakota, 2014):

● Increase in corticotropin leads to increased stress response in the neonate and hyperphagia.

● Decrease in dopamine results in hyperirritability and anxiety.

● Increase in acetylcholine is responsible for diarrhea, vomiting, yawning, sneezing, and sweating.

● Decrease in serotonin leads to sleep deprivation and fragmentation.

● Increase in noradrenaline results in hyperthermia, hypertension, tremors, and tachycardia.

● Other receptors' increase results in hyperalgesia and allodynia.

■ In addition to the items in the previous list, ongoing studies are looking at the role of genetics and epigenetics on NAS/NOWS severity of withdrawal, length of stay, and response to medications. Single-nucleotide polymorphisms in OPRM-1 and COMT have been identified (Mele, 2020; Wachman & Farrer, 2019; Wachman et al., 2013).

DIAGNOSIS

■ Both screening and testing are used to assist with the diagnosis of NAS/NOW in the neonate. A thorough review of the maternal history should occur to determine if substance use occurred during the pregnancy. Many confuse screening with testing, but there is a distinct difference between the two. Screening consists of interviewing the pregnant woman/new mother while testing involves checking for the presence of legal and illegal substances in a biological fluid.

■ **Maternal screening:** This is the first step to determine if there is substance usage/abuse during pregnancy. Questions should include inquiry on prescription medications; over-the-counter medications; nutritional and herbal supplements; legal substances such as alcohol, tobacco, and, in some states, marijuana; and illicit substances such as heroin and cocaine. The American College of Obstetricians and Gynecologists (ACOG) and the American Academy of Family Practice (AAFP) recommend a screening tool validated for use in substance use disorders such as the Parents, Partner, Past, and Present (4 Ps); Tolerance, Annoyance, Cut-Down, Eye-Opener (T-ACE); Alcohol, Smoking, and Substance Involvement Screening Test (ASSIST); Car, Relax, Alone, Forget, Friends, Trouble (CRAFFT); and Alcohol Use Disorders Identification Test–Concise (AUDIT–C; AAFP, 2020; ACOG, 2017).

■ Both ACOG (2017) and AAFP (2020) recommend screening for substance use/ opioid use disorder during pregnancy, and this screening should occur during prenatal visits for all pregnant women. In addition, the substance use of other household members should also be discussed.

■ **Maternal test:** Urine toxicology testing of maternal urine during prenatal visits as well as admittance to the hospital for delivery can help to determine if substance use is occurring.

■ Urine drug tests are not always accurate and can be negative even when a woman is abusing a substance. Reasons for inaccurate test results are:

● Due to fear of losing their baby, women with substance abuse disorder will go to great lengths to hide their problem. Websites sell devices that can be utilized to hide clean urine as well as give instructions on how to beat a urine drug test.

● The drug half-life and the timing of the test will determine if the test is positive or negative.

■ Due to legal implications of profiling, many hospitals and medical practices have begun performing routine urine drug testing on all pregnant women.

■ **Neonatal testing:** Utilized when there is suspicion of exposure to opioids or other substances in utero or a neonate is demonstrating signs associated with NAS/NOWS. The following are the pros and cons of each type of biologic testing available for a neonate.

● Urine: This is easy to obtain but not as accurate as the other tests. Only recent drugs used by the mother will be detected; if the mother is an infrequent user or has not used in the past week, the test can be negative (Hudak et al., 2012; Kocherlakota, 2014; Kwong & Ryan, 1997; Ostrea, 2001; Sutter et al., 2014).

● Hair: More accurate than urine testing, hair tests can detect the past 3 to 4 months of drug usage by the mother. Hair is rarely used in neonates as the quantity of hair needed can be lacking or the mothers object to the shaving of their newborn's head (Kwong & Ryan, 1997; Ostrea, 2001; Vinner et al., 2003).

● Meconium: This is the gold standard and most common form of drug testing in newborns. It detects in utero drug usage for the previous two trimesters. Meconium collection is not always collected and stored correctly, leading to false negatives. To be accurate, the entire column of meconium has to be collected and stored in a specimen cup. When adding meconium to the specimen cup, mix the meconium thoroughly to ensure the metabolites are evenly distributed. The laboratory will only take one small sample (2–5 g) of the entire meconium; if it is not mixed properly, the laboratory could get a sample with no metabolites, leading to a false negative. While the metabolites are stable for 2 weeks at room temperature, it is preferred that it remains refrigerated (Kocherlakota, 2014; Ostrea, 2001). Other reasons meconium is not always accurate are:

• In babies that are not suspected initially of being exposed in utero to substances, part of the meconium will be missing for testing.

• Neonates that pass meconium in utero will also lack having the entire meconium for testing.

• In neonates who room in with their parents, meconium samples can be missed as the parents do not always save the diapers for the staff to collect the meconium and may get rid of it to assure testing cannot be done.

● Umbilical cord: This is a newer method for testing neonates. Umbilical cord testing is highly reliable and can detect the last 4 to 5 months of maternal drug usage (United States Drug Testing Laboratories [USDTL], 2020). The advantage of the cord over meconium is the availability and ease of collection. A 6-inch segment of cord is obtained at the time of birth, drained of blood, cleansed per the laboratory instructions, labeled, sealed, and stored. The cord can be stored for 1 week at room temperature, 3 weeks in the refrigerator, or 1 year in a deep freezer. Institutions that do cord testing often collect all neonates' cords and have them available if the baby starts to show signs of withdrawal. The major disadvantage to testing the cord is that if it is not collected at birth then it cannot be used (USDTL, 2020).

CLINICAL MANIFESTATIONS

■ These signs were first described by Finnegan and MacNew in 1974. Opioid withdrawal affects the central nervous, autonomic nervous, gastrointestinal, and respiratory systems.

Clinical manifestations of NAS/NOWS include (Hudak et al., 2012):

■ Central nervous system
  High-pitched crying
  Irritability
  Tremors

Hyperactive Moro reflex

Sleep disturbances

Increased muscle tone

Skin excoriation

Seizures

■ Autonomic nervous system

Fever

Mottling

Sweating

Yawning

■ Gastrointestinal system

Excessive sucking

Poor feeding

Regurgitation

Vomiting

Loose or watery stool

■ Respiratory system

Tachypnea

Sneezing

Nasal flaring

Nasal stuffiness

ASSESSMENT TOOLS

■ There are a variety of assessment tools available to help with the assessment and treatment of NAS/NOWS that have been developed over the past 50 years. The creation of multiple tools demonstrates the lack of agreement on how to best assess for NAS/NOWS. The majority of the tools have been validated for reliability and sensitivity to diagnose NAS/NOWS.

■ The most commonly used tool, the Finnegan Neonatal Abstinence Scoring Tool (FNAST), is commonly referred to as the Finnegan scoring tool (Bagley et al., 2014; Gomez-Pomar & Finnegan, 2018).

■ The Finnegan currently consists of 21 items that evaluate neurologic, autonomic, gastrointestinal, respiratory, and other signs demonstrated by the neonate that is experiencing withdrawal. The items are scored on a scale of 1 to 5 (Finnegan et al., 1975). There is much confusion on the definition of the items on the Finnegan tool.

■ A newer, simpler method of assessing and caring for the NAS/NOWS neonate is the Eat Sleep Console (ESC) method. This method looks at three key indicators to determine how the baby is doing. The three indicators are: Is the baby eating at least 1 ounce of food or breastfed well? Is the baby sleeping more than or equal to 1 hour? and Can the baby be consoled within 10 minutes? (Grossman et al., 2018).

■ All the assessment tools are subjective in nature, so it is essential that nurses be trained on the proper use of the tool. The FNAST and the ESC have programs available to help with the training of the healthcare provider. One method for obtaining reliability in assessment is to have nurses do dual scoring on an infant at least two times/day. This helps to maintain the inter-rater reliability achieved when training is done.

TREATMENT

■ Because NAS/NOWS can mimic other diseases such as hypoglycemia, hypocalcemia, hypomagnesemia, and sepsis, it is important to do laboratory work to differentiate NAS/NOWS from other diseases.

■ Once the diagnosis of NAS/NOWS is established, the initial treatment should always begin with nonpharmacologic interventions before advancing to pharmacologic treatment. In many instances, nonpharmacologic interventions are all that will be needed.

■ Nonpharmacologic interventions (Edwards & Brown, 2016; Mangat et al., 2019):

● Minimize environmental stimulation—maintain low lighting and decreased noise levels; do not use TV or mobiles

● Swaddling in a flexed position with hands midline against the chest and legs loosely swaddled in lumbar flexion to decrease sensory stimulation

● Clustering cares to give neonate extended periods of quiet and rest

● Rooming in with the mother

● Skin-to-skin care (kangaroo mother care) with mother or other family members

● Avoid abrupt changes in the neonate's environment—move the baby's position slowly, handling gently, and keeping the neonate close to the body to increase security

● Approach the baby slowly and purposefully with a soft voice and gentle touch

● Limit all stimulation at first signs of distress

● Prone positioning in the acute phase of withdrawal and placing supine in a safe sleep environment once the neonate is stable in preparation for home

● Rocking of the baby—slow and gentle with vertical preferred over horizontal rocking; do not talk to the neonate while rocking

- Pacifiers for nonnutritive sucking
- Hand containment during cares to provide boundaries; involve mom with this when she is present
- Music: initially soft shushing, humming, or singing of simple lullabies
- Feedings:
  - Breastfeeding should be encouraged for all mothers who are in a treatment program and are HIV negative; this policy is recommended by the American Academy of Pediatrics (AAP), Academy of Breastfeeding Medicine, and ACOG (ACOG, 2017; Chantry et al., 2015; Hudak et al., 2012).
  - Breastfeeding has been shown to decrease length of stay, decrease medication usage, and increase attachment (McQueen et al., 2011; Pritham et al., 2012; Short et al., 2016).
  - For mothers who are unable to or choose not to breastfeed their infant, a high-calorie formula is recommended. Studies have shown that high-calorie feeds (24 Kcal/oz) decrease the length of stay and medication usage. No difference was found in length of stay and medication usage with the use of low-lactose formula compared to regular formula (Hall et al., 2014, 2015; Kaplan et al., 2020). Studies have not demonstrated any benefits to the use of partially hydrolyzed formulas (Alsaleem et al., 2020).
  - Neonates with feeding difficulties may consider doing small frequent feedings or doing gavage feeds.
- During feedings:
  - To help with preparation for sucking, offer firm support to the neonate's feet and place your hand on the neonate's chest. This will help maintain flexion of the neonate.
  - Apply firm pressure to the neonate's palate to increase and improve quality of sucking.
  - Avoid talking to the infant while feeding so the infant can focus on feeding.
- Relaxation bath
- Acupuncture
- Massage therapy
- Aromatherapy using mother's scent only

■ Pharmacologic treatment:
- In cases where nonpharmacologic treatments do not work, medication-assisted treatment should be initiated. The AAP recommends using medication from the same class of drug the infant was exposed to in utero (Hudak et al., 2012).
- Opioids morphine and methadone are the most common replacement medications for babies, but buprenorphine is becoming an alternative for opioid replacement (Kraft et al., 2017).

- In neonates whose mothers were polysubstance abusers (those using barbiturates, benzodiazepines, amphetamines, antidepressants, sedatives, antipsychotics), the use of clonidine or phenobarbital may be needed (Kocherlakota, 2014).

- Common medications, routes, and dosage used in treatment of NAS are:

  - Morphine: 0.04 mg/kg/dose po q3h to q4h. Increase by 0.04 mg/kg to maximum dose of 0.2 mg/kg/day.

  - Methadone: 0.05 to 0.1 mg/kg/dose po q6h, increase by 0.05 mg/kg as needed or q 4 hours. Maximum dose 1 mg/kg/day.

  - Buprenorphine: 5.3 mcg/kg/dose sublingual q8h, increase by 25% increments as needed. Maximum dose 60 mcg/kg/day.

  - Clonidine: Initial dose: 0.5 to 1.0 mcg/kg po q6h, followed by 0.5 to 1.25 mcg/kg/dose q4h to q6h. Maximum dose: 1 mcg/kg q3h.

  - Phenobarbital: Loading dose: 10 mg/kg po divided into two doses every 4 to 6 hours. Maintenance dose: 5 mg/kg/day po divided into dose every 12 hours.

- No matter the pharmacologic treatment used, it is important to develop and adhere to an NAS medication protocol as it decreases length of stay and medication for the neonate (Hall et al., 2015).

NONJUDGMENTAL NURSING CARE

■ When caring for a neonate with NAS/NOWS, you will also be interacting and caring for the mother of the neonate. Women with substance use disorders face many stigmas from healthcare providers (Recto et al., 2020). It is important as a care provider that you confront your feelings regarding neonates that are exposed to substances in utero.

■ When caring for the mother–infant dyad, it is important to remember these:

- Over 40% of the mothers who have a substance use/opioid use disorder are survivors of a major trauma such as child abuse, sexual abuse, or both (Konkoly-Thege et al., 2017).

- Substance use/opioid use disorder is a chronic disease of the brain. The mothers deserve the same respect we give any patient family member with a chronic disease.

- The mother did not decide to have a substance use/opioid use disorder after becoming pregnant.

- The mother has a distrust of the healthcare system due to being treated poorly by judgmental healthcare providers, requiring you to work hard to develop a therapeutic relationship with her.

- To better care for the mother and infant, educate yourself on trauma-informed care (see Chapter 10).

■ Caring for the NAS/NOWS neonate requires the following:

- Careful ongoing physical assessments, as well as documentation of fluid and electrolyte status
- Documentation of the neonate's tolerance to stimuli
- Ensure the scoring tool utilized by your institution remains reliable through inter-rater reliability testing.
- If the infant is receiving pharmacotherapy, assure the medication is given on time.
- When working with the mother, assure her that all information provided is clear and concise with guidelines for expected behaviors.
- Provide education to the mother on the infant's behavior, emphasizing that the behavior is not a reflection of her. Discuss that the neonate is withdrawing and the behavior is the result of the withdrawal. Put it into perspective for her by asking her how she felt when she experienced withdrawal—let her know the baby is feeling that way, too.
- Acknowledge to yourself that caring for this mother–infant dyad is difficult, time-consuming, and exhausting. It involves being flexible, having patience, expending energy, and taking a nonjudgmental attitude. Take breaks as you need them.

DISCHARGE PREPARATION

■ Preparing for discharge prior to the actual day of discharge is essential to assure a successful transition from the hospital to home for any neonate, especially those diagnosed with NAS/NOWS due to their higher risk for adverse outcomes after discharge (Patrick et al., 2020).

■ The AAP statement on NOWS (Patrick et al., 2020) recommends the following in preparation for discharge:

- Do not discharge home on pharmacotherapy, but if needed, the neonate needs a structured close follow-up plan
- No clinical signs of withdrawal for 24 to 48 hours after discontinuation of pharmacotherapy
- Education to parents/caregivers on signs of NAS/NOWS, care of the normal newborn including but not limited to bathing, thermoregulation, sleep patterns, feeding, and emphasizing safe sleep
- A follow-up appointment made prior to discharge with primary care provider for 48 hours after discharge
- Early intervention referral
- Plan of safe care coordinating with child protective services
- Home health nurse referral
- Early start referral
- Testing completed: hepatitis C, HIV, and referral to pediatric infectious disease expert if needed

● NAS/NOWS follow-up clinic or developmental behavioral pediatrician referral

DEVELOPMENTAL OUTCOMES

■ Long-term effects of NAS/NOWS are not completely known at the time of publication, as data is limited.

■ Studies are currently being done to determine long-term effects, but the studies are confounded by other factors such as low-socioeconomic factors, poor nutrition, poor parenting skills, and poor prenatal care, which can also affect the development of the growing child. In addition, many children are lost to follow-up if the parents feel their child is meeting their developmental milestones (Oei, 2018).

■ Developmental outcomes that children with NAS/NOWS have demonstrated as they grew are:

● Visual disturbances such as nystagmus, strabismus, refractive errors, reduced visual acuity, and cerebral visual impairment (Hamilton et al., 2010; Spiteri-Cornish et al., 2013; Sundelin-Wahlsten & Sarman, 2013)

● Cognitive deficits such as verbal and perceptual abilities and poorer scores on the Columbia Mental Maturity Scale have been reported (Grossman & Berkwitt, 2019; Lizcano-MacMillan, 2019)

● Poor psychomotor outcomes after 12 months of age (Maguire et al., 2016; Rosen & Johnson, 1982; Strauss et al., 1976)

● Decreased school performance when compared to children who have no in utero exposure (Oei et al., 2017)

● Increased mortality (Cohen et al., 2015; Kahila et al., 2007)

REFERENCES

Alsaleem, M., Berkelhamer, S. K., Wilding, G. E., Miller, L. M., & Reynolds, A. M. (2020). Effects of partially hydrolyzed formula on severity and outcomes of neonatal abstinence syndrome. *American Journal of Perinatology, 37*(11), 1177–1182. https://doi.org/10.1055/s-0039-1692684

American Academy of Family Physicians. (2020). *Opioid use disorder (OUD): Screening.* www.aafp.org/family-physician/patient-care/clinical-recommendations/all-clinical-recommendations/oud.html

American College of Obstetricians and Gynecologists. (2017). Opioid use and opioid use disorder in pregnancy. Committee Opinion 711. *Obstetrics & Gynecology, 130*(2), 488–489. https://doi.org/10.1097/AOG.0000000000002229

American Psychiatric Association. (n.d.). Opioid use disorder. https://www.psychiatry.org/patients-families/addiction/opioid-use-disorder

American Psychiatric Association. (2013). Introduction. In *Diagnostic and statistical manual of mental disorders* (5th ed.). https://doi.org/10.1176/appi.books.9780890425596.Introduction

Bagley, S. M., Wachman, E. M., Holland, E., & Brogly, S. B. (2014). Review of the assessment and management of neonatal abstinence syndrome. *Addiction Science and Clinical Practice, 9*(1), 19. https://doi.org/10.1186/1940-0640-9-19

Chantry, C. J., Eglash, A., & Labbok, M. (2015). ABM position statement on breastfeeding—Revised 2015. *Breastfeeding Medicine, 10*(9), 407–411. https://doi.org/10.1089/bfm.2015.29012.cha

Cohen, M. C., Morley, S. R., & Coombs, R. C. (2015). Maternal use of methadone and risk of sudden neonatal death. *Acta Peaediatric, 104*(9), 883–337. https://doi.org/10.1111/apa.13046

Edwards, L., & Brown, L. F. (2016). Nonpharmacologic management of neonatal abstinence syndrome: An integrative review. *Neonatal Network, 35*(5), 305–313. https://doi.org/10.1891/0730-0832.35.5.305

Finnegan, L. P., Cron, R. E., Connaughton, J. F., & Emich, J. P. (1975). Assessment and treatment of abstinence in the infant of the drug-dependent mother. *International Journal of Clinical Pharmacology and Biopharmacy, 12* (1–2), 19–32.

Finnegan, L. P., & MacNew, B. A. (1974). Care of the addicted infant. *American Journal of Nursing, 74*(4), 685–693. https://journals.lww.com/ajnonline/Abstract/1974/04000/Care_of_the_Addicted_Infant.51.aspx

Gomez-Pomar, E., & Finnegan, L. P. (2018). The epidemic of neonatal abstinence syndrome, historical references of its origins, assessment and management. *Frontiers in Pediatrics, 6*(33), 1–8. https://doi.org/10.3389/fped.2018.00033

Grossman, M., & Berkwitt, A. (2019). Neonatal abstinence syndrome. *Seminars in Perinatology, 43*, 173–186. https://doi.org/10.1053/j.semperi.201901.007

Grossman, M. R., Lipshaw, M. J., Osborn, R. R., & Berkwitt, A. K. (2018). A novel approach to assessing infants with neonatal abstinence syndrome. *Hospital Pediatrics, 8*(1), 1–6. https://doi.org/10.1542/hpeds.2017-2018

Hall, E. S., Wexelblatt, S. L., Crowley, M., Grow, J. L., Jasin, L. R., Klebanoff, M. A., McClead, R. E., Meinzen-Derr, J., Mohan, V. K., Stein, H., Walsh, M. C., & on behalf of the OCHNAS Consortium. (2014). A multicenter cohort study of treatments and hospital outcomes in neonatal abstinence syndrome. *Pediatrics, 134*(2), e527–534. https://doi.org/10.1542/peds.2013-4036

Hall, E. S., Wexelblatt, S. L., Crowley, M., Grow, J. L., Jasin, L. R., Klebanoff, M. A., McClead, R. E., Meinzen-Derr, J., Mohan, V. K., Stein, H., Walsh, M. C., & on behalf of the OCHNAS Consortium. (2015). Implementation of neonatal abstinence syndrome weaning protocol: A cohort study. *Pediatrics, 136*(4), e803–e810. https://doi.org/10.1542/peds.2015.1141

Hamilton, R., McGlone, I., MacKinnon, J. R., Russell, H. C., Bradnam, M. S., & Mactier, H. (2010). Ophthalmic, clinical and visual electrophysiological findings in children born to mothers prescribed methadone in pregnancy. *British Journal of Ophthalmology, 94*(6), 696–700. https://doi.org/10.1136/bjo.2009.169284

Hirai, A. H., Ko, J. Y., Owens, P. L., Stocks, C., & Patrick, S. W. (2021). Neonatal abstinence syndrome and maternal opioid-related diagnoses in the US, 2010–2017. *JAMA, 325*(2), 146–155. https://doi.org/10.1001/jama.2020.24991

Hudak, M. L, Tan, R. C., the Committee on Drugs, & Committee on Fetus and Newborn. (2012). Neonatal drug withdrawal. *Pediatrics, 129*(2), e540–e560. https://doi.org/10.1542/peds.2011-3212

Kahila, H., Saisto, T., Kivitie-Kallio, S., Haukkamaa, M., & Hlmesmaki, E. (2007). A prespective study on buprenorphine use during pregnancy: Effects on maternal and neonatal outcome. *Acta Obstetricia Gynecologica Scandanavia, 86*(2), 185–190. https://doi.org/10.1080/00016340601110770

Kaplan, H. C., Kuhnell, P., Walsh, M. C., Crowley, M., McClead, R. E., Wexelblatt, S., Ford, S., Provost, L. P., Lannon, C., Macaluso, M., & for the Ohio Perinatal Collaborative. (2020). Orchestrated testing of formula type to reduce length of stay in neonatal abstinence syndrome. *Pediatrics, 146*(4), e20190914. https://doi.org/10.1542/peds.2019-0914

Ko, J. Y., Patrick, S. W., Tong, V. T., Pate, R., Lind, J. N., & Barfield, W. D. (2016). Incidence of neonatal abstinence syndrome—28 states, 1999–2013. *Morbidity Mortality Weekly Report, 65*(31), 799–802. https://doi.org/10.15585/mmwr.mm6531a2

Kocherlakota, P. (2014). Neonatal abstinence syndrome. *Pediatrics, 134*, e547–e561. https://doi.org/10.1542/peds.2013-3524

Konkoly-Thege, B., Horwood, L., Slater, L., Tan, M. C., Hodgins, D. C., & Wild, T. C. (2017). Relationship between interpersonal trauma exposure and addictive behaviors: A systematic review. *British Medical Journal Psychiatry, 17*(1), 164. https://doi.org/10.1186/s12888-017-1323-01

Kraft, W. K., Adeniyi-Jones, S. C., Chervoneva, I., Greenspan, J. S., Abatemarco, D., Kaltenbach, K., & Ehrlich, M. E. (2017). Buprenorphine for the treatment of neonatal abstinence syndrome. *New England Journal of Medicine, 376*(24), 2341–2348. https://doi.org/10.1056/NEJMoa1614835

Kwong, T. C., & Ryan, R. M. (1997). Detection of intrauterine illicit drug exposure by newborn drug testing. *Clinical Chemistry, 43*(1), 235–242. https://doi.org/10.1093/clinchem/43.1.235

Lizcano-MacMillan, K. D. (2019). Neonatal abstinence syndrome: Review of epidemiology, care models, and current understanding of outcomes. *Clinics Perinatology, 46*, 817–832. https://doi.org/10.106/j.cip.2019.08.012

Maguire, D. J., Taylor, S., Armstrong, K., Shaffer-Hudkins, E., Germain, A. M., Brooks, S. S., Cline, G. J., & Clark, L. (2016). Long-term outcomes of infants with neonatal abstinence syndrome. *Neonatal Network, 35*(5), 227–286. https://doi.org/10.1891/0730-0832.35.5.277

Mangat, A. K., Schmolzer, G. M., & Krafft, W. K. (2019). Pharmacological and nonpharmacological treatment of neonatal abstinence syndrome (NAS). *Seminars in Perinatology, 24*(2), 133–141. https://doi.org/10.1016/j.siny.2019.01.009

McQueen, K. A., Murphy-Oikonen, J., Gerlach, K., & Montelpare, W. (2011). The impact of feeding method on neonatal abstinence scores of Methadone-exposed infants. *Advances in Neonatal Care, 11*(4), 282–292. https://doi.org/10.1097/ANC.0b013e318225a30c

Mele, C. (2020). Genomics and neonatal opioid withdrawal syndrome. *Journal of Pediatric Nursing, 50*, 128–130. https://doi.org/10.1016/j.pedn.2019.10.009

Oei, J. L. (2018). Adult consequences of prenatal drug exposure. *Internal Medicine Journal, 48*, 25–31. https://doi.org/10.1111/imj.13658

Oei, J. L., Melhuish, E., Uebel, H., Azzam, N., Breen, C., Burris, L., Hilder, L., Bajuk, B., Abel-Latif, M. E., Ward, M., Feller, J. M., Falconer, J., Clews, S., Eastwood, J., Li, A., & Wright, I. M. (2017). Neonatal abstinence syndrome and high school performance. *Pediatrics, 139*(2), e20162651. https://doi.org/10.1542/peds.2016-2651

Ostrea, E. M. (2001). Understanding drug testing in the neonate and the role of meconium analysis. *Journal of Perinatal and Neonatal Nursing, 14*(4), 61–82. https://doi.org/10.1097/00005237-200103000-00006

Patrick, S. W., Barfield, W. D., Poindexter, B. B., the Committee on Drugs, Committee on Fetus and Newborn, & American Academy of Pediatrics. (2020). Neonatal opioid withdrawal syndrome. *Pediatrics, 146*(5), e2020029074. https://doi.org/10.1542/peds.2020-029074

Patrick, S. W., Davis, M. M., Lehmann, C. U., & Cooper, W. O. (2015). Increasing incidence and geographic distribution of neonatal abstinence syndrome: United States 2009 to 2012. *Journal of Perinatology, 35*(8), 650–655. https://doi.org/10.1038/jp.2015.36

Patrick, S. W., Schumacher, R. E., Benneyworth, B. D., Krans, E. E., McAllister, J. M., & Davis M. M. (2012). Neonatal abstinence syndrome and associated health care expenditures: United States, 2000–2009. *JAMA, 307*(18), 1934–1940. https://doi.org/10.1001/jama.2012.3951

Pritham, U. A., Paul, J. A., & Hayes, M. J. (2012). Opioid dependency in pregnancy and length of stay for neonatal abstinence syndrome. *Journal of Obstetric, Gynecology and Neonatal Nursing, 41*(2), 180–190. https://doi.org/10.1111/j.1552-6909.2011.01330.x

Recto, P., McGlothen-Bell, K., & McGrath, J. (2020). The role stigma in the nursing care of families impacted by neonatal abstinence syndrome. *Advances in Neonatal Care, 20*(5), 354–363. https://doi.org/10.1097/ANC.0000000000000778

Rosen, T. S., & Johnson, H. L. (1982). Children of methadone-maintained mothers: Follow-up to 18 months of age. *Journal of Pediatrics, 101*(2), 192–196. https://doi.org/ 10.1016/S0022-3476(82)80115-7

Short, V. L., Gannon, M., & Abatemarco, D. J. (2016). The association between breastfeeding and length of hospital stay among infants diagnosed with neonatal abstinence syndrome: A population based study of in-hospital births. *Breastfeeding Medicine, 11*(7), 343–349. http://doi.org/10.1089/bfm.2016.0084

Spiteri-Cornish, K., Hrabovsky, M., Scott, N. W., Myerscough, E., & Reddy, A. R. (2013). The short and long-term effects on the visual system of children following exposure to maternal substance misuse in pregnancy. *American Journal Ophthamology, 156*(1), 190–194. https://doi.org/10.1016/j.ajo.2013.02.004

Strahan, A. E., Guy, G. P., Jr., Bohm, M., Frey, M., & Ko, J. Y. (2019). Neonatal abstinence syndrome incidence and healthcare costs in the United States, 2016. *JAMA Pediatrics, 174*(2), 200–202. https://doi.org/10.1001/jamapediatrics.2019.4791

Strauss, M. E., Starr, R. H., Ostrea, E. M., Chavez, C. J., & Stryker, J. C. (1976). Behavioural concomitants of prenatal addiction to narcotics. *Journal of Pediatrics, 89*(5), 842–846. https://doi.org/10.1016/S0022-3476(76)80822-0

Substance Abuse and Mental Health Services Administration. (2019). *The national survey on drug use and health: 2019.* Substance Abuse and Mental Health Services Administration.https:// www.samhsa.gov/data/sites/default/files/reports/rpt29392/Assistant-Secretary-nsduh 2019_presentation/Assistant-Secretary-nsduh2019_presentation.pdf

Sundelin-Wahlsten, V., & Sarman, I. (2013). Neurodevelopmental development of pre-school-age children born to addicted mothers given opiate maintenance treatment with buprenorphine during pregnancy. *Acta Paediatrica, 102*(5), 544–549. https://doi.org/ 10.1111/apa.12210

Sutter, M. B., Leeman, L., & Hsi, A. (2014). Neonatal opioid withdrawal syndrome. *Obstetrics, Gynecology Clinics of North America, 41*(2), 317–334. https://doi.org/10.1016/j.ogc.2014.02.010

Tolia, V. N., Patrick, S. W., Bennett, M. M., Murthy, K., Sousa, J., Smith, P. B., Clark, R. H., & Spitzer, A. R. (2015). Increasing incidence of the neonatal abstinence syndrome in U.S. Neonatal ICUs. *New England Journal of Medicine, 372*(22), 2118– 2126. https://doi .org/10.1056/NEJMsa1500439

United States Drug Testing Laboratories. (2020). *Frequently asked questions.* https://www .usdtl.com/faq

United States Food and Drug Administration. (2016). *Neonatal opioid withdrawal syndrome and medication-assisted treatment with methadone and buprenorphine.* https://www.fda.gov/ Drugs/DrugSafety/ucm503630.htm

Villapiano, N. L. G., Winkelman, T. N. A., Kozhimannil, K. B., Davis, M. M., & Patrick, S. W. (2017). Rural and urban differences in neonatal abstinence syndrome and maternal opioid use, 2004 to 2013. *JAMA Pediatrics, 171*(2), 1940196. https://doi.org/10.1001/ jamapediatrics.2016.3750

Vinner, E., Vignau, J., Thibault, D., Codaccioni, X., Brassart, C., Humbert, L., & Lhermitte, M. (2003). Neonatal hair analysis contribution to gestational drug exposure profile and predicting a withdrawal syndrome. *Therapeutic Drug Monitoring, 25*(4), 421–432. https:// doi.org/10.1097/00007691-200308000-0000

Wachman, E. M., & Farrer, L. A. (2019). The genetics and epigenetics of neonatal abstinence syndrome. *Seminars in Fetal and Neonatal Medicine, 24*(2), 105–110. https://doi.org/ 10.1016/j.siny.2019.01.002

Wachman, E. M., Hayes, M. J., Brown, M. S., Paul, J., Harvey-Wilkes, K., Terrin, N., Huggins, G. S., Aranda, J. V., & Davis, J. M. (2013). Association of OPRM-1 and COMT single nucleotide polymorphisms with hospital length of stay and treatment of neonatal absti-nence syndrome. *JAMA, 309*(17), 1821–1827. https://doi.org/10.1001/jama.2013.3411

14

Palliative Care

CAROLE KENNER

OVERVIEW

Integral to the care of medically fragile neonates is the reality that not all will survive. Perinatal palliative care is an interdisciplinary, coordinated care plan that supports quality of life and decreases suffering while incorporating cultural beliefs and the family's values (American College of Obstetricians & Gynecologists [ACOG], 2019). Perinatal death refers to fetal deaths after 20 weeks' gestation and live births with only brief survival (Barfield & The Committee on Fetus and Newborn, 2016). Neonatal palliative care is rendered to those infants who experience life-threatening illnesses and may die. Quality of life through symptom management and pain relief is key to providing palliative and end-of-life care (Catlin et al., 2015). This chapter defines and discusses perinatal and neonatal palliative care.

BACKGROUND AND INCIDENCE

Advanced genetic testing and technology affords families the opportunity to know before birth if there is a neonatal problem. If this problem poses a threat to life, palliative care interdisciplinary teams can work with families to prepare for this birth (Kenner et al., 2015). Palliative care may begin in the prenatal period and then continue for infants born with life-limiting conditions or who develop life-limiting conditions during their neonatal hospitalization.

Pediatric palliative care is needed by approximately 21.6 million children (Downing et al., 2018). Most of these children reside in low- and middle-income countries where little or no access to such care exists (Downing et al., 2018). Yet palliative care is part of the Sustainable Development Goal (SDG) #3 that addresses Good Health and Well-Being and is included in universal healthcare (UHC) in many countries (Downing et al., 2018). The leading causes for infant mortality globally and in the United States include congenital anomalies, prematurity, low birthweight, and maternal complications (Centers for Disease Control and Prevention [CDC], n.d.-a). The U.S. neonatal mortality rate was 5.7 per 1,000 live births in 2018 (CDC, n.d.-a). In 2018, 8.28% births were low birthweight, and 10.02% were preterm (CDC, n.d.-b).

Palliative care is focused on interventions aimed at improving quality of life and maximizing comfort. The World Health Organization (WHO, 2018) states that palliative care is "a crucial part of integrated, people-centered" care. It is just as vital as disease management or curative care. This type of care often creates mortal distress for families and health professionals alike because crucial conversations must include options that often run counter to one's beliefs and values. Two such scenarios involve compassionate extubation and the withdrawal of artificial nutrition and hydration (Garten & Buhrer, 2019).

RECOMMENDED INTERVENTIONS

■ Palliative care should be offered at any period in which the infant's life may be limited—prenatally, at the time of birth, after the birth, initially in the labor and delivery suite, in the NICU, and at home following discharge.

■ When a prenatal diagnosis is made, palliative care should be offered while the fetus is in utero. Parents should be supported throughout the decision-making process. Options for terminating or continuing the pregnancy should be offered in a balanced manner, and family decisions should be supported by the healthcare team.

■ When continuing the pregnancy is chosen, an advocate or coordinator of care for a family should be identified prenatally to assist with (a) helping families navigate the healthcare system, (b) coordinating care conferences between the healthcare team and family, (c) answering questions, and (d) assisting parents with a birth plan that is appropriate. A birth plan is a written document available to all stakeholders outlining parental wishes about the pregnancy, labor, birth, and postnatal period.

■ Provision of care and services should be coordinated among interdisciplinary team members. Recommendations should be made as a team through consensus to avoid fragmentation in communication and care. Should any party wish to change the agreed-upon plan, the interdisciplinary team must all meet to reassess whether changes should be made.

■ Parents are part of the caregiving team and should participate in the decision-making process. Family conferences are essential to caregivers' understanding of families' needs, hopes, and goals for their infant.

■ Appropriate family support services should be provided, including those of perinatal social workers, hospital chaplains and clergy, mental health specialists, and hospital palliative care team members to provide emotional and spiritual support; a child life specialist or family support specialist to support the infant's siblings; and a lactation consultant to assist mothers who want to breastfeed their infant or donate breast milk at the end of life and to help mothers with lactation suppression (Carroll et al., 2020).

■ Initial training, availability of written protocols, annual competencies, and support services should be available for all staff members. Debriefing for staff is essential after a difficult death.

ASSESSMENT

Neonatal nurses spend more time with families than any other health professional (Kenner, 2016; Schroeder & Lorenz, 2018). They are in a unique position to understand the wants and needs of the family and their infant. Nurses are key to clear, concise communication among the healthcare team including families (Kenner, 2016). Nurses play an instrumental role in shifting the focus of treatment from curative to one of comfort and compassion.

Comprehensive assessment in the physical, psychological, social, spiritual, and cultural domains should recur on a regular basis. Experts in pain and symptom management are essential partners in the care. The treatment plan may be twopronged disease management and amelioration of pain and suffering to promote the highest quality of life possible (Carter, 2018).

A document for the healthcare team to use and refer to should be created to avoid fragmentation of care and provide continuity of care.

DIAGNOSIS AND PLANNING

Diagnostic information should be offered in a timely and compassionate manner. Since prognosis may be uncertain and an infant may live longer than expected, a treatment plan can be developed prenatally. A treatment plan is a written document available to all stakeholders stating fetal/neonatal diagnoses and anticipated treatments necessary to keep the infant comfortable as assessment dictates (i.e., breathing, pain, feeding). Palliative care is appropriate for neonates with a wide range of life-limiting conditions, including severe prematurity and its accompanying complications, birth-related trauma or complex congenital anomalies, and whether the condition will result in death during the infant's first few hours of life or after several years.

Written information should be given to parents that complements palliative care interventions, such as (a) referrals to community resources, counselors, community members, and other parents; (b) what to expect during the dying process; and (c) who to contact when death occurs.

When an infant with a potentially life-limiting condition is being transported to a tertiary care center, parents should be informed that palliative care may be the focus of care, as parents may believe that transport means cure when in fact transport may be indicated to confirm a diagnosis.

When a decision has been made to pursue palliative care interventions, the proper focus of palliative care should be maintained.

- Active orders should be reviewed to determine whether they should be continued when palliative care is initiated.

- Pain and distressing symptoms, such as gasping or seizures, should be treated in consultation with a neonatal pharmacist, with the least invasive route considered the desired method of delivery (i.e., buccal, dermal, or rectal delivery if intravenous access is no longer desired or available).

■ Comfort measures including holding and kangaroo mother care or skin-to-skin care should be encouraged.

■ A validated instrument to measure infant pain and sedation should be used.

End-of-life care should give attention to the following concerns:

■ Care should be provided in a private location with or near nursing staff with the goal of keeping the family members together.

■ If possible, the environment should have a "home away from home" feel to facilitate comfort and privacy.

■ Alarms and pagers of those in attendance should be turned off. Light levels should be adjusted for family comfort.

■ Routine measurement of vital signs and laboratory analyses should cease.

■ Pain assessments to identify infant distress should be performed frequently.

■ Pain medication should be offered frequently in standardized doses based on the infant's weight.

■ No painful assessments (e.g., heel sticks, measurement of blood gases) should be made.

■ Appropriate access to medications (intravenous, rectal, buccal, or topical) should be given.

■ Offering small amounts of oral fluids such as drops of breast milk and lip lubrication as a comfort measure is appropriate.

■ Infants should be bathed, dressed, and held.

■ Infants should be taken outside into the sunlight if possible.

■ Spiritual and mental health support should be offered to the family.

■ Family and friends should be welcomed, and visiting restrictions should be waived.

■ Memory-making activities should be encouraged, including taking family photographs (by lay or professional photographers), making handprints and footprints, cutting locks of hair, and holding special spiritual or religious ceremonies. However, some cultures do not support these activities, so be sure that the family's values and beliefs are considered.

■ Know the family's wishes about compassionate extubation, discontinuation of life supports, and the withdrawal of artificial nutrition and hydration.

■ If the family is not available, nurses should hold and comfort the infant.

■ Family should be accompanied by staff when leaving the hospital.

TRANSITIONS TO HOME AND PRIMARY CARE

When palliative care includes the removal of life-sustaining technology in the hospital or at home, support from a hospice or palliative care organization should be provided. Before life-sustaining technology is removed, a plan should be in place for the eventuality that the infant continues to breathe independently. When ventilator support of an infant is discontinued, caregivers should attend to the following concerns:

■ The infant's parents should decide who will be present.

■ Vasopressors should be discontinued.

■ The infant should be weaned from neuromuscular blocking agents prior to the removal of life-sustaining technology.

■ Nurses should explain as much of the process to the parents as the parents wish to hear.

■ The infant should be held by a parent or family members, or, if the parents and family do not wish to hold the infant, by a staff member. (Some parents may find it difficult to hold a dying infant.)

■ Gentle suction may be performed, and the endotracheal tube may be removed.

■ Tape and additional lines may be removed.

■ Medication such as morphine should be given if respiratory discomfort exists; oxygen therapy may be used as a comfort measure based on assessment and parental wishes.

■ Medications to treat respiratory distress or to prevent discomfort should be given in standardized dosages based on the infant's weight and may be repeated if necessary. (Bolus medications in larger than normal doses are not appropriate.)

Hospital personnel should have a relationship with a local hospice or palliative care organization to offer seamless continuity of care. Where local hospices do not provide pediatric care, pediatric home health agencies and a primary care pediatrician may oversee the palliative care needs. Infants who are discharged with life-limiting illnesses should have a plan of care, including necessary resources and a portable non-resuscitation plan to avoid unnecessary resuscitation.

The provision of whether the infant who continues to live will receive artificial nutrition and hydration should be discussed. Artificial feeding and hydration are viewed as a life-extending technology (Garten & Buhrer, 2019). If the infant only receives comfort care, survival may be days to weeks during which time the family can provide unencumbered infant care.

BEREAVEMENT

Bereavement interventions can be offered by nursing staff and identified community services. Support may include:

■ Giving the parents a gift such as a stuffed teddy bear to take home (which allows them to leave the hospital without empty arms)

■ Calling the family the next day

■ Sending the family a card, email, or letter from the staff; if possible, personalize the message and send it signed by the team

■ Contacting the family on anniversaries of the infant's birth or death, as the family wishes (by telephone, card, text, or email)

■ Introducing the family to a member of a local or online support group or organization

■ Providing a brochure about bereavement, including support contacts

■ Paying attention to sibling needs and supportive services

■ Archiving infant photographs for a period to allow parents to consider if they wish to have them

■ Conducting follow-up meetings where family members can ask questions or express their perceptions of the care they received

■ Holding an annual memorial event for bereaved families in memory of their babies

EVALUATION

Palliative care will help the family to cope, relieve infant suffering and pain, and increase the quality of life while easing the transition from curative to palliative, and finally bereavement, care.

Written documentation reflects the need for physician management, skilled nursing care, and interdisciplinary support. Appropriate diagnoses and accurate procedural coding ensures reimbursement of palliative care measures. Assessment of quality indicators through regular and systematic measurements from patients (i.e., patient satisfaction) and other stakeholders (outcomes related) should be conducted.

This chapter contains portions of the National Association of Neonatal Nursing Position Statement #3051, 2015, Palliative Care for Neonates, used with permission. (National Association of Neonatal Nurses, 2015).

REFERENCES

American College of Obstetricians & Gynecologists. (2019). *Perinatal palliative care.* https://www.acog.org/clinical/clinical-guidance/committee-opinion/articles/2019/09/perinatal-palliative-care

Barfield, D., & The Committee on Fetus and Newborn. (2016). Standard terminology for fetal, infant, and perinatal deaths. *Pediatrics, 137*(5), e20160551. https://doi.org/10.1542/peds.2016-0551

Carroll, K., Noble-Carr, D., Sweeney, L., & Waldby, C. (2020). The "lactation after infant death (AID) framework": A guide for online health information provision about lactation after stillbirth and infant death. *Journal of Human Lactation, 36*(3), 480–491. https://doi.org/10.1177/0890334420926946

Carter, B. S. (2018). Pediatric palliative care in infants and neonates. *Children (Basel), 5*(2), 21. https://doi.org/10.3390/children5020021

Catlin, A., Brandon, D., Wool, C., & Mendes, J. (2015). NANN position statement: Palliative and end-of-life care for newborns. *Advances in Neonatal Care, 15*(4), 239–240. https://doi .org/10.1097/ANC.0000000000000215

Centers for Disease Control and Prevention. (n.d.-a). *Reproductive health: Infant mortality.* https://www.cdc.gov/reproductivehealth/maternalinfanthealth/infantmortality.htm

Centers for Disease Control and Prevention. (n.d.-b). *Infant health.* https://www.cdc.gov/ nchs/fastats/infant-health.htm

Downing, J., Boucher, S., Daniels, A., & Nkosi, B. (2018). Paediatric palliative care in resource-poor countries. *Children (Basel), 52,* 27. https://doi.org/10.3390/children5020027

Garten, L., & Buhrer, C. (2019). Pain and distress management in palliative neonatal care. *Seminars in Fetal and Neonatal Medicine, 24*(4), 101008. https://www.sciencedirect.com/ science/article/pii/S1744165X19300381

Kenner, C. (2016). The role of neonatal nurses in palliative care. *Newborn and Infant Nursing Reviews, 16*(2), 74–77. https://doi.org/10.1053/j.nainr.2016.03.009

Kenner, C., Press, J., & Ryan, D. (2015). Recommendations for palliative and bereavement care in the NICU: A family-centered integrative approach. *Journal of Perinatology, 35,* S19–S23. https://doi.org/10.1038/jp.2015.145

National Association of Neonatal Nurses. (2015). *Palliative and end-of-life care for newborns and infants. Position Statement #3063.* NANN.

Schroeder, K., & Lorenz, K. (2018). Nursing and the future of palliative care. *Asia Pacific Journal of Oncology Nursing, 5*(1), 4–8. https://doi.org/10.4103/apjon.apjon_43_17

World Health Organization. (2018). *Palliative care. Palliative care is focused on interventions aimed at improving quality of life and maximizing comfort.* WHO (2014) states that, in the case of life-limiting conditions, palliative care should begin at the same time that curative care begins.

Transition to Home and Primary Care

MARINA V. BOYKOVA, CAROLE KENNER, AND DEB DISCENZA

OVERVIEW

The transition from hospital to home for infants and their families who experienced a NICU stay consists of two major components:

■ Transition of infant to primary healthcare settings for medical and developmental follow-up care

■ Parental transition to independent caregiving and parenting

These two major transitions can influence the infant's health to a great extent. The provision of care postdischarge should be carefully coordinated using an integrated team approach. This chapter addresses each of these transitions. This next section focuses on postdischarge care.

BEFORE DISCHARGE

Before NICU infants can be discharged home, they have to meet the following criteria:

■ They must be physiologically stable and have mature respiratory control.

■ Oral feedings should be sufficiently established to support appropriate growth.

■ They must be able to maintain normal body temperature in a homelike environment without supplemental heat (American Academy of Pediatrics [AAP], Committee on Fetus and Newborn, 2008). For most NICU term infants, these criteria will usually be satisfied before discharge, but it can be challenging for prematurely born infants. Most preterm infants achieve physiologic milestones by 34 to 36 weeks' postconceptual age; however, feeding and respiratory control milestones are achieved last (Bakewell-Sachs et al., 2009; Lau, 2020).

● For infants who are in the NICU, a weight gain of 15 to 30 g/d must continue for several days prior to discharge (up to 1 week), and it should occur in an open environment (crib; Sherman et al., 2016).

● Available evidence suggests that preterm infants can be safely discharged home while weighing about 2.2 to 2.5 kg (Edwards et al., 2021), considering that the criteria mentioned previously are satisfied.

● Preterm infants should be able to keep body temperature in normal range for at least 48 hours when clothed appropriately (Sherman et al., 2016).

● Observation for up to 7 days without apnea/bradycardia before discharge is recommended as apneic episodes are common in preterm infants (Eichenwald & Committee on Fetus and Newborn, 2016; Lorch et al., 2011; Nivamat, 2016).

● Hearing screening should be performed before discharge in any NICU infant (Joint Committee on Infant Hearing, 2020). The auditory brainstem response (ABR, automated or not) is preferable so the auditory neuropathy is not missed (Delaney, 2020). If the first hospital examination was abnormal, a follow-up appointment with an audiologist should be planned before discharge.

● The first ophthalmic examination should also be done in the hospital before discharge: infants between 4 and 6 weeks of chronologic age or between 31 and 33 weeks' postmenstrual age should be evaluated for the signs of retinopathy of prematurity (ROP; Fierson et al., 2018).

● Age-appropriate immunizations also should be performed before discharge in infants with a prolonged hospital stay. Stable preterm and term infants should begin immunizations at the usual chronological age of 6 to 8 weeks (Kilpatrick et al., 2017). An updated immunization schedule (including catch-up schedule) is available at the AAP website: www.aap.org/en-us/advocacy-and-policy/aap-health-initiatives/immunizations/Pages/Immunization-Schedule.aspx.

Please see Chapter 19 for more information.

TIMING OF THE FOLLOW-UP APPOINTMENTS

■ For preterm/high-risk infants and infants with an early discharge from the maternity unit (<48 hours after delivery), the first appointment with the primary care provider should occur in the first 24 to 48 hours after discharge (Kilpatrick et al., 2017).

■ The following appointments with primary care providers for high-risk infants should occur in accordance with the individual needs of the infant (Kilpatrick et al., 2017).

■ Some of the high-risk infants should be examined weekly or semimonthly in the immediate period after discharge (Kilpatrick et al., 2017).

MONITORING GROWTH OF AN INFANT

Length, head circumference, and weight must always be considered together for proper infant growth assessment. Growth and body composition should be evaluated simultaneously as well.

■ Frontal-to-occipital head circumference in preterm infants should be increasing by 0.7 to 1 cm/wk (in term infants 0.5 cm) in the immediate postnatal period; by 12 to 18 months of age the increase in head circumference should decline to 0.1 to 0.4 cm/mo (Sherman et al., 2016).

■ The increase in crown-to-heel length should be approximately 0.8 to 1.1 cm/wk in preterm infants (0.7–0.75 in term infants), and by the age of 12 to 18 months, it should decline to 0.75 to 1.5 cm/mo (Sherman et al., 2016).

■ Many preterm infants will grow slower than term infants; recently developed tools such as INTERGROWTH-21st postnatal growth standards can be used to assess physical growth of preterm infants up to 64 weeks' postmenstrual age (Appendix D; Crippa et al., 2020; Gordova & Belfort, 2020; Villar et al., 2015, 2018).

■ The weight gain of 15 to 40 g/d should continue during the first 3 to 4 months of life and then decline to 5 to 15 g/d by age 12 to 18 months (Sherman et al., 2016).

■ For larger and healthier infants, energy intake at approximately 110 kcal/kg/d and protein about 3 g/kg/d can be sufficient for adequate growth (Ruys et al., 2021).

■ For preterm infants, high energy (i.e., 120–130 kcal/kg/d) and high protein (>3 g/100 kcal) may be required in the first weeks of life (up to 32–34 weeks' post-conceptional age). It is then recommended to discontinue such diet to prevent excess fat mass and decrease possible risks for cardiometabolic diseases later in life. A higher protein-to-energy (P:E) ratio (i.e., >2.5–3.0 g/100 kcal) may improve growth and body composition in the short term; close monitoring of the infant's growth pattern is a must (Ruys et al., 2021).

■ Multinutrient human milk (HM) fortification, iron, vitamins, folate, and vitamin D supplementation are often necessary for adequate weight gain and growth, especially for breastfed preterm infants (Crippa et al., 2020). Two HM fortifications are recommended: (1) adjustable fortification when protein adequacy is monitored twice weekly and controlled by blood urea nitrogen (BUN), which should be no lower than 10 mg/dL, and (2) targeted HM fortification when macronutrients in HM are analyzed and milk is supplemented according to the results (Arslanoglu et al., 2019).

■ Protein fortification of breast milk beyond term age should only be considered if the increase in growth is not steady (Ruys et al., 2021).

■ HM feeding in preterm infants is associated with better body composition (i.e., fat-free mass deposition) despite slower weight gain (compared to formula feedings), which may lead to better metabolic and neurodevelopmental outcomes (Cerasani et al., 2020).

■ Postdischarge preterm formulas (energy and protein enriched; 74–77 kcal, P:E 2.7–2.8) or breast milk fortification may be used until 40 to 52 weeks of post-conceptional age (up to 6 months) in presence of low growth velocity (Faienza et al., 2019); individualized nutritional care is warranted.

■ The infants with specific conditions or dependence on technology will have differing needs than the average NICU graduate. Such infants include late preterm infants (34–37 weeks of gestation), term and preterm infants who have had surgery, and infants with chronic lung diseases (CLDs) or congenital heart defects (CHDs). Depending on the exact condition, the infant may require more calories/protein due to the work of breathing or digestive problems. Infants with CLD/CHD may require 120 to 150 kcal/kg/d plus increased protein intake as well as fluid restriction and regular electrolyte monitoring. Again, an individualized nutritional approach is warranted, and rapid catch-up growth of exacerbation of failure to thrive should be avoided (Crippa et al., 2020).

■ Semisolid foods can be introduced while breastfeeding is continued, approximately after 17 weeks of age (4–6 months; Grimshaw et al., 2013). If the introduction/acceptance of semisolid food is problematic, attention should be paid to the intake of micronutrients (Crippa et al., 2020).

■ Neonatal intestinal dysbiosis can be detrimental for the health outcomes of the infant: minimizing unnecessary antibiotics use and exposure and routine administration of prebiotics and probiotics should be considered for NICU graduates and, especially, for preterm infants (Underwood et al., 2020).

MONITORING DEVELOPMENT OF AN INFANT

The neurodevelopmental, behavioral, and sensory status of infants should be assessed several times (by qualified professionals and if the parent has any concerns) during the first year for early identification of problems and timely referral for the appropriate early interventions (EIs; AAP, 2020; Kilpatrick et al., 2017). Purdy and Melwak (2012) and Walker et al. (2012) have suggested the following "red flags" for high-risk infant follow-up:

■ Apgar score at 5 minutes of less than 4

■ Intraventricular hemorrhage more than Grade II, hydrocephalus

■ Hypoxic–ischemic encephalopathy, abnormal neurologic examination (tremors, hypo/hypertonia), seizures

■ Hyperbilirubinemia close to exchange transfusion levels

■ Severe infections (sepsis, meningitis)

■ Hypoglycemia requiring treatment

■ Persistent pulmonary hypertension, extracorporeal membrane oxygenation, use of inhaled nitric oxide

■ Discharge on apnea monitor and caffeine

■ Infant of substance-abusing mother

■ Infants who underwent major and minor surgeries (for conditions such as diaphragmatic hernia, major heart defects, pyloric stenosis, inguinal hernia)

Physical Examinations

■ Infant physical examination and measurements are recommended at 1, 2, 4, 6, 9, and 12 months; in early childhood, these evaluations should take place at 15, 18, 24, and 30 months of age, and then at 3 and 4 years of age (AAP, 2020). High-risk infants may require more frequent follow-up than recommended for healthy infants.

Developmental Screening

■ Developmental screening using validated and standardized tools is recommended at 9, 18, and 24 or 30 months of age (AAP, 2020; Centers for Disease Control and Prevention [CDC], 2021a). More information on the available tools, developmental milestones through the first 5 years of life, and resources for healthcare professionals and families can be found at the CDC (2020) and U.S. Department of Health and Human Services (2020) websites (see the reference list). The CDC also lists EI services by state at www.cdc.gov/ncbddd/actearly/parents/states.html. Parents should be supplied with information at discharge as well as at follow-ups with the pediatrician and/or developmental team.

Ophthalmic/Vision Screening

■ Infants less than 1,500 g or younger than 32 weeks, as well as infants with an unstable clinical course, should have retinal screening (Fierson et al., 2018). The first fundal examination for infants older than 22 weeks of gestation should occur between 4 and 6 weeks of chronologic age or between 31 and 33 weeks postmenstrual age (which might happen in the NICU). Follow-up appointments should occur in 1- to 3-week intervals based on the initial examination findings.

■ Regardless of the initial examination, follow-up ophthalmologic examinations should occur within 4 to 6 months after discharge as NICU infants are at risk for numerous visual disorders. More information on ROP diagnostics and treatment can be found in the recently revised policy statement from the AAP (Fierson et al., 2018).

Hearing Screening

■ An infant should be evaluated at 1 and 3 months of age; follow-up appointments should be planned based on the findings and individual needs of an infant. If the follow-up examination confirms hearing loss, an infant should begin receiving EI services as soon as possible, preferably by the age of 3 months and at least by 6 months, which is beneficial for appropriate language development (Joint Committee on Infant Hearing, 2020; U.S. Department of Health and Human Services, 2021; Vohr et al., 2008).

■ Evaluation by an audiologist every 6 months for the first 3 years of life is recommended (Joint Committee on Infant Hearing, 2020). Children at risk (even without a NICU stay) should have a full hearing test by 2 to 2.5 years of age (CDC, 2021b).

Screening for Metabolic Bone Disease

■ Also referred to as osteopathy, osteopenia, and rickets of prematurity, metabolic bone disease (MBD) should be considered in preterm, low birthweight, and chronically ill infants.

■ Screening tests, despite being not completely indicative of MBD, include serum levels of alkaline phosphatase (ALP), phosphorus, calcium, and parathyroid hormone (PTH), as well as tubular reabsorption of phosphorus (TRP) and vitamin D level (25-hydroxyvitamin D or 25(OH)D; Rayannavar & Calabria, 2020).

■ ALP should be measured in all preterm infants (especially in those exclusively breastfed) every 1 to 2 weeks starting at 4 to 6 weeks of age and 2 to 4 weeks postdischarge; mineral supplementation is recommended when APL levels are higher than 800 to 1,000 IU/L (Faienza et al., 2019). Phosphorus levels lower than 1.8 mmol/L (5.5 mg/dL) correlate with MBD (Rayannavar & Calabria, 2020).

■ Vitamin D deficiency is defined as serum concentration of 25(OH)D less than 12 ng/mL (30 nmol/L); and vitamin D insufficiency is defined as 12 to 20 ng/mL (30–50 nmol/L) of 25(OH)D (Munns et al., 2016; Rayannavar & Calabria, 2020).

■ Children with malabsorptive disorders, children with long-term use of seizure medications, and infants who are exclusively breastfed (especially when the mother has vitamin D deficiency) may require closer monitoring and increased doses of vitamin D supplement as catabolism of vitamin D is increased with these conditions (Rayannavar & Calabria, 2020).

■ Vitamin D supplementation: 400 IU are recommended in the first 12 months. Beyond 12 months of age, children should receive 600 IU, which usually comes in their diet (or can be supplemented if needed so). Up to 2,000 IU/d is needed for the treatment of nutritional rickets (Munns et al., 2016).

■ Vitamin D supplementation should be carried out carefully under the supervision of a primary care provider. Vitamin D toxicity is defined as hypercalcemia and serum 25(OH)D >250 nmol/L, with hypercalciuria and suppressed PTH (Munns et al., 2016).

■ For infants 0 to 6 and 6 to 12 months of age, the adequate calcium intake is 200 mg/d and 260 mg/d, respectively (Munns et al., 2016).

■ Dual-energy x-ray absorptiometry (DEXA) and quantitative ultrasound (QUS) are preferred methods of screening in the asymptomatic phase of MBD (Faienza et al., 2019).

In addition, in high-risk infants postdischarge, periodic evaluation of electrolyte status, acid–base balance, and blood tests should be performed; it is important to monitor for low levels of hemoglobin, hematocrit, potassium, and calcium as well as for other components to prevent possible development of various health problems (such as apnea, anemia, and MBD). Some other additional issues (discussed in the text that follows) should be addressed as well.

Respiratory Syncytial Virus

■ Immunoprophylaxis with palivizumab (Synagis Swedish Orphan Biovitrum AB—Sobi, Stockholm, Sweden) is recommended in the first year of life for premature infants and infants with CHD to reduce the frequency and severity of the respiratory syncytial virus (RSV) infection (seasonal prevalence October/November and March/May, depending on the hemisphere; Anderson et al., 2017; Fergie et al., 2020). It is recommended that all infants 32 weeks of gestational age (GA) or younger and infants at 32 to 35 weeks of GA with additional risk factors (i.e., CHD) should be considered for RSV immunoprophylaxis (Krilov & Anderson, 2020).

■ It is important when getting Synagis that families understand that compliance for all doses is key to the best possible protection for the infant. If there is a challenge in getting time off of work, transportation, and more, there should be a discussion and connection to resources that can assist with such matters to ease the parent's burden.

■ With the rules around handwashing, as well as no illness or smoking, in the NICU, parents will adapt to those rules and will dutifully carry them into the home setting when instructed appropriately. The issue, however, is the family and friends who are not part of this NICU environment are likely to tell the new parents that they are being overprotective. It is recommended that doctors and nurses provide a letter to families to help them educate others coming into the sphere of the discharged infant.

Gastroesophageal Reflux

■ Mild physiological reflux does not require antireflux medications and may be treated with nonpharmacological measures (such as food thickening and infant positioning). Histamine-2 receptor antagonists and proton pump inhibitors (e.g., omeprazole) are not recommended for physiological reflux (AAP, 2019).

■ Antireflux medications can be used for gastroesophageal reflux (GER) disease (when severe respiratory exacerbations, erosive esophagitis, and growth restriction occur), but evidence is controversial for acid neutralization drugs (i.e., omeprazole) and prokinetics (i.e., Reglan or metoclopramide, Baclofen or gablofen) due to increased rates of pneumonia/gastroenteritis/enterocolitis (Eichenwald & Committee on Fetus and Newborn, 2018; Reinhart et al., 2020; Slaughter et al., 2016).

Car Seat Safety and Screening

■ Car seat tolerance screening should be performed on all infants born <37 weeks' GA, regardless of associated comorbidities, for 90 to 120 minutes within 24 to 48 hours before discharge. Preterm infants (including late preterm) may have desaturations, bradycardia,s and obstructive apnea when placed in their car seat; supplemental oxygen might be needed for safe discharge from a hospital (Magnarelli et al., 2020). Car beds are recommended for preterm infants. The Children's Hospital of Philadelphia has sound information on car seat safety for a newborn and child up to the age of 2 years (available at www.chop.edu/centers-programs/car-seat-safety-kids/car-seat-safety-by-age/newborn-2-years#.Vwb6OnqRy6Y).

■ After discharge, traveling in a car with high-risk infants should be postponed as long as possible and performed only when it cannot be avoided.

COVID-19

■ At present, preliminary data suggest that novel SARS-CoV-2 virus infection (aka COVID-19) might increase the risk of severe maternal illness and preterm birth (Woodworth et al., 2020). Breastfeeding appears to be safe as well as skin-to-skin contact, indicating no separation of mothers is needed (Amatya et al., 2020; Sánchez-Luna et al., 2021). Findings from recent small studies suggest that COVID-19 infection in infants seems to be less dangerous than RSV in terms of respiratory problems (Ozdemir et al., 2020). However, more research on COVID-19 in neonates and mothers/families is warranted.

CARE FOR PARENTS POSTDISCHARGE

Parental Preparedness and Education

Preparing parents for the transition to home while still in the hospital is vital to the infant's and family's health and well-being following discharge and especially for families with limited English proficiency (Gupta et al., 2019; Obregon et al., 2019).

■ Before discharge, parents, especially mothers as key caregivers, must be evaluated for their own readiness to take over the care of their infant (Gupta et al., 2019).

■ Appropriate parental education regarding feeding, medicine administration (e.g., inhalers), and home use of oxygen and humidifiers (if prescribed) should be done before discharge.

■ Parents should also receive education regarding cardiopulmonary resuscitation and car seat safety.

■ The information about major developmental milestones for an infant should be given as well, preferably in printed form.

■ In-hospital education before discharge improves parental compliance with follow-up visits (Brachio et al., 2020).

Parental Emotional and Psychosocial Well-Being After Discharge

High-risk and preterm births, infant hospitalization, and specific needs of initially sick or prematurely born infants bring tremendous stress on parents.

■ Many parents of high-risk infants often suffer from posttraumatic stress or post-traumatic stress disorder (PTSD or PTS) that can be detrimental to the infant and parent's health (Schecter et al., 2020). Symptoms of PTS include recurrent memories, flashbacks of traumatic events, changes in thinking or mood with very negative tones, avoidance behaviors, trouble sleeping, overreaction to situations, outbursts of anger, and distractibility; such emotions and behaviors are usually centered on situations that bring back bad memories related to infant hospitalization. It is recommended to screen parents for PTS, so timely and appropriate professional support could be provided if needed (Moreyra et al., 2021).

■ Parents of NICU infants also often suffer from depression that has been shown to affect infant development. Parents might also have prominent anxiety and worries about their infant after discharge that are related to possible illnesses, repeated readmissions, and the development of their infants in the future (O'Donovan & Nixon, 2019). It is recommended to screen parents for depressive symptoms and other emotional disorders before and after discharge, especially those with previous mental health disorders (Hawes et al., 2016; Hynan et al., 2020). Advising parents of the developmental consequences and the importance of getting treatment and of self-care can make a big difference for that infant. Parents postdischarge often report physical exhaustion, sleep deprivation, and tiredness related to caring for an infant with specific needs, numerous appointments, and many treatments. Information about respite care should be given to parents if necessary.

■ Separation from an infant (while gaining adequate weight/respiratory control in the NICU) should be considered as a factor influencing parental well-being and parental role development before and after discharge. Active engagement of parents in direct infant care while in the NICU helps to promote parental role development. Attention should be given to the style of parenting in these parents, as they might be prone for overprotective behaviors, compensatory parenting, and vulnerable child syndrome. Parenting disturbances might influence infant development (or even cause the child to have behavioral problems in the future; Neel et al., 2018, 2019) and the use of healthcare services postdischarge (e.g., overuse of emergency departments). In severe cases, a parent may require professional support from a counselor or a psychologist.

■ Parenting an infant who survived a life-threatening condition is a challenging task. There is a resource for parents who have infants and children with disabilities called Parent Training and Information Centers, which can be found at www.parentcenterhub.org/find-your-center.

■ Health professionals postdischarge should also consider the social consequences of having a medically fragile infant. Parents might suffer from social isolation due to infant vulnerability and parental willingness to protect their infant from possible infections (such as RSV infection; Baraldi et al., 2020).

■ In some instances, social stigmatization may occur depending on the cultural characteristics of the family and surrounding communities. Health professionals also should be careful with stigmatization produced by themselves and should not put labels on such parents and infants (such as "former preemie," "parent of preemie"), but rather treat these vulnerable families with dignity and support. It is important to provide parents with the information about parental support groups available such as Alliance for Black NICU Families (www.blacknicufamilies.org), European Foundation for the Care of Newborn Infants (EFCNI) (www.efcni.org), GLO Preemies (https://GloPreemics. org), Hand to Hold (https://handtohold.org/nicu-family-support), NICU Parent Network (https://nicuparentnetwork.org), Preemie World (https:// preemieworld.com), and Preemie Crystal Ball Health (https://crystalballhealth. com/about-us).

■ Preterm birth and NICU experience may dramatically change family dynamics and marital relationships (Baraldi et al., 2020). In some cases, professional counseling for families might be needed.

■ Financial consequences of having a medically vulnerable infant can be large. With the increasing costs of healthcare, parents should be advised on the availability of helpful resources in order to decrease their healthcare costs and out-of-pocket expenses (such as their ability to cover some expenses with Medicaid). Providing parents with such information will also help improve parental adherence with recommendations for infant health checkups and promote the use of specialized services (speech/language therapy, occupational/physical therapy, EI programs).

■ Appropriate information about primary care providers and referral options should be given to parents at the time of discharge, to enhance parental adherence with recommendations for infant's health checks, continuation of needed treatments, or adjustment/discontinuation of medications. Often, several healthcare specialists should be involved in the postdischarge care of a high-risk infant. These specialists are nutritionists, dieticians, developmental specialists, speech/language and occupational therapists, pediatric surgeons, pulmonologists, and neurologists; collaborative efforts in NICU follow-up care are pivotal (Litt et al., 2020). Parents should be provided with information on how to get referral to these healthcare providers.

■ Transition to home programs should be focusing on socioenvironmental medical risk factors. Contacting parents in the nearest period after discharge, even by telephone call, will help to develop trust, decrease parental anxiety and worry, and prevent unneeded use of healthcare (i.e., overuse of emergency rooms and readmissions; Hintz et al., 2019; Liu et al., 2018; Vohr et al., 2017). Establishing trustful relationships and honest communication are the keys. Regular contacts with parents are recommended as the means of improving care for infants and parents postdischarge. Transition to a home screening tool is available (Boykova, 2018) and can be used for assessment of transitional problems parents might have after NICU discharge. The instrument demonstrated adequate psychometric properties and is available upon request.

CONCLUSION

This chapter highlights the common issues regarding follow-up care for high-risk infants and parents who are making the transition from the NICU to home and to community-based primary care practices. The recommended screening and follow-up care are outlined. The following strategies can be recommended to help parents and families during the transition to home: discharge teaching and information giving; clear communication and coordinated continuity of care postdischarge; adequate social and professional support; and timely health and developmental screenings. Continuity and coordination of care postdischarge is of vital importance for infant health/development and family well-being.

REFERENCES

Amatya, S., Corr., T. E., Gandhi, C., Glass, K. M., Kresch, M. J., Mujsce, D. J., Oji-Mmuo, C. N., Mola, S. J., Murray, Y. L., Palmer T. W., Singh, M., Fricchione, A., Arnold, J., Prentice, D., Bridgeman, C. R., Smith, B. M., Gavigan, P. J., Ericson, J. E., Miller, J. R., . . . Kaiser, J. R. (2020). Management of newborns exposed to mothers with confirmed or suspected COVID-19. *Journal of Perinatology, 40*(13), 987–996. https://doi.org/10.1038/s41372-020-0695-0

American Academy of Pediatrics. (2019). *Choosing wisely: Ten things physicians and patients should question.* https://www.choosingwisely.org/wp-content/uploads/2015/02/AAP-Choosing-Wisely-List.pdf

American Academy of Pediatrics. (2020). *Recommendations for preventive pediatric health care.* https://downloads.aap.org/AAP/PDF/periodicity_schedule.pdf

American Academy of Pediatrics & American College of Obstetrics and Gynecology. (2017). *Guidelines for perinatal care* (8th ed.).

American Academy of Pediatrics, Committee on Fetus and Newborn. (2008). Hospital discharge of the high-risk neonate. *Pediatrics, 122*(5), 1119–1126. https://doi.org/10.1542/peds.2008-2174

Anderson, E. J., Carosone-Link, P., Yogev, R., Yi, J., & Simões, E. A. F. (2017). Effectiveness of palivizumab in high-risk infants and children: A propensity score weighted regression analysis. *The Pediatric Infectious Disease Journal, 36,* 699–704. https://doi.org/10.1097/INF.0000000000001533

Arslanoglu, S., Boquien, C., King, C., Lamireau, D., Tonetto, P., Barnett, D., Bertino, E., Gaya, A., Gebauer, C., Grovslien, A., Moro, G., Weaver, G., Wesolowska, A. M., & Picaud, J. C. (2019). Fortification of human milk for preterm infants: Update and recommendations of the European Milk Bank Association (EMBA) working group on human milk fortification. *Frontiers in Pediatrics, 7,* 76. https://doi.org/10.3389/fped.2019.00076

Bakewell-Sachs, S., Medoff-Cooper, B., Escobar, G. J., Silber, J. H., & Lorch, S. A. (2009). Infant functional status: The timing of physiologic maturation of premature infants. *Pediatrics, 123*(5), e878–e886. https://doi.org/10.1542/peds.2008-2568

Baraldi, E., Allodi, M. W., Smedler, A. C., Westrup, B., Löwing, K., & Ådén, U. (2020). Parents' experiences of the first year at home with an infant born extremely preterm with and without post-discharge intervention: Ambivalence, loneliness, and relationship impact. *International Journal of Environmental Research and Public Health, 17*(24), 9326. https://doi.org/10.3390/ijerph17249326

Boykova, M. (2018). Transition from hospital to home in parents of preterm infants: Revision, modification, and psychometric testing of the questionnaire. *Journal of Nursing Measurement, 26*(2), 296–310. http://doi.org/10.1891/1061-3749.26.2.296

Brachio, S. S., Farkouh-Karoleski, C., Abreu, A., Zygmunt, A., Purugganan, O., & Garey, D. (2020). Improving neonatal follow-up: A quality improvement study analyzing in-hospital interventions and long-term show rates. *Pediatric Quality and Safety, 6*(5), 1–7. https://doi.org/10.1097/pq9.0000000000000363

Centers for Disease Control and Prevention. (2020, June 10). *Learn the signs. Act early: CDC's developmental milestones.* https://www.cdc.gov/ncbddd/actearly/milestones/index.html

Centers for Disease Control and Prevention. (2021a). *Developmental monitoring and screening.* https://www.cdc.gov/ncbddd/childdevelopment/screening.html

Centers for Disease Control and Prevention. (2021b, February 11). *Screening and diagnosis of hearing loss.* https://www.cdc.gov/ncbddd/hearingloss/screening.html

Cerasani, J., Ceroni, F., De Cosmi, V., Mazzocchi, A., Morniroli, D., Roggero, P., Mosca, F., Agostoni, C., & Giannì, M. L. (2020). Human milk feeding and preterm infants' growth and body composition: A literature review. *Nutrients, 12*, 1155. https://doi.org/10.3390/nu12041155

Crippa, B. L., Morniroli, D., Baldassarre, M. E., Consales, A., Vizzari, G., Colombo, L., Mosca, F., & Giammi, M.L. (2020). Preterm's nutrition from hospital to solid foods: Are we still navigating by sight? *Nutrients, 12*, 3646. https://doi.org/10.3390/nu12123646

Delaney, A. (2020). *Newborn hearing screening.* https://emedicine.medscape.com/article/836646-overview

Edwards, E. M., Greenberg, L. T., Ehret, D. E. Y., Lorch, S. A., & Horbar, J. D. (2021). Discharge age and weight for very preterm infants: 2005–2018. *Pediatrics, 147*(2), e2020016006. https://doi.org/10.1542/peds.2020-016006

Eichenwald, E., & Committee on Fetus and Newborn. (2016). Apnea of prematurity. *Pediatrics, 137*(1), e20153757. https://doi.org/10.1542/peds.2015-3757

Eichenwald, E., & Committee on Fetus and Newborn. (2018). Diagnosis and management of gastroesophageal reflux in preterm infants. *Pediatrics, 142*, e20181061. https://doi.org/10.1542/peds.2018-1061

Faienza, M. F., D'Amato, E., Natale, M. P., Grano, M., Chiarito, M., Brunetti, G., & D'Amato, G. (2019). Metabolic bone disease of prematurity: Diagnosis and management. *Frontiers in Pediatrics, 7*, 143. https://doi.org/10.3389/fped.2019.00143

Fergie, J., Goldstein, M., Krilov, L. R., Wade, S., Kong, A. M., & Brannman, L. (2020). Update on respiratory syncytial virus hospitalizations among U.S. preterm and term infants before and after the 2014 American Academy of Pediatrics policy on immunoprophylaxis: 2011–2017. *Human Vaccines and Immunotherapeutics, 17*, 1–10. https://doi.org/10.1080/21645515.2020.1822134.

Fierson, W. M., & American Academy of Pediatrics Section on Ophthalmology, American Academy of Ophthalmology, American Association for Pediatric Ophthalmology and Strabismus, and American Association of Certified Orthoptists. (2018). Screening examination of premature infants for retinopathy of prematurity. *Pediatrics, 142*(6), e20183061. https://doi.org/10.1542/peds.2018-3061

Gordova, E. G., & Belfort, M. B. (2020). Updates on assessment and monitoring of the postnatal growth of preterm infants. *NeoReviews, 21*(2), e98–e108. https://doi.org/10.1542/neo.21-2-e98

Grimshaw, K., Maskell, J., Oliver, E., Morris, R., Foote, K., Mills, E. N. C., Roberts, G., & Margetts. B. M. (2013). Introduction of complementary foods and the relationship to food allergy. *Pediatrics, 132*(6), e1529–e1538. https://doi.org/10.1542/peds.2012-3692

Gupta, M., Pursley, D. M., & Smith, V. C. (2019). Preparing for discharge from the neonatal intensive care unit. *Pediatrics, 143*(6), e20182915. https://doi.org/10.1542/peds.2018-2915

Hawes, K., McGowan, E., O'Donnell, E., Tucker, R., & Vohr, B. (2016). Social emotional factors increase risk of postpartum depression in mothers of preterm infants. *Journal of Pediatrics, 179*, 61–67. http://doi.org/10.1016/j.jpeds.2016.07.008

Hintz, S. R., Gould, J. B., Bennett, M. V., Lu, T., Gray, E. E., Jocson, M. A. L., Fuller, M., & Lee, H. C. (2019). Factors associated with successful first high-risk infant clinic visit for very low birth weight infants in California. *Journal of Pediatrics, 210*, 91–98. https://doi .org/10.1016/j.jpeds.2019.03.007

Hynan, M. T., Cicoo, R., & Hatfield, B. (2020). *IFCDC-recommendations for best practice reducing & managing pain & stress in newborns & families. Developmental care standards for infants in intensive care.* https://nicudesign.nd.edu/nicu-care-standards/

Joint Committee on Infant Hearing, American Academy of Audiology, American Academy of Pediatrics, American Speech-Language-Hearing Association and Directors of Speech and Hearing Programs in State Health and Welfare Agencies. (2020). Year 2000 Position Statement: Principles and guidelines for early hearing detection and intervention programs. *Pediatrics, 106*(4), 798–817. https://doi.org/10.1542/peds.106.4.798

Kilpatrick, S. J., Papile, L.-A., & Macones, G. A. (2017). *Guidelines for perinatal care* (8th ed.). American Academy of Pediatrics.

Krilov, L. R., & Anderson, E. J. (2020). Respiratory syncytial virus hospitalizations in US preterm infants after the 2014 change in immunoprophylaxis guidance by the American Academy of Pediatrics. *Journal of Perinatology, 40*(8), 1135–1144. https://doi.org/10.1038/ s41372-020-0689-y

Lau, C. (2020). To individualize the management care of high-risk infants with oral feeding challenges: What do we know? What can we do? *Frontiers in Pediatrics, 8*, 296. https://doi .org/10.3389/fped.2020.00296

Litt, J. S., Edwards, E. M., Lainwala, S., Mercier, C., Montgomery, A., O'Reilly, D., Rhein, L., Woythaler, M., Hartman, T., & on behalf of the New England Follow-up Network. (2020). Optimizing high-risk infant follow-up in nonresearch-based paradigms: The New England follow-up network. *Pediatric Quality and Safety, 2*, e287. https://doi.org/10.1097/ pq9.0000000000000287

Liu, Y., McGowan, E., Tucker, R., Glasgow, L., Kluckman, M., & Vohr, B. (2018). Transition Home Plus Program reduces Medicaid spending and health care use for high-risk infants admitted to the neonatal intensive care unit for 5 or more days. *Journal of Pediatrics, 200*, 91–97. https://doi.org/10.1016/j.jpeds.2018.04.038

Lorch, S. A., Srinivasan, L., & Escobar, G. J. (2011). Epidemiology of apnea and bradycardia resolution in premature infants. *Pediatrics, 128*(2), e366–e373. https://doi.org/10.1542/ peds.2010-1567

Magnarelli, A., Solanki, N. S., & Davis, N. L. (2020). Car seat tolerance screening for late-preterm infants. *Pediatrics, 145*(1), e20191703. https://doi.org/10.1542/peds.2019-1703

Moreyra, A., Dowtin, L. L., Ocampo, M., Perez, E., Borkovi, T. C., Wharton, E., Simon, S., Arme, E. G., & Shaw, R. J. (2021). Implementing a standardized screening protocol for parental depression, anxiety, and PTSD symptoms in the Neonatal Intensive Care Unit. *Early Human Development, 154*. https://doi.org/10.1016/j.earlhumdev.2020.105279

Munns, C., Shaw, M., Kiely, M., Specker, B. L., Thacher, T. D., Ozono, K., Michigami, T., Tiosano, D., Mughal, M. Z., Mäkitie, Q., Ramos-Abad, L., Ward, L., DiMeglio, L. A., Atapattu, N., Cassinelli, H., Braegger, C., Pettifor, J. M., Seth, A., Idris, H. W., . . . , Högler, W. (2016). Global consensus recommendations on prevention and management of nutritional rickets. *Journal of Clinical Endocrinology and Metabolism, 101*(2), 394–415. https://doi.org/10.1210/jc.2015-2175

Neel, M. L., Slaughter, J. C., Stark, A. R., & Maitre, N. L. (2019). Parenting style associations with sensory threshold and behaviour: A prospective cohort study in term/preterm infants. *Acta Paediatrica, 108*, 1616–1623. https://doi.org/10.1111/apa.14761

Neel, M. L. M., Stark, A. R., & Maitre, N. L. (2018). Parenting style impacts cognitive and behavioural outcomes of former preterm infants: A systematic review. *Child: Care, Health and Development, 44,* 507–515. https://doi.org/10.1111/cch.12561

Nivamat, D. J. (2016). *Apnea of prematurity.* http://emedicine.medscape.com/article/974971-overview

Obregon, E., Martin, C., Frantz, I, III, Ptel, P., & Smith, V. (2019). Neonatal intensive care unit discharge preparedness among families with limited English proficiency. *Journal of Perinatology, 39,* 135–142. https://doi.org/10.1038/s41372-018-0255-z

O'Donovan, A., & Nixon, E. (2019). "Weathering the storm:" Mothers' and fathers' experiences of parenting a preterm infant. *Infant Mental Health Journal, 40,* 573–587. https://doi.org/10.1002/imhj.21788

Ozdemir, S. A., Soysal, B., Calkavur, S., Yildirim, T. G., Kıymet, E., Kalkanli, O., Çolak, R., & Devrim, I. (2020). Is respiratory syncytial virus infection more dangerous than COVID 19 in the neonatal period? *Journal of Maternal-Fetal & Neonatal Medicine.* https://doi.org/10.1080/14767058.2020.1849125

Purdy, I. B., & Melwak, M. A. (2012). Who is at risk? High-risk infant follow-up. *Newborn and Infant Nursing Reviews, 12*(4), 221–226.

Rayannavar, A., & Calabria, A. C. (2020). Screening for metabolic bone disease of prematurity. *Seminars in Fetal and Neonatal Medicine, 25,* 101086. https://doi.org/10.1016/j.siny.2020.101086

Reinhart, R. M., McClary, J. D., Zhang, M., Marasch, J. L., Hibbs, A. M., & Nock, M. L. (2020). Reducing antacid use in a level IV NICU: A QI project to reduce morbidity. *Pediatric Quality and Safety, 3,* e303. https://doi.org/10.1097/pq9.0000000000000303

Ruys, C. A., van de Lagemaat, M., Rotteveel, J., Finken, M. J., & Lafeber, H. N. (2021). Improving long-term health outcomes of preterm infants: How to implement the findings of nutritional intervention studies into daily clinical practice. *European Journal of Pediatrics, 180,* 1–9. https://doi.org/10.1007/s00431-021-03950-2

Sánchez-Luna, M., Colomer, B. F., de Alba Romero, C., Allen, A. A., Souto, A. B., Longueira, F. C., Badía, M. C., Pradell, Z. G., López, M. G., Herrera, M., Bautista, C. R., García, L. S., Flores, E. Z., & on behalf of the SENEO COVID-19 Registry Study Group. (2021). Neonates born to mothers with COVID-19: Data from the Spanish Society of Neonatology Registry. *Pediatrics, 147*(2), e2020015065. https://doi.org/10.1542/peds.2020-015065

Schecter, R., Pham, T., Hua, A., Spinazzola, R., Sonnenklar, J., Li, D., Papaioannou, H., & Milanaik, R. (2020). Prevalence and longevity of PTSD symptoms among parents of NICU infants analyzed across gestational age categories. *Clinical Pediatrics, 59*(2), 163–169. https://doi.org/10.1177/0009922819892046

Sherman, M. P., Lauriello, N. F., & Aylward, G. P. (2016). *Follow-up of the NICU patient.* http://emedicine.medscape.com/article/1833812-overview#a1

Slaughter, J., Stenger, M., Reagan, P., & Jadcherla, S. (2016). Neonatal H2-receptor antagonist and proton pump inhibitor treatment at US children's hospitals. *Journal of Pediatrics, 174,* 63–70. https://doi.org/10.1016/j.jpeds.2016.03.059

Underwood, M. A., Mukhopadhyay, S., Lakshminrusimha, S., & Bevins, C. L. (2020). Neonatal intestinal dysbiosis. *Journal of Perinatology, 40,* 1597–1608. https://doi.org/10.1038/s41372-020-00829-2

U.S. Department of Health and Human Services, Office of Early Childhood Development. (2020, November 3). *Birth to 5: Watch me thrive!* https://www.acf.hhs.gov/ecd/child-health-development/watch-me-thrive

U.S. Department of Health and Human Services, National Institute on Deafness and Other Communication Disorders. (2021, February 11). *Your baby's hearing screening.* https://www.nidcd.nih.gov/health/your-babys-hearing-screening

Villar, J., Giuliani, F., Barros, F., Roggero, P., Zarco, I. A. C., Rego, M. A. S., Ochieng, R., Gianni, M. L., Rao, S., Lambert, A., Ryumina, I., Britto, C., Chawla, D., Ismail, L. C., Ali, S. R., Hirst, J., Teji, J. S., Abawi, K., Asibey, J., ... Kennedy, S. (2018). Monitoring the postnatal growth of preterm infants: A paradigm change. *Pediatrics, 141*(2), e20172467. https://doi.org/10.1542/peds.2017-2467

Villar, J., Giuliani, F., Bhutta, Z. A., Bertino, E., Ohuma, E. O., Ismail, L. C., Barros, F. C., Altman, D. G., Victora, C., Noble, J. A., Gravett, M. G., Purwar, M., Pang, R., Lambert, A., Papageorghiou, A. T., Ochieng, R., Jaffer, Y. A., Kennedy, S. H., & International Fetal and Newborn Growth Consortium for the 21(st) Century (INTERGROWTH-21(st)). (2015). Postnatal growth standards for preterm infants: The preterm postnatal follow-up study of the INTERGROWTH-21st Project. *Lancet, 3*(11), e681–e691. https://doi.org/10.1016/S2214-109X(15)00163-1

Vohr, B., Jodoin-Krauzyk, J., Tucker, R., Johnson, M. J., Topol, D., & Ahlgren, M. (2008). Early language outcomes of early-identified infants with permanent hearing loss at 12 to 16 months of age. *Pediatrics, 122*(3), 525–544. https://doi.org/10.1542/peds.2007-2028

Vohr, B., McGowan, E., Keszler, L., Alksninis, B., O'Donnell, M., Hawes, K., & Tucker, R. (2017). Impact of a transition home program on rehospitalization rates of preterm infants. *Journal of Pediatrics, 181*, 86–89. http://doi.org10.1016/j.jpeds.2016.10.025

Walker, K., Holland, A. J., Halliday, R., & Badawi, N. (2012). Which high-risk infants should we follow-up and how should we do it? *Journal of Paediatrics and Child Health, 48*(9), 789–793. https://doi.org/10.1111/j.1440-1754.2012.02540.x

Woodworth, K. R., Olsen, E. O., Neelam, V., Lewis, E. L., Galang, R. R., Oduyebo, T., Aveni, K., Yazdy, M. M., Harvey, E., Longcore, N. D., Barton, J., Fussman, C., Siebman, S., Lush, M., Patrick, P. H., Halai, U.-A., Valencia-Prado, M., Orkis, L., Sowunmi, S., . . ., COVID-19 Pregnancy and Infant Linked Outcomes Team (PILOT). (2020). Birth and infant outcomes following laboratory-confirmed SARS-COV-2 infection in pregnancy—SET-NET, 16 jurisdictions. *Morbidity and Mortality Weekly Reports, 69*, 1635–1640. http://doi.org/10.15585/mmwr.mm6944e2external icon

Common Procedures, Diagnostic Tests, Lab Values, and Drugs

Common Procedures, Diagnostic Tests, and Lab Values

COMMON PROCEDURES

Overview

This chapter outlines the most common procedures done in a NICU. The content presents basic information on each procedure. Members of the healthcare team should operate under their individual scope of practice as well as institutional guidelines/policy and procedures.

BLOOD DRAWS

STEPHANIE R. SYKES AND JODI A. ULLOA

Blood draws in the newborn are performed to obtain serum or whole blood specimens for laboratory testing. Blood may be drawn by capillary blood draw from heelstick, venipuncture, arterial puncture, or from a central catheter. Before obtaining any specimen, the patient's identity should be confirmed by institutional protocol confirming correct patient by name, medical record number, and date of birth.

CAPILLARY BLOOD DRAW FROM HEEL

The goal is to obtain a capillary blood specimen from a heel puncture.

Clinical Indications

Heel capillary blood draw is indicated to obtain small quantities of blood for capillary blood testing, point-of-care glucose screen, newborn screening test (blood spot test), or routine blood testing.

Clinical Contraindications

Heel capillary blood draw is contraindicated if the perfusion is poor, if the heel has been traumatized, if adequate flow cannot be obtained after puncture, or if a large quantity of blood is needed for a lab test. Excessive squeezing of the heel results in trauma and can alter the integrity of the specimen for testing. Any method of blood drawing is contraindicated in the newborn with a known or suspected bleeding diathesis as establishing hemostasis may be difficult.

Equipment for Capillary Blood Draw From Heel

- Personal protective equipment (PPE)
- Heel warmer
- Facility-approved antiseptic
- Newborn or premature size lancet
- Appropriate specimen collection container for ordered lab work (verify amount of blood needed and collection containers prior to starting the procedure)
- 2 × 2 gauze
- Appropriate skin covering for gestational age to apply to site postprocedure

Steps

- Wash hands.
- Don gloves.
- Use developmentally appropriate techniques to assist in decreasing painful stimuli such as containment, oral sucrose or breast milk with a pacifier, sensorial saturation, or put the infant to the mother's breast.
- Activate the heel warmer and wrap the heel warmer around the heel.
- Remove the heel warmer after the heel is adequately warmed.
- Cleanse the area of the heel to be punctured with facility-approved antiseptic.
- Puncture either the outer or inner lateral aspect of the heel with a lancet.
- Wipe away the first drop with a sterile 2 × 2 gauze.
- Gently squeeze the foot to produce blood flow from the punctured site.
- Obtain the specimen.
- Cover the puncture site with clean gauze and apply gentle pressure for hemostasis.
- Apply appropriate skin covering for gestational age over the puncture site.

Assessment and Care Postprocedure

- Examine the punctured heel for trauma and persistent bleeding from the puncture site.

Complications

■ Skin trauma and scarring

■ Excessive blood loss

■ Pain

■ Infection

Documentation

Document the site of puncture, specimen obtained including total amount of blood drawn, visible trauma or residual bleeding from the site (if any), and infant tolerance to procedure including prepain and postpain scores per institutional policy.

BLOOD DRAW FROM VENIPUNCTURE

Clinical Indications

This procedure is indicated if volume needed is greater than 1 mL from the infant or if laboratory testing guidelines require venous blood.

Clinical Contraindications

Any method of blood drawing is contraindicated in the newborn with a known or suspected bleeding diathesis as establishing hemostasis may be difficult. Venipuncture is also contraindicated if the skin is not intact, if infection is present, or if the vessel is potentially needed for central line or peripheral intravenous (PIV) catheterization.

Equipment for Venipuncture

■ PPE

■ Facility-approved antiseptic

■ Appropriate gauge butterfly needle (23 or 25 gauge)

■ Syringe size based on total amount of blood to be collected or specific to lab ordered (blood gas syringe)

■ Appropriate specimen collection containers for ordered lab work (verify amount of blood needed and collection containers prior to starting the procedure)

■ 2 × 2 gauze

■ Appropriate skin covering for gestational age to apply to site postprocedure

Steps

■ Wash hands.

■ Don gloves.

■ Use developmentally appropriate techniques to assist in decreasing painful stimuli such as containment, oral sucrose or breast milk with a pacifier, or sensorial saturation. Swaddle the infant with the extremity to be punctured exposed or have an additional assistant hold the infant.

■ Cleanse the site over the vein with facility-approved antiseptic.

■ Insert the butterfly needle at a 45° angle into the vein with the bevel pointed up.

■ Once blood appears in the butterfly tubing, draw the desired volume into the syringe.

■ Remove the needle and apply pressure to the puncture site with 2 × 2 gauze until hemostasis is attained.

■ Apply appropriate skin covering for gestational age over the puncture site.

Assessment and Care Postprocedure

Evaluate puncture site/extremity for residual bleeding, trauma, and peripheral circulation.

Complications

■ Cellulitis
■ Phlebitis
■ Hematoma
■ Pain
■ Nerve damage

Documentation

Record the site punctured, size of needle used, amount of blood drawn, residual bleeding, trauma, and peripheral circulation, as well as infant tolerance of procedure including prepain and postpain scores per institutional policy.

BLOOD DRAW FROM ARTERIAL PUNCTURE

Definition

Recommended arteries for arterial puncture in the infant population include the radial, ulnar, and the posterior tibial arteries.

Clinical Indications

Arterial puncture is indicated when drawing arterial blood gases, when specific laboratory tests require arterial sampling, when large quantities of blood are necessary for sampling, or when capillary or venous sampling are not obtainable.

Clinical Contraindications

Arterial punctures are contraindicated for infants with coagulation disorders, thrombocytopenia, circulatory compromise of the extremity, infection at the site of the procedure, or if the artery is necessary for cannulation to establish a peripheral arterial line; in those cases, it should not be punctured for a one-time lab. Arteries should be used for one puncture for each procedure to avoid increased risk of hematoma or damage to the artery. The ulnar artery should be used only if other alternative arteries are not available because of increased risk of impaired circulation to the hand and proximity of the ulnar and median nerves. Avoid the use of brachial arteries, which can result in brachial nerve damage; temporal arteries, which can result in temporal nerve damage; or femoral arteries, which can result in osteomyelitis of the hip joint.

Equipment for Blood Draw From Arterial Puncture

■ PPE

■ Facility-approved antiseptic

■ Appropriate gauge butterfly needle (23 or 25 gauge)

■ Syringe size based on total amount of blood to be collected or specific to lab ordered (e.g., blood gas syringe)

■ Appropriate specimen collection containers for ordered lab work (verify amount of blood needed and collection containers prior to starting the procedure)

■ 2 × 2 gauze

■ Appropriate skin covering for gestational age to apply to site postprocedure

■ Transilluminator light (optional)

Steps

■ Wash hands.

■ Don gloves.

■ Use developmentally appropriate techniques to assist in decreasing painful stimuli such as containment, oral sucrose or breast milk with a pacifier, or sensorial saturation. Swaddle the infant with the extremity to be punctured exposed or have an additional assistant hold the infant.

■ Locate the artery using palpation of the pulse or a transillumination device (optional).

■ Perform a modified Allen test to confirm collateral circulation if either radial or ulnar arteries are to be used.

■ Cleanse the site over the vein with facility-approved antiseptic.

■ Insert the butterfly needle at a 30° angle for superficial arteries and 45° angle if deeper artery with the bevel pointed up.

■ Once blood appears in the butterfly tubing, draw the desired volume into the syringe.

■ Remove the needle and apply pressure to the puncture site with 2 × 2 gauze for at least 1 to 2 minutes or until hemostasis is attained.

■ Apply appropriate skin covering for gestational age over the puncture site.

■ Monitor for bleeding.

Assessment and Care Postprocedure

Evaluate circulation distal to the puncture site, site for bleeding, and surrounding area for evidence of trauma.

Complications

■ Hematoma

■ Unintended blood loss

■ Pain

■ Infection

■ Nerve damage

Documentation

Record the site punctured, result of the Allen test (if used), size of needle used, amount of blood drawn, residual bleeding, trauma, and peripheral circulation as well as infant tolerance of procedure, including preprocedure and postprocedure pain scores per institutional policy.

BLOOD DRAW FROM A CENTRAL OR PERIPHERAL ARTERIAL CATHETER

Definition

Blood samples can be drawn from indwelling arterial catheters with emphasis on aseptic technique and minimizing stress or trauma to the infant and vessels. Newer closed central catheter systems allow for blood sampling while maintaining the system integrity.

Clinical Indications

Critically ill infants or when frequent and multiple arterial blood sampling is necessary for treatment or monitoring.

Clinical Contraindications

Rapid blood withdrawal from catheters in premature infants has been associated with changes in cerebral blood flow. Indwelling catheters in infants have been associated with frequent blood sampling and iatrogenic anemia.

Equipment for Blood Draw From a Central or Peripheral Arterial Catheter

■ PPE

■ Facility-approved antiseptic for cleaning access ports of indwelling catheters

■ Syringe size based on total amount of blood to be collected or specific to lab ordered (e.g., blood gas syringe)

■ Appropriate specimen collection containers for ordered lab work (verify amount of blood needed and collection containers prior to starting the procedure)

Steps

■ Wash hands.

■ Don gloves.

■ Close the stopcock, connect the syringe to the catheter access port or stopcock, interrupt infusion, open the stopcock or access port to the syringe, and draw back the catheter manufacturer-specified volume to clear the line, then close the stopcock or access port. Disconnect this syringe and discard this specimen.

■ Connect the specimen-collecting syringe to the stopcock or access port, open the stopcock or access port, and withdraw the required blood specimen volume. Close the stopcock or access port.

■ Flush residual blood from the catheter as follows:

   ● Connect the syringe with flush, open the stopcock, and slowly flush the line to clear it of residual blood, OR

   ● If using a closed system, follow manufacturer guidelines for flushing the catheter and line to clear it of residual blood.

   ● Resume fluid infusion.

Assessment and Care Postprocedure

Verify that the line is infusing with fluid without residual blood or air in line.

Complications

■ Iatrogenic blood loss

■ Air embolism

■ Bloodstream infection

■ Vessel thrombosis

■ Infiltration

Documentation

Document volume of specimen obtained, lab specimens sent, and complications, if any.

INTRAVASCULAR CANNULATION

STEPHANIE R. SYKES AND JODI A. ULLOA

INSERTION OF PERIPHERAL INTRAVENOUS CATHETER

Definition

Insertion of an appropriately sized plastic cannula of various sizes into a peripheral vein.

Clinical Indications

Peripheral intravenous (PIV) catheters are inserted when there is a need for intravenous (IV) access for administration of medications, fluids, parenteral nutrition, or blood products (Legemaat et al., 2016).

Clinical Contraindications

Contraindications include decreased circulation of the surrounding tissue or compromised skin integrity.

Equipment for Insertion of Peripheral Intravenous Catheter

■ Heel warmer (if needed to increase circulation to extremity)

■ Swaddling blanket

■ Gloves

■ Pacifier

■ Sucrose

■ Facility-approved antiseptic

■ 22- to 26-gauge IV catheter

■ T-connector

■ 3 mL syringe with normal saline to flush catheter

■ Tourniquet

■ Transparent bioocclusive dressing

■ Catheter securement device or adhesive tape to secure catheter per facility protocol

■ Sterile 2 × 2 gauze

■ Cotton balls, arm board if needed

■ Transilluminator or procedure light to visualize vein if needed

Steps

■ Wash hands and don gloves.

■ Swaddle as necessary using developmentally appropriate techniques or obtain assistance to stabilize the infant during the procedure.

■ Flush the T-connector with saline flush and keep connections sterile.

■ Identify the vein with optional use of procedural light or transilluminator: plantar surface of hand or foot, scalp, forearm, or leg. Veins on the hands and feet are often easier to see and access (Hugill, 2016). A warm compress may be used to increase circulation to extremity prior to visualization per facility protocol.

■ Apply a tourniquet proximal to the vein to increase venous congestion and dilate the vein.

■ Cleanse the skin over the vein.

■ Insert the catheter bevel up. Once blood flashes into the catheter reservoir, thread the plastic part of the catheter into the vein and retract the needle.

■ Remove the tourniquet.

■ Connect the T-connector and flush the catheter with normal saline to verify patency.

■ Once the catheter is inserted and flushes easily, secure with the transparent dressing and tape.

■ Use the other securing or limb-stabilizing devices if needed to protect the PIV from dislodging.

■ If unable to flush or the tissue proximal to the catheter tip becomes distended with fluid during flushing, apply pressure above the catheter tip and pull the catheter out, applying pressure to the insertion site for hemostasis.

■ If the initial attempt is unsuccessful, attempt again with a new catheter in an alternative location following the previous steps.

Assessment and Care Postprocedure

Verify the patency of the PIV immediately after insertion, after securing, and before attaching infusion equipment. Monitor the integrity of the surrounding skin and insertion site at least hourly to avoid excessive extravasation of infusate into the surrounding tissue. Monitor for signs of phlebitis or other evidence of infection. Ensure proper anatomical position of extremity if an immobilization device is utilized.

Complications

■ Infiltration

■ Phlebitis

■ Accidental placement in artery

■ Infection

■ Impaired skin integrity from tape or securement devices or from warm compress

■ Hematoma

■ Air embolism

Documentation

Document the site of insertion, number of attempts, infant's tolerance, blood loss, and complications, if any.

CHEST NEEDLE ASPIRATION

STEPHANIE R. SYKES AND JODI A. ULLOA

Definition

This is the emergent percutaneous insertion of a needle for the removal of fluid, blood, or air from the pleural space, which is most often the first step for evacuation of a clinically significant pneumothorax or effusion. The patient may need placement of a chest tube if the air or fluid reaccumulates (Ramasethu & Seo, 2020, chapter 41). An anterior approach is preferred for emergency evacuation, as this position will not interfere with the placement of an indwelling drainage tube on the lateral chest if needed.

Clinical Indications

Clinical indications include signs of cardiorespiratory compromise or failure in the presence of life-threatening air or fluid accumulations in the pleural space.

Clinical Contraindications

Clinical contraindications include impaired skin integrity at the site, coagulopathy, or small air or fluid collections without clinical compromise that may self-resolve.

Equipment for Chest Needle Aspiration

■ Needle (#23- or #25-gauge butterfly needle or #20-, #22-, or #24-gauge angiocath)

■ Facility-approved antiseptic

■ T-connector

■ Three-way stopcock

■ Extension tubing

■ 10 to 60 mL syringe

■ Pain control/sedation as indicated

■ Personal protective equipment (PPE) including sterile gloves

■ Sterile 2 × 2 gauze

■ Sterile drapes

■ Positioning aids (such as blanket rolls)

Steps

■ Locate and assemble supplies.

■ Perform a time-out at the bedside to verify patient name, medical record number, and correct site.

■ Provide adequate ventilator support as needed; closely monitor cardiorespiratory status and vital signs during procedure.

■ Provide adequate pain control +/– sedation if needed.

■ Place the patient in a supine position with the positioning aid under the affected side.

■ Maintain thermoregulation and monitor vital signs/oxygen saturation during the procedure.

■ Assemble equipment (if using an angiocath, attach the T-connector to the end of the IV catheter and the three-way stopcock to the end of the T-connector. The aspiration syringe can be attached to the stopcock. If using the butterfly needle, attach the stopcock to the end of the tubing and the syringe to the stopcock for aspiration).

■ Locate landmarks at the second to third intercostal space, midclavicular line.

■ Wash hands, don sterile gloves, and organize supplies in a sterile fashion.

■ Drape the patient.

■ Cleanse the area.

■ Insert the needle firmly into the identified space perpendicular to the chest wall and above the upper border of the third rib, advancing it until a "pop" is felt.

■ Use the syringe to aspirate air and/or fluid from the pleural space.

■ Secure the needle in place with dressing and monitor for reaccumulation of air or fluid.

Assessment and Care Postprocedure

Monitor vital signs and oxygen saturations. Set up for chest tube insertion if needed.

Complications

■ Bleeding

■ Infection

■ Pain

■ Nerve injury

Documentation

- Date and time of the procedure
- Indications
- Equipment used
- Vital signs prior to and following procedure
- Pain control measures (medication/comfort care)
- Number of attempts
- Patient tolerance to procedure
- Anterior-posterior (AP) chest x-ray results prior to and following procedure

CHEST TUBE INSERTION

STEPHANIE R. SYKES AND JODI A. ULLOA

Definition

Placement of a tube is done to remove air or fluid from the pleural space with negative pressure setup using water seal or suction. Air is most effectively removed by an anteriorly placed chest tube. Fluid is most effectively removed by a posteriorly placed chest tube.

Clinical Indications

Clinical indications include presence of a tension pneumothorax with cardiorespiratory compromise or drainage of large pneumothorax, drainage of pleural effusion, obtaining fluid for diagnostic purposes (empyema), or for postoperative drainage after tracheal or esophageal surgery (Ramasethu & Seo, 2020, chapter 41).

Clinical Contraindications

Clinical contraindications include impaired skin integrity at site, uncorrected coagulopathy, or small air or fluid collections that may self-resolve without intervention.

Equipment for Chest Tube Insertion

- Facility-approved antiseptic
- Personal protective equipment (PPE) including sterile gown and gloves; hat and mask
- Prepackaged chest tube tray (may vary depending on facility)
- Sterile drapes

▪ Commonly used chest tube options

- Pigtail catheter with natural coil, nonlocking using modified Seldinger technique.

  • Pigtail catheter (natural coil): size 6 or 8 Fr (<28 weeks), 8 Fr (>28 weeks)

  • Introducer and J-shaped guidewire (inserted in a sleeve)

  • Needle (size varies with different manufacturers, may be 18–24 gauge)

  • Dilator

  • Adaptor for external end of the catheter to connect to pleural drainage device

  • Optional: syringe

- Chest tube with safety color change indicator: polyurethane catheter with a blunt safety cannula

- Connecting tube

- Syringe

▪ Sterile water (to clean off cleaning solution following procedure)

▪ Pain medications and/or sedation as indicated

▪ Positioning aids (blanket rolls)

▪ Pleural evacuation drainage system

▪ Adhesive tape and occlusive dressing appropriate for gestational age to secure tube postprocedure

Steps

▪ Locate and assemble supplies.

▪ Perform a time-out at the bedside to verify patient name, medical record number, and correct site.

▪ Provide adequate ventilator support as needed; closely monitor cardiorespiratory status and vital signs during procedure.

▪ Provide adequate pain control; consider sedation if needed.

▪ Position the patient with positioning aids such as a blanket roll to elevate the affected side of the chest (approximately 45°–60°) and secure arm above head with shoulder internally rotated and abducted.

▪ Locate the site (second to third intercostal space at the midclavicular line or fourth to fifth intercostal space at the midaxillary line). A horizontal line from the nipple can be used to identify the fourth intercostal space.

▪ Wash hands, don sterile PPE, and organize supplies in a sterile fashion.

▪ Cleanse the area and allow to dry.

▪ Drape the area from the third to eighth ribs.

■ May administer subcutaneous lidocaine to anesthetize the area per facility protocol and formulary.

■ To insert pigtail catheter (Cook Incorporated, 2019):

● Optional additional step: attach a syringe applying negative pressure until a lack of resistance is felt and air or fluid is evacuated while inserting introducer needle (Ramasethu & Seo, 2020, chapter 41).

● Insert the tip of the introducer needle into the skin in fourth intercostal space between anterior and midaxillary lines above the upper border of the fifth rib.

● Advance the introducer needle slowly, perpendicular to the chest wall.

● Stabilize the introducer needle with one hand, remove the syringe, and insert the guidewire through the introducer needle.

● Advance the guidewire until the depth marker on the guidewire is visible at the hub of the introducer needle.

● Carefully remove the introducer needle, maintaining stability of the guidewire at the chest wall.

● Place the dilator over the guidewire and insert the dilator into the chest wall in a slow twisting motion to dilate the tract. Advance the dilator only far enough to dilate the skin tract and parietal pleura (about 1 cm in the preterm and 2 cm in the term infant).

● Carefully remove the dilator, maintaining stability of the guidewire at chest wall.

● Insert the pigtail catheter over the guidewire which requires uncoiling the pigtail catheter and holding it straight with one hand while advancing it onto the guidewire. Advance the pigtail catheter into the chest wall toward the apex of the lung, visualizing that all of the side holes of the pigtail catheter are inserted at the chest wall. The pigtail catheter will coil into a loop inside the pleural space.

● Carefully remove the guidewire, maintaining stability of the pigtail catheter at the chest wall.

● Attach the adaptor at the external end of the pigtail catheter and immediately connect it to the pleural evacuation drainage system.

● Secure the chest tube in place with adhesive tape and occlusive dressing appropriate for gestational age.

● Suturing the catheter in place is typically not necessary, as there is no skin incision to close and the skin and catheter stays secure with an occlusive dressing.

■ To insert a chest tube with a safety color indicator (e.g., Turkel:)

● Confirm that the blunt safety cannula, housed within the sharp beveled hollow needle, is functioning properly by the color change indicator displaying green.

● Hold the blunt safety cannula firmly near the insertion site to prevent unintended movement as the blunt safety cannula can float freely on the sharp beveled hollow needle.

- Insert the blunt safety cannula into the fourth intercostal space between the anterior and midaxillary lines above the upper border of the fifth rib.
- When the blunt safety cannula meets the skin and subcutaneous tissue, the spring-loaded cannula will recede into the needle, exposing the sharp needle tip; this is indicated by change of the color indicator from green to red. When the distal end of the device enters the pleural space and a lack of resistance is felt, the spring-loaded blunt safety cannula will automatically advance forward and the color indicator will change back from red to green.
- Slide the chest tube off the needle to the desired depth in the chest wall (approximately 2–3 cm), then gently remove the needle assembly.
- Immediately attach the external end of the chest tube to the closed suction system to water seal or wall suction.
- Secure the chest tube in place with adhesive tape and occlusive dressing appropriate for gestational age.
- Suturing the catheter in place is typically not necessary, as there is no skin incision to close and the skin and catheter stays secure with an occlusive dressing.

Assessment and Care Postprocedure

■ Continue to monitor cardiorespiratory status including vital signs and oxygen saturations.

■ Obtain follow-up chest x-ray to assess for correct placement of chest tube and reevaluation of air leak or effusion. Monitor for additional pain management and complications.

Complications

■ Trauma including hemorrhage or damage to cardiothoracic organs
■ Nerve damage
■ Misplacement of tube
■ Infection
■ Pain
■ Equipment malfunction
■ Subcutaneous air leakage through pleural opening

Documentation

■ Date and time of the procedure
■ Time-out performed
■ Location (site of entry)

■ Clinical indications

■ Equipment used (including size of the chest tube)

■ Vital signs prior to and following procedure

■ Pain control measures (medication/comfort care)

■ Number of attempts

■ Patient tolerance to procedure/complications (if any)

■ Fluid/air removal; activity in drainage system (bubbling, drainage type and amount, fluctuation of fluid levels)

■ Blood loss (if any)

■ AP chest x-ray results and physical exam findings prior to and following procedure

OROTRACHEAL INTUBATION

STEPHANIE R. SYKES AND JODI A. ULLOA

Definition

This involves the placement of an endotracheal tube (ETT) into the trachea between the glottis and carina in order to provide mechanical ventilation. Alternative devices (oral airway, nasal tube, laryngeal mask airway [LMA], or tracheostomy) may be used by specialists in the case of a difficult or complex airway.

Clinical Indications

Clinical indications include for respiratory failure that is unresponsive to noninvasive respiratory support, to alleviate upper airway obstruction or subglottic stenosis, to administer surfactant, to maintain the airway during procedures requiring moderate to deep sedation, or when a congenital diaphragmatic hernia is prenatally suspected or confirmed.

Clinical Contraindications

Clinical contraindications include known congenital anomalies that would require a specialist to perform intubation such as otolaryngologist or anesthesiologist or in situations where the patient has an advance directive that identifies that no artificial airway should be placed.

Equipment for Orotracheal Intubation

■ Sterile suction catheter (8 or 10 French to clear oral secretions)

■ Wall suction regulator with canister and tubing

■ ETT, see Table 16.1

■ Laryngoscope handle with appropriate-sized blade and light source

■ Resuscitation bag and mask or T-piece resuscitator for ventilation

■ Oxygen source

■ Stylet (optional)

■ Gloves

■ End-tidal CO_2 detector

■ Securement device (commercially available device or adhesive tape)

■ Pulse oximeter with heart rate (HR) monitor

■ Preprocedural medication considerations: vagolytic, analgesic +/– sedative, and neuromuscular block per facility protocol

Steps

■ Prepare and check the working order of all equipment prior to beginning procedure.

■ Review patient history including risk factors for difficult airway. If suspected, assure that alternative devices and/or specialized personnel are readily available.

■ Don appropriate Personal protective equipment (PPE) per facility protocol.

■ Place the patient supine in a "sniffing" position: head midline with neck slightly extended (may use shoulder roll).

TABLE 16.1 Endotracheal Tube Length for Neonatal Intubation

GESTATIONAL AGE (WEEKS)	DEPTH OF INSERTION AT LIPS (CM)	WEIGHT (G)	ET TUBE SIZE (ID, MM)
23–24	5.5	500–600	Size 2.5
25–26	6.0	700–800	<1,000 g or <28 weeks
27–29	6.5	900–1,000	Size 3.0
30–32	7.0	1,100–1,400	1,000–2,000 g or 28–34 weeks
33–34	7.5	1,500–1,800	Size 3.5
35–37	8.0	1,900–2,400	>2,000 g or >34 weeks
38–40	8.5	2,500–3,100	
41–43	9.0	3,200–4,200	33.5–4.0

Source: Weiner, G. (2016). *Textbook of neonatal resuscitation* (7th ed.). American Academy of Pediatrics. Reprinted by permission from the American Academy of Pediatrics. Shaded table adapted from Kempley, S. T., Moreira, S. W., & Petrone, F. L. (2008). Endotracheal tube length for neonatal intubation. *Resuscitation, 77*(3), 369–373. https://doi.org/10.1016/j.resuscitation.2008.02.002

- Suction the oropharynx to clear secretions.
- Administer premedications based on facility protocol.
- Continually monitor the HR and oxygen saturation throughout the procedure. Provide adequate ventilation to prexygenate prior to intubation attempt.
- Open the patient's mouth, hold the laryngoscope with the left hand, and gently insert the blade into the patient's mouth, sweeping the tongue to the side to visualize the oropharynx.
- Lift the blade vertically (avoid rocking motions) to visualize the glottis by vertically lifting the epiglottis.
- Gentle external pressure may be needed over the thyroid cartilage to visualize vocal cords.
- Pass the ETT along the right side of the mouth and through the cords as they open during inspiration.
- Advance the tube into the trachea to the appropriate level (see Table 16.1).
- Withdraw the laryngoscope blade from the mouth and begin positive-pressure ventilation (PPV).
- Confirm correct placement of ETT by use of end-tidal CO_2 detector, auscultation of lung fields for breath sounds and symmetry, visualization of condensation in ETT, adequate chest rises with ventilation, and stability of vital signs.
- Secure the ETT with the securing device.
- Obtain a chest x-ray to confirm the proper placement of the ETT.

Assessment and Care Postprocedure

Provide continued respiratory support and monitoring. Use blood gas analysis and serial x-rays based on patient condition.

Complications

- Tracheal perforation
- Esophageal perforation
- Improper tube position including right mainstem or esophageal intubation
- ETT obstruction
- ETT dislodgement
- Gum, lip, or oral mucosal trauma
- Cardiovascular instability including bradycardia
- Trauma to oropharynx
- Vocal cord injury

■ Laryngospasm
■ Cardiac arrest or death

Documentation

The procedure note should describe the indication for the procedure, method, medications administered, equipment used, confirmation of proper ETT placement including radiographic findings, patient tolerance of the procedure, and family notification.

UMBILICAL CATHETER INSERTION

STEPHANIE R. SYKES AND JODI A. ULLOA

Definition

Umbilical artery and umbilical vein catheters are often inserted into sick and premature newborns admitted to intensive care nurseries to facilitate vascular access for lab testing, continuous blood pressure or venous pressure monitoring, and/or infusion of intravascular fluids or medications.

Clinical Indications

■ **An umbilical artery catheter** is indicated in infants who require arterial blood gas monitoring, central blood pressure monitoring, and frequent blood sampling for laboratory specimens.

■ **An umbilical vein catheter** is indicated for emergency vascular access in infants in the delivery room during resuscitation. An umbilical vein catheter is also indicated for infants less than 14 days old in the NICU who require uninterrupted glucose or medication infusions or IV fluids/parenteral nutrition solutions with specific osmolality or concentration requirements contraindicated in a peripheral venous site (Lewis & Spirnack, 2020). Umbilical venous catheter is also indicated for use in premature infants to avoid difficult access to small and friable peripheral veins and avoidance of noxious procedures associated with obtaining peripheral venous access.

Clinical Contraindications

■ **Umbilical artery catheter contraindications:** Evidence of local-lower extremity vascular compromise, peritonitis, necrotizing enterocolitis, omphalitis, omphalocele, and acute abdomen etiology.

■ **Umbilical vein catheter contraindications:** Peritonitis, necrotizing enterocolitis, omphalitis, and omphalocele.

Equipment for Insertion of Umbilical Catheters

■ Cardiorespiratory monitor

■ Radiant warmer

■ Standardized measurement graphs for appropriate length placement of umbilical arterial and venous catheters are available

■ Personal protective equipment (PPE) including sterile gloves, sterile gown, mask, and hat for all personnel performing or directly assisting with the procedure

■ PPE including hat and mask for all personnel in immediate vicinity of procedure

■ Immobilizing materials appropriate for gestation of infant (options: diaper with tape for across legs, gauze with tape or safety pins, or soft straps for extremities)

■ Optional use of commercial umbilical catheter insertion tray or individual components:

- Measuring tape
- Facility-approved antiseptic
- Sterile umbilical tape
- Sterile curved hemostats
- Toothed iris forceps
- Nontoothed curved iris forceps
- Scissors
- Straight forceps
- Needle holder
- Sterile drapes
- Sterile scalpel
- Umbilical catheters: 3.5 French for infants less than 1,200 g and 5 French for infants greater than 1,200 g with optional dual lumen catheter for insertion in umbilical venous catheter
- Sterile three-way stopcocks with Luer Lock for each catheter port with optional neutral closure device for second port of dual lumen umbilical venous catheter
- Sterile 3 mL syringes (optional one sterile heparinized blood gas syringe)
- Sterile saline flush (optional heparinized saline flush)
- Sterile 2 × 2 or 4 × 4 gauzes
- 3.0 or 4.0 silk suture with needle

Steps

■ Make external measurements as necessary to estimate length of catheters to be inserted for one of both umbilical catheters.

■ Immobilize infant extremities to prevent movement and reduce possible contamination of insertion site.

■ Put on cap and masks.

■ Prepare a sterile field with an open commercial tray or sterile towel and place all catheters, instruments, syringes, or components on the sterile field.

■ Open sterile gloves and gown packages, maintaining sterility.

■ Prepare hands for major procedure as follows: remove all jewelry from hands and arms; clean nails and scrub hands including between fingers, wrist, forearms, and elbows using antiseptic preparation for at least 4 to 5 minutes; rinse forearms and hands, keeping them elevated above elbows; dry hands followed by forearms using sterile towels provided in the sterile gown package.

■ Put on sterile gown with assistant.

■ Put on sterile gloves without contaminating external surface of the gloves.

■ Have assistant hold the saline vials for the inserter to aspirate saline and fill 3 mL syringes.

■ Attach stopcock/s to hub of catheter/s and fill system with saline solution, removing all air and then turn stopcock/s to off position.

■ Have assistant hold the umbilical cord vertical with a straight hemostat to allow inserter to apply adequate antiseptic on and around the cord.

■ Prepare the umbilical cord and surrounding area with antiseptic solution approximately 5 cm around base of cord.

■ Tie the umbilical tape loosely around the base of the umbilicus above the skin if able to control bleeding once umbilical clamp is removed.

■ Inserter cuts the cord horizontally approximately 1.5 to 2 cm above the base of the umbilicus using the sterile scalpel while assistant continues to hold with a straight hemostat. The assistant then removes the cord with clamp and discards away from the sterile field.

■ Drape the procedure area with sterile towels covering approximately 80% area immediately surrounding the infant.

■ Utilize sterile gauze to blot away any bleeding from the umbilical vessels.

■ Control excessive bleeding with gentle tension on the umbilical tie around the base of the cord.

■ Identify the umbilical vessels (two arteries, one vein). Umbilical artery is usually thick walled and smaller, whereas umbilical vein is usually thin walled and larger in diameter.

■ Grasp the cord stump with toothed forceps to provide stability for catheter/s insertion.

■ Umbilical arteries usually need to be dilated prior to catheter insertion by introducing points of the curved iris forceps into the lumen with the points closed, gently opening while in the lumen and then repeatedly probing gently to a depth up to 0.5 to 1 cm to facilitate catheter insertion.

■ Insert appropriately sized catheter/s into the umbilical vessels to predetermined length.

■ Gently aspirate catheters for blood to verify intraluminal placement.

■ If no blood return, catheter/s may be outside vessels into false channel and should be immediately removed.

■ Secure catheters temporarily by looping over abdomen or bedside infant on sterile drapes for radiographic confirmation of correct tip location of catheter/s.

■ Obtain radiographic confirmation with inserter, maintaining sterile field and security of catheter/s during testing.

■ Umbilical arterial catheter tip should be between thoracic 6 to thoracic 9 for high position and lumbar 3 to lumbar 5 for low positioning (Kumar et al., 2012).

■ Umbilical venous catheter tip should be in the inferior vena cava (IVC) at the level of the diaphragm.

■ Advancement of catheter/s to appropriate length measurements based on radiographic measurements can only be done during the initial sterile insertion procedure. Withdrawing catheter/s to appropriate length measurements based on radiographic measurements should only be done using sterile technique. Repeat radiographic testing is recommended after repositioning any umbilical catheter/s.

■ Suture the catheter/s using the 3.0 or 4.0 sterile sutures, noting the insertion length.

■ Loosen the umbilical tie around the base of the cord and observe for bleeding from umbilicus.

■ Withdraw blood for ordered specimens; best practice is to obtain blood cultures while the sterile field is maintained during the catheter/s insertion procedure.

■ Flush the catheter/s every 5 minutes with a small amount of heparinized saline to maintain patency until ordered solution to infuse through catheter/s is infusing.

■ Transducer and IV catheter tubing to catheter/s should be completely primed with ordered solution, free from air, and attached using sterile technique.

■ Clean the excess antiseptic from the skin around the umbilicus.

■ Secure the catheter/s to the infant using facility-recommended devices following best practices based on gestational age and skin integrity.

■ Remove all restraints and sterile drapes from infant.

■ Discard used supplies and equipment in appropriate facility containers.

Assessment and Care Postprocedure

Monitor circulation, maintain continuous infusion, and use appropriate care to maintain the sterility of the connections and prevent exposure to contaminated surfaces. Umbilical arterial catheters are recommended for use for up to 7 days and umbilical venous catheters are recommended for use for 7 to 14 days.

Complications

■ Umbilical vessel/s perforation

■ Umbilical vessel/s thrombus or occlusions

■ Catheterization of the urachus

■ Bleeding from umbilical vessel/s

■ Catheter-related thromboembolism in distal blood vessel/s

■ Incision of the peritoneum

■ Central line blood-related stream infection

■ Pericardial, pleural, or peritoneal effusions

■ Internal breakage or accidental dislodgement of catheter/s while in patient

■ Mispositioned catheter tips for umbilical catheter/s have increased risk of complications and should be avoided

Documentation

Document informed consent (if applicable), insertion length for catheter/s (including any adjustments of catheter insertion length), patient tolerance, and complications, if any.

URINARY CATHETER INSERTION

STEPHANIE R. SYKES AND JODI A. ULLOA

Definition

Urinary catheters are medical devices used for straight bladder catheterization either for a one-time urine sample, relief of urinary retention, or for strict continuous monitoring of urine output.

Clinical Indications

Urinary catheters are inserted into the bladder via the urethra to obtain a urine specimen, relieve urinary retention, evaluate the presence of urine, obtain a sterile urine specimen for culture, or inject contrast for an image study of the urinary system. Indwelling catheters are used to monitor continuous urine output or when bladder function may be compromised by medications or obstructions to normal urination.

Clinical Contraindications

Clinical contraindications include urinary tract infection, congenital anomalies of urinary tract, preexisting ureteral trauma, or uncorrected bleeding diathesis.

Equipment for Urinary Catheter Insertion

■ Urinary catheter, silicone or polyurethane, should be soft and of the appropriate size (3.5–8 French). For infants less than 1,000 g, use a 3.5 French catheter; for infants who are 1,000 to 1,800 g, use a 5 French catheter; and for infants over 1,800 g, use an 8 French catheter.

■ Sterile specimen cup/receptacle for one-time catheterization

■ A sterile closed drainage system if using indwelling catheters

■ Sterile towel

■ Facility-approved antiseptic

■ Water-soluble lubricant

■ Normal saline wipes

■ Sterile gloves

■ Use developmentally appropriate techniques to assist in decreasing painful stimuli such as containment, oral sucrose or breast milk with a pacifier, or sensorial saturation. Swaddle the infant with the extremity to be puncture exposed or have an additional assistant hold the infant.

Steps

■ Prepare equipment.

■ Wash hands.

■ Place the infant supine on a flat surface with adequate thermal support.

■ Swaddle the upper body and/or obtain assistance of someone to contain the infant and provide a pacifier with optional sucrose.

■ Remove the diaper and place a pad or clean diaper under the buttocks.

■ Gently abduct the thighs in a frog position to fully expose the perineum.

■ Don sterile gloves.

■ Place the catheter tip in the sterile lubricant.

■ Place one sterile drape under the baby and one drape over the thighs and abdomen.

■ Expose the urethra.

● In the male newborn, if uncircumcised, retract the foreskin with the nondominant hand to reveal the meatus.

● In the female newborn, spread the labia majora with the nondominant hand to reveal the urethral meatus superior to the vaginal opening.

■ Cleanse the exposed urethral opening area with facility-approved aseptic solution.

■ Maintaining sterile technique, insert it into the urethra meatus, advancing until urine flow is evident in the tubing. If obstruction is encountered, do not attempt to force it through the obstruction.

● Insert the catheter a maximum of 2 in. (5 cm) in a male newborn who is less than 750 g and 2.3 in. (6 cm) in a male who weighs more than 750 g.

● Insert the catheter a maximum of 1 in. (2.5 cm) in a female newborn who is less than 750 g and 2 in. (5 cm) in a female who weighs more than 750 g.

■ Once the catheter is in place, obtain a sterile specimen or connect to the closed drainage system.

■ If the catheter is intended to be indwelling, secure with adhesive tape and occlusive dressing appropriate for gestational age to secure tube postprocedure.

Assessment and Care Postprocedure

Note the length of the catheter extending from the meatus. Assess the perineum for trauma, and the urine flow if using an indwelling catheter. Assess for evidence of blood or stool in the urine or if urine is leaking around the catheter.

Complications

■ Development of a catheter-associated urinary tract infection (CAUDI)

■ Trauma to the urethra or bladder

■ Pain and discomfort to infant

Documentation

Document the length of the catheter used and how far it is inserted in centimeters, tolerance of the procedure, securing of indwelling catheter, amount of specimen collected and labeled, and lab assays requested.

REFERENCES

Cook Incorporated. (2019, September). *Fuhrman pleural/pneumopericardial drainage set: Instructions for use.* https://www.cookmedical.com/data/IFU_PDF/C_T_PPD_REV4.PDF

Hugill, K. (2016). Vascular access in neonatal care settings: Selecting the appropriate device. *British Journal of Nursing, 25*(3), 171–176. https://doi.org/10.12968/bjon.2016.25.3.171

Kumar, P. P., Kumar, C. D., Nayak, M., Shaikh, F., Dusa, S., & Venkatalakshmi, A. (2012). Umbilical arterial catheter insertion length: In quest of a universal formula. *Journal of Perinatology, 32,* 604–607. https://doi.org/10.1038/jp.2011.149

Legemaat, M., Carr, P. J., van Rens, R. M., van Dijk, M., Poslawsky, I. E., & van den Hoogen, A. (2016). Peripheral intravenous cannulation: Complication rates in the neonatal population: A multicenter observational study. *Journal of Vascular Access, 17*(4), 360–365. https://doi.org/10.5301/jva.5000558

Lewis, K., & Spirnak, P. W. (2020, February). *Umbilical vein catheterization*. StatPearls. https://www.ncbi.nlm.nih.gov/books/NBK549869/

Ramasethu, J., & Seo, S. (Eds.). (2020). *MacDonald's atlas of procedures in neonatology* (6th ed.). Lippincott Williams & Wilkins.

Additional Resources

Soares, B. N., Pissarra, S., Rouxinol-Dias, A. L., Costa, S., & Guimaraes, H. (2017). Complications of central lines in neonates admitted to a level III neonatal intensive care unit. *Journal of Maternal-Fetal & Neonatal Medicine, 31*(20), 2770–2776. https://doi.org/10.1080/14767058.2017.1355902

Wei, Y., Lee, C., Cheng, H., Tsao, L., & Hsiao, C. (2014). Pigtail catheters versus traditional chest tubes for pneumothoraces in premature infants treated in a neonatal intensive care unit. *Pediatrics and Neonatology, 55*, 376–380. https://doi.org/10.1016/j.pedneo.2014.01.002

Weiner, G. (2016). *Textbook of neonatal resuscitation* (7th ed.). American Academy of Pediatrics.

PERIPHERALLY INSERTED CENTRAL CATHETER

ELIZABETH L. SHARPE

Definition

A peripherally inserted central catheter (PICC) is a long catheter inserted into a peripheral vein, then threaded to place the catheter tip at the superior vena cava (SVC) or inferior vena cava (IVC). For catheters inserted into the veins of the upper extremity or scalp, the optimal catheter tip location for central placement is in the SVC (Gorski et al., 2021; Infusion Nurses Society [INS], 2016; U.S. Food and Drug Administration [FDA], 1989; Wyckoff & Sharpe, 2015). For catheters inserted into the veins in the lower extremities, the optimal catheter tip location for central placement is in the IVC between the right atrium and diaphragm (Wyckoff & Sharpe, 2015).

■ A midline catheter is a long catheter inserted into a peripheral vein, then threaded to place the tip (avoid tip placement in a joint):

● Below the axilla if inserted in an upper extremity

● The external jugular vein above the clavicle if inserted in a scalp vein

● Below the inguinal crease if inserted in a lower extremity

Clinical Indications

The Centers for Disease Control and Prevention (O'Grady et al., 2021) recommend that patients who require in excess of 6 days of therapy should be considered for more than a peripheral intravenous (PIV) device, that is, a midline catheter or PICC or other centrally placed catheter. Early assessment for vascular access needs supports minimizing the number of attempts and trauma to the patient and increased availability of sites and success.

Clinical indications for long-term venous access include:

■ Hyperosmolar medications (>600 mOsm/L)

- Parenteral nutrition
- Prolonged IV therapy
- Irritant or vesicant medications

Clinical Contraindications

General contraindications include:

- Uncontrolled bacteremia or fungemia
- Family withholding consent
- Coagulopathy or thrombocytopenia
- Inability to identify an appropriate vein

Specific site selection considerations include:

- Fracture and/or birth injury
- Decreased venous return
- Skin breakdown
- Site or vessel needed for another purpose

Some examples of situations where the site may be needed for another purpose include when an infant is a candidate for a ventricular reservoir or ventriculoperitoneal shunt and scalp vessels should be avoided. Similarly, for a cardiac catheterization or an extracorporeal membrane oxygenation (ECMO) candidate, the right upper extremity should be avoided. In infants with congenital heart defects, consider the anticipated sequence and surgical sites of intended future surgeries.

Equipment

- Hat, mask
- Sterile gown
- Sterile gloves
- Sterile tape measure
- Sterile tourniquet
- Sterile drapes for maximum sterile barrier precautions
- Catheter for peripherally inserted central tip location (PICC catheter)
- Introducer—over the needle or sheath introducer appropriate to catheter size and type
- Scissors and/or trim tool
- Sterile forceps
- Skin antiseptic (chlorhexidine gluconate or povidone-iodine)

■ Sterile flush solution

■ Sterile 10 mL syringes (two)—or may use prefilled 0.9% sodium chloride

■ Sterile extension tubing (Luer lock)

■ Sterile gauze

■ Sterile water or saline—for topical application

■ Sterile skin-closure strips or adhesive padded foam

■ Transparent dressing and stabilization device (if available)

Steps

Personnel inserting central venous catheters should receive specialized training upon their hire, annually thereafter, and when this task is added to their job responsibilities.

■ Evaluate characteristics, needs, and duration of intended therapy to confirm indications.

■ Discuss with the family and obtain informed consent.

■ Evaluate patient history and treatment plan for site selection contraindications.

■ Perform physical assessment for vein selection utilizing vascular visualization equipment as available such as transilluminator, near infrared, and ultrasound technology.

■ Determine the catheter insertion length by measuring the following:

  ● For the upper extremity or scalp vessels to the SVC: Measure the distance from the intended insertion site along the vein track to the right clavicular head and to the third intercostal space.

  ● For lower extremity vessels to the IVC: Measure the distance from the intended insertion site along the vein track to the right of the umbilicus then to the xiphoid.

■ Gather the central line kit, catheter, introducer, sterile gloves, maximum sterile barriers, antiseptic, and other needed supplies.

■ Prepare the patient for the procedure, including pharmacologic and developmental comfort measures.

■ Don hair covering and mask.

■ Perform hand hygiene.

■ Prepare a sterile field and assemble equipment.

■ Prepare the catheter by flushing and trimming to the premeasured length.

■ Position the patient as developmentally appropriate.

■ Prepare the insertion site by disinfecting the skin with an antimicrobial agent. Allow the antiseptic to dry on the skin according to the manufacturer's directions. Chlorhexidine gluconate or povidone-iodine may be used. Chlorhexidine may be used with caution in premature infants or infants younger than 2 months of age. These products may cause irritation or chemical burns.

■ Utilize maximum sterile barrier precautions to isolate the extremity or insertion site.

■ Apply a sterile tourniquet.

■ Insert the introducer bevel up at a 15° to 30° angle and observe for blood return. Remove the needle if using an over-the-sheath introducer.

■ Remove the tourniquet.

■ Place the catheter in the introducer lumen using nontoothed or sheathed forceps and thread catheter in small increments.

■ Remove the introducer per manufacturer's directions.

■ Apply gentle pressure to the site as needed until bleeding stops.

■ Verify the inserted catheter length and amount of any externally lying catheter.

■ If a catheter with stylet is used, remove the stylet slowly at this time.

■ Aspirate to confirm blood return and flush to confirm patency.

■ Attach extension tubing if not part of the catheter apparatus, with care to eliminate air entry into the tubing.

■ Secure the catheter temporarily with skin-closure tapes placed over the securement disc or hub while awaiting radiographic confirmation.

■ Confirm the catheter tip location in SVC or IVC.

■ Reposition the catheter if not in SVC or IVC.

■ Obtain radiographic reconfirmation of the catheter tip location.

■ Remove povidone-iodine from the skin using sterile saline or water and allow to dry.

■ Secure the catheter to the skin and apply a sterile transparent occlusive dressing.

■ Document the procedure, including any repositioning, radiographic confirmation, premedication, and catheter specifics including brand and lot number, trimmed length, inserted length, and patient tolerance.

Assessment and Care Postprocedure

■ Assess the condition of the insertion site hourly including an evaluation of dressing integrity, erythema, leakage, and length of externally lying catheter.

■ Confirm that the catheter tip location (central or midline) correlates to accommodate the properties of the infusate (osmolarity, irritant, or vesicant).

■ Limit dextrose concentration to D12.5% or less if the catheter tip location is not in a central tip location in SVC or IVC.

■ Change the dressing when it becomes loose, nonocclusive, moist, and soiled, if there is exposed catheter, or according to manufacturer's directions for dressing and any additional materials beneath the dressing or according to facility protocol.

■ Maintain adequate minimum infusion rates to minimize risk of occlusion (0.5–1 mL/hr).

■ Flush with a 10 mL syringe or following manufacturer's directions (INS, 2016).

■ If heparin locking, flush with 1 mL normal saline or 1 mL of 10 units/mL heparin every 6 hours and before and after administration of each medication.

Complications

■ Central line-associated bloodstream infection (CLABSI) is a laboratory-confirmed bloodstream infection where the central line was in place for more than 2 days prior to development of the infection and not related to another site.

■ Occlusion may be partial or complete. Slowing flow or increased resistance are initial signs and a solution-specific clearing agent may be indicated.

■ Malposition occurs when the catheter tip becomes external or internal to the intended central catheter tip location. This is a risk for pleural and pericardial effusion, and vessel damage indicates reevaluation of the medications and IV therapy to be infused.

■ Dislodgement occurs when the catheter becomes partially or completely removed. Partial dislodgement indicates reevaluation of the catheter tip location and infusate properties. Use of an appropriate securement device and hourly monitoring of the catheter and site promote prevention and early detection.

Documentation

■ Indication for the procedure

■ Consent and parent education

■ Correct patient identification

■ Patient preparation including pain management strategies and response

■ Site preparation including type of antiseptic and removal, if indicated

■ Brand, type, gauge/size, lot number, and number of lumens of catheter

■ Style, size of introducer

■ Utilization and removal of stylet

■ Description of procedure including visualization technology utilized

■ Insertion site

■ Number of attempts

■ Length of catheter and, if trimmed, original length and trimmed length

■ Inserted length of catheter and externally lying catheter

■ Securement method including stabilization and dressing type

■ Initial radiographic/imaging confirmation

■ Any repositioning performed and final radiographic confirmation of catheter tip location

■ Complications encountered and management

■ Patient tolerance of procedure

■ Date, time, and name of clinician performing the procedure

In addition to patient-specific documentation in the health record, some institutions require completion of a standardized tool or procedural checklist for adherence to specific bundle practices. Some of these components include hand hygiene, maximum sterile barrier precautions, chlorhexidine for skin antisepsis, and continued daily evaluation of line necessity.

REFERENCES

Gorski, L. A., Hadaway, L., Hagle, M. E., Broadhurst, D., Clare, S., Kleidon, T., Meyer, B. M., Nickel, B., Rowley, S., Sharpe, E., & Alexander, M. (2021, January–February 1). Infusion therapy standards of practice, 8th edition. *Journal of Infusion Nursing, 44*(Suppl. 1), S1–S224. https://doi.org/10.1097/NAN.0000000000000396

Infusion Nurses Society. (2016). *Policies and procedures for infusion therapy: Neonate to adolescent* (2nd ed.). Infusion Nurses Society.

O'Grady, N. P., Alexander, M., Burns, L. A., Dellinger, E. P., Garland, J., Heard, S. O., Lipsett, P. A., Masur, H., Mermel, L. A., Pearson, M. L., Raad, I. I., Randolph, A., Rupp, M. E., & Healthcare Infection Control Practice Advisory Committee. (2021) *Guidelines for the prevention of intravascular catheter-related infections, 2011* (3rd ed.). https://www.cdc.gov/infectioncontrol/pdf/guidelines/bsi-guidelines-H.pdf

U.S. Food and Drug Administration Task Force. (1989). *Precautions necessary with central venous catheters. FDA Drug Bulletin.* U.S. Government Printing Office.

Wyckoff, M., & Sharpe, E. (2015). *Peripherally inserted central catheters guidelines for practice* (3rd ed.). National Association of Neonatal Nurses.

ADVANCED RESPIRATORY TECHNOLOGIES

LISA A. LUBBERS AND WAKAKO M. EKLUND

High-Frequency Ventilation

High-frequency ventilation (HFV) has been used frequently when infants are unable to ventilate/oxygenate sufficiently on conventional mechanical ventilation (CMV). HFV is a mode of ventilation which utilizes small Vt, often less than the infant's anatomic dead space, with rapid rates. This unique mode allows the infant to receive ventilatory support with lower peak airway pressures, all the while achieving adequate oxygenation and ventilation. With the use of small Vt and lower peak airway pressure, HFV also enables alveolar recruitment and distribution of medications, such as nitric oxide (iNO: used to treat persistent pulmonary hypertension of the newborn (PPHN), electively dilates the pulmonary vasculature, allowing for optimal gas exchange) while decreasing volutrauma or barotrauma to the fragile lungs (Goldsmith et al., 2017).

The two most commonly used HFV devices are:

■ High-frequency jet ventilation (HFJV), which delivers high-velocity pulses of pressurized gas to the infant's airway with passive exhalation (4–10 Hz, 240–600 cycles/min)

■ High-frequency oscillatory ventilation (HFOV), which moves the gas back and forth at the opening of the airway at a high frequency (3–20 Hz, 180–1,200 cycles/min)

These two types promote distribution (convective flow) and diffusion of respiratory gases while eliminating CO_2 effectively. The theory is HFV optimizes lung expansion while using low tidal volumes and lower inspiratory pressures, thus preventing lung injury and the development of long-term pulmonary sequelae commonly called bronchopulmonary dysplasia or chronic lung disease. The fact that HFV optimizes the lung expansion with the use of small tidal volume and lower inspiratory pressure gave hopes to prevent lung injury, thus preventing the development of bronchopulmonary dysplasia. Current evidence does not suggest that elective (versus rescue) use of HFV is superior to CMV (Cools et al., 2015). No study compared the superiority of HFOV versus HFJV in decreasing mortality and morbidity (Ethawi et al., 2016); thus, HFV is most likely applicable when severe respiratory failure is noted using the CMV.

Noninvasive High-Frequency Oscillatory Ventilation

Noninvasive high-frequency oscillatory ventilation (nHFOV) has become increasingly recognized as the novel approach for its noninvasive nature. Prolonged use of an endotracheal tube (ETT) has the risk of harming subglottic tissues, leading to stenosis or edema, complicating extubation later in many neonates. The nHFV addresses the disadvantages of mechanical ventilation that require intubation. This mode delivers HFV to neonates using nasal prongs or nasopharyngeal tubes. Increasing popularity is observed in this method; however, evidence is still emerging at the time of this writing (Chan et al., 2017).

Neurally Adjusted Ventilatory Assist

Neurally adjusted ventilatory assist (NAVA) is a novel approach which adjusts ventilator pressure based on the infant's actual diaphragmatic electrical activity measured by the esophageal electrodes attached to a uniquely designed feeding tube. NAVA can improve the diaphragm's ability to increase tidal volume or maintain the current tidal volume with less effort required by the infant. NAVA has shown to be effective in synchronizing the positive pressure with the spontaneous respiration. However, NAVA relies on rather mature respiratory control, so its impact on premature neonates is not fully explored (Goldsmith et al., 2017). Cochrane review states that effectiveness of the synchronization may lead to adequate gas exchange at a lower peak airway pressure, which in turn may prevent occurrences of barotrauma or air leaks (Rossor et al., 2017). However, paucity of evidence prevents definitive recommendations for NAVA over other triggered ventilation. One randomized controlled trial reviewed in this

Cochrane review indicates that NAVA did not demonstrate significant difference in duration of mechanical ventilation or rates of bronchopulmonary dysplasia, pneumothorax, or intraventricular hemorrhage (Rossor et al., 2017).

PROCEDURES NECESSARY TO TREAT RESPIRATORY CONDITIONS

LISA A. LUBBERS AND WAKAKO M. EKLUND

ENDOTRACHEAL INTUBATION

Definition

This involves the placement of an orotracheal or nasotracheal tube designed for neonatal airway management into the trachea between the glottis and the level of carina to provide artificial ventilation.

Clinical Indications

Intubation is often required during neonatal resuscitation in the delivery room or after admission to the NICU to treat the respiratory conditions including administration of surfactant. Intubation can be completed either nasally or orally. Oral intubation is preferred in most cases, and clinicians are likely more accustomed to perform the intubation orally.

■ To provide respiratory support through mechanical ventilation
■ To obtain sputum sample for culture
■ To clear the trachea of meconium when indicated (routine endotracheal suctioning is not recommended)
■ To alleviate airway obstruction or subglottic stenosis
■ To administer surfactant

Equipment (Figure 16.1)

■ Sterile suction catheter (10 or 12 French to clear oral secretions) connected to the suction canister and apparatus (continuous suction set at 80–100 mmHg)
■ Endotracheal tube (ETT; 2.5, 3.0, 3.5, or 4.0 mm based on the weight of the neonate; Table 16.2)
■ Laryngoscope handle with appropriate-sized blade and light source (No. 1 for term, No. 0 for preterm, No. 00 for very low-birthweight infants)
■ Bag and mask or T-piece resuscitator for ventilation with appropriate size mask
■ Oxygen source (when need of intubation is evident, adjust the oxygen concentration as appropriate from 21% to >40%)

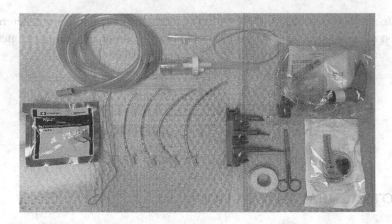

FIGURE 16.1 Items needed for intubation. Suction apparatus not shown.

TABLE 16.2 Endotracheal Tube Size and Placement

INFANT'S WEIGHT (KG)	TUBE SIZE (MM)	INSERTION DEPTH (CM)
<1	2.5	<7
1–2	3	7–8
2–3	3.5	8–9
>3	3.5–4	>9

Source: Data from the American Heart Association Emergency Cardiac Care Committee and Subcommittees. (1992). Guidelines for cardiopulmonary resuscitation and emergency cardiac care. Emergency Cardiac Care Committee and Subcommittees. American Heart Association, Part 1, Introduction. *JAMA, 268*(16), 2171–2183. https://doi.org/10.1001/jama.1992.03490160042024; Kattwinkel, J. (2011). *Neonatal resuscitation textbook* (6th ed.). American Academy of Pediatrics and American Heart Association.

▓ Stylet (proper placement of stylet to not allow the tip of stylet to extend past the end of the ETT is critical)

▓ Gloves

▓ CO_2 detector (document the confirmation of successful intubation revealed by the color change of the CO_2 detector)

▓ Securing device (tape or other ETT securement)

▓ Meconium aspirator (as condition requires)

▓ Pulse oximeter with heart rate (HR) monitor (recommended to place on neonate when infant requires resuscitation with supplemental oxygen) as well as electronic cardiac monitoring (ECG) when neonates' HR is low initially and requires close monitoring (HR is the primary indicator for an effective positive-pressure ventilation (PPV) when it is indicated)

▓ Preprocedural pain management if route and time available

Steps

■ Prepare and check all equipment and supplies prior to delivery.

■ Place the infant supine in a "sniffing position." An additional neck roll to place under the infant's neck may allow better visualization of the cords that are often positioned anteriorly in neonates. Avoid hyperextension of the neck.

■ Suction the oropharynx to clear secretions if needed.

■ Provide artificial ventilations until the heart rate, oxygen saturation, and color are stable and monitor throughout the procedure.

■ Hold the laryngoscope with your left hand and gently insert the blade into the neonate's mouth (see Figure 16.2).

■ Sweep the tongue to the side to visualize the field.

■ Lift the blade to visualize the glottis by lifting the epiglottis. The lifting motion is not directly lifting the handle up toward the ceiling but rather lifting the lower jaw up and forward, pointing the laryngoscope handle slightly toward the foot of the bed. Avoid rocking the laryngoscope blade against the mandible as this can cause damage to fragile tissues (see Figure 16.3).

■ Gentle external pressure may be applied by the assistant over the cricoid cartilage to enhance the visualization of the vocal cords.

■ Pass the ETT along the right side of the mouth and through the cords as they open during inspiration while maintaining the visualization of the cord.

■ Advance the tube into the trachea to the appropriate level (# kg of weight + 6 [e.g., 2 kg, then 8 cm]; see Table 16.2).

■ Use a CO_2 detector to confirm placement and document the confirmation. Auscultate for equal breath sounds to ensure that the tube is not too far in the right main stem. Mist in the tube is another positive sign; however, the CO_2 detector is considered to be the confirmation. For infants who were depressed with low HR, auscultating for increasing HR as PPV is initiated is important.

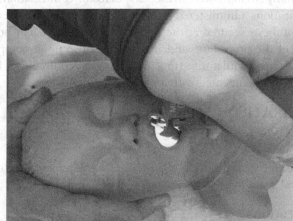

FIGURE 16.2 How the left hand holds the blade in the infant's mouth.

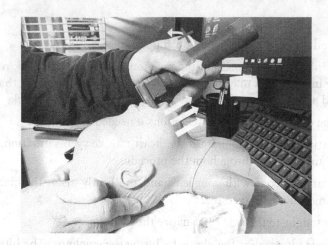

FIGURE 16.3 How the blade should be lifted to visualize the glottis.

■ Secure the ETT with tape or a securing device available at the facility.

■ Obtain a chest x-ray to confirm the proper placement of the ETT and evaluate the lung fields to evaluate the current treatment as well as to consider further interventions.

Assessment and Care Postprocedure

Monitor for infant's tolerance; any need for oxygen adjustment; and any complications, including tracheal perforation, esophageal perforation, improper tube position, tube obstruction, or dislodgement. Provide continued respiratory support and monitoring. Use blood gas analysis serial x-rays as indicated. The importance of nursing assessment during this phase is paramount.

Documentation

The procedure notes should describe the rationale for the procedure, who performed it, how many attempts were made, CO_2 detector confirmation, route (orally or nasally), medications administered if any, equipment and size used, centimeter mark where the tube is secured at the lip, confirmation of equal breath sounds, infant tolerance of the procedure, and infant's response upon completion of the procedure. Vital signs, ventilator settings, and oxygen requirements following the procedure should be documented with a plan for further care.

NEEDLE ASPIRATION

Definition

This involves the emergent insertion of a needle for the removal of fluid, blood, or air from the plural space to allow reexpansion of the lungs.

Clinical Indications

Clinical indications include general conditions and symptoms of cardiorespiratory compromise or failure, as well as the size of the air leak (pneumothorax) or fluid accumulation in pleural space (pleural effusion) as evidenced on x-ray. If the air leak or fluid leak is small and the infant is not symptomatic, needle aspiration may not be immediately indicated.

Clinical Contraindications

Considerations must be cautiously made regarding the infant's skin integrity at the site and coagulation status prior to performing this invasive procedure. Possible complications include pain, bleeding, infection, and nerve injury. The risk factors for therapeutic needle thoracentesis are less than 1% of all neonates undergoing this procedure.

Equipment

- Needle (#23- to #25-gauge butterfly needle or #22- to #24-gauge angiocath)
- Cleaning solution (2% chlorhexidine, povidone-iodine)
- Sterile water (to clean off cleaning solution following procedure)
- T-connector
- Three-way stopcock
- 30- to 60-mL syringe (if small baby, 20-mL syringe may be sufficient; larger baby can accumulate large volume of air)
- Local anesthetics (most frequently lidocaine without epinephrine is used)
- Sterile gloves
- Sterile 2 × 2 gauze
- Sterile drape
- Positioning aids (blanket rolls)

Steps

- Place the patient in a supine position with the positioning aid to elevate the affected side up for air accumulation or place the infant in the supine or affected side slightly lower for fluid accumulation.
- Maintain thermoregulation and monitor vital signs/oxygen saturation during the procedure.
- Assemble equipment (if using an angiocath, attach the T-connector to the end of the IV catheter and the three-way stopcock to the end of the T-connector. The aspiration syringe can be attached to the stopcock. If using the butterfly needle, attach the stopcock to the end of the tubing and the syringe to the stopcock for aspiration). See Figure 16.4.
- Locate landmarks at the second or third intercostal space, midclavicular line, or fourth to sixth intercostal space for a posterior placement at the anterior axillary line. When fluid accumulation is suspected, a posterior approach at the anterior axillary line in lower intercostal space is preferred. Nipple line is a landmark for the fourth intercostal space.

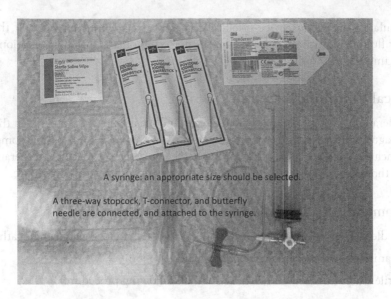

FIGURE 16.4 Equipment needed for needle aspiration.

■ Wash hands, don sterile gloves, and organize supplies in a sterile fashion.

■ Drape the patient.

■ Cleanse the area and provide local anesthetic in addition to nonpharmacologic comfort measures. Lidocaine needs to be injected deep in the muscles to achieve the local anesthesia.

■ Insert the needle firmly into the identified space, advancing it until a "pop" is felt. If using an IV catheter, thread off the sheath. Hold steady and ensure the connection to the tubing, T-connector, and the syringe.

■ Use the syringe to aspirate air and/or fluid from the plural space.

■ If using the catheter (not the needle), you may consider securing the catheter in place with a clear occlusive dressing and monitor for an accumulation of air leak. This allows the procedure to be repeated without reinserting the catheter/needle. Do not recommend leaving the butterfly needle in place because it can repoke the expanding lungs.

Assessment and Care Postprocedure

■ Monitor vital signs, work of breathing, breath sounds, skin color, and oxygen saturations. Repeat chest x-ray may be ordered.

■ Set up for chest tube insertion if reaccumulation of the air or fluid persists.

Documentation

■ Date, time, and who performed the procedure

■ Indications

- Equipment used and size
- Vital signs prior to and following procedure
- Pain control measures (medication/comfort care)
- Number of attempts and the amount of air/fluid that was evacuated during the procedure
- Patient tolerance to procedure and response after the procedure (work of breathing, saturation, RR)
- Chest anterior-posterior (AP) results prior to and following procedure

REFERENCES

Chan, J., Jones, L. J., Osborn, D. A., & Abdel-Latif, M. E. (2017). Non-invasive high-frequency ventilation in newborn infants with respiratory distress. *Cochrane Database of Systematic Reviews, 2017*(7), CD012712. https://doi.org/10.1002/14651858.CD012712

Cools, F., Offringa, M., & Askie, L. M. (2015). Elective high frequency oscillatory ventilation versus conventional ventilation for acute pulmonary dysfunction in preterm infants. *Cochrane Database of Systematic Reviews* (3), CD000104. https://doi.org/10.1002/14651858.CD000104.pub4

Ethawi, Y. H., Abou Mehrem, A., Minski, J., Ruth, C. A., & Davis, P. G. (2016). High frequency jet ventilation versus high frequency oscillatory ventilation for pulmonary dysfunction in preterm infants. *Cochrane Database of Systematic Reviews* (5), CD010548. https://doi.org/10.1002/14651858.CD010548.pub2

Goldsmith, J. P., Karotkin, E. H., Keszler, M., & Suresh, G. K. (2017). *Assisted ventilation of the neonate: An evidence-based approach to newborn respiratory care* (6th ed.). Elsevier.

Rossor, T. E., Hunt, K. A., Shetty, S., & Greenough, A. (2017). Neurally adjusted ventilatory assist compared to other forms of triggered ventilation for neonatal respiratory support. *Cochrane Database of Systematic Reviews* (10), CD012251. https://doi.org/10.1002/14651858.CD012251.pub2

Additional Reading

Weiner, G. M., & Zaichkin, J. (2016). *Neonatal resuscitation textbook* (7th ed.). American Academy of Pediatrics and American Heart Association. https://ebooks.aappublications.org/content/textbook-of-neonatal-resuscitation-nrp-7th-ed

THERAPEUTIC HYPOTHERMIA WITH WHOLE BODY COOLING

GEORGIA R. DITZENBERGER AND SUSAN TUCKER BLACKBURN

OBJECTIVE

The objective is to provide controlled active therapeutic hypothermia using whole body cooling for eligible neonates with hypoxic–ischemic encephalopathy. Please note this guideline does not include passive cooling techniques. These guidelines only pertain to the achievement, maintenance, and resolution of controlled active therapeutic hypothermia.

GENERAL INFORMATION

■ Whole body cooling therapy will be provided to newborns meeting eligibility criteria. The neonatologist or pediatric neurologist will evaluate the newborn and determine whether the newborn meets the criteria for whole body cooling.

■ Continuous monitoring of cardiac, respiratory, and arterial blood pressure (via umbilical arterial catheter) is essential during all phases.

■ The newborn will undergo whole body cooling therapy to achieve and maintain an esophageal temperature of 33.5 °C (range 33 °C–34 °C).

■ Cooling therapy is a 72-hour period of maintaining the esophageal body temperature at 33.5 °C (range 33 °C–34 °C).

■ On completion of 72 hours of body cooling, the newborn will be rewarmed over a 6-hour period.

■ A physician or neonatal nurse practitioner (NNP) must complete the whole body cooling order set in the electronic chart to initiate this protocol.

■ A physician or NNP must complete the rewarming order set in the electronic chart to initiate rewarming the newborn.

■ Risks to newborn:
  ● Blood pressure changes: either hypotension or hypertension
  ● Respiratory pattern changes; may require ventilator support
  ● Abnormal clot formation
  ● Skin breakdown, fat necrosis
  ● Metabolic acidosis

EQUIPMENT

■ Equipment and supplies:
  ● Radiant warmer
  ● Electric cooling unit with a probe adapter cable and one set of connecting hoses
  ● One newborn-sized (22 in. × 33 in.) cooling blanket
  ● Two single-patient-use esophageal probes (one for esophageal temperature and one for skin temperature monitoring)
  ● Distilled/sterile water
  ● Tape to secure esophageal probe

Steps

■ Electric cooling unit setup; follow manufacturer's guidelines:

● Fill the water reservoir, monitor the water level while unit is in use, and add water as needed.

● Connect the hoses.

● Be sure the power switch is OFF prior to inserting the power plug into a grounded receptacle.

● Once the unit is plugged into a grounded receptacle, turn the unit on.

● Press and hold the test lights button:

• Observe that all lights function properly.

• Confirm the audible alarm sounds are functioning.

● Place a blanket on the radiant warmer.

● The blanket should be flat and the two hose clamps OPEN to allow the blanket to fill.

● Water will begin to circulate into the blanket.

• Check for leaks.

• Do not use pins or sharp objects on the blanket.

● After the blanket has filled, check the level of water in the reservoir; refill as needed to keep the green line on the float visible.

● Do not overfill the reservoir.

■ Precool the blanket before the newborn is placed on the blanket:

● Operate the electric cooling unit in the manual control mode.

● Change the temperature scale by pressing the Celsius/Fahrenheit button to display "Celsius."

● Set the temperature desired to 33.5 °C.

● The unit will cool as required to bring the blanket temperature to the set point.

■ Temperature probes:

● Esophageal probe insertion:

• Soften the esophageal probe prior to insertion by placing it in warm water for a few minutes.

• Do not use lubricants.

• Nasal placement of the probe is preferred.

• Position the esophageal temperature probe in the lower third of the esophagus.

• Measure the distance from the nares to the ear to the sternum minus 2 cm.

• Mark the probe with an indelible pen before inserting.

• Secure the probe by taping it to the newborn's nose.

- Probe position may be confirmed with the next routine chest radiographic examination.
- Connect the esophageal probe to the probe adapter cable and plug into the probe jack on the electric cooling unit skin probe.
- Position over the abdomen; affix to skin with a radiant warmer temperature probe reflective patch.
- Skin temperature probe and cable are compatible with the cardiorespiratory monitor and are connected directly into the monitor's temperature module.

■ Cooling the newborn:

- Place the newborn directly on the cooling blanket on the radiant warmer in the supine position:
  - The newborn's entire head and body should be resting on the cooling blanket.
  - There should be nothing between the newborn and the cooling blanket (no receiving blankets, cloth diapers, gel pads, etc.).
- The radiant warmer must be OFF.
- Any other exogenous heat source must be OFF.
- Change the electric cooling unit to automatic control mode:
  - Make sure the SET POINT is 33.5 °.
  - The unit will cool as required to bring the newborn's esophageal temperature to the SET POINT.

■ Maintain the SET POINT at 33.5 °:

- This is the desired esophageal temperature for the next 72 hours.
- Once the newborn's esophageal temperature reaches the SET POINT of 33.5 °, a single blanket layer, such as a thin receiving blanket, may be used between the newborn and the cooling blanket to minimize soiling the cooling blanket.
- Patient temperature display will flash until the newborn's temperature is within 1 °C of the SET POINT.
- Expect some fluctuation around the SET POINT; it should not be more than ±1 °C.

■ Monitor temperatures:

- Record the esophageal, skin, axillary, and blanket water temperatures in the electronic patient record.
- Temperatures should be recorded:
  - Every 15 minutes for 2 hours.
  - Then, every hour for 4 hours.
  - Then every 2 hours until completion of the 72 hours of cooling.

■ Assess skin integrity, perfusion, vital signs, and potential complications every hour.

REWARMING THE NEWBORN

■ Verify the rewarming order set is in the electronic patient chart:

- The newborn is rewarmed gradually, increasing the esophageal temperature at a rate of 0.5 °C per hour over a 6-hour period.
  - Every hour, increase the electric cooling unit SET POINT by 0.5 °C.
  - During rewarming, temperatures should be recorded every hour until the skin temperature is stable at 36.5 °C.

■ At the end of the 6-hour rewarming period, turn on the radiant warmer skin control 0.5 °C higher than the newborn's current skin temperature.

■ Continue to increase the radiant warmer skin control by 0.5 °C every hour until the newborn's axillary temperature is 36.5 °C.

- Avoid rewarming any faster than 6 hours.
- Avoid axillary temperatures greater than 37 °C.

■ Remove the cooling blanket from beneath the newborn.

■ Remove the esophageal probe and discard.

RESUSCITATION AND STABILIZATION

SUSAN M. ORLANDO AND JANA L. PRESSLER

DEFINITION OF RESUSCITATION

"Resuscitation" refers to emergency lifesaving procedures to bring someone who is unconscious or close to death back to a viable condition. Resuscitative efforts are completed to revive someone when the heart has stopped beating and/or they have stopped breathing. Permanent brain damage or death can occur within minutes of the heart stopping or breathing stopping, indicating that the individual needs immediate actions to restore their life.

Resuscitation is short for *cardiopulmonary resuscitation* (CPR). CPR is a combination of chest compressions and rescue breathing. Chest compressions keep oxygen-rich blood flowing until the heartbeat can be adequately restored. Rescue breathing is a way of providing oxygen to the lungs until breathing can be restored. Guidelines for CPR have been established by the International Liaison Committee on Resuscitation (ILCOR) for neonates, children, and adults. "Newborn" or "newly born" refers to an infant who is within the *first minutes to hours after birth* (Perlman et al., 2010). Traditionally, a "neonate" is defined as an infant during their first 28 days postnatally. Infancy begins at birth and extends through 12 months of age.

NEONATAL RESUSCITATION

The majority of newly born infants transition from fetal to neonatal life and breathe spontaneously at birth. A small percentage will require assistance to establish effective respiratory efforts. Approximately 5% to 10% of newborns require some degree of CPR at birth (e.g., stimulation to breathe), with approximately 3% of babies born in a hospital reportedly requiring assisted ventilation (Perlman et al., 2015). Cardiac compressions and administration of epinephrine are required for those few infants who fail to respond to effective positive-pressure ventilation (PPV).

It is critical that the knowledge and skills required to effectively complete CPR techniques successfully be taught to all neonatal care providers. Although oftentimes newborns' needs for CPR are predictable, newborns' needs for CPR also occur without warning. Knowing this vital fact can alert caregivers of CPR's primary importance, especially in healthcare facilities that do not routinely provide neonatal intensive care.

■ Providers must be able to translate resuscitation knowledge into action and know when and how to perform the necessary skills to restore breathing and circulation.

■ Individual competency in resuscitation can be achieved through opportunities to practice hands-on skills.

■ Team competencies in performing neonatal resuscitation can be achieved using simulated resuscitation scenarios to practice team member communication and roles.

■ Ongoing competency evaluation and utilization of a quality improvement framework to evaluate performance and outcomes are essential to achieve optimal outcomes.

CLINICAL INDICATIONS

CPR is an emergency procedure required to preserve intact brain function when a person's heart has stopped beating and/or a person has stopped breathing. CPR is indicated for any unresponsive neonate who is not breathing or is breathing only in agonal gasps. If a neonate has a pulse but is not breathing (respiratory arrest), artificial respirations are needed.

■ Ineffective or absent respiratory effort is the primary reason why neonates require resuscitation at birth. Most of these infants have a normal heart but fail to establish or sustain adequate respiratory efforts.

Stabilization of vital signs is required when a person's heart is not performing well enough to adequately circulate oxygenated blood and/or a person is not breathing adequately such that they are receiving sufficient oxygen and exhaling carbon dioxide (CO_2).

■ All neonates who need full resuscitation must subsequently be brought to a stabilized condition.

■ A neonate might not require full resuscitation, yet still need to have their vital signs stabilized. Or a neonate might require resuscitation and need postresuscitation stabilization.

CLINICAL CONTRAINDICATION

Noninitiation of Resuscitation

The delivery of extremely premature infants and infants having severe congenital anomalies raises questions about whether and to what extent to initiate resuscitation in the delivery room.

■ Some infants with severe anomalies and/or chromosomal abnormalities have little or no chance of survival and will not benefit from resuscitation at birth.

■ Resuscitation of neonates born extremely preterm at the limits of viability may not improve the chances of survival with or without severe disability. Efforts to sustain life in these cases can result in unacceptable pain and suffering.

The American Medical Association (AMA) Code of Medical Ethics (AMA, 2010) provides a framework to guide decision-making in neonatal resuscitation. Providers must consider several factors in deciding what is best for each neonate. These factors include:

■ The chance that resuscitation will be successful

■ The risk and benefits of treatment (resuscitation) compared to no treatment

■ The degree to which resuscitation will extend the neonate's life

■ The pain and suffering associated with resuscitation

■ The expected quality of life for the neonate with and without the treatment

Successful management of younger, smaller, and sicker newborns is advancing on an ongoing and steady basis. To complicate the decision of which neonates should receive further attempts to resuscitate, antenatal information might be incomplete and/or unreliable. In situations of uncertain prognosis, including uncertain gestational age, resuscitation options include a trial of resuscitation and then discontinuation after a thorough assessment of the infant. In cases not highly likely to result in survival or survival without severe disability, initiation of resuscitation at the time of delivery does not mandate continued resuscitation and stabilization.

■ Noninitiation of resuscitative support and subsequent withdrawal of resuscitative support are considered to be ethically equivalent.

■ Subsequent withdrawal of resuscitative support allows care providers more time to assimilate complete clinical information and provide counseling to the infant's family.

Discontinuation of Resuscitation

Discontinuation of resuscitative efforts might be undertaken when life-sustaining measures are no longer in the neonate's best interest. Ongoing evaluation and discussion with parents and the healthcare team should guide continuation versus withdrawal of support. Failure to respond to maximal resuscitative efforts beyond 20 minutes is associated with poor neurodevelopmental outcomes, risk of severe disability, and high mortality. Globally, the International Consensus on CPR and Emergency Cardiovascular Care Science With Treatment Recommendations (CoSTR) conclude that local discussions take place to formulate guidelines consistent with local resources and outcome data (Wyckoff et al., 2020).

ETHICS

National and local protocols should direct the procedures that are followed. It is imperative that resuscitation procedures, protocols, policies, and neonatal outcomes be reviewed regularly by the primary neonatal care providers with updates shared as needed pertaining to changes made in resuscitation, delivery room, and intensive care practices.

SETTING

A clean and warm environment is best for conducting any infant resuscitations. Not all neonatal resuscitations are performed in the delivery room. Out of hospital births may result in an immediate need for neonatal resuscitation in the ED. Specific perinatal risk factors can predict that certain infants will require resuscitation; however, not all infants' resuscitation needs are predictable. Thus, to be prepared and safe, it is important to maintain the cleanliness and warmth of all hospital settings in case an infant's needs warrant resuscitation.

EQUIPMENT

No equipment is needed to initiate basic CPR of a neonate or infant. However, supplemental oxygen, an appropriately sized oxygen mask with a ventilation device, an oxygenation saturation monitor, a stethoscope, an endotracheal tube (ETT), a laryngoscope handle and blade, venous access supplies, and medications are needed as required to expedite and facilitate optimal neonatal resuscitation. A radiant warmer may be sufficient to maintain normal body temperature in late-preterm and term infants. However, supplemental warming methods such as plastic wrapping or bags, thermal mattresses, caps, and warm blankets may be required to maintain normothermia during resuscitation of newly born preterm infants.

■ Wherever deliveries occur, a complete inventory of resuscitation equipment and supplies should be maintained and accessible at all times.

SUPPLIES

The Seventh Edition of the Neonatal Resuscitation Program (NRP) in the *Textbook of Neonatal Resuscitation* presents a checklist of supplies and equipment useful for resuscitation (see Table 16.3). Supplies and equipment are listed according to each step of the resuscitation process.

TABLE 16.3 Neonatal Resuscitation Supplies and Equipment

PURPOSE	SUPPLIES AND EQUIPMENT
Warm	Preheated warmer
	Warm towels or blankets
	Temperature sensor and sensor cover for prolonged resuscitation
	Hat
	Plastic bag or plastic wrap (<32 weeks' gestation)
	Thermal mattress (<32 weeks' gestation)
Clear Airway	Bulb syringe
	10F or 12F suction catheter attached to wall suction, set at 80 to 100 mmHg
	Meconium aspirator
Auscultate	Stethoscope
Ventilate	Flowmeter set at 10 L/min
	Oxygen blender set to 21% (21%–30% if <35 weeks' gestation)
	PPV device
	Term- and preterm-sized masks
	8F feeding tube and large syringe
Oxygenate	Equipment to give free-flow oxygen
	Pulse oximeter with sensor and cover
	Target oxygen saturation table
Intubate	Laryngoscope with size-0 and size-1 straight blades (size-00 optional)
	Stylet (optional)
	Endotracheal tubes (sizes 2.5, 3.0, 3.5)
	Carbon dioxide (CO_2) detector

(continued)

TABLE 16.3 Neonatal Resuscitation Supplies and Equipment (*continued*)

PURPOSE	SUPPLIES AND EQUIPMENT
Intubate (*cont.*)	Measuring tape and/or endotracheal tube insertion depth table
	Waterproof tape or tape-securing device
	Scissors
	Laryngeal mask (size 1) and 5 mL syringe
Medicate	Access to:
	1:10,000 (0.1 mg/mL) epinephrine
	Normal saline
	Supplies for placing emergency umbilical catheter and administering medications
	Electronic cardiac (ECG) monitor leads and ECG monitor

PPV, positive-pressure ventilation.

Source: Weiner, G. M., Zaichkin, J., American Academy of Pediatrics, & American Heart Association. (2016). *Textbook of neonatal resuscitation (NRP)* (7th ed.). American Academy of Pediatrics, p. 25. Reprinted by permission from the American Academy of Pediatrics.

Personal protective equipment (PPE) should be available for personnel use during a neonatal resuscitation.

■ Standard universal precautions should be followed carefully, particularly in situations where blood and body fluids are likely to be present.

■ Personnel should wear gloves and other appropriate protective barriers when handling newly born infants during resuscitation.

STEPS TO RESUSCITATION

The international consensus recommendations for resuscitation (Perlman et al., 2015; Wyckoff et al., 2015) formulated the basis of the current algorithm and procedures used in neonatal resuscitation. The NRP developed by the American Academy of Pediatrics (AAP) and the American Heart Association (AHA) is based on the best available scientific evidence reviewed and summarized in the 2015 International Consensus of CPR and Emergency CoSTR. There is insufficient new evidence to warrant a change to the current algorithm.

Neonatal Resuscitation Algorithm

The AHA/AAP Neonatal Resuscitation algorithm provides a road map to guide a provider through the initial assessment and steps of resuscitation. Under ideal conditions, the plan for newborn resuscitation starts prior to the delivery with preparation of the family, resuscitation team, and equipment. A concise flowchart identifies the actions required to effectively resuscitate a newly born infant based on assessment of general condition, heart rate (HR), respiratory effort, and oxygenation. These actions are identified in the flowchart in Figure 16.5.

Preparation for Resuscitation

The mother/baby:

■ What perinatal risk factors are present?

■ What is the gestational age?

■ Is the amniotic fluid clear?

■ Is this a singleton or multiple birth?

The team:

■ Are additional personnel required for this resuscitation?

■ Who will serve as the team leader for the resuscitation?

■ What is the assigned role for each team member?

The equipment

■ Is the necessary resuscitation equipment present and ready for use?

■ Is additional equipment or supplies needed?

Initial Assessment and Actions Within the First 60 Seconds

■ What is the infant's status immediately at birth?

● A term infant with good tone and normal respiratory effort can remain with the mother and receive routine care.

• Routine care includes providing warmth, positioning to keep the airway clear, drying the infant, and continuing observation and assessment.

● A preterm infant or a nonvigorous infant requires warmth to maintain body temperature, positioning to support a patent airway, clearance of secretions when necessary, drying, and stimulation if their respiratory effort is not adequate.

■ What is the infant's response to clearing the airway, drying, and stimulation?

● When labored breathing or cyanosis persists, the focus should be on clearing the airway, evaluation of oxygen saturation status, and provision of oxygen, if needed. Continuous positive airway pressure (CPAP) should be considered at this time.

● If the infant is gasping, experiencing apnea, or their HR is below 100 bpm, begin PPV at a rate of 40 to 60 breaths per minute and initiate use of an oxygen saturation monitor to evaluate the need for supplemental oxygen. Place the sensor on the infant's right hand or wrist. Use of an HR monitor should be considered at this time.

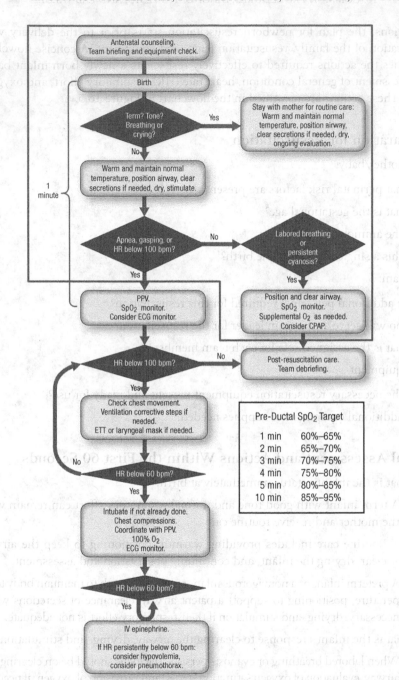

FIGURE 16.5 Newborn resuscitation algorithm.

CPAP, continuous positive airway pressure; ETT, endotracheal tube; HR, heart rate; PPV, positive-pressure ventilation; SpO₂, oxygen saturation.

Source: Weiner, G. M., Zaichkin, J., American Academy of Pediatrics, & American Heart Association. (2016). *Textbook of neonatal resuscitation (NRP)* (7th ed.). American Academy of Pediatrics, p. 34. Reprinted by permission from the American Academy of Pediatrics.

- An oxygen saturation monitor (pulse oximeter) with a reliable signal is required to guide the initiation and titration of supplemental oxygen.
  - The pulse oximeter may not function when the newborn has poor perfusion or a low HR. Use an ECG monitor to display heart rate.
  - Targets for preductal oxygen saturation for the first 10 minutes of life are as follows:

    | 1 minute | 60% to 65% |
    | 2 minutes | 65% to 70% |
    | 3 minutes | 70% to 75% |
    | 4 minutes | 75% to 80% |
    | 5 minutes | 80% to 85% |
    | 10 minutes | 85% to 90% |

■ Is the infant's HR above or below 100 bpm following initiation of PPV?

- When the infant has responded to PPV and the HR is above 100 bpm, begin postresuscitation care.
- When the HR is below 100 bpm with PPV, assess the infant for adequate chest rise with ventilation and take corrective steps.
  - Does the mask require adjustment?
  - Is the head in a neutral or slightly extended position?
  - Is the airway open and clear?
  - Is more positive pressure required to move the chest?
  - Would an alternate airway improve ventilation?
    - An ETT placed between the vocal cords provides the most reliable airway to deliver effective artificial ventilation.
    - A skilled provider is required to perform the intubation procedure.
    - A CO_2 detector should be used to confirm the placement of the ETT in the trachea by the presence of exhaled CO_2 when effective ventilation is delivered.
    - A laryngeal mask airway (LMA) can be used as an alternative method for establishing an airway, especially if the bag-mask ventilation is ineffective for the newborn or attempts at tracheal intubation have been unsuccessful.
    - Infant size may prohibit use of the LMA since the smallest size may be too big for a preterm infant.
  - Could the airway be obstructed by meconium, blood, or other thick secretions resulting in ineffective ventilation?
    - Connect a meconium aspirator to the ETT to clear the airway. Apply suction to the tube to remove the obstruction.

- Repeat the suction procedure as needed to relieve the obstruction and allow effective ventilation.

- Continue with the steps of resuscitation.

■ Is the HR above or below 60 once effective ventilation has been established?

● An HR below 60 despite 30 seconds of effective PPV indicates more aggressive intervention is needed.

● Endotracheal intubation should precede initiation of chest compressions.

● Chest compressions should be initiated and coordinated with PPV to deliver three compressions and one ventilation (3:1 ratio) every 2 seconds.

● The neonate should receive a total of 90 compressions and 30 breaths each minute.

● The chest is compressed by encircling the chest and placing the thumbs side by side or one on top of the other in the middle of the sternum just below the nipple line.

● Avoid compressing the xyphoid or moving the thumbs onto the infant's ribs.

● The depth of chest compression is determined by the anterior-posterior (AP) diameter of the chest. The correct depth of insertion is one third of the AP diameter of the chest.

■ Is the infant's condition improving after initiation of coordinated chest compressions and PPV?

● Assess the HR after delivering 60 seconds of coordinated compressions and ventilation.

● The HR can be assessed using an ECG monitor, a stethoscope, or a pulse oximeter having a reliable signal.

● Chest compressions can be stopped when the HR is 60 bpm and rising while ventilation continues at 40 to 60 breaths per minute.

● Administration of epinephrine is indicated when the HR is not rising after 60 seconds of coordinated compressions and effective ventilation.

  • The recommended concentration of epinephrine for neonatal use is 1:10,000 (0.1 mg/mL).

  • The recommended dose of epinephrine is 0.1 to 0.3 mL/kg for IV administration.

  • The umbilical vein is the recommended and preferred route for emergency administration of epinephrine.

  • The intraosseous (IO) route can be used as an alternate route of administration of epinephrine when the umbilical vein cannot be cannulated.

  • The dose of epinephrine is the same for drug delivery via the umbilical vein or the IO route.

- Epinephrine can be delivered via the ETT if there is no IV or IO access, but a higher dose will be required to produce the desired effect.
- Epinephrine should be given rapidly followed by a normal saline flush to ensure no medication remains in the tubing.
- Repeat doses of epinephrine can be administered every 3 to 5 minutes.

■ What should be done after administering epinephrine to an infant receiving coordinated chest compressions and ventilation and the HR is low?

- Assess the infant's response to epinephrine and determine if the HR remains below 60 bpm.

- Assess the infant for signs of shock:
  - Volume expansion is indicated when there are signs of shock in an infant who has not responded to resuscitation interventions.
  - Prepare normal saline 10 mL/kg for administration via the umbilical vein or IO route.

- Does the infant have a history of blood loss?
  - Emergency management of acute blood loss includes transfusion of O Rh-negative blood.

- Evaluate for other life-threatening conditions:
  - Consider pneumothorax; and also
  - Evaluate for anomalies that cause airway obstruction or lung compression.

Recent Resuscitation Updates

The 2019 recommended neonatal resuscitation guidelines required no change in the 2015 Neonatal Resuscitation Algorithm Update. The 2019 guideline update was based on two evidence reviews conducted as guided by the International Liaison Committee on Resuscitation Neonatal Life Support Task Force (ILCOR, 2006; Perkins et al., 2017). The International Liaison systematic reviewers plus content experts comprehensively reviewed scientific literature on the appropriate initial oxygen concentration used during neonatal resuscitation of term and late-preterm (>35 weeks' gestation) and preterm newborns (<35 weeks' gestation). The reviewers concluded that:

■ The initial use of 21% oxygen is acceptable for term and late-preterm newborns receiving respiratory support at birth.

■ 100% oxygen should not be used for these newborns because it has been shown to be associated with excessive mortality.

■ Between 21% and 30% oxygen is reasonable at the beginning of a resuscitation for preterm newborns receiving respiratory support at birth.

■ Subsequent oxygen titration completed should be based on saturation goals (Hingley et al., 2020).

In October 2020, resuscitation and stabilization guidelines for neonates were updated formally to reflect the most recent pertinent scientific findings. These neonatal guidelines were published in *Pediatrics* as part 5 of the 2020 AHA Guidelines for CPR and Emergency Cardiovascular Care (Aziz et al., 2021). Developing skills and practicing PPV were emphasized.

■ Effective PPV is the main intervention needed by neonates who require further intervention to help them breathe, including neonates who are apneic, bradycardic, or breathing ineffectively.

■ Both individual caregiver and caregiver team training were noted as critical to ensuring that PPV is implemented correctly to neonates.

■ The recent guidelines that follow form the basis of the AAP/AHA NRP, Eighth Edition, which will become available in June 2021 with full implementation expected by January 2022. An overview of differences between the 7th and 8th editions can be found at https://downloads.aap.org/DOICH/Integrate%20 8th%20Edition%20into%20NRP%207th%20Edition.pdf.

Delayed Cord Clamping

■ For all term and preterm neonates not requiring resuscitation, a 30- to 60-second delay has been added for clamping the umbilical cord. However, the umbilical cord should be clamped immediately and clamping not delayed if the placental circulation is disrupted (e.g., placental abruption; Fogarty et al., 2017; Weiner et al., 2016).

Body Temperature Maintenance

■ For small preterm neonates, hypothermia has been found to be consistently associated with severe morbidities and higher mortality (Wyckoff et al., 2015). As a result, it is recommended that delivery room temperatures be kept at 23 °C to 25 °C (74 °F–77 °F; Jia et al., 2013).

■ For preterm neonates born at <32 weeks' gestation, a combination of techniques, including plastic wrapping, thermal mattresses, radiant warmers, neonatal head caps, and warmed humidified gases, for resuscitation are now formally recommended. Newborns known not to be asphyxiated should have their axillary temperatures maintained at 36.5 °C to 37.5 °C (97.7 °F–99.5 °F) (Wyckoff et al., 2015).

Suctioning

■ Suctioning of newborns should be performed only if the airway is obstructed or if PPV is needed (Perlman et al., 2010; Weiner et al., 2016).

■ In nonvigorous neonates born having meconium-stained amniotic fluid (MSAF), intubation and endotracheal suctioning should only be completed for those who require it for ventilation or who are experiencing an airway obstruction (Chettri et al., 2015; Jia et al., 2013; Perlman et al., 2015; Singh et al., 2019).

Heart Rate Assessment

■ Current recommendations for assessing HR during resuscitation advise using a three-lead ECG for rapid and accurate assessment when PPV is initiated. The preferred method of HR assessment once chest compressions begin is the ECG (Weiner et al., 2016).

■ A rising HR remains the cardinal indicator of successful ventilation (Weiner et al., 2016; Wyckoff et al., 2015).

Positive-Pressure Ventilation

■ PPV is indicated for neonates who are apneic or gasping and when their HR is <100 beats/min.

■ PPV can also be initiated in spontaneously breathing neonates whose HRs are greater than 100 beats/min and do not maintain oxygen saturations with the target range, despite CPAP or free-flowing oxygen.

■ During PPV, the continued recommendation is to start with a positive inspiratory pressure of 20 to 25 cm H_2O. Also, a positive end-expiratory pressure (PEEP) of 5 cm H_2O is recommended. To achieve this PEEP goal with self-inflating bags, a PEEP valve is required (Wyckoff et al., 2015).

Endotracheal Intubation

■ Endotracheal intubation is indicated for ineffective PPV, prolonged PPV, or for special circumstances—such as an abnormal airway anatomy.

■ When a neonate needs chest compressions, intubation is strongly recommended (Escobedo et al., 2019).

Supplemental Oxygen

■ Room air (21% O_2 at sea level) is recommended at the initiation of resuscitation for neonates born at greater than 35 weeks' gestation.

■ In healthy term neonates, supplemental oxygen should be used as needed to achieve saturation targets using pulse oximetry (Welsford, Nishiyama, Shortt, Isayama, et al., 2019).

■ For preterm neonates less than 35 weeks' gestation, beginning resuscitation with 21% to 30% supplemental O_2 is recommended and titrating to saturation targets that are similar to those used for term infants (Weiner et al., 2016; Welsford, Nishiyama, Shortt, Isayama, et al., 2019; Wyckoff et al., 2015).

Chest Compressions

■ When a neonate's HR remains less than 60 beats/min after at least 30 seconds of PPV, chest compressions are indicated.

■ When chest compressions are begun, supplemental O_2 can be increased until the neonate's HR recovers and then supplemental O_2 can be weaned afterward as soon as appropriate (Perlman et al., 2015; Weiner et al., 2016; Wyckoff et al., 2015).

Epinephrine

■ Epinephrine administered through either the IV or IO route is indicated when a neonate's HR is <60 beats/min after 60 seconds of chest compressions coordinated with PPV using 100% O_2 (Weiner et al., 2016; Wyckoff et al., 2015).

■ After the June 2021 NRP update is published, a new resuscitation quality improvement (RQI) program for NRP focused on PPV is planned to be introduced. This RQI program is being codeveloped by the AHA and Laerdal Medical (https://bit.ly/2GKTwnT).

ASSESSMENT AND CARE POSTRESUSCITATION

■ Because there are considerable assessments and reassessments completed during resuscitation, coordination between and among resuscitation care providers is critical.

■ At least one care provider should oversee the overall resuscitative event.

■ Another care provider should keep a written record of events that have taken place and the neonate's response.

■ Additional help should be requested when needed. Referral or tertiary centers should be called for advice and/or assistance with transport.

■ Termination of resuscitation is difficult and should follow local protocols and medical direction.

DOCUMENTATION

■ Procedure notes should be written for all procedures completed.

■ All lab results should be listed and/or noted as pending.

■ All working diagnoses should be noted.

■ All plans for additional diagnostics and therapeutic interventions should be noted.

■ Informed consent(s) should be included, if any consents were needed as part of the resuscitation.

■ Parent(s) should have seen/touched the neonate before or following the resuscitation.

■ Staff consultations should be written and included in the medical record.

■ Any pertinent information regarding heritable and familial conditions should be noted.

■ Notification of any referring physicians and the mother's obstetrician should be noted.

■ The family's religious preference should be noted.

DEFINITION OF STABILIZATION

Stabilization refers to a state where vital signs are within normal limits. In order to transition a neonate to a steadfast and stable state—such that their HR and breathing are within normal limits—interventions that require a variety of supplies and equipment might be needed. Because there are so many different interventions required for stabilizing a particular condition or set of conditions, only a general discussion of stabilization is presented here.

STABILIZATION OR CONTINUING CARE AFTER RESUSCITATION

As part of stabilization, ongoing and/or supportive care, monitoring, and appropriate diagnostic evaluation are necessary after resuscitation. Once adequate ventilation and circulation are established, the neonate should be maintained within, or transferred to, an environment where close monitoring and ongoing care can be provided.

Postresuscitation monitoring should include monitoring of temperature, HR, respiratory rate, arterial oxygen saturation, administered oxygen concentration, and blood gas analysis at regular intervals and as indicated. Blood pressure should be assessed and documented. Blood glucose also should be assessed during stabilization after resuscitation.

A chest radiograph may help identify the underlying causes of the arrest or detect respiratory complications. Additional care might include treatment of hypotension with volume expanders or vasopressors, treatment of possible infections, and initiation of appropriate fluid therapy. Some infants with hypoxic–ischemia encephalopathy may require time-sensitive therapeutic hypothermia treatment be initiated within the first hours after resuscitation.

Further information about specific stabilizing caregiving is accessible from the S.T.A.B.L.E. Program resource (Karlsen, 2013). The S.T.A.B.L.E. Program for neonatal caregivers was developed to meet the educational needs of healthcare providers who deliver stabilization care to neonates. S.T.A.B.L.E. education is very helpful in reducing infant morbidity and mortality. It is useful in postresuscitations, pretransports, and at other times when a neonate's condition is unstable in one or more body systems. S.T.A.B.L.E. is the most widely used neonatal education program to focus exclusively on stabilization care of sick infants. Based on a mnemonic, S.T.A.B.L.E. stands for the six assessment and care modules in the program: sugar and safe care, temperature, airway, blood pressure, lab work, and emotional support. A seventh module, quality improvement, stresses the professional responsibility of improving and evaluating care provided to sick infants.

S.T.A.B.L.E. (Karlsen, 2013) endorses recommendations pertinent to six areas.

1. *Sugar and safe care* that reviews the importance of establishing IV access. Neonates are at risk for developing hypoglycemia. IV fluid administration must be monitored to determine hydration and glucose status. Safe patient care that eliminates and prevents errors is a top priority.

2. *Temperature* reviews special thermal needs of infants, including avoiding hyperthermia and selective cerebral hypothermia, as a protection against brain injury in the asphyxiated infant.

3. *Airway* reviews evaluation of respiratory distress, basic chest x-ray evaluation, useful initial ventilator settings, and respiratory treatments. Any supplementary oxygen administered should be regulated by blending oxygen and air, using oximetry measured from the right upper extremity to guide titration of the blend delivered; if supplemental oxygen is unavailable and PPV is required, use room air.

4. *Blood pressure* reviews risk for hypovolemic, cardiogenic, and septic shock in infants and how to assess and treat shock.

5. *Lab work* focuses on neonatal infection, the complete blood count, and initial antibiotic treatment for suspected infection.

6. *Emotional support* reviews the crisis surrounding the birth of a sick neonate and how to support the infant's family.

REFERENCES

American Medical Association. (2010). *Council on ethical and judicial affairs* (2010–2011 ed.). Code of medical ethics. Current Opinions with Annotations. American Medical Association (Opinion 2.215).

Aziz, K., Lee, H. C., Escobedo, M. B., Hoover, A. V., Kamath-Rayne, B. D., Kapadia, V. S., Magid, D. J., Niermeyer, S., Schmölzer, G. M., Szyld, E., Weiner, G. M., Wyckoff, M. H., Yamada, N. K., & Zaichkin, J. (2021). Part 5: Neonatal Resuscitation 2020 American Heart Association Guidelines for Cardiopulmonary Resuscitation and Emergency Cardiovascular Care. *Pediatrics, 147*(Suppl. 1), e2020038505E. https://doi.org/10.1542/peds.2020-038505E

Chettri, S., Adhisivam, B., & Bhat, B. V. (2015). Endotracheal suction for nonvigorous neonates born through meconium stained amniotic fluid: A randomized controlled trial. *Journal of Pediatrics, 166*(5), 1208–1213. https://doi.org/10.1016/j.jpeds.2014.12.076

Escobedo, M. B., Shah, B. A., Song, C., Makkar, A., & Szyld, E. (2019). Recent recommendations and emerging science in neonatal resuscitation. *Pediatric Clinics of North America, 66*(2), 309–320. https://doi.org/10.1016/j.pcl.2018.12.002

Fogarty, M., Osborn, D. A., Askie, L., Seider, A. L., Hunter, K., Lui, K., Simes, J., & Tarnow-Mordi, W. (2017). Delayed vs early umbilical cord clamping for preterm infants: A systematic review and meta-analysis. *American Journal of Obstetrics & Gynecology, 218*(1), 1–18. https://doi.org/10.1016/j.ajog.2017.10.231

Hingley, S., Booth, A., Hodgson, J., Langworthy, K., Shimizu, N., & Maconochie, I. (2020). Concordance between the 2010 and 2015 Resuscitation Guidelines of International Liaison Committee of Resuscitation Councils (ILCOR) members and the ILCOR Consensus of Science and Treatment Recommendations (CoSTRs). *Resuscitation, 151*, 111–117. https://doi.org/10.1016/j.resuscitation.2020.04.001

International Liaison Committee on Resuscitation. (2006). The International Liaison Committee on Resuscitation (ILCOR) consensus on science with treatment recommendations for pediatric and neonatal patients: Pediatric basic and advanced life support. *Pediatrics, 117*(5), e955–e977. https://doi.org/10.1542/peds.2006-0206

Jia, Y. S., Lin, Z. L., Lv, H., Li, Y-M., Green, R., & Lin, J. (2013). Effect of delivery room temperature on the admission temperature of premature infants: A randomized controlled trial. *Journal of Perinatology, 33*(4), 264–267. https://doi.org/10.1038/jp.2012.100

Karlsen, K. (2013). *The S.T.A.B.L.E. program, learner/provider manual: Post-resuscitation/pretransport stabilization care of sick infants—guidelines for neonatal healthcare providers* (6th ed.). S.T.A.B.L.E.

Perkins, G. D., Neumar, R., Monsieurs, K. G., Lim, S. H., Castren, M., Nolan, J. P., Nadkarni, V., Montgomery, B., Steen, P., Cummins, R., Chamberlain, D., Aickin, R., de Caen, A., Wang, T.-L., Stanton, D., Escalante, R., Callaway, C. W., Soar, J., Olasveengen, T., … Bossaert, L. (2017). The International Liaison Committee on Resuscitation-Review of the last 25 years and vision for the future. *Resuscitation, 121,* 104–116. https://doi.org/10.1016/j.resuscitation.2017.09.029

Perlman, J. M., Wyllie, J., Kattwinkel, J., Atkins, D. L., Chameides, L., Goldsmith, J. P., Guinsburg, R., Hazinski, M. F., Morley, C., Richmond, S., Simon, W. M., Singhal, N., Szyld, E. Tamura, M., Valaphi, S., & Neonatal Resuscitation Chapter Collaborators. (2010). Part 11: Neonatal resuscitation: 2010 international consensus on cardiopulmonary resuscitation and emergency cardiovascular care science with treatment recommendations. *Circulation, 122*(16 Suppl. 2), S516–S538. https://doi.org/10.1161/CIRCULATIONAHA.110.971127

Perlman, J. M., Wyllie, J., Kattwinkel, J., Wyckoff, M. H., Aziz, K., Guinsburg, R., Kim, H.-S., Liley, H. G., Mildenhall, L., Simon, W. M., Szyld, E., Tamura, M., Velaphi, S., & Neonatal Resuscitation Chapter Collaborators. (2015). Part 7: Neonatal resuscitation: 2015 international consensus on cardiopulmonary resuscitation and emergency cardiovascular care science with treatment recommendations. *Circulation, 132*(16 Suppl. 1), S204–S241. https://doi.org/10.1161/CIR.0000000000000276

Singh, S. N., Saxena, S., Bhriguvanshi, A., Kumar, M., Chandrakanta, & Sujata. (2019). Effect of endotracheal suctioning just after birth in non-vigorous infants born through meconium stained amniotic fluid: A randomized controlled trial. *Clinical Epidemiology and Global Health, 7*(2), 165–170. https://doi.org/10.1016/j.cegh.2018.03.006

Weiner, G. M., Zaichkin, J., American Academy of Pediatrics, & American Heart Association. (2016). *Textbook of neonatal resuscitation (NRP)* (7th ed.). American Academy of Pediatrics.

Welsford, M., Nishiyama, C., Shortt, C., Isayama, T., Dawson, J. A., Weiner, G., Roehr, C. C., Wyckoff, M. H., & Rabi, Y. (2019). Room air for initiating term newborn resuscitation: A systematic review with meta-analysis. *Pediatrics, 143,* e20181825. https://doi.org/10.1542/peds.2018-1825

Welsford, M., Nishiyama, C., Shortt, C., Weiner, G., Roehr, C. C., Isayama, T., Dawson, J. A., Wyckoff, M. H., & Rabi, Y. (2019). Initial oxygen use for preterm newborn resuscitation: A systematic review with meta-analysis. *Pediatrics, 143,* e20181828. https://doi.org/10.1542/peds.2018-1828

Wyckoff, M. H., Aziz, K., Escobedo, M. B., Kapadia, V. S., Kattwinkel, J., Perlman, J. M., Simon, W. M., Weiner, G. M., & Zaichkin, J. G. (2015). Part 13: Neonatal resuscitation: 2015 American Heart Association guidelines update for cardiopulmonary resuscitation and emergency cardiovascular care (reprint). *Pediatrics, 136*(Suppl. 2), 196–218. https://doi.org/10.1161/CIR.0000000000000267

Wyckoff, M. H., Wyllie, J., Aziz, K., de Almeida, M. F., Fabres, J., Fawke, J., Guinsburg, R., Hosono, S., Isayama, T., Kapadia, V. S., Kim, H.-S., Liley, H. G., McKinlay, C. J. D., Mildenhall, L., Perlman, J. M., Rabi, Y., Roehr, C. C., Schmölzer, G. M., Szyld, E., . . ., Neonatal Life Support Collaborators. (2020). Neonatal Life Support: 2020 international consensus on cardiopulmonary resuscitation and emergency cardiovascular care science with treatment recommendations. *Circulation, 142*(16, Suppl. 1), S185–S221. https://doi.org/10.1161/CIR.0000000000000895

Diagnostic Tests

SAMUAL L. MOONEYHAM

OVERVIEW

Care of the neonate typically involves numerous diagnostic procedures and tests to identify dysfunction related to birth, prematurity, illness, or congenital malformations. This chapter highlights the commonly used methods for developing a medical or surgical diagnosis in the newborn and infant.

DIAGNOSTIC IMAGING IN INFANTS

Diagnostic imaging in newborns and infants is unique. The disease entities and the diagnostic imaging needed are different in the neonate than the older child or adult. Concerns over positioning, exposure factors, and methods of immobilization make imaging somewhat challenging in the neonate.

CONDITIONS REQUIRING DIAGNOSTIC IMAGING

Pathologic conditions commonly encountered in adults often are not found in infants, and many abnormal conditions are exclusive to the newborn period. Examples of these pathologic conditions are the congenital abnormalities of the newborn, such as atresias of the gastrointestinal (GI) tract, severe or critical congenital heart defects (CCHD), surgical causes of respiratory distress, spina bifida, and bilateral choanal atresia. These lesions, which are lethal if left untreated, often are symptomatic in the first days after birth. Medical problems related to premature and postmature birth, intrauterine growth disturbances, nonlethal developmental defects, genetic abnormalities, and perinatal asphyxia are of greatest concern in the newborn period. In addition, malignant tumors, such as neuroblastoma and Wilms' tumor, may appear in the newborn period and up to approximately 4 years of age. Certain infections, such as cytomegalovirus (CMV), toxoplasmosis, and syphilis, have a distinct radiographic and ultrasonographic presentation if exposure occurred in utero rather than in the neonatal period (Martin et al., 2020).

ANATOMIC PROPORTIONS

The anatomic proportions of infants are very different from those of adults, and the younger the infant, the more marked the differences. It is important to take the differences into consideration when interpreting the diagnostic imaging. It is important that not only the area in question but the whole of the area in question appear in the imaging field.

As shown in Figure 17.1, the newborn's head is large in proportion to the body, and the cranial vault is large in proportion to the area of the face. The neck is short, and the diaphragm is high. The kidneys are low, about midway between the diaphragm and symphysis pubis. The abdomen is large because of the relative size of the liver and stomach. The pelvic cavity is very small, and the bladder extends above the symphysis pubis. The chest, pelvis, and limbs are much small in proportion to the abdomen. The lungs may appear wider or longer and higher than

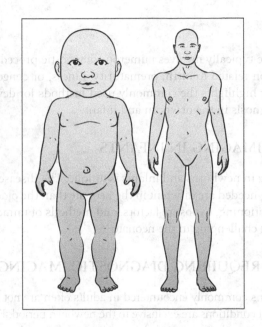

FIGURE 17.1 Proportional anatomic differences between a neonate and an adult.

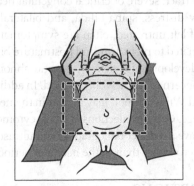

FIGURE 17.2 Neonatal radiographs should be limited to only the area of interest. Total body radiographs should be avoided. The top box (light dashed lines) defines the area of interest for an anteroposterior (AP) chest radiograph. The bottom box (heavy dashed lines) defines the area of interest for an AP abdominal film. The gonad shield has been omitted for illustrative purposes.

expected in the thoracic cavity when an anteroposterior (AP) image is taken. The diaphragm is located just below the level of the nipples. A lateral view may make the lungs appear extended from the posterior aspect.

The newborn's abdomen bulges laterally wider than the pelvis, and the bulge contains abdominal organs displaced by the large liver and stomach. This abdominal area must be included if an accurate image is to be taken. Irradiation should encompass the smallest possible body area. Often the field is too large, particularly in premature infants and newborns, and results in the appearance of other body parts in the film (Figure 17.2).

REFERENCE

Martin, R., Fanaroff, A., & Walsh, M. (2020). *Neonatal-perinatal medicine* (11th ed.). Elsevier.

TYPES OF DIAGNOSTIC IMAGING

The four major diagnostic imaging methods used in neonatal care are x-ray (roentgenologic), radionuclide, ultrasonographic, and MRI. This chapter discusses each of these imaging modalities in relation to the biophysical principles responsible for producing the image, the potential risks of the procedure, and the nursing care of the newborn or infant undergoing such an examination. Table 17.1 summarizes the types of diagnostic imaging commonly used for neonates.

X-Ray Imaging (Roentgenology)

The principles of conventional radiography have not changed since the discovery of x-rays in the late 1800s. However, the equipment and techniques have become far more sophisticated; current radiographic methods include tomography, fluoroscopy, CT, and digital radiography.

Roentgenologic Biophysical Principles

When an x-ray beam is directed toward a part of the body, differential absorption of the x-ray photons by different types of body tissue occurs. Bone and metal fragments absorb x-ray photons and therefore appear white on the radiographic film, whereas air-containing structures, such as lungs and gas-filled bowel, absorb few x-ray photons and appear black. Soft tissues and blood vessels appear as intermediate shades of gray.

A radiograph gives a two-dimensional projection of three-dimensional structures. This simple imaging technique can distinguish only among air, fat, and tissues with densities approximately equal to those of water or metals, but it continues to be enormously valuable and is still the diagnostic imaging method most often used in neonatal care.

TABLE 17.1 Diagnostic Imaging Methods Commonly Used for Neonates

TECHNIQUE	INDICATIONS AND ADVANTAGES	LIMITATIONS	POTENTIAL RISKS	COMMENTS	COST
Roentgenologic Techniques					
Radiographic imaging	Most frequently used initial diagnostic screening mode	Detects only four different levels of photon absorption (air, fat, water, and mineral); two-dimensional (2D) projection of three-dimensional (3D) structures	Ionizing radiation; thermal stress of cool film plate	Proper positioning of infant is essential; child must be monitored during procedure	$
Xeroradiographic imaging	Used to evaluate soft tissue structures	Tissue structures defined by relative amounts of air, fat, water, and minerals; seldom used since advent of newer diagnostic imaging methods	Higher level of ionizing radiation than with routine radiographs	Proper positioning of infant is essential; child must be monitored during procedure	$$
Fluoroscopic imaging	Used to evaluate motion or function of cardiovascular, GI, and GU systems; may be used to guide therapeutic or diagnostic procedures	Images rely on greater radiation and/or movement of contrast material; improper diagnostic sequencing may delay informational yield; contrast material may have physiologic consequences	Much higher level of ionizing radiation than with routine radiographs; thermal stress of cool radiology environment	Proper positioning of infant is essential; child must be monitored during procedure	$$-$$$$

CT	Used to provide detailed, superior characterization of various soft tissue densities that cannot be detected by conventional radiographs	Motion artifact may cause blurring of scans; radiation dose depends on scan time; contrast material may have physiologic consequences	Ionizing radiation; thermal stress of cool environment	Proper positioning of infant is essential; child must be monitored during procedure	$$$
Ultrasound imaging	Does not use ionizing radiation but rather uses sound waves to depict anatomic and functional motion of tissue; sound waves can be directed in a beam in a variety of planes; portable; different graphic displays are available	Ultrasound technique is operator dependent; does not provide as much information on organ function such as urography; reveals less anatomic detail than CT; scan is adversely affected by the presence of bone and air	Thermal stress may occur with application of cool scanning gel to infant's skin; there are no known deleterious effects from clinical use of ultrasound imaging	Proper positioning of infant is essential; child must be monitored during procedure	$
Radionucleotide imaging	Used to trace anatomic proportions and a wide range of physiologic functions in virtually every organ in the body; amount of ionizing radiation emitted by injected agent is significantly less than the amount required for corresponding radiograph	Diagnostic yield depends on uptake of radionucleotide by different organs; radionucleotides are rarely organ specific; limited anatomic resolution	Thermal stress during nucleotide scanning	Proper positioning of the infant is essential; maximum radiation exposure is not always the organ of interest; child must be monitored during procedure	$$

(continued)

TABLE 17.1 Diagnostic Imaging Methods Commonly Used for Neonates (*continued*)

TECHNIQUE	INDICATIONS AND ADVANTAGES	LIMITATIONS	POTENTIAL RISKS	COMMENTS	COST
PET and SPECT	Both techniques have greater sensitivity and qualifications of the distribution and density of radioactivity to depict the "metabolic" function of tissue; 3D imaging is possible with computer reconstruction; dose of nucleotide is the same; artifactual lesions can be eliminated; amount of ionizing radiation emitted by injected agents (carbon 11, oxygen 15, nitrogen 13) is significantly less than the amount required for corresponding radiograph	PET scanning requires access to a cyclotron to produce the positrons used in scans	Thermal stress during nucleotide scanning	Proper positioning of infant is essential; child must be monitored during procedure	$$$$$
MRI	Uses magnetic fields and radio waves to produce images; the region of the body scanned can be controlled electronically, and hardware does not limit scanning sites; scans are free of high-intensity artifacts; newer scanning techniques can quantify many pathologic conditions	Availability and cost; limited use in unstable infants on life support; monitoring equipment must be free from interference with magnetic field	Does not use ionizing radiation to produce images; limited access to infant during procedure	Proper positioning is essential; must be monitored during procedure	$$$$$

GI, gastrointestinal; GU, genitourinary; PET, positron emission tomography; SPECT, single photon emission computed tomography.

564

CT

CT scanning obtains cross-sectional images rather than the shadow images of conventional radiography. Conventional radiography is based on variable attenuation of the x-ray beam as it passes through tissue. Conventional radiographs cannot produce a detailed characterization of various soft tissue densities. Bone is the densest, absorbs most of the x-rays, and appears white; air is the least dense and appears black; soft tissues are displayed as intermediate shades of gray. CT detects density changes in very small tissue areas. It allows identification of the subarachnoid space, white and gray matter, and ventricles. CT demonstrates tissue structure with precise clarity. CT permits two-dimensional visualization of entire anatomic sections of tissue, which aids the determination of the extent of the disease or malformation. Anatomic and physiologic information can be visualized despite overlying gas and bone. Bolus injection of contrast material allows excellent visualization of vascular structures.

As good as CT is as an imaging modality, it is still not a radiologic microscope; CT does have its drawbacks. It also uses ionizing radiation, and because the computers require a cool room for proper equipment performance, the neonate's environment is altered significantly, a circumstance that must be considered.

Radiographic Contrast Agents

Plain radiography can differentiate only four kinds of body tissue: tissue containing gas (lung and bowel), fatty tissue, tissue containing calcium (bone or pathologic calcifications), and tissues of water density (solid organs, muscle, and blood). To demonstrate blood vessels that are in solid organs or surrounded by muscle or to demonstrate other hollow structures, artificial radiographic contrast agents must be introduced. Administration may be by injection, enema, or swallowing.

Negative contrast media absorb less radiation than adjacent soft tissues and therefore cast a darker radiographic image. Gases such as air, oxygen, and carbon dioxide can be used as negative contrast media. Positive contrast media use elements with a high atomic number, which absorb much more radiation than surrounding soft tissues and therefore cast a lighter image. Barium and iodine are the two elements currently used. Barium sulfate, a relatively stable, nontoxic compound, is the major contrast agent used for outlining the walls of the GI tract.

Iodine-containing salts that are excreted by the kidneys are used for a wide variety of urographic and angiographic studies. The kidneys also excrete the newer nonionic, iodine-containing media. Because of their lower osmolality, these agents are less painful than iodine-containing salts. Some of the radiopharmaceuticals used in neonatal imaging include Technetium 99m sulfur or tin colloid, albumin microspheres, pertechnetate, diethylenetriaminepentaacetic acid (DTPA), hepatoiminodiacetic acid (HIDA), iodine 131, xenon 131, krypton 81m, and thallium 201.

Factors Affecting Radiographic Quality

Several factors determine the technical quality of a radiograph, including film exposure, phase of respiration, motion, tube angulation, and infant positioning. If one of these factors is unsatisfactory, the film may be misinterpreted. When nurses understand these factors, the technical quality of radiographs is improved.

Film Exposure

If the film is underexposed, the dorsal disc spaces are lost and the lungs and other structures have a homogeneous, "whitewashed" appearance. If the film is overexposed, lungs have a black, "burned out" appearance, and it is difficult to see the pulmonary vasculature.

Phase of Respiration

The phase of respiration at the time the film is obtained affects the appearance of the radiograph considerably (Figure 17.3). On an expiratory film, the heart may appear enlarged and the lung fields opaque, with the diaphragm at the level of the seventh rib. On an inspiratory film, the diaphragm is at the eighth rib, the cardiothymic diameter is normal, and the pulmonary vascularity is prominent. The right hemidiaphragm is slightly higher than the left.

Motion

If the infant moves just as the radiograph is made, the resulting film is blurred. Movement blur on diagnostic images can be prevented by fast imaging and adequate immobilization.

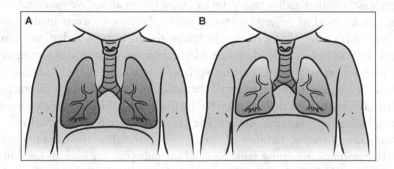

FIGURE 17.3 Differences in appearance between inspiration (A) and expiration (B) in a neonatal chest radiograph. On full inspiration, the diaphragm is located at the eighth rib, and the lungs appear larger and darker. During expiration, the diaphragm is at or above the seventh rib, and the lung fields appear smaller and lighter. The heart size may also appear larger on expiratory films.

Speed

A short exposure time is essential for obtaining clear images. This can be achieved by limiting the duration of exposure to the energy source and by increasing the use of computed imaging.

Immobilization

The nursing staff is primarily responsible for ensuring adequate immobilization during diagnostic imaging. Inadequate immobilization is an important cause of poor quality in neonatal images. Proper immobilization techniques improve image quality and may be less traumatic than manual restraint alone. An immobilization board may be required, or tape, foam rubber blocks and wedges, towels, diapers, or clear plastic acetate sheets may be used.

Physical risks to neonates are associated with immobilization. Infants lie still only when they are very ill. Otherwise, they greatly resent being forcibly restrained, especially in an unusual position.

Tube Angulation

Another factor is angulation of the x-ray tube, along with improper field limitation. Often on neonatal films, the infant's chest appears mildly lordotic, with the medial clavicular ends projected on or above the dorsal vertebrae. This results in a rather peculiar chest configuration. The preossified anterior arcs of the upper ribs are positioned superior to the posterior arcs (Figure 17.4). The lordotic projection tends to increase the apparent transverse cardiac diameter, making it difficult to determine the size of the heart. When the x-ray tube is angled cephalad, when the x-ray beam is centered over the abdomen, or when an irritable infant has arched, the back lordotic projections can occur. If the x-ray beam is centered over the head or in a downward position, the anterior rib arcs are angulated sharply downward.

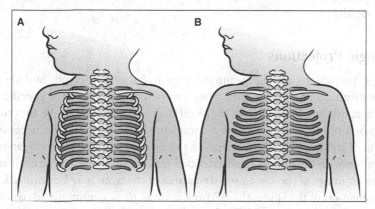

FIGURE 17.4 Skeletal position in a normally positioned radiograph (A) and in a film obtained with cephalad positioning of the x-ray (B).

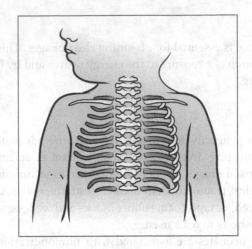

FIGURE 17.5 Skeletal configuration in a film obtained with the infant rotated to the right.

Infant Positioning

If the infant is rotated, the view is distorted, potentially leading to a misinterpretation of the film (Figure 17.5). The direction and degree of rotation can be estimated by comparing the lengths of the posterior arcs of the ribs from the costovertebral junction to the lateral pleural line at a given level. Another measurement for determining the degree of rotation is the distance from the medial aspect of the clavicles to the center of the vertebral body at the same level. The distance is greater on the side toward which the infant is rotated. On a lateral view, rotation can be readily determined by observing the amount of offset between the anterior tips of the right and left sets of ribs.

Before any chest film is interpreted, these factors must be systematically evaluated. Through experience, this evaluation becomes automatic, and the film can be scanned rapidly.

Radiologic Projections

Radiologic projections are the geometric views of the radiograph, and they vary among institutions and radiologists. They can be customized to the specific infant or clinical condition. For example, the skull may require a simple AP film to make the diagnosis of a fracture, whereas a complete skull series may be necessary for evaluation of congenital malformations. In the neck and upper airway, a lateral film in inspiration with the infant's head extended may be sufficient for the evaluation of stridor, or an image of the soft tissue structures of the neck may be required.

For evaluation of the spine, the AP projection is most commonly used. Oblique views of the spine usually are difficult to obtain in infants because it is difficult to position and immobilize babies. Also, the diagnostic information gained does not outweigh the risk of the greater radiation exposure required to obtain such views. For evaluation of congenital hip dysplasia, an AP view of the entire pelvis and both hips is required. Gonadal exposure should be minimized with proper shielding during radiographic examination of the hips. Assessment of skeletal maturation in the infant requires an AP film of the left hemiskeleton or long bone films.

Chest radiographs are the most frequently performed diagnostic imaging procedure in the NICU. In most cases, an AP projection from a supine position is satisfactory for evaluating the infant's chest, heart, lung fields, endotracheal tube, line placement, and pneumothorax (air leak complications related to mechanical ventilation). The cross-table view allows verification of the pleural chest tube being placed anteriorly or posteriorly. Lateral decubitus is used to evaluate small pneumothorax and small pleural fluid collection; these can be hard to see on an AP view. Upper right shows abdominal perforation, which shows free air under the diaphragm (rarely used). Lateral projections of the chest often are poorly positioned, have diminished technical quality, and require greater radiation exposure of the infant. For the experienced radiographer, an AP film in the supine position is sufficient in most cases.

Abdominal x-ray films also are frequently obtained in the NICU. Because the infant's abdomen is relatively cylindric, a lateral view provides more information than it does in an older child or adult. AP views define the gas pattern, intestinal displacement, some masses, ascites, and placement of lines such as umbilical catheters or intestinal tubes. The cross-table lateral view is useful for suspected abdominal perforation. The left lateral decubitus reveals intra-abdominal air (Gomella et al., 2020).

A Few General Principles

1. Exposure time should be kept short to prevent movement blur and limit the radiation dose.

2. Radiographic technicians should be knowledgeable about factors and variables that affect exposure so repeat films occasioned by poor technique can be avoided.

3. Every possible precaution should be taken to ensure that the first attempt produces a film of diagnostic quality.

4. Before a repeat is done, the film should be shown to the radiologist or neonatologist who requested it; although the quality may not be ideal, it may provide sufficient information.

Radiation exposure can also be reduced by using ultrasounds or MRIs. If radiologic imaging is the best diagnostic approach for the infant's condition, it may be important to "customize" the examinations, to limit the area examined, and to reduce the number of follow-up films.

Plain films should be obtained first. Then, if indicated, a dye contrast study (e.g., excretory urograph) should be performed, because the contrast material is rapidly eliminated from the body. Barium contrast studies are performed after the others because (a) barium interferes with any nuclear scintigraphic scans, body computed tomograms, and ultrasonographic scans, and (b) barium is slowly eliminated from the GI tract, which delays further diagnostic evaluation.

If GI and genitourinary (GU) imaging are both to be performed, the GU examination should be scheduled first. Although each institution has its own policies in preparation for a GU examination, such as excretory urography, the infant should be kept on nothing by mouth (NPO) status for no longer than 3 hours; this can be accomplished by withholding the early morning feeding and scheduling the examination for 8 a.m. No preparation is necessary for excretory urography in infants with abdominal masses, trauma, or GU emergencies. If the infant has impaired renal function, the radiologist and the neonatologist should discuss the condition thoroughly so that the risks of this procedure are minimized. For an infant who has been feeding, the baby is prepared for a GI contrast study by keeping the child on NPO status for no longer than 3 hours before the examination. If the entire GI tract is to be examined, do the lower GI first. No colon preparation is necessary and can be dangerous in some abdominal conditions.

Collaborative Care

Radiation Protection

Any radiation is considered harmful to the infant, and all efforts must be made to reduce radiation exposure without forgoing diagnostic information. Reduction of radiation exposure should be the goal for sites that are sensitive genetically (gonads) and somatically (eyes, bone marrow). Methods of reducing radiation exposure include performing examinations only when they are clinically indicated, selecting the appropriate imaging modality, using the lowest radiation dose that achieves an image of diagnostic quality, avoiding repeat examinations, reducing the number of films obtained, using appropriate projections with tight field limitation, ensuring proper positioning and immobilization, and shielding the gonads.

If the gonads are not within the area of interest, gonadal exposure depends on the adequacy of field limitation. The maximum gonadal dose occurs when the gonads are unshielded and exposed to the primary x-ray beam. This dose declines rapidly as the distance from the gonads to the primary beam increases. The gonads should be shielded whenever they are within 5 cm of the primary x-ray beam.

Contact gonadal shields are easy to make from 0.5 mm thick lead rubber sheets, and they should be sized for gender and age (Figure 17.6; Swischuk, 1997, 2003). In males, proper positioning of the shield avoids obscuration of any bony detail of the pelvis if the upper edge of the shield is placed just below the pubis and if the testicles have descended into the scrotum. In females, the position of the ovaries varies with bladder distention. Because of their anatomic location, the ovaries cannot be shielded without obscuring lower abdominal and pelvic structures. The lower margin of the gonad shield should be placed at the level of the pubis, and the upper margin should cover at least the lower margin of the sacroiliac joints (Hilton & Edwards, 2006; Swischuk, 1997, 2003).

Radiation Safety

Portable radiologic examinations are the most common form of diagnostic imaging routinely performed in the NICU. During these procedures, there is a tendency for all the nurses to leave the room when an exposure is being produced; consequently, other

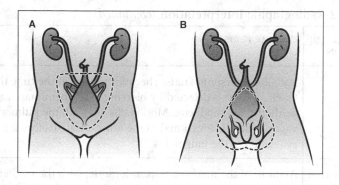

FIGURE 17.6 Anatomic placement of gonad shield for female infants (A) and for male infants (B).

infants may be left unattended for that short period. Because of this practice, parents have expressed fear about their infants facing environmental radiation hazards.

It appears that if certain basic radiation precautions are observed, nurses and other NICU personnel need not leave the room during x-ray exposures. However, staff members should stay 30 cm (1 foot) or farther from the infant being radiographed. Care must be taken to ensure that if a horizontal beam film is obtained (e.g., in a cross-table lateral projection), no one is in the direct x-ray beam; this is because the radiation dose in the primary beam is considerably higher than in the scattered portion. When a horizontal beam is used, it should not be directed at any other patient or person. Any employee within 30 cm (1 foot) of the incubator or one who is holding the infant for the exposure should wear a lead apron and gloves. Table 17.2 summarizes the process of systematic interpretation of radiographic images in the neonate.

TABLE 17.2 Radiographic Interpretation

TECHNICAL EVALUATION	CHARACTERISTICS
Film density and contrast	The intravertebral disc spaces should be visible through the cardiothymic silhouette. Underexposed films appear whitish with progressive loss of spaces; overexposed films have a "burned out" appearance with loss of pulmonary vascular markings.
Phase of respiration	The respiratory phase affects the appearance of the lung fields. During expiration, the cardiothymic silhouette appears larger, and the lung fields appear more opaque; the hemidiaphragms usually are at the level of the seventh rib. During inspiration, the cardiothymic silhouette is normal, pulmonary vascularity is seen, and the lung fields are clear. Adequate inspiration puts the right hemidiaphragm at the level of the posterior eighth rib; the right hemidiaphragm usually is slightly higher than the left during basal breathing.

(continued)

TABLE 17.2 Radiographic Interpretation (continued)

TECHNICAL EVALUATION	CHARACTERISTICS
Motion	Radiology personnel must check for motion at the time the film is taken. Motion is detected by blurring of the hemidiaphragms and cardiothymic silhouette. Motion obscures all fine pulmonary vascular detail, which makes the films unsatisfactory for evaluation of the lung fields.
Tube angulation and patient positioning	AP films of the newborn appear lordotic, with the medial ends of the clavicles projecting on or above the second dorsal vertebra.
	If the tube has been angled cephalad, the lordosis is exaggerated, with the anterior arcs of the ribs positioned superior to the posterior arcs. The cardiothymic silhouette appears larger because the view is through the transverse diameter of the heart. This occurs if the infant arches during the procedure or if the beam has been centered over the abdomen. Caudad angulation of the beam over the head results in distortion of the chest, with the anterior rib arcs angled sharply downward in relation to the posterior arcs.
Rotation of the patient	Assessment of rotation is critical in determining whether mediastinal shift is present. Lateral rotation may lead to the false impression of a mediastinal shift. The trachea shifts toward the side of the rotation, and the contours of the heart are altered. The direction and degree of rotation are estimated by comparing the lengths of the posterior arcs of the ribs on both sides. The side with the longest posterior arc is the side to which the patient is rotated. Rotation also results in unequal lengths of the clavicles when they are measured from the medial aspects to the center of the vertebral body at the same level. The patient is rotated to the side with the longer clavicle.
Heart size and pulmonary vascularity	These features are difficult to determine in the newborn in the first 24 hours of life because of the dynamic cardiovascular alterations that occur during this period. Changes in the transitional circulation are associated with an increase in pulmonary blood flow and in blood return to the left atrium, a decrease in blood return and lower pressure in the right atrium, and changes in systemic and pulmonary arterial pressures. The newborn's heart size is relatively larger in the first 48 to 72 hours because of those rapid changes. Heart size can be accurately assessed only during basal breathing, because the size is

TABLE 17.2 Radiographic Interpretation (*continued*)

TECHNICAL EVALUATION	CHARACTERISTICS
	significantly altered during phases of the cardiac cycle and during hyperexpansion of the lung. After the first 24 hours, a cardiothoracic ratio above 0.6 is the upper limit of normal. Fetal lung fluid is reabsorbed, and the air spaces are filled with air on inspiration. The resorption of lung fluid enhances the appearance of the pulmonary lymphatics, resulting in an apparent increase in vascularity at birth. Transient tachypnea of the newborn is characterized by perihilar streaky infiltrates with increased pulmonary vascularity and good lung inflation.
Cardiothymic silhouette	The cardiac configuration is difficult to determine in the newborn largely because of the variation in size and shape of the thymus. The aortic knob and main pulmonary artery are obscured by the thymus, which frequently has a wavy border. A tuck may be seen in the left lobe of the thymus at the lateral margin of the right ventricle, a feature called a "sail sign." The apex of the heart has a more cephalad position and assumes a more caudal position over time. The elevation of the apex is due to the relative right ventricular hypertrophy of the fetus. After birth, as the left ventricle becomes more prominent, the cardiac apex descends. The thymus involutes rapidly under the stress of delivery and over the next 2 weeks of life may enlarge slightly.
Aeration of the lungs	Satisfactory inspiration positions the hemidiaphragms at the posterior arcs of the eighth rib. Expansion and radiolucency of the right and left sides are equal. If the sides are not comparable, a right and left lateral decubitus film should be obtained to evaluate for fluid levels or air. The lungs may bulge slightly through the ribs. On lateral projection, the hemidiaphragms should be smoothly domed. The AP and transverse diameters of the chest vary with age and disease. In a normal newborn, the AP and transverse diameters are equal. Over time, the transverse diameter increases, giving the chest cavity an oblong appearance. Air-trapping diseases produce a more rounded configuration, whereas hypoaeration results in a more flattened AP diameter. With hypoaeration, the right hemidiaphragm is located at the seventh rib, the posterior arcs have a more downward slope, and the transverse diameter of the chest is reduced. Laterally, hypoaeration results in increased doming of the diaphragm. With hyperaeration, the hemidiaphragm is located below the level of the ninth rib, the diaphragm is flattened, and the posterior rib arcs are horizontal. Hyperaeration also results in greater bulging of the lungs through the intercostal spaces and an increased diameter of the upper thorax.

(*continued*)

TABLE 17.2 Radiographic Interpretation (*continued*)

TECHNICAL EVALUATION	CHARACTERISTICS
Pulmonary infiltrates	Films should be evaluated for areas of increased pulmonary lucency or density. The characteristics and distribution of densities may lead to a diagnosis. Infiltrates should be described with regard to their distribution (unilateral, bilateral) and nature (alveolar, reticulated, diffuse, nondiffuse, patchy, streaky).
Mediastinal shift	The examiner evaluates for mediastinal shift by determining if the trachea, heart, and mediastinum are in normal position. In general, the shift occurs toward the side with the diminished lung volume or away from the hemithorax with the increased lung volume. Rotation of the patient must first be excluded.
Liver size	The edges of the liver should be clearly defined, and the size of the organ should correlate well with the size determined by palpation, especially when the intestines are filled with air. If insufficient gas is present in the abdomen, the size of the liver cannot be determined. Atelectasis obscures the upper margin of the liver. Radiographically, the size of the liver is not altered by the phase of respiration, as it is during palpation. Liver size may vary with progression of right-sided heart failure. The position of the liver may be altered by congenital malformations such as situs inversus.
Abdominal gas pattern	Swallowing air produces gas in the stomach. The gas pattern must be interpreted in light of the infant's history. In the newborn, stomach air is present, with progression of air through the small bowel at 3 hours of life and rectal air by 6 hours. With bowel obstruction, gaseous distention progresses until at some point the bowel is blocked; beyond that point, there is a paucity of air or a gasless bowel. Lack of haustra in the colon makes it possible to distinguish the small and large bowels on the radiograph. A gasless abdomen may be seen with prolonged GI decompression, severe dehydration, acidosis, oversedation, brain injury, diaphragmatic hernia, midgut volvulus, and esophageal atresia. Marked aerophagia may be due to mechanical ventilation, tracheoesophageal fistula, necrotizing enterocolitis, and mesenteric vascular occlusion. Free peritoneal air rises to the highest level and outlines superior structures; therefore, it is best demonstrated on a left lateral decubitus film.
Catheter and tube positions	All catheter and tube positions should be evaluated and reported each time a radiograph is made. The position of these devices may provide clues to the underlying disease, and malpositioning of tubes and catheters may be life-threatening. The trachea is positioned to the right in the midmediastinum, anterior, and slightly to the right of the esophagus. The carina is located at T_4.

TABLE 17.2 Radiographic Interpretation (*continued*)

TECHNICAL EVALUATION	CHARACTERISTICS
	In the right aortic arch, the trachea is found slightly to the left of the vertebral column. Endotracheal tubes optimally are placed in the midtrachea. If the tip is too low (below T_4) or too high (above the thoracic inlet), ventilation is suboptimal. Inadvertent esophageal intubation has occurred when the tip of the tube is below T_4 but is still in the midline or when the trachea can be visualized apart from the tube. Nasogastric (NG) tube placement should be reported. NG tubes may be too short (seen in the distal esophagus) or too long (seen in the duodenum or jejunum), or they may be coiled in the esophagus (tracheoesophageal atresia). The location of vascular catheters must be evaluated. Central catheters should be placed with the tip in the superior part of the inferior cava. Umbilical artery catheters ideally should be located in the high (thoracic) (T_6–T_9) or low (lumbar) (L3–L5) position, away from major arterial branches. Umbilical venous catheters should be positioned with the tip in the inferior vena cava and not in a hepatic branch.
Bony structures	The skeleton should be evaluated, especially the general configuration of the thoracic cage. Normally, over time, the cephalic portion of the thoracic cage becomes rounded and the transverse diameter increases. Hyperaeration exaggerates cephalic rounding and the horizontal position of the rib arcs. Hypoaeration reduces the diameter of the upper thorax and increases the inferior slope of the rib arcs (bell-shaped thorax). The radiograph must be evaluated for fractures, dislocations, hypodensities, or other lucencies. Persistent elevation of the scapula and an ipsilateral elevated diaphragm (which occur secondary to phrenic nerve injury) may accompany Erb's palsy. Scans should be done for vertebral, rib, and other bony anomalies. Rib aplasia is associated with hemivertebrae, and complete or partial aplasia of the clavicles may be a manifestation of chromosomal abnormality. The proximal humeri can yield information related to congenital infections such as in rubella, syphilis, and CMV infection. The bone density should be evaluated in relation to film penetration.

REFERENCES

Gomella, T. L., Eyal, F. G., & Bany-Mohammed, F. (2020). *Neonatology: Management, procedures, on-call problems, diseases, and drugs* (8th ed.). McGraw-Hill.

Hilton, S., & Edwards, D. K., III. (2006). *Practical pediatric radiology* (3rd ed.). Saunders Elsevier.

Swischuk, L. E. (1997). *Differential diagnosis in pediatric radiology* (3rd ed.). Lippincott Williams & Wilkins.

Swischuk, L. E. (2003). *Imaging of the newborn, infant, and young child* (5th ed.). Lippincott Williams & Wilkins.

ULTRASONIC IMAGING

With neonates, ultrasonography frequently is used in the evaluation and treatment of internal anatomic structures. Ultrasonography:

■ Emits no ionizing radiation and has no known deleterious somatic or genetic effects; therefore, follow-up may be repeated at will.

■ Waves can be directed as a beam.

■ Sound waves obey laws of reflection and refraction.

■ Waves are reflected by objects of small size.

■ Used in a variety of transverse, longitudinal, sagittal, or oblique planes.

■ Considerably less costly than either CT or MRI.

■ Equipment is easily portable.

■ Examination is relatively painless and well tolerated.

■ Sedation is rarely required.

■ Relies on acoustic impedance of tissue to demonstrate anatomy.

■ Is diagnostically accurate.

Disadvantages of ultrasonography:

■ Operator dependent.

■ Does not provide as much information on organ function as urography.

■ Limited value as a screening procedure for "acute abdominal distress"; rather, the examination should focus on a particular area of interest.

■ CT is superior in demonstrating the extent of disease, because ultrasonography demonstrates a smaller area of interest and less anatomic detail.

■ Bone, excessive fat, and gas artifacts adversely affect ultrasonography (Bushong, 2013).

Because of these drawbacks, certain parts of the body, such as the brain, must be imaged through an ultrasound "window," such as the anterior fontanel. In addition, because sound waves are poorly propagated through a gaseous medium, the transducer must have airless contact with the surface being examined, and parts of the body that contain large amounts of air are difficult to examine.

Ultrasonography also is useful as a diagnostic imaging method because it is reflected at tissue interfaces. A principle called "sonic momentum" describes the velocity of sound transmitted through tissue.

The major patterns of ultrasound reflection are anechoic, echoic, and mixed. An anechoic structure, which is described as sonar lucent, is a structure in which the acoustic medium is homogeneous and the sound waves are unimpeded. An anechoic structure may be fluid filled (bladder), cystic (hydronephrosis), or solid (lymphoma), as long as the tissue is homogeneous. Cystic structures usually have sharp echogenic margins anteriorly and posteriorly. Echoic structures are inhomogeneous and reflect sound waves. These tissues generally are solid and have a variety of densities (typical Wilms' tumor) or may be cystic (hemorrhagic Wilms' tumor). A mixed pattern of reflections has the combined qualities of anechoic and echoic tissues. In addition, ribs and calculi may cause imaging artifacts on an ultrasonographic image.

When the tissue interface is moving (e.g., the movement of red blood cells in a vessel), the reflected ultrasound wave has a shifted frequency directly proportional to the velocity of the reflecting blood cells, in accordance with a principle called the "Doppler effect." If the movement of the blood cells is toward the transducer, the frequency of the reflected wave is higher than the transmitted frequency. Conversely, movement of blood away from the transducer results in a lower frequency of the reflected wave (Bushong, 2013). The difference between the transmitted frequency and the reflected frequency is called the Doppler shift. It is the principle of sound frequency shifts that allows the application of the mathematic relationship between the velocity of the target and the Doppler frequency to calculate flow. This is used most commonly in the echocardiographic evaluation of the heart and in cerebral blood flow determinations (Bushong, 2013).

Biologic Effects of Ultrasonography

Ultrasonic imaging was introduced into obstetric practice in 1966. Since that time, despite the widespread use of this imaging modality and the use of multiple scans during an individual pregnancy, no injuries or adverse fetal outcomes occur when the ultrasound is used appropriately.

Indications for ultrasonography in neonatal intensive care commonly include evaluation of brain parenchyma and ventricular size, myocardial function and structure, cholelithiasis, choledochal cysts, intestinal duplication, renal neoplasms, urinary tract dilation and duplication, pelvic masses, and skeletal anomalies of the spine and hips (Martin et al., 2020).

Collaborative Care

The care of a neonate undergoing a diagnostic ultrasound examination ensures that any disruption of the infant's microenvironment is minimal. The infant's temperature can be maintained more easily if the ultrasound examination can be performed by using the transducer in the incubator.

MRI

The theoretic basis for MRI is a development of research conducted since the 1940s for studying atomic nuclear structure, which resulted in the awarding of the Nobel Prize for physics in 1952 to Edward Purcell and Felix Block. In addition to the advances in atomic nuclear research, other developments were necessary, such as superconductivity and advances in computer programming, before this concept could be applied to diagnostic imaging. The MRI:

1. Like ultrasonography, does not use ionizing radiation to produce the image but rather uses magnetic fields and radio waves.

2. Depends on three separate molecular parameters that are sensitive to changes in structure and bioactivity rather than on x-ray photon interaction with tissue electrons as in CT.

3. The region of the body imaged is not limited by the gantry geometry, as it is with CT, but can be controlled electronically, allowing imaging in transverse planes and in true sagittal, coronal, and oblique planes.

4. Are free of the high-intensity artifacts produced in CT scans by sharp, dense bone, or metallic surgical clips.

The principal disadvantages of MRI are its high cost and limited availability.

Biophysical Principles

All particles in an atom have either a positive or a negative charge, or a "spin," like a tiny spinning top. The total spin of the protons and neutrons on the nucleus is the sum of the individual spins. In MRI, the strong magnetic field is imposed to align the molecular magnetic dipoles, and radio frequency pulses then are applied. The known specific frequency of these radio waves displaces the net magnetic moment by an amount determined by the strength and duration of the pulse. The frequency is directly proportional to the strength of the magnetic field and is known as the resonant frequency. After the pulse, the protons emit radio frequencies as they return to their original orientation. Therefore, the frequency of signals emitted by the protons after the application with radio frequency waves reflects their position in the tissue.

After each radio frequency pulse, the net magnetic force of the sample is reduced; therefore, too rapid a radio frequency repetition depletes the magnetization of the tissue, and an image cannot be produced. Hence, radio frequency pulses are sequenced with a certain time interval to allow the magnetic force to be reestablished.

The interval between the application of a radio frequency pulse and the emitted signal depends on the alignment and synchronization of magnetic dipoles. A strong magnetic force results in a long interval for the emitted signal after the pulse.

The third variable that affects image resolution with MRI is spin density. "Spring density" refers to the strength of the signal received before it deteriorates. This strength is proportional to the number of nuclei within the detection volume of the scanner. Spin density is an indication of hydrogen concentration in the tissue.

The spatial resolution of an MRI scan compares favorably to that obtained with CT. If the object scanned is of high tissue contrast, a lesion as small as 1 mm can be defined. As more data are collected on this imaging modality, even greater spatial resolution and enhanced three-dimensional images are being obtained.

MRI is better able than CT to detect differences between low-contrast structures. The difference in T1 and T2 MRI between biologic tissues frequently is 10% or more. The MRI has become the diagnostic imaging mode of choice for certain neurologic conditions such as multiple sclerosis, cerebral infarctions, and periventricular leukomalacia. MRI may be useful in the early diagnosis of periventricular leukomalacia.

Safety of MRI

MRI scanning uses three kinds of fields associated with the imaging process: (a) a static, moderately strong magnetic field; (b) a switched, weaker magnetic field gradient; and (c) radio frequency waves.

The hazards of MRI relate primarily to any ferromagnetic objects (e.g., tools, oxygen cylinders, watches, bank cards, pens, and paper clips) that are accelerated toward the center of the magnetic field. The magnetic propulsion of these objects can result in projectile damage; therefore, any patient with a pacemaker or an extensive metal prosthesis should be excluded from this imaging technique. In addition, MRI has not been fully tested with pregnant women.

REFERENCES

Bushong, S. C. (2013). *Radiologic science for technologists: Physics, biology, and protection* (10th ed.). Elsevier Mosby.

Martin, R., Fanaroff, A., & Walsh, M. (2020). *Neonatal-perinatal medicine* (11th ed.). Elsevier.

CARDIAC PROCEDURES

Electrocardiography

Electrocardiography is a noninvasive diagnostic tool used with neonates. It is most useful in the diagnosis and management of cardiac arrhythmias or in conjunction with other diagnostic measures to evaluate cardiac function, specifically the circulatory demands placed on individual heart chambers. It is not as useful if significant ventricular enlargement is present.

Echocardiography

Echocardiography, another noninvasive diagnostic procedure, commonly is used in the evaluation of the structure and function of the heart. This information can be important not only in the preoperative assessment of cardiac defects but also in the postoperative evaluation of procedures. High-frequency sound waves send vibrations to the structures in the heart, which reflect energy, which is transmitted into a visual image. Echocardiography may be used prenatally as early as 11 weeks' gestation.

Single-dimension echocardiography allows the evaluation of anatomic structures, including valves, chambers, and vessels. Two-dimensional echocardiography provides more in-depth information about relationships between the heart and the great vessels (Flanagan et al., 2005).

Doppler echocardiography is used in various forms in the evaluation of characteristics of blood flow through the heart, valves, and great vessels. It can measure not only cardiac output but also flow velocity changes, as demonstrated in stenotic lesions. Regurgitation through insufficiently functioning valves can also be identified. Doppler studies can be used to show regurgitation through insufficiently functioning valves or to identify shunting, as through a patent ductus arteriosus (Bocks et al., 2020).

Cardiac Catheterization

With the advent of more sophisticated echocardiography, especially Doppler echocardiography, cardiac catheterization is used increasingly as a therapeutic modality. The use of radiopaque dye allows clarification of congenital heart disease and helps to provide data that cannot be obtained from echocardiography.

Immobilization and constant monitoring of the neonate are required during cardiac catheterization. The infant must be restrained to maintain supine positioning. Electrocardiographic electrodes must also be placed to provide constant monitoring of vital signs. Sedation may be considered to maintain proper positioning during the procedure.

A local anesthetic is administered at the insertion site. A radiopaque catheter is inserted into an arm or leg vessel by percutaneous puncture or cut-down. Under fluoroscopy, the catheter is visualized and passed into the heart. Contrast medium is injected through the catheter to allow visualization of the various cardiac structures. Selected chambers and vessels of the heart can be evaluated for size and function. Intracardiac pressures and oxygen saturations can also be measured during this procedure. Balloons during catheterization can be used during a septostomy, angioplasty, and valvuloplasty (Friedman, 2020).

After the necessary information has been obtained, the catheter is carefully removed. If a cut-down was performed, the vessel is ligated and the skin is sutured. Pressure should be applied over a percutaneous puncture site to enhance clot formation. For continued bleeding problems, pressure dressings may be applied to the insertion site; these must be checked frequently for active bleeding. After cardiac catheterization, the vital signs should be measured frequently and compared with precatheterization baseline values. Evaluation of localized bleeding or of signs of hypotension resulting in changes in heart rate and blood pressure is essential. Assessment of the insertion site and affected extremity for bleeding, color, peripheral pulses, temperature, and capillary refill should continue for at least 24 hours after the procedure. In addition, the nurse must monitor for complications of catheterization, including hypovolemia (as a result of bleeding or fluid loss during the procedure), infection, thrombosis, or tissue necrosis.

REFERENCES

Bocks, M. L., Boe, B. A., & Galantowicz, M. E. (2020). Neonatal management of congenital heart disease. In R. Martin, A. Fanaroff, & M. Walsh (Eds.), *Neonatal-perinatal medicine* (11th ed., pp. 1472–1495). Elsevier.

Flanagan, M. F., Yeager, S. B., & Weingling, S. N. (2005). Cardiac disease. In M. G. MacDonald, M. D. Mullett, & M. K. Seshia (Eds.), *Avery's neonatology pathophsyiolgy & management of the newborn* (6th ed., pp. 633–709). Lippincott Williams & Wilkins.

Friedman, S. H. (2020). Cardiac embryology. In R. Martin, A. Fanaroff, & M. Walsh (Eds.), *Neonatal-perinatal medicine* (11th ed., pp. 1352–1368). Elsevier.

GENETIC TESTING

Chromosome Analysis

High-Resolution Karyotyping and Banding

Analysis of chromosome composition can assist in identification of various genetic disorders. A blood specimen is obtained from the infant and used to harvest an actual set of chromosomes. During active cell division, usually during metaphase, the chromosomes are photographed and then arranged in pairs by number. The chromosomes are also separated into regions, bands, and subbands. The end result, a karyotype with banding, is evaluated for the appropriate number of pairs, chromosome size, and structure. Abnormal genes on the chromosomes can also cause genetic disorders, such as Duchenne muscular dystrophy, an X-linked recessive disorder.

High-resolution karyotype is widely used for infants with multiple congenital anomalies. This test consists of analysis of chromosomes from white blood cells. The cells are cultured and stimulated to divide, and then cell division is halted with a mitotic inhibitor in the prometaphase stage. In this stage, the chromosomes are at their longest length, and the stained band observed can reach 800 to 900 base pairs (bp). This test can take up to 2 weeks (Gomella et al., 2020).

Fluorescence In Situ Hybridization

Chromosomes can be further analyzed using fluorescence in situ hybridization (FISH) to detect syndromes that are not visible to the naked eye. The FISH process allows fluorescent-coated DNA probes to detect submicroscopic chromosomal deletions. It can be used with interphase and metaphase cells. This test is faster than high-resolution karyotyping (but still could take up to several weeks to complete). This test can provide a quick diagnosis for infants with trisomy 13, 18, 21, or Turner syndrome (Gilmore, 2020; Gomella et al., 2020; Martin et al., 2020).

Bone marrow cells may be analyzed for chromosomes if a more rapid evaluation is required. Skin fibroblast analysis is required when an infant has been transfused, making lymphocyte analysis inaccurate. In cases such as stillbirth, tissue biopsy specimens can be used for chromosome testing.

Sweat Chloride Test

The sweat chloride test is used to evaluate for and confirm the diagnosis of cystic fibrosis. If the level is 60 mmol/L or higher, a diagnosis is reached while levels less than 30 mmol/L cystic fibrosis are ruled out (National Heart, Lung, and Blood Institute, 2021). Sweat tests can be inaccurate if an inadequate amount of sweat is produced, if the sweat evaporates, or if the patient has edema. Genetic testing for a mutation in the cystic fibrosis transmembrane conductance regulator (CFTR) genes is used along with the sweat chloride (National Heart, Lung, and Blood Institute, 2021).

Comparative Genomic Hybridization or Chromosomal Microarray Analysis

The comparative genomic hybridization (CGH) and chromosomal microarray analysis (CMA) detects chromosomal deletions or duplication; this cytogenetic technique is relatively new. CGH/CMA compares reference standard DNA to the patient's DNA through a florescent technique. This test compares hundreds of regions across the entire genome to assess for the number of differences. It commonly assesses for microdeletion and microduplication, subtelomeric, and pericentromeric regions (Gomella et al., 2020).

NEWBORN SCREENING

Every infant born in a hospital in the United States undergoes newborn screening. Newborn screening is done before leaving the hospital, usually about day 1 or 2. Some states require follow-up at about 2 weeks. All states are required to screen for 26 health conditions according to the March of Dimes (MOD; 2021). In addition, the MOD recommends that each state screen for 31. Some states are known to screen for 50 or more. For more information on newborn screens, please see www.marchofdimes.org/baby/newborn-screening-tests-for-your-baby.aspx (MOD, 2021).

REFERENCES

Gilmore, A. (2020). Genetic aspects of perinatal disease and prenatal diagnosis. In R. Martin, A. Fanaroff, & M. Walsh (Eds.), *Neonatal-perinatal medicine* (11th ed., pp. 198–216). Elsevier.

Gomella, T. L., Cunningham, M. D., & Eyal, F. G. (2020). *Neonatology: Management, procedures, on-call problems, diseases, and drugs* (8th ed.). McGraw-Hill.

March of Dimes. (2021). *Newborn screening test for your baby.* https://www.marchofdimes.org/baby/newborn-screening-tests-for-your-baby.aspx

Martin, R., Fanaroff, A., & Walsh, M. (Eds). (2020). *Neonatal-perinatal medicine* (11th ed.). Elsevier.

National Heart, Lung, and Blood Institute. (2021). *Cystic fibrosis.* https://www.nhlbi.nih.gov/health-topics/cystic-fibrosis

GASTROINTESTINAL PROCEDURES

Barium Enema

A barium enema is used in the evaluation of the structure and function of the large intestine. The diagnosis of disorders such as Hirschsprung disease and meconium plug syndrome can easily be supported by the use of this procedure.

For the enema procedure, either air or a contrast solution (e.g., barium sulfate) is instilled and a series of films are taken under fluoroscopy. The infant must be well restrained, starting in the supine position. As the contrast solution is instilled, its flow through the bowel is observed as the infant's position is changed. A series of abdominal x-ray films should be taken once the bowel has been filled with contrast solution. Follow-up films may also be necessary to document evacuation of the contrast solution from the bowel. Evaluation of the bowel is essential after this procedure to prevent constipation or obstruction. Assessment of bowel elimination is an important nursing concern after barium enema.

Upper Gastrointestinal Series With Small Bowel Follow-Through

As with the barium enema, barium sulfate or some other water-soluble contrast solution is used for the upper GI series with small bowel follow-through. However, the contrast solution is swallowed so that the upper GI tract can be examined. The three main areas examined are (a) the esophagus (for size, patency, reflux, and presence of a fistula or swallowing abnormality), (b) the stomach (for anatomic abnormalities, patency, and motility), and (c) the small intestine (for strictures, patency, and function).

Follow-up x-ray films may be desirable to evaluate both the emptying ability of the stomach and intestinal motility as the contrast material moves through the small bowel. Again, care of the infant includes assessment of temperature and cardiac and respiratory status throughout the procedure. The nurse should be alert for reflux or vomiting, which can be accompanied by aspiration. Evacuation of contrast material from the bowel remains a concern after upper GI series with small bowel follow-through and should be monitored by the nurse. It is also possible for fluid to be pulled out of the vascular compartment and into the bowel, resulting in hypotension. It is imperative that the healthcare team assess the infant for signs of these complications.

Rectal Suction Biopsy

Rectal biopsy is a procedure commonly used to help determine the presence or absence of ganglion cells in the bowel (the latter condition is seen in Hirschsprung disease). Before a rectal biopsy, it is essential to obtain bleeding times, prothrombin time, partial thromboplastin time, and platelet counts, as well as a spun hematocrit, to ensure that the infant is in no danger of excessive bleeding.

The infant is positioned supine with the legs held toward the abdomen. Small specimens of rectal tissue from the mucosal and submucosal levels are excised with a suction blade apparatus inserted through the anus into the bowel. The section of the pathology department that deals with the composition of ganglion cells evaluates the specimens.

Care of the infant after rectal suction biopsy should focus on assessments for bleeding or intestinal perforation. These assessments should include evaluation of vital signs for increased heart rate or decreased blood pressure, fever, persistent guaiac-positive stools, or frank rectal bleeding.

Liver Biopsy

Open or closed liver biopsy may be required for neonates. Open liver biopsy is a surgical procedure that requires general anesthesia, whereas a closed liver biopsy may be done using local anesthesia. As with the rectal biopsy, coagulation studies are essential, including bleeding time, platelet count, and spun hematocrit. Preoperative care may include sedation of the infant, requiring frequent monitoring of vital signs. Throughout the procedure, assessment of vital signs is essential for identifying changes in hemodynamics or respiratory status. After the procedure, assessment of vital signs for signs and symptoms of hemorrhage is essential. Indications of hemorrhage include decreases in the hemoglobin and hematocrit, which makes laboratory monitoring an important element of postbiopsy care. The biopsy site must be evaluated for signs of active bleeding, ecchymosis, swelling, or infection.

GENITOURINARY PROCEDURES

Cystoscopy

Cystoscopy permits direct visualization of the urinary structures, including the bladder, urethra, and urethral orifices, allowing diagnosis of abnormalities in the structure of the bladder and urinary tract.

Cystoscopy is performed using general anesthesia. Preparation of the urethral opening with an antiseptic solution is followed by sterile draping. The lubricated cystoscope is inserted through the urethra, and the urinary structures are examined.

As with any patient who has had anesthesia, postprocedural care includes vital sign assessment. However, particular attention should be paid to assessing for adequate urinary output, the presence of hematuria, and signs of infection (Pagana & Pagana, 2018).

Excretory Urography and Intravenous Pyelography

Excretory urography and intravenous pyelography complement cystoscopic evaluation because they allow the examiner not only to evaluate structures but also to focus on the function of those structures. The intravenous route injects small amounts of contrast media, and as the contrast material is excreted through the urinary system, a sequence of x-ray films is taken. The configuration of organs and the rate of excretion of the contrast media are reflected in these films.

Excretory urography and intravenous pyelography are relatively safe for use in neonates and should cause no postprocedural complications.

Voiding Cystourethrogram

The purpose of a voiding cystourethrogram is to visualize the lower urinary tract after instillation of contrast media through urethral catheterization. The infant's bladder is emptied after catheterization and then filled with the contrast media. Serial films under fluoroscopy in a variety of positions are taken during voiding. After voiding, additional films are obtained. Pathologic results of a voiding cystourethrogram demonstrate residual urine in the bladder, such as with a neurogenic bladder, posterior valve obstructions, or vesicourethral reflux.

As with cystoscopy, the infant should be evaluated for hematuria; the baby also should be checked for signs of infection (fever, cloudy or sedimented urine, foul-smelling urine) in the event of contaminated catheterization.

Electroencephalography

An electroencephalographic examination records the electrical activity of the brain. Numerous electrodes are placed at precise locations on the infant's head to record electrical impulses from various parts of the brain. This procedure can be important for diagnosing lesions or tumors, for identifying nonfunctional areas of the brain, or for pinpointing the focus of seizure activity.

The infant may require sedation during this procedure to prevent crying or movement. As much equipment as is safely possible should be removed to reduce electrical interference. Also, calming procedures, such as reducing light stimulation or warming the environment, may help quiet the infant during electroencephalography. The infant should be closely observed throughout the procedure for any signs of seizure activity.

RESPIRATORY PROCEDURES

Pulse Oximetry

Pulse oximetry is a widely used, noninvasive method of monitoring arterial blood oxygen saturations (SaO_2). The SaO_2 is the ratio of oxygenated hemoglobin to total hemoglobin. A single probe, attached to an infant's extremity or digit, uses light emitted at different wavelengths, which is absorbed differently by saturated and unsaturated hemoglobin. The change in the light during arterial pulses is used to calculate the oxygen saturation. Pulse oximetry saturations reflect a more accurate measure of actual hemoglobin saturation.

Proper placement of the probe should be assessed regularly, because movement, environmental light, edema, and diminished perfusion can reduce the accuracy of readings. The probe should be rotated every few hours to prevent skin breakdown at the site.

Bronchoscopy

Bronchoscopy of the newborn is performed to visualize the upper and lower airways and to collect diagnostic specimens. The procedure can be done in the NICU using a flexible bronchoscope, or it can be performed under general anesthesia in the operating room using either a flexible or rigid bronchoscope. The flexible bronchoscope is preferable for examining the lower airways of an intubated patient or for examination of a patient with mandibular hypoplasia. A rigid bronchoscope is more advantageous in situations requiring removal of foreign bodies and for evaluation of patients with H-type tracheoesophageal fistula (TEF), laryngotracheoesophageal clefts, and bilateral abductor paralysis of the vocal cords. Examination of structures by direct visualization provides the opportunity to identify congenital anomalies, obstructions, masses, or mucus plugs and to evaluate stridor or respiratory dysfunction.

Bronchoscopy done at the bedside requires the nurse to assist with positioning, sedation, and monitoring of vital signs. Whether the infant undergoes flexible or rigid bronchoscopy, respiratory, and cardiovascular monitoring should be continued in the immediate postprocedural period. Possible complications related to these procedures include bronchospasm, laryngeal spasms, laryngeal edema, or pneumothorax or bradycardia resulting in hypoxia.

SUMMARY

Marked technical advances over the past two decades have produced a variety of imaging methods for the diagnosis, treatment, and evaluation of neonates. Sizable expenditures have been directed toward improving image presentation and quality on the assumption that a trained clinical eye can make diagnostic use of the data provided. Investigations are useful only insofar as they reduce the diagnostic uncertainty. The final product of any radiologic imaging procedure is not a set of photographic pictures but a diagnostic opinion that should be beneficial to management of the infant. Before initiating any imaging method, physicians should consider whether further information is really needed, and they should select the imaging technique that will give the required information with sufficient reliability and with minimal risk to the patient. The value of any diagnostic imaging examination must be balanced against the potential hazards. In addition to care of the newborn during and after a procedure, nursing care of newborns and infants undergoing diagnostic procedures requires a knowledge of the expected outcomes and methods so that the best result possible is obtained. Nurses also must be knowledgeable about normal values for the laboratory tests commonly used in the care of newborns and infants.

REFERENCE

Pagana, K. D., & Pagana, T. J. (2018). *Mosby's manual diagnostic and laboratory tests* (6th ed.). Mosby.

EXPANDED NEWBORN SCREENING: CRITICAL CONGENITAL HEART DISEASE

WAKAKO M. EKLUND

The aim of performing an expanded newborn screening prior to discharge from the hospital is to identify certain treatable diseases during the early days of the newborn's life. The goal of the early screening efforts is to make early interventions possible to improve the outcome. These screenings are generally intended for healthy newborns, both late term to term, and not typically for NICU patients. The late-term to term newborn experiences a relatively short hospitalization in any global region, during which time some of the critical conditions, such as critical congenital heart disease (CCHD), would not often become symptomatic, thus causing a delay in diagnosis.

HISTORY OF CRITICAL CONGENITAL HEART DISEASE SCREENING IN THE UNITED STATES

In September 2010, the U.S. Health and Human Services Secretary's Advisory Committee on Heritable Disorders in Newborn and Children (SACHDNC) recommended that CCHD screening be added to the Recommended Uniform Screening Panel (RUSP) in addition to the blood sampling for multiple metabolic or genetic diseases and hearing screening (Kemper et al., 2011; Mahle et al., 2009; Mahle et al., 2012). This recommendation was made based on major studies that were conducted primarily in Europe (de-Wahl Granelli et al., 2009; Ewer et al., 2012; Riede et al., 2010; Thangaratinam et al., 2012). As a result of the collaboration by SACHDNC, the American College of Cardiology, the American Academy of Pediatrics, and the American Heart Association, CCHD screening was implemented in the United States (Kemper et al., 2011).

By 2018, CCHD screening was legislated in all U.S. states and became a standard of care (Dlidewell et al., 2019). Prenatal ultrasound and postnatal physical examination have been completed routinely; however, they do not always capture critical conditions early or prior to discharge home.

GLOBAL LANDSCAPE: CRITICAL CONGENITAL HEART DISEASE SCREENING

This screening method has become a standard of care in high-resource countries during the last decade and has been increasingly implemented not only in North America or Europe with positive outcomes but attempts have also been made to implement the practice in other global regions, such as Asia, the Middle East, or South America (Al Mazrouei et al., 2013; AlAql et al., 2020; de-Wahl Granelli et al., 2014; Hom & Martin, 2014; Mahle et al., 2009; Riede et al., 2010; Sola et al., 2020; Zhao et al., 2014). Robust discussions have been ongoing more recently among the policy makers, researchers, and professionals in developing regions to increase awareness for CCHD screening or to conduct pilot studies in the mid- to low-resource regions (El Idrissi Slitine et al., 2020; Hom & Martin, 2020). However, numerous barriers against the universal implementations are identified by those who understand the regions where resources are limited. Some of the barriers include the lack of human resources, hospitals with limited or low-quality equipment, a high rate of homebirths, challenges in gaining national support, and, importantly, limited access to pediatric cardiology for confirmation of the diagnosis or cardiac surgery services. Neonatal transport infrastructure may not be well established in these regions to accommodate the newborns who are identified as needing treatment in a timely manner (Hom & Martin, 2020; Kumar, 2016).

RELEVANCE TO NURSES

The education related to CCHD screening aimed at early detection is essential knowledge for nurses and other healthcare members, primarily because earlier detection is linked to improved outcomes for patients with CCHD. Undetected CCHD cases are associated with high mortality and morbidity (Eckersley et al., 2016; Thangaratinam et al., 2012). As the primary staff who perform CCHD screening globally, nurses play an important role in its early detection.

INCIDENCE

The congenital heart defects (CHDs), which are the most commonly occurring birth defects, contribute to death both during infancy as well as later in life (Centers for

Disease Control and Prevention [CDC], 2020). During 1999 to 2006, 41,494 CHD-associated deaths were reported in the United States. Out of this number, 27,960 deaths occurred primarily due to the CHD. Nearly half (48%) of the 27,960 deaths occurred before 1 year of age, demonstrating the significant impact of CHD. As for the critical congenital cases, 2 in every 1,000 newborns are diagnosed with CCHD (Plana et al., 2018).

SIGNIFICANCE

When the CCHDs are not recognized early, the conditions become life-threatening and potentially lethal upon closure of the ductus arteriosus or other causes related to the physiological changes in the postnatal period (Kemper et al., 2011). Earlier identification and initiation of treatment allows the infants to avoid the consequences of hypoperfusion, such as potential organ damage (Mahle et al., 2009). The delayed diagnosis leads to severe hemodynamic collapse and shock, leaving the infants in poorer preintervention condition. This unfortunately leads to poorer postintervention outcomes (Brown et al., 2006). Timing of treatment initiation is critical to achieve optimal outcome (Eckersley et al., 2016; Thangaratinam et al., 2012).

One study reported (Peterson, Ailes, et al., 2014) that nearly 30% of the babies with CCHD were not diagnosed until they were older than 3 days of age. This report underscores the importance of CCHD screening, which utilizes easy-to-use, cost-effective equipment to evaluate the saturation reading to detect possible signs of CCHD (or, a slight decrease in oxygen saturation).

NURSING ASSESSMENT

Prenatal ultrasounds and postnatal physical examination alone have limitations in identifying CCHD early. The most important clinical information that should be remembered by every nurse is that infants with CCHD may appear healthy, as a subtle decrease in oxygen saturation is often not detectable by visual assessment, and no other symptoms may exist. Bedside nurses must be aware that, based on the type of structural defects, the newborn's presentation and resultant morbidity and mortality may differ. Some newborns with certain critical defects may present with a significant murmur or cyanosis, which allows easier recognition and further evaluation, such as echocardiography. Unfortunately, not all the cardiac defects present with recognizable murmur, vital sign changes, cyanosis, or other abnormal assessment findings. This occurs more often when they have ductal-dependent CHD during the period while the ductus is patent; however, significant cardiovascular collapse can occur quickly at ductal closure.

In the United States or worldwide, where routine discharges from the hospital after birth occur as early as 24 to 48 hours or even earlier after birth, physiologic changes related to the defects do not present until after the hospital discharge. The benefit of recognizing the potential problem postnatally, and prior to discharge, is especially emphasized in regions where family of ill infants reside at a distance away from regional referral centers, or when a prenatal ultrasound was not always performed as a part of routine prenatal care.

WHY PULSE OXIMETRY IS IMPORTANT FOR CRITICAL CONGENITAL HEART DISEASE: CURRENT EVIDENCE

A pulse oximetry device, which is familiar to most in healthcare, is the recommended tool to use. This device is painless to the babies, simple for anyone to use, and found to be relatively inexpensive when equipment and labor cost are considered; however, this is debatable depending on in which region of the globe one is practicing (Peterson, Grosse, et al., 2014; Reeder et al., 2015). Pulse oximetry is used to detect a possible decrease in oxygen saturation. Many cases of CCHD are accompanied by hypoxemia that is not visually detectable but is detectable by pulse oximetry, during the early days of life (Mahle et al., 2009). Prior to the United States achieving the nationwide CCHD screening mandate, it was reported that the states where the screening policies were implemented saw a reduction of early CCHD-associated death by 33% (Abouk et al., 2017). A Cochrane systematic review (Barreto, 2019; Plana et al., 2018) states that the CCHD screening with the use of pulse oximetry is an evidence-based approach of screening to increase the early identification of infants with CCHD. This review analyzed 19 studies including 436,758 infants, demonstrating CCHD screening to have moderate sensitivity (76.3%) and high specificity (99.9%). As a result, it reports that out of 10,000 healthy-appearing infants, both late-preterm and term, CCHD would be found in six of them. Additionally, implementing the CCHD screening will identify five of them; however, it may miss one. Moderate sensitivity translates to 14 false positives among the 10,000 infants who may be identified as high risk but actually do not have CCHD. The review concludes that there is a significant value in CCHD screening in asymptomatic newborns prior to discharge from the hospital.

CRITICAL CONGENITAL HEART DISEASE DEFINED: TARGETED DEFECTS

In the United States, for purposes of CCHD screening, CCHD is defined as a CHD that requires surgical or catheter intervention within the first year of life (Mahle et al., 2009).

The primary screening targets include the following seven CHDs based on the physiology of the lesions which would be expected to present with a low saturation (Kemper et al., 2011; Mahle et al., 2009; Mahle et al., 2012).

■ Hypoplastic left heart syndrome

■ Pulmonary atresia

■ Tetralogy of Fallot

■ Total anomalous pulmonary venous return

■ Transposition of the great arteries

■ Tricuspid atresia

■ Truncus arteriosus

Several other defects are also highly critical; however, they were not included in this target list. The other defects include a coarctation of the aorta (CoA), an interrupted aortic arch, double outlet right ventricle, or Ebstein's anomaly. This is due primarily to the fact that these conditions do not often present early with lower oxygen saturation; therefore, it is less likely to detect these lesions early (Mouledoux et al., 2017). CoA is the most difficult condition to diagnose early. Even with the screening, half or greater are still missed (Liberman et al., 2014; Mouledoux & Walsh, 2013; Peterson, Ailes, et al., 2014). The clinicians must remain aware of the difficulty of identifying CoA by continuing with a thorough physical examination. The critical need to assess the pulses in the lower extremities of each newborn prior to discharge and at postdischarge checkups cannot be overemphasized. Newborns with delayed CoA diagnosis have presented with symptoms such as tachypnea, cyanosis, murmur, poor feeding, respiratory distress, or circulatory collapse in need of rigorous resuscitation, or even death. The age of diagnosis for the missed CoA in the state of Tennessee in 2011 ranged from 7 to 30 days of life (Mouledoux & Walsh, 2013).

Bedside nurses who educate the parents at the time of discharge must inform the parents that the fact of passing CCHD screening does not rule out the presence of potential CCHD entirely, and that vigilance and observations are still important. The parents must be informed of danger signs and symptoms and the need to seek immediate care for further evaluation. Nurses' role in providing education to the parents or the caretaker of the infants is highly critical.

RECOMMENDED REGIONAL POLICY FOR THE CRITICAL CONGENITAL HEART DISEASE SCREENING

Based on the U.S. Health and Human Services Department's Recommendations, in the United States by 2018, all states have enacted legislation to make CCHD screening a mandatory aspect of newborn screening. Numerous other countries have also implemented CCHD screening as the standard of care. Readers are encouraged to follow the local/regional guidelines and recommendations as regional needs may vary widely. It is critically important that every nurse who works with newborns is informed of the potential of CCHD among healthy-appearing infants, and the policies and protocols in place at the institution where they work. The staff who perform CCHD screening is predominantly nursing staff in the United States and likely in many other regions globally. Nurses play an important role in the cardiac assessment of the newborns.

NECESSARY EQUIPMENT AND THE SAMPLE PROTOCOL

Equipment Needed

■ A U.S. Food and Drug Administration (FDA)-approved pulse oximeter (approved for newborn use) that is motion-tolerant

■ Manufacturer-recommended probes that are disposable or reusable

Protocol

■ Follow the manufacturer's recommendation to apply the probe by ensuring that the emitter and the detector portion of the probe are positioned appropriately.

■ The infant should not be cold or crying at the time of screening. (Nursing consideration: Educate the family regarding the importance of CCHD screening and invite the family to assist to soothe the infant.)

■ Screen every infant after 24 hours, or as close to the time of discharge as possible, especially when infants are discharged prior to 24 hours of age. Screening before 24 hours is associated with higher false positives (Plana et al., 2018). Screening an infant between 24 and 48 hours of age is recommended.

Recommended Screening Procedure

A multidisciplinary expert panel consisting of multiple stakeholders reviewed the accumulated evidence and new updated recommendations were made in 2020. The following procedure reflects the updates (Martin et al., 2020).

■ Perform pulse oximetry screening (POS) on both right hand (RH) and one foot (either the right or left).

■ **Pass**: POS reading is >95% in both locations, and a difference of ≤3% is observed.

No need to repeat the screen.

■ **Fail**: POS reading is 89% or less in either the RH or foot.

Refer for immediate assessment and do not wait to retest.

■ **Only retest in 1 hour if**: (1) pulse oximetry reading is 90% to 94% in either RH or foot,

OR

(2) a difference of 4% of more is measured between the RH and foot.

■ **Retest for the second time to obtain a second set of measurements**

● **Fail**: (1) POS is <94% in either the RH or foot or,

(2) POS reading shows >4% difference between the RH and foot.

Refer for immediate assessment. Do not repeat the screening further.

● **Pass:** POS is >95% in RH or foot and the difference between the two is ≤3%.

Provide normal newborn care and do not rescreen.

■ If any clinical findings suggest the possibility of CHDs at any time, even after the infant has passed the screening, obtain further consultation for evaluation of CHDs.

An Alternate Screening Procedure: One Extremity Approach

One extremity method of CCHD screening to test only the foot was evaluated in the state of Tennessee in the United States since 2006, prior to the U.S. Health and Human Services' recommendations. This one extremity method measures the pulse oximetry reading in the foot, and if the result is 97≥%, the infant is considered to have passed the CCHD screening without the need to examine the RH, thus reducing the number of POS significantly.

The rationale for this method includes several important points:

■ Setting the "pass" cutoff for the foot POS to be ≥97% makes it impossible for the RH and foot difference to be ≥3%. This eliminates the practice of checking the RH. In Tennessee, if the POS is 90% to 96% on the foot, an RH exam follows and, based on the results, the procedure commences.

■ This method follows the national recommendation for further evaluation. Based on the data from 2013 to 2014, Tennessee saved over 150,000 unnecessary POS readings while still detecting the predicted number of CCHDs. The approach to examine both RH and foot measurements began with the hope to detect those "difficult to detect" CCHDs, such as CoA or interrupted aortic arch; however, this has not been fully realized to justify the numerous additional POS attempts (Mouledoux et al., 2017; Walsh & Ballweg, 2017). Tennessee still continues to use this method in 2021.

Special Considerations

Perfusion Matters

If there is poor perfusion or vasoconstriction caused by hypothermia or hypotension, an accurate saturation cannot be obtained, potentially leading to false-positive screening. It is recommended that rescreening is performed when infants' condition is optimal for the most accurate saturation measurement.

Altitude Matters

In higher altitude, due to the low partial oxygen pressure, oxygen saturation tends to be lower than at sea level. This leads to higher false-positive rates on CCHD screening, burdening the families, patients, and healthcare systems with a high number of rescreenings or further evaluations. With an effort to reduce false positives, while not increasing the false negatives, Lueth and colleagues made an adjustment to the current guideline and used a lower saturation cutoff (≤85 in RH or foot represents failure), and further incorporated a 26% oxygen hood placed for 20 minutes (in order to mimic the infant's environment to sea-level alveolar oxygen tension) prior to retesting when initial screening showed saturation of 86% to 94% (Lueth et al., 2016). This is the only study so far to have made a specific adjustment to the algorithm for moderately high-altitude settings with positive results; however, the authors suggest the need for further studies.

NICU Patients Do Matter

The current recommendations for the CCHD screening do not include NICU patients. A few studies focused on CCHD screening in the NICU and generally supported the routine screening (Iyengar et al., 2014; Manja et al., 2015; Van Naarden Braun et al., 2017). It is prudent to observe the pulse oximeter reading on inpatients at 24 to 48 hours when stable or once prior to discharge from the hospital. Frequently, NICU may have late-term to term infants who may be admitted for conditions that may not require oxygen (and therefore may not have the continuous pulse oximetry monitoring) such as brief hypoglycemia, hypothermia, or maternal substance use. These infants would benefit from CCHD screening at 24 to 48 hours of age. In any case, the CCHD screening is not intended to minimize or replace a careful physical examination by trained professionals and a thorough history taking to identify risk factors. Family history of previous CHD or maternal risk factors associated with CHD (such as infant of a diabetic mother) are important findings that must be noted. The final physical examination prior to discharge should include the assessment of femoral pulses bilaterally.

CONCLUSION

The presentation of a CCHD may be subtle or completely asymptomatic. The use of pulse oximetry is intended to increase the rate of early detection of CCHDs, which can allow the early initiation of treatment. It is very important that every birthing facility and hospital where births occur institute provisions to address these efforts toward early detection of CCHDs. The staff must be educated to perform the CCHD screening and to understand and follow the algorithm accurately. Staff must also be well aware of the chain of communication when abnormalities are detected.

REFERENCES

Abouk, R., Grosse, S. D., Ailes, E. C., & Oster, M. E. (2017). Association of US state implementation of newborn screening policies for critical congenital heart disease with early infant cardiac deaths. *JAMA, 318*(21), 2111–2118. https://doi.org/10.1001/jama.2017.17627

Al Mazrouei, S. K., Moore, J., Ahmed, F., Mikula, E. B., & Martin, G. R. (2013). Regional implementation of newborn screening for critical congenital heart disease screening in Abu Dhabi. *Pediatric Cardiology, 34*(6), 1299–1306. https://doi.org/10.1007/s00246-013-0692-6

AlAql, F., Khaleel, H., & Peter, V. (2020). Universal screening for CCHD in Saudi Arabia: The road to a 'State of the Art' program. *International Journal of Neonatal Screening, 6*(1), 13. https://doi.org/10.3390/ijns6010013

Barreto, T. (2019). Pulse oximetry screening for critical congenital heart defects in newborns. *American Family Physician, 99*(7), 421–422. https://www.ncbi.nlm.nih.gov/pubmed/30932460

Brown, K. L., Ridout, D. A., Hoskote, A., Verhulst, L., Ricci, M., & Bull, C. (2006). Delayed diagnosis of congenital heart disease worsens preoperative condition and outcome of surgery in neonates. *Heart, 92*(9), 1298–1302. https://doi.org/10.1136/hrt.2005.078097

Centers for Disease Control and Prevention. (2020). *Data and statistics on congenital heart defects.* https://www.cdc.gov/ncbddd/heartdefects/data.html

de-Wahl Granelli, A., Meberg, A., Ojala, T., Steensberg, J., Oskarsson, G., & Mellander, M. (2014). Nordic pulse oximetry screening—Implementation status and proposal for uniform guidelines. *Acta Paediatrica, 103*(11), 1136–1142. https://doi.org/10.1111/apa.12758

de-Wahl Granelli, A., Wennergren, M., Sandberg, K., Mellander, M., Bejlum, C., Inganas, L., Eriksson, M., Segerdahl, N., Agren, A., Ekman-Joelsson, B.-M., Sunnegårdh, J., Verdicchio, M., & Ostman-Smith, I. (2009). Impact of pulse oximetry screening on the detection of duct dependent congenital heart disease: A Swedish prospective screening study in 39,821 newborns. *British Medical Journal, 338*, a3037. https://doi.org/10.1136/bmj.a3037

Dlidewell, J., Grosse, S., Riehle-Colarusso, T., Pinto, N., Hudson, J., Daskalov, R., Gaviglio, A., Darby, E., Singh, S., & Sontag, M. (2019). Actions in support for newborn screening for critical congenital heart disease-United States, 2011–2018. *Morbility and Mortality Weekly Report, 68*, 107–111. http://doi.org/10.15585/mmwr.mm6805a3

Eckersley, L., Sadler, L., Parry, E., Finucane, K., & Gentles, T. L. (2016). Timing of diagnosis affects mortality in critical congenital heart disease. *Archives of Disease in Childhood, 101*(6), 516–520. https://doi.org/10.1136/archdischild-2014-307691

El Idrissi Slitine, N., Bennaoui, F., Sable, C. A., Martin, G. R., Hom, L. A., Fadel, A., Moussaoui, S., Inajjarne, N., Boumzebra, D., Mouaffak, Y., Younous, S., Boukhanni, L., & Maoulainine, F. M. R. (2020). Pulse oximetry and congenital heart disease screening: Results of the first pilot study in Morocco. *International Journal of Neonatal Screening, 6*(3), 53. https://doi.org/10.3390/ijns6030053

Ewer, A. K., Furmston, A. T., Middleton, L. J., Deeks, J. J., Daniels, J. P., Pattison, H. M., Powell, R., Roberts, T. E., Barton, P., Auguste, P., Bhoyar, A., Thangaratinam, S., Tonks, A. M., Satodia, P., Deshpande, S., Kumararatne, B., Sivakumar, S., Mupanemunda, R., & Khan, K. S. (2012). Pulse oximetry as a screening test for congenital heart defects in newborn infants: A test accuracy study with evaluation of acceptability and cost-effectiveness. *Health Technology Assessment, 16*(2), v–xiii, 1–184. https://doi.org/10.3310/hta16020

Hom, L. A., & Martin, G. R. (2014). U.S. international efforts on critical congenital heart disease screening: Can we have a uniform recommendation for Europe? *Early Human Development, 90*(Suppl. 2), S11–S14. https://doi.org/10.1016/S0378-3782(14)50004-7

Hom, L. A., & Martin, G. R. (2020). Newborn critical congenital heart disease screening using pulse oximetry: Value and unique challenges in developing regions. *International Journal of Neonatal Screening, 6*(3), 74. https://doi.org/10.3390/ijns6030074

Iyengar, H., Kumar, P., & Kumar, P. (2014). Pulse-oximetry screening to detect critical congenital heart disease in the neonatal intensive care unit. *Pediatric Cardiology, 35*(3), 406–410. https://doi.org/10.1007/s00246-013-0793-2

Kemper, A. R., Mahle, W. T., Martin, G. R., Cooley, W. C., Kumar, P., Morrow, W. R., Kelm, K., Pearson, G. D., Glidewell, J., Grosse, S. D., & Howell, R. R. (2011). Strategies for implementing screening for critical congenital heart disease. *Pediatrics, 128*(5), e1259–e1267. https://doi.org/10.1542/peds.2011-1317

Kumar, R. K. (2016). Screening for congenital heart disease in India: Rationale, practical challenges, and pragmatic strategies. *Annals of Pediatric Cardiology, 9*(2), 111–114. https://doi.org/10.4103/0974-2069.181499

Liberman, R. F., Getz, K. D., Lin, A. E., Higgins, C. A., Sekhavet, S., Markenson, G. R., & Anderka, M. (2014). Delayed diagnosis of critical congenital heart defects: Trends and associated factors. *Pediatrics, 134*(20), e373–e381. https://doi.org/10.1542/peds.2013-3949

Lueth, E., Russell, L., Wright, J., Duster, M., Kohn, M., Miller, J., Eller, C., Sontag, M., & Rausch, C. M. (2016). A novel approach to critical congenital heart disease (CCHD) screening at moderate altitude. *International Journal of Neonatal Screening, 2*(3), 4. https://www.mdpi.com/2409-515X/2/3/4

Mahle, W. T., Martin, G. R., Beekman, R. H., 3rd, & Morrow, W. R. (2012). Endorsement of Health and Human Services recommendation for pulse oximetry screening for critical congenital heart disease. *Pediatrics, 129*(1), 190–192. https://doi.org/10.1542/peds.2011-3211

Mahle, W. T., Newburger, J. W., Matherne, G. P., Smith, F. C., Hoke, T. R., Koppel, R., Gidding, S. S., Beekman, R. H., 3rd, Grosse, S. D., American Heart Association Congenital Heart Defects Committee of the Council on Cardiovascular Disease in the Young, Council on Cardiovascular Nursing, and Interdisciplinary Council on Quality of Care and Outcomes Research, & American Academy of Pediatrics Section on Cardiology and Cardiac Surgery, and Committee on Fetus and Newborn. (2009). Role of pulse oximetry in examining newborns for congenital heart disease: A scientific statement from the American Heart Association and American Academy of Pediatrics. *Circulation, 120*(5), 447–458. https://doi.org/10.1161/CIRCULATIONAHA.109.192576

Manja, V., Mathew, B., Carrion, V., & Lakshminrusimha, S. (2015). Critical congenital heart disease screening by pulse oximetry in a neonatal intensive care unit. *Journal of Perinatology, 35*(1), 67–71. https://doi.org/10.1038/jp.2014.135

Martin, G. R., Ewer, A. K., Gaviglio, A., Hom, L. A., Saarinen, A., Sontag, M., Burns K. M., Kemper, A. R., & Oster, M. E. (2020). Updated strategies for pulse oximetry screening for critical congenital heart disease. *Pediatrics, 146*(1). https://doi.org/10.1542/peds.2019-1650

Mouledoux, J., Guerra, S., Ballweg, J., Li, Y., & Walsh, W. (2017). A novel, more efficient, staged approach for critical congenital heart disease screening. *Journal of Perinatology*, 37(3), 288–290. https://doi.org/10.1038/jp.2016.204

Mouledoux, J. E., & Walsh, W. F. (2013). Evaluating the diagnostics gap: Statewide incidence of undiagnosed critical congenital heart disease before newborn screening with pulse oximetry. *Pediatric Cardiology*, 34(7), 1680–1686. https://doi.org/10.1007/s00246-013-0697-1

Peterson, C., Ailes, E., Riehle-Colarusso, T., Oster, M. E., Olney, R. S., Cassell, C. H., Fixler, D. E., Carmichael, S. L., Shaw, G. M., & Gilboa, S. M. (2014). Late detection of critical congenital heart disease among US infants: Estimation of the potential impact of proposed universal screening using pulse oximetry. *JAMA Pediatrics*, 168(4), 361–370. https://doi.org/10.1001/jamapediatrics.2013.4779

Peterson, C., Grosse, S. D., Glidewell, J., Garg, L. F., Van Naarden Braun, K., Knapp, M. M., Beres, L. M., Hinton, C. F., Olney, R. S., & Cassell, C. H. (2014). A public health economic assessment of hospitals' cost to screen newborns for critical congenital heart disease. *Public Health Reports*, 129(1), 86–93. https://doi.org/10.1177/003335491412900113

Plana, M. N., Zamora, J., Suresh, G., Fernandez-Pineda, L., Thangaratinam, S., & Ewer, A. K. (2018). Pulse oximetry screening for critical congenital heart defects. *Cochrane Database of Systematic Reviews*, 3, CD011912. https://doi.org/10.1002/14651858.CD011912.pub2

Reeder, M. R., Kim, J., Nance, A., Krikov, S., Feldkamp, M. L., Randall, H., & Botto, L. D. (2015). Evaluating cost and resource use associated with pulse oximetry screening for critical congenital heart disease: Empiric estimates and sources of variation. *Birth Defects Research Part A Clinical and Molecular Teratology*, 103(11), 962–971. https://doi.org/10.1002/bdra.23414

Riede, F. T., Worner, C., Dahnert, I., Mockel, A., Kostelka, M., & Schneider, P. (2010). Effectiveness of neonatal pulse oximetry screening for detection of critical congenital heart disease in daily clinical routine—results from a prospective multicenter study. *European Journal of Pediatrics*, 169(8), 975–981. https://doi.org/10.1007/s00431-010-1160-4 .

Sola, A., Rodriguez, S., Young, A., Lemus Varela, L., Villamayor, R. M., Cardetti, M., Navarrete, J. P., Favareto, M. V., Lima, V., Baquero, H., Forero, L. V., Venegas, M. E., Davila, C., Dieppa, F. D., Germosén, T. M., Barrantes, A. N. O., Castañeda, A. L. A., Morgues, M., Avila, A., . . . Golombek, S. (2020). CCHD screening implementation efforts in Latin American countries by the Ibero American Society of Neonatology (SIBEN). *International Journal of Neonatal Screening*, 6(1), 21. https://doi.org/10.3390/ijns6010021

Thangaratinam, S., Brown, K., Zamora, J., Khan, K. S., & Ewer, A. K. (2012). Pulse oximetry screening for critical congenital heart defects in asymptomatic newborn babies: A systematic review and meta-analysis. *Lancet*, 379(9835), 2459–2464. https://doi.org/10.1016/S0140-6736(12)60107-X

Van Naarden Braun, K., Grazel, R., Koppel, R., Lakshminrusimha, S., Lohr, J., Kumar, P., Govindaswami, B., Giuliano, M., Cohen, M., Spillane, N., Jegatheesan, P., McClure, D., Hassinger, D., Fofah, O., Chandra, S., Allen, D., Axelrod, R., Blau, J., Hudome, S., . . . Garg, L. F. (2017). Evaluation of critical congenital heart defects screening using pulse oximetry in the neonatal intensive care unit. *Journal of Perinatology*, 37(10), 1117–1123. https://doi.org/10.1038/jp.2017.105

Walsh, W., & Ballweg, J. A. (2017). A single-extremity staged approach for critical congenital heart disease screening: Results from Tennessee. *International Journal of Neonatal Screening*, 3(4), 31. https://www.mdpi.com/2409-515X/3/4/31

Zhao, Q. M., Ma, X. J., Ge, X. L., Liu, F., Yan, W. L., Wu, L., Ye, M., Liang, X. C., Zhang, J., Gao, Y., Jia, B., & Huang, G. Y. (2014). Pulse oximetry with clinical assessment to screen for congenital heart disease in neonates in China: A prospective study. *Lancet*, 384(9945), 747–754. https://doi.org/10.1016/S0140-6736(14)60198-7

Common Laboratory Values

SAMUAL L. MOONEYHAM

A wide variety of laboratory tests can be used in both the diagnosis and care of the newborn. The values given in this chapter represent the broader normal ranges, but values in a specific chapter may vary slightly, depending on the range the author considers to be within normal limits. Every attempt has been made to provide consistent diagnostic and laboratory values. However, many hospitals have compiled their own list of acceptable laboratory test values; therefore, specific laboratories should be contacted when evaluating results (see Tables 18.1–18.16). Nurses also must be knowledgeable about normal values for the laboratory tests commonly used in the care of newborns and infants.

TABLE 18.1 Common Electrolyte and Chemistry Values

PARAMETER	NORMAL VALUE
Serum Electrolytes	
Sodium (Na)	136–146 mEq/L
Potassium (K)	3.5–5.5 mEq/L
Chloride (Cl)	96–111 mEq/L
Carbon dioxide (CO_2)	23–33 mEq/L
Serum Chemistries	
Blood urea nitrogen (BUN)	4–15 mg/dL
Calcium (Ca)	8–12 mg/dL
Creatinine (Cr)	Less than 0.6 mg/dL
Glucose (G)	30–90 mg/dL
Magnesium (Mg)	1.6–2.8 mEq/dL
Phosphorus (P)	5.0–8.0 mg/dL

TABLE 18.2 Age-Specific Normal Blood Cell Values in Fetal Samples (26–30 Weeks' Gestation) and Neonatal Samples (28–44 Weeks' Gestation)

AGE	Hb (G/DL)[a]	Hct (%)[a]	MCV (FL)[a]	MCHC (G/DL RBC)[a]	RETICULOCYTES	WBCs (×10³/ML)[b]	PLATELETS (10³/ML)[b]
26–30 weeks' gestation[c]	13.4 (11)	41.5 (34.9)	118.2 (106.7)	37.9 (30.6)	–	4.4 (2.7)	254 (180–327)
28 weeks	14.5	45	120	31.0	(5–10)	–	275
32 weeks	15.0	47	118	32.0	(3–10)	–	290
Term[d] (cord)	16.5 (13.5)	51 (42)	108 (98)	33.0 (30.0)	(3–7)	18.1(9–30)[d]	290
1–3 days	18.5 (14.5)	56 (45)	108 (95)	33.0 (29.0)	(1.8–4.6)	18.9 (9.4–34)	192
2 weeks	16.6 (13.4)	53 (41)	105 (88)	31.4 (28.1)	–	11.4 (5–20)	252
1 month	13.9 (10.7)	44 (33)	101 (91)	31.8 (28.1)	(0.1–1.7)	10.8 (4–19.5)	

[a] Data are mean (number in parenthesis is -2 SD).

[b] Data are mean (number in parenthesis is -2 SD).

[c] In infants younger than 1 month, capillary Hb exceeds venous Hb: at 1 hour old, the difference 3.6 g; at 5 days, 2.2 g; at 3 weeks, 1.1 g.

[d] Mean (95% confidence limits).

Hb, hemoglobin; Hct, hematocrit; MCHC, mean corpuscular hemoglobin concentration; MCV, mean corpuscular volume; RBC, red blood cell; WBCs, white blood cells.

Source: Modified from Costa, K. (2018). Hematology. In H. K. Hughes & L. K. Kahl (Eds.), The Harriet Lane handbook (pp. 364–394). Elsevier.

TABLE 18.3 White Cell and Differential Counts in Premature Infants

	BIRTH WEIGHT					
	UNDER 1,500 G			1,500–2,500 G		
	1 WEEK OLD	2 WEEKS OLD	4 WEEKS OLD	1 WEEK OLD	2 WEEKS OLD	4 WEEKS OLD
Total Count (×10³/mm³)						
Mean	16.8	15.4	12.1	13	10	8.4
Range	6.1–32.8	10.4–21.3	8.7–17.2	6.7–14.7	7.0–14.1	5.8–12.4
Percentage of Total Polymorphs						
Segmented	54	45	40	55	43	41
Unsegmented	7	6	5	8	8	6
Eosinophils	2	3	3	2	3	3
Basophils	1	1	1	1	1	1
Monocytes	6	10	10	5	9	11
Lymphocytes	30	35	41	29	36	38

Source: Data from Klaus, M. H., & Fanaroff, A. A. (Eds.). (2001). *Care of the high-risk neonate* (5th ed.). WB Saunders.

TABLE 18.4 Normal Blood Levels of Coagulation Inhibitors in Newborns (30 Weeks' Gestation to Term)

COAGULATION INHIBITORS	30–36 WEEKS' GESTATION			FULL TERM	
	DAY 1 MEAN (BOUNDARY)	DAY 5 MEAN (BOUNDARY)	DAY 1 MEAN (BOUNDARY)	DAY 5 MEAN (BOUNDARY)	
Antithrombin III (U/mL)	0.38 (0.14–0.62)	0.56 (0.3–0.82)	0.63 (0.39–0.87)	0.67 (0.41–0.93)	
Alpha2-macroglobulin (U/mL)	1.1 (0.56–1.82)	1.25 (0.71–1.77)	1.39 (0.95–1.83)	1.48 (0.98–1.98)	
C1 esterase inhibitor (U/mL)	0.65 (0.31–0.99)	0.83 (0.45–1.21)	0.72 (0.36–1.08)	0.90 (0.6–1.2)	
Alpha1-antitrypsin (U/mL)	0.9 (0.36–1.44)	0.94 (0.42–1.46)	0.93 (0.49–1.37)	0.89 (0.49–1.29)	
Heparin cofactor II (U/mL)	0.32 (0.1–0.6)	0.34 (0.1–0.69)	0.43 (0.1–0.93)	0.48 (0.1–0.96)	
Protein C (U/mL)	0.28 (0.12–0.44)	0.31 (0.11–0.51)	0.35 (0.17–0.53)	0.42 (0.2–0.64)	
Protein S (U/mL)	0.26 (0.14–0.38)	0.37 (0.13–0.61)	0.36 (0.12–0.6)	0.5 (0.22–0.78)	

Source: Modified from Andrew, M., Paes, B., & Johnston, M. (1990). Development of the hemostatic system in the neonate and young infant. American Journal of Pediatric Hematology/Oncology, 12, 97–98. https://doi.org/10.1097/00043426-199021000-00019

TABLE 18.5 Normal Blood Levels of Fibrinolytic Components in Premature and Term Newborns

FIBRINOLYTIC COMPONENT	PREMATURE INFANTS		FULL-TERM INFANTS	
	DAY 1 MEAN (BOUNDARY)	DAY 5 MEAN (BOUNDARY)	DAY 1 MEAN (BOUNDARY)	DAY 5 MEAN (BOUNDARY)
Plasminogen (U/mL)	1.7 (1.12–2.48)	1.91 (1.21–2.61)	1.95 (1.25–2.65)	2.17 (1.41–2.93)
Tissue plasminogen activator (ng/mL)	8.48 (3–16.7)	3.97 (2–6.93)	9.6 (5–18.9)	5.6 (4–10)
Alpha2-antiplasmin (U/mL)	0.78 (0.4–1.16)	0.81 (0.49–1.13)	0.85 (0.55–1.15)	1 (0.7–1.3)
Plasminogen activator inhibitor (U/mL)	5.4 (0–12.2)	2.5 (0–7.1)	6.4 (2–15.1)	2.3 (0–8.1)

Source: Modified from Andrew, M., Paes, B., & Johnston, M. (1990). Development of the hemostatic system in the neonate and young infant. American Journal of Pediatric Hematology/Oncology, 12, 97–98. https://doi.org/10.1097/00043426-199021000-00019

TABLE 18.6 Summary of Normal Urinary Laboratory Values

	AGE OF INFANT	NORMAL VALUE
Calcium	1 week	Under 2 mg/dL
Chloride	Infant	1.7–8.5 mEq/24 hr
Creatinine	Newborn	7–10 mg/kg/d
Glucose[a]	Preterm Full term	60–130 mg/dL 12–32 mg/dL
Glucose (renal threshold)	Preterm Full term	2.21–2.84 mg/mL 2.20–3.68 mg/mL
Magnesium		180 ± 10 mg/1.73 m^2/dL
Osmolality	Infant	50–600 mOsm/kg
Potassium		26–123 mEq/L
Protein		Under 100 mg/m^2/dL
Sodium		0.3–3.5 mEq/dL (6–10 mEq/m^2)
Specific gravity	Newborn	1.006–1.008

[a]Actual blood level.

Source: Ichikawa, I. (1990). *Pediatric textbook of fluids and electrolytes.* Lippincott Williams & Wilkins. Reprinted by permission of Lippincott Williams & Wilkins.

TABLE 18.7 Electrocardiographic Data Pertinent to the Neonate[a]

		AGE			
PARAMETER	BIRTH TO 24 HOURS	1–7 DAYS	8–30 DAYS	1–3 MONTHS
Heart rate (beats/min)	119 (94–145)	133 (100–175)	163 (115–190)	154 (124–190)
PR interval (sec)	0.1 (0.07–0.12)	0.09 (0.07–0.12)	0.09 (0.07–0.11)	0.1 (0.07–0.13)
P-wave amplitude-II	1.5 (0.8–2.3)	1.6 (0.8–2.5)	1.6 (0.8–2.4)	1.6 (0.8–2.4)
QRS duration (sec)	0.065 (0.05–0.08)	0.06 (0.04–0.08)	0.06 (0.04–0.07)	0.06 (0.05–0.08)
QRS axis (degrees)	135 (60–180)	125 (80–160)	110 (60–160)	80 (40–120)
R amplitude V$_{4R}$ (mm)	8.6 (4–14.2)	—	6.3 (3.3–8.5)	5.1 (1.1–10.1)
R amplitude V$_1$ (mm)	11.9 (4.3–21)	—	11.1 (3.3–18.7)	11.2 (4.5–18)
R amplitude V$_5$ (mm)	10.2 (4–18)	10.7 (3.4–19)	11.9 (3.5–27)	13.6 (7.3–20.7)
R amplitude V$_6$ (mm)	3.3 (2.3–7)	5.1 (2.2–13.1)	6.7 (1.7–20.5)	8.4 (3.6–12.9)
S amplitude V$_{4R}$ (mm)	3.8 (0.2–13)	—	1.8 (0.8–4.6)	3.4 (0–9.3)
S amplitude V$_1$ (mm)	9.7 (1.1–19.1)	—	6.1 (0–15)	7.5 (0.5–17.1)
S amplitude V$_5$ (mm)	11.9 (0.24)	6.8 (3.6–16.2)	4.8 (2.7–12.3)	4.7 (2–12.7)
S amplitude V$_6$ (mm)	4.5 (1.6–10.3)	3.3 (0.8–9.9)	2 (0.6–9)	2.4 (0.8–5.8)

[a]Mean (5th–95th percentile).

Source: Data from Fanaroff, A. A., & Martin, R. J. (1987). *Neonatal–perinatal medicine: Diseases of the fetus and infant* (4th ed.). Mosby; Liebman, J., & Plonsey, R. (1977). Electrocardiography. In A. J. Moss, F. H. Adams, & G. C. Emmanouilides (Eds.). *Heart disease in infants, children and*

TABLE 18.8 Acid–Base Status

ARTERIAL BLOOD GAS	NORMAL VALUES
pH	7.35–7.45
paO_2	50–80 mmHg (term) 45–65 mmHg (preterm)
$paCO_2$	35–45 mmHg
HCO_3	20–25 MEq/L
Base excess	0 +/– 4 mEq/L

Note: Always consider weight and gestational age as these values vary accordingly.

TABLE 18.9 Selected Chemistry Values in Preterm and Full-Term Infants

CONSTITUENT	PRETERM INFANT	FULL-TERM INFANT
Alkaline phosphatase (U/L) (mean ± SD)[8]	207 ± 60 to 320 ± 142	164 ± 68
Ammonia (mcg/dL)[1]		90–150
Base, excess (mmol/L)[1]		–10 to –2
Bicarbonate, standard (mmol/L)[2]	18–26	20–26
Bilirubin, total (mg/dL)		
Cord[2]	Under 2.8	Under 2.8
24 hours old	1–6	2–6
48 hours old	6–8	6–7
3–5 days old	10–12	4–6
1 month or older	Under 1.5	Under 1.5
Bilirubin, direct (mg/dL)[2]	Under 0.5	Under 0.5
Calcium, total (mg/dL), week 1[3,4]	6–10	8.4–11.6
Ceruloplasmin (mg/dL)[1]		1–3 months: 5–18

(continued)

TABLE 18.9 Selected Chemistry Values in Preterm and Full-Term Infants (*continued*)

CONSTITUENT	PRETERM INFANT	FULL-TERM INFANT
Cholesterol (mg/dL)		
Cord[2]		45–98
3 days to 1 year old		65–175
Creatine phosphokinase (U/L)		
Day 1[5]		44–1,150
Day 4		14–97
Creatine (mg/dL)	10 days: 1.3 ± 0.07	1–4 days: 0.3–1
	1 month: 0.6 ± 0.05	Over 4 days: 0.2–0.4
Ferritin (mcg/dL)		
Neonate[1]		25–200
1 month old		200–600
2–5 months old		50–200
Over 6 months old		7–142
Gamma-glutamyl transferase (GGT) (U/L)[6]		14–131
Glucose (mg/dL)	20–125	30–125
Under 72 hours old[7,9]	40–125	40–125
Over 72 hours old		357–953
Lactate dehydrogenase (U/L)[6]		1.7–2.4
Magnesium (mg/dL)[4]		275–295 (may be as low as 266)
Phosphorus (mg/dL)		
Birth[4]		4.5–8.7

(*continued*)

TABLE 18.9 Selected Chemistry Values in Preterm and Full-Term Infants (*continued*)

CONSTITUENT	PRETERM INFANT	FULL-TERM INFANT
Day 5		4.2–7.2
1 month old		4.5–6.5
Aspartate aminotransferase (SGOT/ AST) (U/L)[7]		24–81
Alanine aminotransferase (SGPT/ ALT) (U/L)[7]		10–33
Triglycerides (mg/dL)[2]		10–140
Urea nitrogen (mg/dL)[1]	3–25	4–12
Uric acid (mg/dL)[2]		3–7.5
Vitamin A (mcg/dL; mean ± SD; under 10 mcg/dL indicates very low hepatic vitamin A stores)[10]	16 ± 1	23.9 ± 1.8
Vitamin D		
25-hydroxycholecalciferol (ng/mL)[a11,12]		20–60
1,25-dihydroxycholecalciferol (pg/mL)[a, 11,12]		40–90

[a]Serum levels are affected by race, age, season, and diet.

[1]Tietz (1988).

[2]Wallach (1983).

[3]Meites (1975).

[4]Nelson et al. (1987).

[5]Drummond (1979).

[6]Statland (1979).

[7]Cornblath and Schwartz (1976).

[8]Glass et al. (1982).

[9]Heck and Erenberg (1987).

[10]Shenai et al. (1981).

[11]Cooke et al. (1990).

[12]Lichtenstein et al. (1986).

Source: Data from Fanaroff, A. A., & Martin, R. J. (2002). *Neonatal–perinatal medicine: Diseases of the fetus and infant* (7th ed.). Mosby.

TABLE 18.10 Plasma Albumin and Total Protein in Preterm Infants From Birth to 8 Weeks

GESTATION (WEEKS)	26	27	28	29	30	31	32	33	34
Albumin (g/dL)									
Reference range (95% confidence limits)	—	1.18–3.06	1.09–2.87	1.20–2.74	1.63–2.75	1.08–3.20	1.38–3.14	1.44–3.34	0.53–3.87
Corrected age									
26–28 weeks' gestation		2.13	2.10	2.58		2.39			
29–31 weeks' gestation					2.02	2.14	2.44	2.44	2.54
32–34 weeks' gestation								2.35	2.42
Total protein (g/dL)									
Reference range (95% confidence limits)	—	1.28–7.94	3.03–5.03	2.18–5.84	2.64–5.80	3.26–5.66	3.63–5.81	3.57–5.87	3.57–6.59

(continued)

TABLE 18.10 Plasma Albumin and Total Protein in Preterm Infants From Birth to 8 Weeks (*continued*)

GESTATION (WEEKS)	26	27	28	29	30	31	32	33	34
Corrected age									
26–28 weeks' gestation		4.07	4.45	4.84	4.49	4.45			
29–31 weeks' gestation					3.93	4.42	4.70	4.82	4.51
32–34 weeks' gestation								4.54	4.93
Albumin (g/dL)									
Reference range (95% confidence limits)	1.15–3.87	1.96–3.44	1.50–4.10	1.89–4.15	2.07–4.15	2.07–4.05	2.04–3.90	2.08–3.90	
Corrected age									
26–28 weeks' gestation	2.73								

29–31 weeks' gestation				2.82				
32–34 weeks' gestation	2.46	2.38	2.44				3.35	
Total protein (g/dL)								
Reference range (95% confidence limits)	1.52–8.62	3.85–6.91	4.69–6.95	3.32–9.16	4.17–8.25	4.26–8.08	3.73–8.47	3.24–8.76
Corrected age	4.41							
26–28 weeks' gestation				4.55				
29–31 weeks' gestation								
32–34 weeks' gestation	4.78	4.86	4.81				4.96	

Source: Data from Fanaroff, A. A., & Martin, R. J. (2002). Neonatal–perinatal medicine: Diseases of the fetus and infant (7th ed.). Mosby; Reading, R., Ellis, R., & Fleetwood, A. (1990). Plasma albumin and total protein in preterm babies from birth to eight weeks. Early Human Development, 22, 81–87. https://doi.org/10.1016/0378-3782(90)90082-t

TABLE 18.11 Plasma-Serum Amino Acid Levels in Premature and Term Newborns (mcmol/L)

AMINO ACID	PREMATURE (1 DAY)	NEWBORN (16 DAYS; BEFORE FIRST FEEDING)	16 DAYS TO 4 MONTHS
Taurine	105–255	101–181	
OH-proline	0–80	0	
Aspartic acid	0–20	4–12	17–21
Threonine	155–275	196–238	141–213
Serine	195–345	129–197	104–158
Asp + Glut	655–1,155	623–895	
Proline	155–305	155–305	141–245
Glutamic acid	30–100	27–77	
Glycine	185–735	274–412	178–248
Alanine	325–425	274–384	239–345
Valine	80–180	97–175	123–199
Cystine	55–75	49–75	33–51
Methionine	30–40	21–37	31–47

Isoleucine	20–60	31–47	31–47
Leucine	45–95	55–89	56–98
Tyrosine	20–220	53–85	33–75
Phenylalanine	70–110	64–92	45–65
Ornithine	70–110	66–116	37–61
Lysine	130–250	154–246	117–163
Histidine	30–70	61–93	64–92
Arginine	30–70	37–71	53–71
Tryptophan	15–45	15–45	
Citrulline	8.5–23.7	10.8–21.1	
Ethanolamine	10.5–13.4	32.7–72	
Alpha-amino-*n*-butyric acid	0–29	8.7–20.4	
Methylhistidine			

Source: Data from Behrman, R. E. (1977). *Neonatal–perinatal diseases of the fetus and infant* (2nd ed.). Mosby; Dickinson, J. C., Rosenblum, H., & Hamilton, P. B. (1965). Ion exchange chromatography of the free amino acids in the plasma of the newborn infant. *Pediatrics, 36*, 2–13. https://pediatrics.aappublications.org/content/36/1/2; Dickinson, J. C., Rosenblum, H., & Hamilton, P. B. (1970). Ion exchange chromatography of the free amino acids in the plasma of infants under 2,500 gm at birth. *Pediatrics, 45*, 606–613. https://pediatrics.aappublications.org/content/45/4/606; Klaus,

TABLE 18.12 Urine Amino Acid Levels in Normal Newborns (mcmol/L)

AMINO ACID	MCMOL/DAY
Cysteic acid	Tr–3.32
Phosphoethanolamine	Tr–8.86
Taurine	7.59–7.72
OH-proline	0–9.81
Aspartic acid	Tr
Threonine	0.176–7.99
Serine	Tr–20.7
Glutamic acid	0–1.78
Proline	0–5.17
Glycine	0.176–65.3
Alanine	Tr–8.03
Alpha-amino-*n*-butyric acid	0–0.47
Valine	0–7.76
Cystine	0–7.96
Methionine	Tr–0.892
Isoleucine	0–6.11
Tyrosine	0–1.11
Phenylalanine	0–1.66
Beta-aminoisobutyric acid	0.264–7.34
Ethanolamine	Tr–79.9
Ornithine	Tr–0.554

(continued)

TABLE 18.12 Urine Amino Acid Levels in Normal Newborns (mcmol/L) *(continued)*

AMINO ACID	MCMOL/DAY
Lysine	0.33–9.79
1-Methylhistidine	Tr–8.64
3-Methylhistidine	0.11–3.32
Carnosine	0.044–4.01
Arginine	0.088–0.918
Histidine	Tr–7.04
Leucine	Tr–0.918

Source: Data from Fanaroff, A. A., & Martin, R. J. (Eds.). (1997). *Neonatal–perinatal medicine: Diseases of the fetus and infant* (6th ed.). Mosby; Klaus, M. H., & Fanaroff, A. A. (2001). *Care of the high-risk neonate* (5th ed.). WB Saunders; Meites, S. (Ed.). (1997). *Pediatric clinical chemistry: A survey of normals, methods, and instruments.* American Association for Clinical Chemistry.

TABLE 18.13 Cerebrospinal Fluid Values of Healthy Term Newborns

COMPONENT	BIRTH TO 24 HOURS	1 DAY	7 DAYS
		AGE	
Color	Clear or xanthochromic	Clear or xanthochromic	Clear or xanthochromic
Red blood cells (cells/mm^3)	9 (0–1,070)	23 (6–630)	3 (0–48)
Polymorphonuclear leukocytes (cells/mm^3)	3 (0–70)	7 (0–26).	2 (0–5)
Lymphocytes (cells/mm^3)	2 (0–20)	5 (0–16)	1 (0–4)
Protein (mg/dL)	63 (32–240)	73 (40–148)	47 (27–65)
Glucose (mg/dL)	51 (32–78)	48 (38–64)	55 (48–62)
Lactate dehydrogenase (IU/L)	22–73	22–73	22–73

Source: Data from Klaus, M. H., & Fanaroff, A. A. (2002). *Neonatal–perinatal medicine: Diseases of the fetus and infant* (6th ed.). Mosby; Naidoo, B. T. (1968). A history of the Durban Medical School. *South African Medical Journal, 42,* 932; Neches, W., & Platt, M. (1968). Cerebrospinal fluid LDH in 257 children. *Pediatrics, 41,* 1097–1103. https://pediatrics.aappublications.org/content/41/6/1097

TABLE 18.14 Cerebrospinal Fluid Values in Very Low-Birthweight Infants on Basis of Birthweight

	≤1,000 G		1,001–1,500 G	
	MEAN ± SD	RANGE	MEAN ± SD	RANGE
Birthweight (g)	763 ± 115	550–980	1,278 ± 152	1,020–1,500
Gestational age (weeks)	26 ± 1.3	24–28	29 ± 1.4	27–33
Leukocytes/mm^3	4 ± 3	0–14	6 ± 9	0–44
Erythrocytes/mm^3	1,027 ± 3,270	0–19,050	786 ± 1,879	0–9,750
PMN leukocytes (%)	6 ± 15	0–66	9 ± 17	0–60
MN leukocytes (%)	86 ± 30	34–100	85 ± 28	13–100
Glucose (mg/dL)	61 ± 34	29–217	59 ± 21	31–109
Protein (mg/dL)	150 ± 56	95–370	132 ± 3	45–227

MN, mononuclear; PMN, polymorphonuclear.

Source: Modified from Rodriquez, A. F., Kaplan, S. L., & Mason, E. O. (1990). Cerebrospinal fluid values in the very low birth weight infant. *Journal of Pediatrics, 116,* 971–974. https://doi.org/10.1016/s0022-3476(05)80663-8

TABLE 18.15 Cerebrospinal Fluid Values in Very-Low-Birthweight Infants (1,001–1,500 g) by Chronologic Age

| | POSTNATAL AGE (DAYS) | | | | | |
| | 0–7 | | 8–28 | | 29–84 | |
COMPONENT	MEAN ± SD	RANGE	MEAN ± SD	RANGE	MEAN ± SD	Range
Birthweight (g)	1,428 ± 107	1,180–1,500	1,245 ± 162	1,020–1,480	1,211 ± 86	1,080–1,300
Gestational age at birth (wk)	31 ± 1.5	28–33	29 ± 1.2	27–31	29 ± 0.7	27–29
Leukocytes/mm³	4 ± 4	1–10	7 ± 11	0–44	8 ± 8	0–23
Erythrocytes/mm³	407 ± 853	0–2,450	1,101 ± 2,643	0–9,750	661 ± 1,198	0–3,800
PMN (%)	4 ± 10	0–28	10 ± 19	0–60	11 ± 19	0–48
Glucose (mg/dL)	74 ± 19	50–96	59 ± 23	39–109	47 ± 13	31–76
Protein (mg/dL)	136 ± 35	85–176	137 ± 46	54–227	122 ± 47	45–187

PMN, polymorphonuclear.

Source: Modified from Rodriquez, A. F., Kaplan, S. L., & Mason, E. O. (1990). Cerebrospinal fluid values in the very low birth weight infant. Journal of Pediatrics, 116, 971–974. https://doi.org/10.1016/s0022-3476(05)80663-8

TABLE 18.16 Thyroid Function in Full-Term and Preterm Infants

	SERUM T$_4$ CONCENTRATION IN PREMATURE AND TERM INFANTS					SERUM-FREE T$_4$ INDEX IN PREMATURE AND TERM INFANTS				
	ESTIMATED GESTATIONAL AGE (WEEKS)									
	30–31	32–33	34–35	36–37	TERM	30–31	32–33	34–35	36–37	TERM
Cord										
Mean	6.5*	7.5***	6.7***	7.5	8.2			5.6	5.6	5.9
SD	1	2.1	1.2	2.8	1.8			1.3	2	1.1
N	3	8	18	17	17			12	10	14
12–72 hours old										
Mean	11.5***	12.3***	12.4***	15.5**	19	13.1†	12.9†	15.5††	17.1	19.7
SD	2.1	3.2	3.1	2.6	2.1	2.4	2.7	3	3.5	3.5
N	12	18	17	15	6	12	14	14	14	6

(continued)

TABLE 18.16 Thyroid Function in Full-Term and Preterm Infants (continued)

	SERUM T₄ CONCENTRATION IN PREMATURE AND TERM INFANTS					SERUM-FREE T₄ INDEX IN PREMATURE AND TERM INFANTS				
	ESTIMATED GESTATIONAL AGE (WEEKS)									
	30–31	32–33	34–35	36–37	TERM	30–31	32–33	34–35	36–37	TERM
3–10 days old										
Mean	7.7**	8.5***	10***	12.7**	15.9	8.3†	9†	12†††	15.1	16.2
SD	1.8	1.9	2.4	2.5	3	1.9	1.8	2.3	0.7	3.2
N	7	8	9	9	29	6	9	5	4	11
11–20 days old										
Mean	7.5**	8.3***	10.5	11.2	12.2	8†	9.1†††	11.8	11.3	12.1
SD	1.8	1.6	1.8	2.9	2	1.6	1.9	2.7	1.9	2
N	5	11	9	9	8	5	8	8	5	8

21–45 days old									
Mean	7.8***	8***	9.3***	11.4	12.1	8.4‡	9†††	10.9	11.1
SD	1.5	1.7	1.3	4.2	1.5	1.4	1.6	2.8	1.4
N	11	17	13	5	5	11	17	5	5
46–90 days old		30–73 weeks					34–35 weeks		
Mean	9.6				10.2	9.4			9.7
SD	1.7				1.9	1.4			1.5
N	16				17	13			10

*p<.05
**p<.005
***p<.001
†p=.001
††p=.025
†††p=.01
‡p=.005

For comparison of premature and term infants (t test).

Source: Data from Cuestas, R. A. (1978). Thyroid function in healthy premature infants. *Journal of Pediatrics, 92*(6), 963–967. https://doi.org/10.1016/
(0022-3476/78/080378-3

REFERENCES

Cooke, R., Hollis, B., Conner, C., Watson, D., Werkman, S., & Chesney, R. (1990). Vitamin D and mineral metabolism in the very low birth weight infant receiving 400 IU of vitamin D. *Journal of Pediatrics, 116,* 423–428. https://doi.org/10.1016/s0022-3476(05)82837-9

Cornblath, M., & Schwartz, R. (Eds.). (1976). *Disorders of carbohydrate metabolism* (2nd ed.). WB Saunders.

Drummond, L. M. (1979). Creatine phosphokinase levels in the newborn and their use in screening for Duchenne muscular dystrophy. *Archives of Disease in Childhood, 54,* 362–366. https://doi.org/10.1136/adc.54.5.362

Fanaroff, A. A., & Martin, R. J. (2015). *Fanaroff and Martin's neonatal–perinatal medicine: Diseases of the fetus and infant* (10th ed.). Elsevier/Saunders.

Glass, L., Hume, R., Hendry, G. M. A., Strange, R., & Forfar, J. O. (1982). Plasma alkaline phosphatase activity in rickets of prematurity. *Archives of Disease in Childhood, 57,* 373–376. https://doi.org/10.1136/adc.57.5.373

Gomella, T. L., Eyal, F. G., & Bany-Mohammed, F. (2020). *Neonatology: Management, procedures, on-call problems, diseases, and drugs* (8th ed.). McGraw-Hill Professional.

Heck, L. J., & Erenberg, A. (1987). Serum glucose levels in the term neonate during the first 48 hours of life. *Pediatric Research, 110,* 119–122. https://doi.org/10.1016/s0022-3476(87)80303-7

Kenner, C., Altimier, L. B., & Boykova, M. V. (2020). *Comprehensive neonatal nursing care* (6th ed.). Springer Publishing Company.

Lichtenstein, P., Specker, B. L., Tsang, R. C., Mimouni, F., & Gormley, C. (1986). Calcium-regulating hormones and minerals from birth to 18 months of age: A cross-sectional study. I. Effects of sex, race, age, season, and diet on vitamin D status. *Pediatrics, 77,* 883–890. https://pediatrics.aappublications.org/content/77/6/883

Liebman, J., & Plonsey, R. (1977). Electrocardiography. In A. J. Moss, F. H. Adams, & G. C. Emmanouilides (Eds.), *Heart disease in infants, children and adolescents* (2nd ed.). Lippincott Williams & Wilkins.

Martin, R. J., Fanaroff, A. A., & Walsh, M. C. (Eds.). (2020). *Fanaroff & Martin's neonatal-perinatal medicine: Diseases of the fetus and infant* (12th ed.). Elsevier.

Meites, S. (1975). Normal total plasma calcium in the newborn. *Critical Reviews of Clinical Laboratory Science, 6,* 1–18. https://doi.org/10.3109/10408367509151562

Nelson, N., Finnstrom, O., & Larsson, L. (1987). Neonatal reference values for ionized calcium, phosphate, and magnesium: Selection of reference population by optimality criteria. *Scandinavian Journal of Clinical Laboratory Investigations, 47,* 111–117. https://doi.org/10.1080/00365518709168878

Shenai, J. P., Chytil, F., Jhaveri, A., & Stahlman, M. T. (1981). Plasma vitamin A and retinal binding protein in premature and term neonates. *Journal of Pediatrics, 99,* 302–305. https://doi.org/10.1016/s0022-3476(81)80484-2

Statland, B. E. (1979). Fundamental issues in clinical chemistry. *American Journal of Pathology, 95*(1), 243–272. https://www.ncbi.nlm.nih.gov/pmc/articles/PMC2042285

Tietz, N. W. (Ed.). (1988). *Textbook of clinical chemistry.* WB Saunders.

Wallach, J. B. (1983). *Interpretation of pediatric tests.* Little Brown.

19

Common Drugs: Medication Guide

BETH SHIELDS

OVERVIEW

Neonatal patients are not simply "small adults." This unique patient population has a need for specialized care, including the provision of safe and effective medication therapy. With approximately 8% of medications not labeled for use in the neonatal population, weight-based dosing and pharmacokinetic differences must be considered each time a medication is prescribed in this patient population.

MEDICATION GUIDE

Medication guides for commonly used medications in neonatal patients are outlined on the following pages.

TABLE 19.1 Neonatal Parenteral Medications

MEDICATION (GENERIC NAME)	CLINICAL INDICATION	MECHANISM OF ACTION	DOSE/FREQUENCY	COMMON IV COMPATIBILITIES	ADMINISTRATION INSTRUCTIONS/ COMMENTS
Acetaminophen	Analgesia/ antipyretic PDA closure	Inhibits prostaglandin synthesis in the central nervous system	10–15 mg/kg/dose PO/PR q4–6h scheduled or PRN (not to exceed 40–60 mg/kg/day in preterm infants and 90 mg/kg/day in term infants) 15 mg/kg/dose q6h IV (×3 days)	Compatible: dexamethasone, heparin, hydrocortisone, midazolam, morphine, vancomycin	Use with caution in infants with hepatic dysfunction Higher doses required per rectum versus orally
Acyclovir	Herpes simplex (HSV-1, HSV-2) infections	Inhibits viral DNA polymerase	20 mg/kg/dose IV q8h	Compatible: ampicillin, ceftazidime, dexamethasone, fentanyl, fluconazole, gentamicin, heparin Incompatible: dopamine, dobutamine	IV over 60 min
Ampicillin	Treatment of susceptible bacterial infections including sepsis/ meningitis, UTI prophylaxis		100 mg/kg/dose IV/IM ≤7 PND q12h <2 kg and >7 PND q12h >2 kg and >7 PND q6h	Compatible: calcium gluconate, famotidine, heparin Incompatible: dopamine, fentanyl, fluconazole, gentamicin, midazolam sodium bicarbonate	Slow IVP (not more than 100 mg/min) Larger doses for meningitis

Drug	Indication	Mechanism	Dose	Compatibility	Administration
Caffeine citrate	Apnea of prematurity	Central nervous system stimulant	Loading dose: 10 mg/kg/dose IV/PO (×1 dose) Maintenance dose: 7–10 mg/kg/dose IV/PO q24h	Compatible: calcium gluconate, gentamicin heparin, potassium chloride, fentanyl, dopamine, dobutamine, morphine Incompatible: furosemide, lorazepam, oxacillin	Maintenance dose 24 hr after loading dose Loading dose: IV over 30 min Maintenance dose IV: IV over 10–15 min
Ceftazidime	Treatment of susceptible bacterial infections including sepsis/meningitis	Inhibits bacterial wall synthesis	50 mg/kg/dose IV/IM ≤7 days q12h, >7 days and <1 kg q12h, >7 days and >1 kg q8h	Compatible: acyclovir, dobutamine, famotidine, heparin, morphine Incompatible: Fluconazole, midazolam, vancomycin	Central line: slow IVP 3–5 min Peripheral line: IV over 30 min
Chlorothiazide	Diuresis	Thiazide diuretic, inhibits chloride reabsorption in the distal tubule	PO: 10–20 mg/kg/dose q12–24h IV: 1–4 mg/kg/dose q12–24h	Compatible: potassium chloride, sodium bicarbonate Incompatible: ampicillin, gentamicin, vancomycin, oxacillin	IV and PO doses are not equivalent

(continued)

TABLE 19.1 Neonatal Parenteral Medications (continued)

MEDICATION (GENERIC NAME)	CLINICAL INDICATION	MECHANISM OF ACTION	DOSE/FREQUENCY	COMMON IV COMPATIBILITIES	ADMINISTRATION INSTRUCTIONS/ COMMENTS
Dexamethasone	Treatment and prevention of chronic lung disease	Enhance surfactant production, stabilize cell membranes, decrease pulmonary edema	0.5 mg/kg/day divided IV/ PO q12h (×6 doses); based on clinical indication, a variety of prolonged weaning schedules have been used	Compatible: caffeine, famotidine, fluconazole, furosemide, heparin, morphine, potassium chloride, sodium bicarbonate, vancomycin Incompatible: midazolam	Slow IVP over 1–3 min
Dobutamine	Increase myocardial contractility	Direct beta one agonist	2.5–20 mcg/kg/min continuous infusion; start low and titrate to response	Compatible: calcium gluconate, dopamine, epinephrine, morphine, potassium chloride, vancomycin Incompatible: heparin, piperacillin–tazobactam, sodium bicarbonate	Use large vein for IV administration; short half-life, so must be administered via continuous infusion
Dopamine	Hypotension secondary to decreased myocardial contractility	Direct beta agonist and release of norepinephrine from storage, alpha-mediated vasoconstriction	2.5–20 mcg/kg/min continuous infusion; start low and titrate to response	Compatible: epinephrine, gentamicin, heparin, midazolam, morphine, potassium chloride Incompatible: ampicillin, furosemide, sodium bicarbonate	Central line preferred; short half-life, so must be administered via continuous infusion

Drug	Use	Mechanism	Dosing	Compatibility	Comments
Fentanyl	Analgesia, sedation	Binds to opioid mu receptor	Intermittent dosing: 0.5–1 mcg/kg/dose q2–4h scheduled or PRN (titrate to response) Continuous infusion: 0.5–1 mcg/kg/hr (titrate to response)	Compatible: caffeine, dobutamine, epinephrine, furosemide, heparin, midazolam, morphine, potassium chloride	Rapid IVP doses may result in chest wall rigidity Use lower doses in nonventilated and/or opiate naive patients
Fluconazole	Prophylaxis and treatment of fungal infections	Inhibits cytochrome P450 in susceptible fungi, leading to decreased ergosterol and increased cell membrane permeability	Prophylaxis: 3 mg/kg/dose IV/PO (<1 kg infants with central lines) twice weekly (until central line out or patient 42 days of age) Systemic treatment: thrush—6 mg/kg/dose (×1) loading dose followed by 3 mg/kg/dose q24h Systemic treatment: 12 mg/kg/dose IV/PO q24h (consider larger loading dose)	Compatible: dexamethasone, dobutamine, gentamicin, heparin, hydrocortisone, midazolam, morphine, potassium chloride, vancomycin Incompatible: ampicillin, ceftriaxone, furosemide	IV over 60 min

(continued)

TABLE 19.1 Neonatal Parenteral Medications (continued)

MEDICATION (GENERIC NAME)	CLINICAL INDICATION	MECHANISM OF ACTION	DOSE/FREQUENCY	COMMON IV COMPATIBILITIES	ADMINISTRATION INSTRUCTIONS/ COMMENTS
Furosemide	Diuresis	Loop diuretic; inhibits resorption of sodium and chloride in the ascending loop of Henle	IV: 1 mg/kg/dose q8–24h PO: 1–2 mg/kg/dose q8–24h	Compatible: calcium gluconate, dexamethasone, dopamine, fentanyl, heparin Incompatible: dobutamine, gentamicin	Slow IVP; maximum rate 0.5 mg/kg/min
Gentamicin	Treatment of susceptible bacterial infections including sepsis, UTI	Inhibits cellular protein synthesis by binding to ribosomal subunits, inhibiting bacterial cell wall membranes	<700 g: 3 mg/kg/dose IV q36h 700–2,500 g: 3 mg/kg/dose IV q24h >2,500 g: 4 mg/kg/dose IV q24h All infants >34 weeks PCA: 4 mg/kg/dose IV q24h	Compatible: acyclovir, clindamycin, dopamine, famotidine, fentanyl, fluconazole, midazolam, morphine Incompatible: ampicillin, furosemide	IV over 30 min Prelevel (trough): immediately prior to dose (goal <1.5 mcg/ mL) Postlevel (peak): 60 min post end of 30-min infusion (6–10 mcg/mL)

Ibuprofen Lysine	Medical closure of PDA	Inhibit prostaglandin synthesis	≤32 wk GA and birthweight 500–1,500 g 10 mg/kg/dose (×1) initial dose Followed by 5 mg/kg/dose at 24 and 48 hrs after the first dose	<u>Compatible</u>: potassium chloride, sodium bicarbonate <u>Incompatible</u>: caffeine, furosemide, midazolam	IV over 15 min, monitor urine output prior to each dose
Indomethacin	Medical closure of PDA	Inhibit prostaglandin synthesis	0.2 mg/kg/dose IV (×1 dose) followed by two additional doses q12h (subsequent doses based on postnatal age) <48 hr: 0.1 mg/kg/dose 2–7 days: 0.2 mg/kg/dose >7 days: 0.25 mg/kg/dose	<u>Compatible</u>: furosemide, potassium chloride, sodium bicarbonate <u>Incompatible</u>: calcium gluconate, dobutamine, dopamine, fentanyl, gentamicin	IV over 30 min; monitor urine output, serum creatinine, and platelets prior to each dose
Midazolam	Sedation, amnesia	Binds to GABA receptor; inhibitory neurotransmitter	Intermittent dosing IV: 0.05–0.1 mg/kg/dose Continuous infusion: 0.03–0.1 mg/kg/hr Intranasal: 0.2 mg/kg/dose preprocedural	<u>Compatible</u>: calcium gluconate, dobutamine, dopamine, fluconazole, gentamicin <u>Incompatible</u>: ampicillin, dexamethasone, furosemide, sodium bicarbonate	Use lower doses in nonventilated and/or benzodiazepine-naive patients

(continued)

TABLE 19.1 Neonatal Parenteral Medications (*continued*)

MEDICATION (GENERIC NAME)	CLINICAL INDICATION	MECHANISM OF ACTION	DOSE/FREQUENCY	COMMON IV COMPATIBILITIES	ADMINISTRATION INSTRUCTIONS/ COMMENTS
Morphine	Analgesia, sedation	Binds to opiate receptors in the central nervous system	Intermittent dosing IV: 0.05–0.1 mg/kg/dose q4–8h scheduled or PRN Continuous infusion: 0.01–0.03 mg/kg/hr	<u>Compatible</u>: ampicillin, fluconazole, furosemide, midazolam, vancomycin <u>Incompatible</u>: phenobarbital, sodium bicarbonate	Use lower doses in nonventilated and/or opiate-naive patients Oral doses are typically higher than IV doses
Vancomycin	Treatment of susceptible bacterial infections including sepsis, pneumonia in skin and soft tissue	Inhibits cell wall synthesis by binding to cell wall precursors	<29 weeks PCA: 20 mg/kg/dose IV q24h 29–31 weeks PCA: 20 mg/kg/dose IV q18h >31–37 weeks PCA: 20 mg/kg/dose IV q12h >37 weeks PCA: 15 mg/kg/dose IV q8h	<u>Compatible</u>: calcium gluconate, dopamine, fentanyl, sodium bicarbonate	IV over 60 min Prelevel: immediately prior to dose 10–15 mcg/mL (lower trough concentrations can achieve desired AUC/MIC value based on specific infection)

GA, gestational age; GABA, gamma-aminobutyric acid; IM, intramuscular; IVP, intravenous push; PCA, postconceptional days; PDA, patent ductus arteriosus; PND, postnatal days; PO, orally; PR, rectally; PRN, as needed; q, every; UTI, urinary tract infection; AUC, area under the curve; MIC, minimum inhibitory concentration.

TABLE 19.2 Neonatal Emergency Parenteral Medications

MEDICATION (GENERIC NAME)	DOSAGE RANGE	CONCENTRATION	COMMENTS
Adenosine	0.1 mg/kg/dose	3 mg/mL	Administer rapid bolus over 1–2 sec; follow each bolus with normal saline flush
Atropine	0.02 mg/kg/dose	0.1 mg/mL	Some recommend no minimum dose in those less than 5 kg
Calcium gluconate	100 mg/kg/dose	100 mg/mL	Dilute with an equal volume of dextrose 5% in water injection prior to administration; may be given slow IVP through the central line during an arrest; for peripheral line, infuse over 60 min
Epinephrine (1:10,000)	0.01 mg/kg/dose	0.1 mg/mL	
Sodium bicarbonate	1–2 meq/kg/dose	0.5 meq/mL	

IVP, intravenous push.

TABLE 19.3 Recommended Immunization Schedule for Birth Through 18 Months (Based On Chronologic Age): United States, 2021

(Alternative schedule exists for catch-up immunizations—see the following table for specific recommendations.)

(Primary series as defined by immunizations given through 6 months of age)

√ = recommended administration age

VACCINE	BIRTH	1–2 MONTHS	2 MONTHS	4 MONTHS	6 MONTHS	6–18 MONTHS
HepB	√	√				√
DTaP			√	√	√	√[a]
Hib			√	√	√[b]	√[c]
PCV13			√	√	√	√[c]
IPV			√	√		√
RV (RV1 or RV5)			√	√	√[d]	

DTaP, diptheria, tetanus, and acellular pertussis; HepB, hepatitis B vaccine; Hib, haemophilus influenza type b; IPV, inactivated polio vaccine; PCV13, pneumococcal conjugate vaccine 13; RV, rotavirus vaccine: RV1 (Rotarix), RV5 (Rotateq).

[a]Fourth dose at 15–18 months.

[b]Two- or three-dose primary series depending on vaccine used in primary series (ActHIB, Hiberix, or Pentacel is a total four-dose series and PediavaxHib a total three-dose series.)

[c]Fourth dose at 12–15 months.

[d]RV5 only; RV1 is a two-dose primary series.

TABLE 19.4 Combination Vaccines (Vaccine Availability Will Vary With Formulary/Contracts)

(Use of combination vaccines generally preferred over separate injections of its equivalent component vaccines.)				
COMBINATION VACCINE BY BRAND NAME	HepB	DtaP	Hib	IPV
Pediarix	√	√		√
Pentacel		√	√	√
Kinrix Quadracel		√		√

DTaP, diptheria, tetanus, and acellular pertussis; HepB, hepatitis B vaccine; Hib, haemophilus influenza type b; IPV, inactivated polio vaccine.

TABLE 19.5 Recommended Catch-Up Immunization Schedule for Birth Through 18 Months (Based On Chronologic Age): United States, 2021

	MINIMUM INTERVAL BETWEEN DOSES 1 AND 2	MINIMUM INTERVAL BETWEEN DOSES 2 AND 3	ADDITIONAL COMMENTS
HepB	4 weeks	8 weeks (at least 16 weeks after the first dose)	Minimum age for the final dose is 24 weeks
DTaP	4 weeks	4 weeks	Minimum interval to doses 3 and 4 and 4 and 5 is 6 months
Hib	4 weeks if the first dose is before 12 months 8 weeks if the first dose is between 12 and 14 months	4 weeks if less than 12 months of age and first dose at less than 7 months 8 weeks if less than 12 months of age and the first dose at 7–11 months OR age 12–59 months and the first dose before the first birthday and the second dose at less than 15 months of age	If the first dose is at 15 months or older, no further doses

(continued)

TABLE 19.5 Recommended Catch-Up Immunization Schedule for Birth Through 18 Months (Based On Chronologic Age): United States, 2021 *(continued)*

	MINIMUM INTERVAL BETWEEN DOSES 1 AND 2	MINIMUM INTERVAL BETWEEN DOSES 2 AND 3	ADDITIONAL COMMENTS
PCV13	4 weeks if the first dose is before 12 months of age 8 weeks if the first dose is administered at or after 12 months of age	4 weeks if current age is less than 12 months and previous dose at less than 7 months of age 8 weeks if the previous dose is between 7 and 11 months of age OR 12 months of age or older and first dose before 12 months	No further doses for healthy children if the first dose is at 24 months or older
IPV	4 weeks	4 weeks (provided under 4 years of age)	
RV (RV1 or RV5)	4 weeks, maximum age for the first dose is 14 weeks, 6 days	4 weeks	Maximum age for the final dose is 8 months, 0 days

DTaP, diptheria, tetanus, and acellular pertussis; HepB, hepatitis B vaccine; Hib, haemophilus influenza type b; IPV, inactivated polio vaccine; PCV13, pneumococcal conjugate vaccine 13; RV, rotavirus vaccine: RV1 (Rotarix), RV5 (Rotateq).

REFERENCES

Centers for Disease Control and Prevention. (2021). *Advisory Committee on Immunization Practices (ACIP)*. https://www.cdc.gov/vaccines/acip/index.html

Centers for Disease Control and Prevention. (2021a). *Recommended child and adolescent immunization schedule for ages 18 years or younger.* https://www.cdc.gov/vaccines/schedules/downloads/child/0-18yrs-child-combined-schedule.pdf

Centers for Disease Control and Prevention. (2021b). *Advisory Committee on Immunization Practices (ACIP)Table 2. Catch-up immunization schedule for person ages 4 months–18 years who start late or who are more than 1 month behind, United States, 2021.* https://www.cdc.gov/vaccines/schedules/hcp/imz/catchup.html

Kroger, A., Bahta, L., & Hunter, P. (2021, May 4). *General best practice guidelines for immunization.* https://www.cdc.gov/vaccines/hcp/acip-recs/general-recs/index.html

Taketomo, C. K., Hodding, J. H., & Kraus, D. M. (2021). *Pediatric and neonatal dosage handbook* (28th ed.). Lexi-Comp.

IV

Appendices

Appendices

A

Common Abbreviations

CAROLE KENNER

25OHD	25-hydroxyvitamine D
4Ps	Parents, Partner, Past, and Present
AAFP	American Academy of Family Practice
AAP	American Academy of Pediatrics
AASM	American Academy of Sleep Medicine
ABE	acute bilirubin encephalopathy
ABG	arterial blood gas
ABR	auditory brainstem response
ACE	angiotensin-converting enzyme
ACE	adverse childhood experience
ACOG	American College of Obstetricians and Gynecologists
ADLs	activities of daily living
AED	automated external defibrillator
aEEG	amplitude-integrated electroencephalogram
AFP	alpha-fetoprotein
AHA	American Heart Association
AIDS	acquired immunodeficiency syndrome
ALP	alkaline phosphatase
AMA	American Medical Association
AOP	apnea of prematurity
AP	anteroposterior
ARC	Australian Resuscitation Council
ARF	acute renal failure
ARPKD	autosomal recessive polycystic kidney disease
ART	antiretroviral therapy
AS	aortic stenosis
ASD	atrial septal defect
ASD	autism spectrum disorder
ASSIST	Alcohol, Smoking, and Substance Involvement Screening Test
ATN	acute tubular necrosis
AUDIT–C	Alcohol Use Disorders Identification Test–Concise

AV	atrioventricular
BG	blood gas
BPD	bronchopulmonary dysplasia
BPS	bronchopulmonary sequestration
BUN	blood urea nitrogen
C	centigrade or Celsius
C3	cervical vertebra at location three
C5	cervical vertebra at location five
C7	cervical vertebra at location seven
CAT	computed axial tomography
CAUDI	catheter-associated urinary tract infection
CBC	complete blood count
cc	cubic centimeter
CCAM	cystic adenomatous malformation
CCHD	critical congenital heart disease
CCK	cholecystokinin
CDC	Centers for Disease Control and Prevention
CDH	congenital diaphragmatic hernia
CFTR	cystic fibrosis transmembrane conductance regulator
CFU	colony-forming units
CGH	comparative genomic hybridization
CHARGE	coloboma, heart defects, atresia of the choanae, retardation of growth and development, genital/urinary abnormalities, ear abnormalities, and/or hearing deficit
CHD	congenital heart disease
CHF	congestive heart failure
CIC	clean intermittent catheterization
CL	chloride
CLABSI	central line-associated bloodstream infection
CLAP	chicken pox, lyme disease, acquired immunodeficiency syndrome, parvovirus B9
CLAR	Council of Latin America for Resuscitation
CLD	chronic lung disease
cm	centimeter
CMA	chromosomal microarray
CMV	cytomegalovirus
CNS	central nervous system
CO_2	carbon dioxide
COA	coarctation of the aorta
CoE	center of expertise
COINN	Council of International Neonatal Nurses, Inc.
CoSTR	Cardiovascular Care Science with Treatment Recommendations
COVID-19	coronavirus disease 2019

CPAM	congenital pulmonary airway malformation
CPAP	continuous positive airway pressure
CPC	choroid plexus cauterization
CPM	congenital pulmonary malformation
CPR	cardiopulmonary resuscitation
CRAFFT	car, relax, alone, forget, friends, trouble
CRIES	crying, requires increased oxygen administration, increased vital signs, expression, sleeplessness
CRP	C-reactive protein
CSF	cerebrospinal fluid
CT	computed tomography
CVC	central venous catheter
CVL	central venous line
CVP	central venous pressure
CXR	chest x-ray
D	daily
DA	ductus arteriosus
DAT	direct antiglobulin test
dB	decibel
DEXA	dual-energy x-ray absorptiometry
DIC	disseminated intravascular coagulation
dL	deciliter
DMSA	dimercaptosuccinic acid
DNA	deoxyribonucleic acid
DPS	developmental participating skills
DTaP	diphtheria tetanus and acellular pertussis
DTPA	diethylenetriaminepentaacetic acid
DV	ductus venous
EA	esophageal atresia
EBF	erythroblastosis fetalis
EBM	expressed breast milk
ECD	endocardial cushion defect
ECG	electrocardiogram
ECMO	extracorporeal membrane oxygenation
EEG	electroencephalogram
EI	early intervention
EKG	electrocardiogram
ELBW	extremely low birthweight
ELS	extrapulmonary sequestration
EM	errors of metabolism
EMR	electronic medical record
ENS	enteric nervous system
EOS	early-onset sepsis

ERC	European Resuscitation Council
ESC	Eat, Sleep, Console
ESPGHAN	European Society for Pediatric Gastroenterology, Hepatology, and Nutrition
ETT	endotracheal tube
ETV	endoscopic third ventriculostomy
EVD	external ventricular device
FAPSBA	folic acid-preventable spina bifida and anencephaly
FCC	family-centered care
FDA	U.S. Food and Drug Administration
FeNa	fractional excretion of sodium
FFP	fresh frozen plasma
FICare	family integrated care
FISH	fluorescence in situ hybridization
FLACC	face, legs, activity, cry, consolability
FNAST	Finnegan Neonatal Abstinence Scoring Tool
FNI	family nurture intervention
FO	foramen ovale
FOC	frontal-occipital circumference
FR	French
FRC	function residual capacity
FTC	foot candle
g	gram
G6PD	glucose-6-phosphate dehydrogenase
GA	gestational age
GABA	gamma-aminobutryic acid
GDM	gestational diabetes mellitus
GER	gastroesophageal reflux
GERD	gastroesophageal reflux disease
GFR	glomerular filtration rate
GI	gastrointestinal
GJ	gastrojejunal
GLANCE	global alliance for newborn care
GM-IVH	germinal matrix intraventricular hemorrhage
G.R.A.C.E.	gathering attention, recalling intention, attuning to self and other, considering what will serve in the moment, engaging and ending
GU	genitourinary
H2	histamine-2
HAEC	Hirschsprung-associated enterocolitis
HALs	hospital-acquired infections
Hb	hemoglobin
HBV	hepatitis B vaccine
HC	head circumference

Hct	hematocrit
HepB	hepatitis B
HFNC	high-flow nasal cannula
Hg	mercury
Hib	hemophilus influenza type B
HIDA	hepatoiminodiacetic acid
HIE	hypoxic–ischemic encephalopathy
HIV	human immunodeficiency virus
HLHS	hypoplastic left heart syndrome
HM	human milk
HPA	hypothalamic pituitary adrenal
HSFC	Heart and Stroke Foundation of Canada
HSV-1	herpes simplex virus 1
HSV-2	herpes simplex virus 2
HUS	head ultrasound
HVAC	heating, ventilation, and air-conditioning
I&O	intake and output
IC	intracranial
ICP	increased intracranial pressure
ICU	intensive care unit
IDC	integrative developmental care
IDM	infant of a diabetic mother or idiopathic diabetes mellitus
IEM	inborn errors of metabolism (or errors of metabolism)
IFCDC	infant family-centered developmental care
IgA	immunoglobulin A
IgB	immunoglobulin B
IgD	immunoglobulin D
IgE	immunoglobulin E
IgM	immunoglobulin M
IHPS	infantile hypertrophic pyloric stenosis
IL	interleukin
ILCOR	International Liaison Committee on Resuscitation
ILS	intrapulmonary sequestration
IM	intramuscular
iNO	inhaled nitrous oxide
IO	intraosseous
IPAT	Infant Position Assessment Tool
IPHS	intraparenchymal hemorrhages
IPV	inactivated polio vaccine
IR	interventional radiologist
IRF	intrinsic renal failure
IU	international unit
IUGR	intrauterine growth restriction

IV	intravenous
IVC	inferior vena cava
IVH	intraventricular hemorrhage
IVIG	intravenous immunoglobulin
IVP	intravenous push
IWL	insensible water loss
J	jejunostomy
K	potassium
KC	kangaroo care
kcal	kilocalorie
kg	kilogram
KMC	kangaroo mother care
L	left
L	liter
L3	lumbar vertebrae at location three
L5	lumbar vertebra at location five
LCT	long-chain triglyceride
LES	lower esophageal sphincter
LFT	liver function test
LGA	large for gestational age
LGEA	long-gap esophageal atresia
LHR	lung area-to-head circumference ratio
LLSB	lower left sternal border
LMA	laryngeal mask airway
LOS	late-onset sepsis
LP	lumbar puncture
MAS	meconium aspiration syndrome
MBD	metabolic bone disease
MBS	modified barium swallow
mcEq	microequivalent
mcg	microgram
MCH	mean corpuscular hemoglobin
MCHC	mean corpuscular hemoglobin concentration
mcmol	micromol
MCT	medium-chain triglyceride
MCV	mean corpuscular volume
MD	medical doctor
mEq	milliequivalents
mg	milligram
MII	multichannel intraluminal impedance
MII-pH	multichannel intraluminal impedance-potential of hydrogen
min	minute
MKD	multicystic kidney disease

mL	milliliter
mmol	millimoles
mo	month
mOsm	milliosmoles
M/P	milk-to-plasma ratio
MRI	magnetic resonance imaging
MRS	magnetic resonance spectroscopy
MSAF	meconium-stained amniotic fluid
NA	sodium
NALS	neonatal advanced life support
NANN	National Association of Neonatal Nurses
NAS	neonatal abstinence syndrome
NAVA	neurally adjusted ventilatory assist
NC	nasal cannula
NEC	necrotizing enterocolitis
NICU-MT	neonatal intensive care unit music therapists
NIDCAP	newborn individualized developmental care and assessment program
NG	nasogastric
NGT	nasogastric tube
NIH	National Institutes of Health
NIPPV	noninvasive positive pressure ventilation
NMD	neuronal migration disorder
NNS	nonnutritive sucking
NOWS	neonatal opioid withdrawal syndrome
NP	nurse practitioner
NPI	neuroprotective interventions
NPO	nothing per os (by mouth)
NRC	noise reduction coefficients
NREM	nonrapid eye movement
NS	normal saline
NS	nutritive sucking
NSAID	nonsteroidal anti-inflammatory drug
NTD	neural tube defect
NTE	neutral thermal environment
NZRC	New Zealand Resuscitation Council
O/E LHR	expected lung-to-head ratio
OFC	occipital frontal circumference
OG	orogastric
OR	operating room
ORL	otolaryngology
oz	ounce
PA	pulmonary artery

PaCO$_2$	partial arterial pressure of carbon dioxide
PaO$_2$	partial arterial pressure of oxygen
PAPVR	partial anomalous pulmonary venous return
PCA	postconceptional day
PCO$_2$	partial pressure of carbon dioxide
PCV 13	pneumococcal conjugate vaccine 13
PDA	patent ductus arteriosus
PDR	physicians' desk reference
P:E	protein to energy
PEEP	positive end-expiratory pressure
PEG	percutaneous endoscopic gastrostomy
PET	positron emission tomography
PFO	patent foramen ovale
PG	phosphatidylglycerol
PGE	prostaglandin E
pH	potential of hydrogen
PHVD	posthemorrhagic ventricular dilatation
PICC	peripherally inserted central catheter
PIE	pulmonary interstitial emphysema
PIPP	premature infant pain profile
PIV	peripheral intravenous
PMI	point of maximal intensity
PND	postnatal day
PO	per os (by mouth)
PO$_2$	partial pressure of oxygen
POD	postoperative day
POPPI	psychological outcomes, preventative psychological intervention
POS	pulse oximetry screening
PPB	pleuropulmonary blastoma
PPE	personal protective equipment
PPHN	persistent pulmonary hypertension
PPI	proton pump inhibitor
PPV	positive pressure ventilation
PR	per rectum (or rectally)
PRBC	packed red blood cells
PRN	pro re nata (as needed)
PROM	prolonged rupture of membranes
PS	pulmonary stenosis
PTH	parathyroid hormone
PTS	posttraumatic stress
PTSD	posttraumatic stress disorder
PTSS	posttraumatic stress symptoms
PUV	post-urethral valves

PVC	polyvinyl chloride
PVHI	periventricular hemorrhagic infarction
PVL	periventricular leukomalacia
PVR	pulmonary vascular resistance
q	every
QRS	Q wave, R wave, S wave
QUS	quantitative ultrasound
R	right
RBC	red blood cell
RCSA	Resuscitation Council of Southern Africa
RCT	randomized controlled trial
RDS	respiratory distress syndrome
REM	rapid eye movement
RH	relative humidity
RH	right hand
RID	relative infant dose
RN	registered nurse
RNA	ribonucleic acid
ROP	retinopathy of prematurity
RQI	resuscitation quality improvement
RSV	respiratory syncytial virus
RT-PCR	reverse transcription polymerase chain reaction
RUSP	recommended uniform screening panel
RV	rotavirus vaccine
RV	1-rotarix
RV	5-rotateq
S1	sacral vertebra at location one
S2	second heart sound
SACHDNC	Secretary's Advisory Committee on Heritable Disorders in Newborn and Children
SAH	subarachnoid hemorrhage
SAIE	subacute infective endocarditis
SAM	sympathetic adrenal medullary
SAMHSA	Substance Abuse and Mental Health Services Administration
SARS-CoV2	Severe Acute Respiratory Syndrome Coronavirus 2
SBS	short bowel syndrome
SDF	supported diagonal flexion
SDG	sustainable development goal
SEM	systolic ejection murmur
SFRs	single-family rooms
SIDS	sudden infant death syndrome
SIP	spontaneous intestinal perforation
SiPAP	sign positive airway pressure

SP-A	surfactant protein A
SP-B	surfactant protein B
SPECT	single photon emission computed tomography
SpO_2	peripheral capillary oxygen saturation
spp	species plurali
SSB	suck, swallow, breathe
SSC	skin-to-skin contact
SSP	safe sleep practices
SSRIs	selective serotonin receptor inhibitors
S.T.A.B.L.E.	sugar, temperature, airway, blood pressure, lab work, and emotional support
SUID	sudden unexpected infant death
SVC	superior vena cava
T1	thoracic vertebra at location one
T6–T9	thoracic vertebra at location six through nine
TA	tricuspid atresia
TA	truncus arteriosus
T-ACE	Tolerance, Annoyance, Cut-down, Eye-opener
TBS	tracheobronchoscopy
TcB	transcutaneous bilirubin
TEF	tracheoesophageal fistula
TEWL	transepidermal water loss
TGA	transposition of the great arteries
TIP	trauma informed professional
TN	Tennessee
TOF	tetralogy of Fallot
TORCHES	toxoplasma gondii, rubella, cytomegalovirus, herpes
TPA	tissue plasminogen activator
TPH	transplacental hemorrhage
TRP	tubular reabsorption of phosphorus
TSB	total serum bilirubin
TTN	transient tachypnea of the newborn
TV	tidal volume
UAC	umbilical arterial catheter
UGI	upper gastrointestinal
UHC	universal healthcare
ULSB	upper left sternal border
UNCRC	United Nations Convention on the Rights of the Child
UNICEF	United Nations International Children's Emergency Fund
UPJ	ureterovesical junction
US	ultrasound
USDHHS	U.S. Department of Health and Human Services
UTI	urinary tract infection

UVC   umbilical venous catheter

VACTERL   vertebral defects, anal atresia, cardiac defects, tracheoesophageal fistula, esophageal defects, renal and limb abnormalities

VAP   ventilator-associated pneumonia

VATER   vertebral defects, anal atresia, tracheosophageal fistula, renal and radial-thumb side dysplasia

VCUG   voiding cystourethrogram

VP   ventricular peritoneal

VQ   ventilation/perfusion ratio

VS   vital signs

VSD   ventricular septal defect

Vt   volume in a section or the lung-tidal volume

WBC   white blood cell

WHO   World Health Organization

wk   week

WMI   white matter injury

wt   weight

X   times

x-ray   x-radiation for diagnostic images

Expected Increases in Weight, Length/Height, and Head Circumference in the First Year of Life

PARAMETER	AGE (MONTHS)	EXPECTED INCREASE
Weight	Birth to 3	25–35 g/d
	3–6	12–21 g/d
	6–12	10–13 g/d
Length/height	Birth to 12	25 cm/y
OFC	Birth to 3	2 cm/mo
	4–6	1 cm/mo
	7–12	0.5 cm/mo

OFC, occipito frontal circumference.

Source: Data from Ditmyer, S. (2004). Hydrocephalus. In P. J. Allen & J. A. Vessey (Eds.), *Primary care of the child with a chronic condition* (4th ed., pp. 543–560). Mosby; Grover, G. (2000). Nutriitional needs. In C. D. Berkowitz (Ed.), *Pediatrics: A primary care approach* (2nd ed.). Saunders.

Conversion Table to Standard International (SI) Units

COMPONENT	PRESENT UNIT	×	CONVERSION FACTOR	=	SI UNIT
Clinical Hematology					
Erythrocytes	per mm^3		1		10^6/L
Hematocrit	%		0.01		(1)vol RBC/ vol whole blood
Hemoglobin	g/dL		10		g/L
Leukocytes	per mm^3		1		10^6/L
Mean corpuscular hemoglobin concentration (MCHC)	g/dL		10		g/L
Mean corpuscular volume (MCV)	mc/m^3		1		fL
Platelet count	10^3/mm^3		1		10^9/L
Reticulocyte count	%		10		10^{-3}
Clinical Chemistry					
Acetone	mg/dL		0.1722		mmol/L
Albumin	g/dL		10		g/L
Aldosterone	ng/dL		27.74		pmol/L

(continued)

COMPONENT	PRESENT UNIT	×	CONVERSION FACTOR	=	SI UNIT
Ammonia (as nitrogen)	mcg/dL		0.7139		mcmol/L
Bicarbonate	mEq/L		1		mmol/L
Bilirubin	mg/dL		17.1		mcmol/L
Calcium	mg/dL		0.2495		mmol/L
Calcium ion	mEq/L		0.50		mmol/L
Carotenes	mcg/dL		0.01836		mcmol/L
Ceruloplasmin	mg/dL		10		mg/L
Chloride	mEq/L		1		mmol/L
Cholesterol	mg/dL		0.02586		mmol/L
Complement, C_3 or C_4	mg/dL		0.01		g/L
Copper	mcg/dL		0.1574		mcmol/L
Cortisol	mcg/dL		27.59		nmol/L
Creatine	mg/dL		76.25		mcmol/L
Creatinine	mg/dL		88.40		mcmol/L
Digoxin	ng/mL		1.281		nmol/L
Epinephrine	pg/mL		5.458		pmol/L
Fatty acids	mg/dL		10		mg/L
Ferritin	ng/mL		1		mcg/L
□-Fetoprotein	ng/mL		1		mcg/L
Fibrinogen	mg/dL		0.01		g/L
Folate	ng/mL		2.266		nmol/L
Fructose	mg/dL		0.05551		mmol/L

COMPONENT	PRESENT UNIT	×	CONVERSION FACTOR	=	SI UNIT
Galactose	mg/dL		0.05551		mmol/L
Gases					
PO$_2$	mmHg (= torr)		0.1333		kPa
PCO$_2$	mmHg (= torr)		0.1333		kPa
Glucagon	pg/mL		1		ng/L
Glucose	mg/dL		0.05551		mmol/L
Glycerol	mg/dL		0.1086		mmol/L
Growth hormone	ng/mL		1		mcg/L
Haptoglobin	mg/dL		0.01		g/L
Hemoglobin	g/dL		10		g/L
Insulin	mcg/L		172.2		pmol/L
	mU/L		7.175		pmol/L
Iron	mcg/dL		0.1791		mcmol/L
Iron-binding capacity	mcg/dL		0.1791		mcmol/L
Lactate	mEq/L		1		mmol/L
Lead	mcg/dL		0.04826		mcmol/L
Lipoproteins	mg/dL		0.02586		mmol/L
Magnesium	mg/dL		0.4114		mmol/L
	mEq/L		0.50		mmol/L
Osmolality	mOsm/kg H$_2$O		1		mmol/kg H$_2$O
Phenobarbital	mg/dL		43.06		mcmol/L

(continued)

COMPONENT	PRESENT UNIT	×	CONVERSION FACTOR	=	SI UNIT
Phenytoin	mg/L		3.964		mcmol/L
Phosphate	mg/dL		0.3229		mmol/L
Potassium	mEq/L		1		mmol/L
	mg/dL		0.2558		mmol/L
Protein	g/dL		10		g/L
Pyruvate	mg/dL		113.6		mcmol/L
Sodium ion	mEq/L		1		mmol/L
Steroids					
17-hydroxy-corticosteroids	mg/24 hr		2.759		mcmol/day
17-ketosteroids	mg/24 hr		3.467		mcmol/day
Testosterone	ng/mL		3.467		nmol/L
Theophylline	mg/L		5.550		mcmol/L
Thyroid tests					
Thyroid-stimulating hormone	mcU/mL		1		mU/L
Thyroxine (T_4)	mcg/dL		12.87		nmol/L
Thyroxine free	ng/dL		12.87		pmol/L
Triiodothyronine (T_3)	ng/dL		0.01536		nmol/L
Transferrin	mg/dL		0.01		g/L
Triglycerides	mg/dL		0.01129		mmol/L
Urea nitrogen	mg/dL		0.3570		mmol/L
Uric acid (urate)	mg/dL		59.48		mcmol/L

(continued)

COMPONENT	PRESENT UNIT	×	CONVERSION FACTOR	=	SI UNIT
Vitamin A (retinol)	mcg/dL		0.03491		mcmol/L
Vitamin B12	pg/mL		0.7378		pmol/L
Vitamin C (ascorbic acid)	mg/dL		56.78		mcmol/L
Vitamin D					
Cholecalciferol	mcg/mL		2.599		nmol/L
25 OH-cholecalciferol	ng/mL		2.496		nmol/L
Vitamin E (alphatocopherol)	mg/dL		23.22		mcmol/L
d-xylose	mg/dL		0.06661		mmol/L
Zinc	mcg/dL		0.1530		mcmol/L
Energy	kcal		4.1868		kJ (kilojoule)
Blood pressure	mmHg (= torr)		1.333		mbar

Source: Modified from Young, D. S. (1987). Implementation of SI units for clinical laboratory data. Style specifications and conversion tables. *Annuals of Internal Medicine, 106,* 114.

International Standards for Newborn Weight, Length, and Head Circumference by Gestational Age and Sex

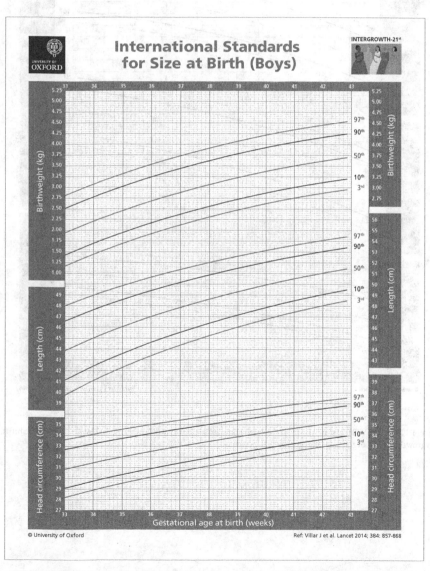

Source: INTERGROWTH-21st newborn size at birth standards. Courtesy of Intergrowth-21st © 2009–2021. https://intergrowth21.tghn.org/articles/category/global-perinatal-package

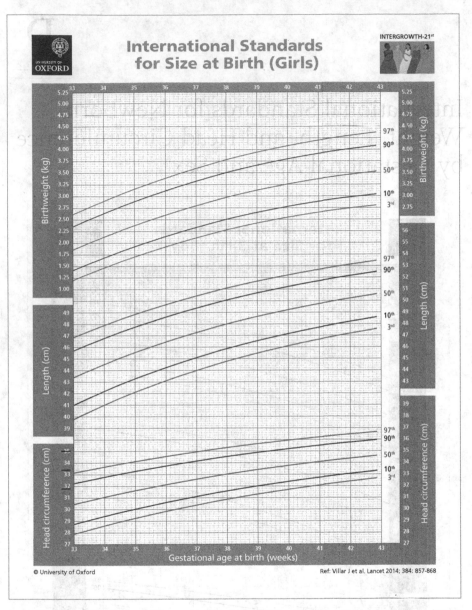

Source: INTERGROWTH-21st newborn size at birth standards. Courtesy of Intergrowth-21st © 2009–2021. https://intergrowth21.tghn.org/articles/category/global-perinatal-package

WEB AND OTHER RESOURCES (SELECTED)

BILIRUBIN

BiliTool™: www.BiliTool.org
Cochrane Library: www.cochranelibrary.com
PICK (Parents of Infants and Children With Kernicterus): pic-k.org

BREASTFEEDING

Baby Friendly USA: www.babyfriendlyusa.org/news/
    the-ten-steps-passed-the-tipping-point-and-moving-forward
Global Breastfeeding Collective: www.who.int/nutrition/topics/
    global-breastfeeding-collective/en
IBCLC: International Board of Certified Lactation Consultants: iblce.org
International Lactation Consultant Association (ILCA): ilca.org/neo-bfhi
La Leche League International: www.llli.org/resources

CARDIAC SYSTEM

American Academy of Pediatrics Website. Newborn Screening for CCHD.
    Answers and Resources for Primary Care Pediatricians: www.aap.org/
    en-us/advocacy-and-policy/aap-health-initiatives/PEHDIC/Pages/
    Newborn-Screening-for-CCHD.aspx
Centers for Disease Control and Prevention (CDC). Congenital Heart Defects.
    Information for Health Care Providers: www.cdc.gov/ncbddd/heartdefects/
    hcp.html
Tennessee Department of Health. Protocol for Critical Congenital Heart
    Disease (CCHD) Screening: https://www.tn.gov/content/dam/tn/health/
    documents/CCHD_Screening_Protocol_Algorithm.pdf

FAMILY-CENTERED CARE

Infant Family Centered Developmental Care (IFCDC): Developmental Care Standards for Infants in Intensive Care: nicudesign.nd.edu/nicu-care-standards

Institute for Patient and Family Centered Care: www.ipfcc.org

HEARING

American Speech-Language-Hearing Association (ASHA): www.asha.org/practice-portal/professional-issues/childhood-hearing-screening

Centers for Disease Control and Prevention (CDC). Hearing Loss in Children: Parent's Guide: www.cdc.gov/ncbddd/hearingloss/parentsguide/understanding/newbornhearingscreening.html

HYDROCELES

Mayo Clinic Web: www.mayoclinic.org/diseases-conditions/hydrocele/basics/definition/con-20024139

INFANT MENTAL HEALTH

World Association for Infant Mental Health: https://waimh.org

Zero to Three: Infant and Early Childhood Mental Health: www.zerotothree.org/espanol/infant-and-early-childhood-mental-health

INFECTIONS

Centers for Disease Control and Prevention (CDC). Evaluation and Management of Neonates at Risk for COVID-19: www.cdc.gov/coronavirus/2019-ncov/hcp/caring-for-newborns.html

Sepsis Alliance: www.sepsisalliance.org/sepsis_and/children

World Health Organization (WHO). *Pocket Book of Hospital Care for Children: Second Edition: Guidelines for the Management of Common Childhood Illness*: www.who.int/maternal_child_adolescent/documents/child_hospital_care/en

INTERNATIONAL GROWTH CURVES

International Growth Curves: intergrowth21.tghn.org

KANGAROO MOTHER CARE

Healthy Newborn Network: www.healthynewbornnetwork.org/topic/
kangaroo-mother-care-kmc
Kangaroo Mother Care: kangaroomothercare.com

LOW RESOURCE COUNTRIES' RESOURCES

medicalguidelines.msf.org/viewport/EssDr/english/glucose-10-dextrose
-10-16688182.html#:~:text=%E2%80%93%20If%20ready%2Dmade%20
10%25,obtain%20a%2010%25%20glucose%20solution
www.bsuh.nhs.uk/wp-content/uploads/sites/5/2016/09/Glucose
-concentration-guide.pdf

NEONATAL RESUSCITATION AND LIFE SUPPORT PROGRAMS

American Academy of Pediatrics: Life Support Programs: www
.aap.org/en-us/continuing-medical-education/life-support/pages/life
-support.aspx

PARENT SUPPORT

Alliance for Black NICU Families: www.blacknicufamilies.org
European Foundation for the Care of Newborn Infants: www.efcni.org
Miracle Babies Foundation: www.miraclebabies.org.au
NICU Parent Network (NPN): nicuparentnetwork.org
Preemie Crystal Ball: crystalballhealth.com
Preemie World: preemieworld.com

PICC LINE

Association for Vascular Access: www.avainfo.org
Infusion Nurses Society (INS): www.ins1.org
PICC Placement in the Neonate NEJM (*New England Journal of Medicine*):
www.youtube.com/watch?v=BgQOZDvm2FE

POSITIONING

Developmentally Supportive Infant Positioning-Supine: Philips Healthcare:
www.youtube.com/watch?v=MfwaGLUj9PA

Wiley, F., Raphael, R., & Ghanouni, P. (2019). NICU positioning strategies to reduce stress in preterm infants: A scoping review. *Early Child Development and Care*. www.tandfonline.com/doi/abs/10.1080/03004430.2019.1707815?journalCode=gecd20

PROFESSIONAL NEONATAL NURSING ASSOCIATIONS

Academy of Neonatal Nurses (ANN): www.academyonline.org
Alliance for Global Neonatal Nursing (ALIGNN): Comprised of ANN, AWHONN, C4HN, COINN, and NANN: malamaonakeiki.org/media/pdf/alignn.pdf
Association of Neonatal Nurses-Kenya (ANNK): no website
Association of Women's Health, Obstetric and Neonatal Nurses (AWHONN): www.awhonn.org
Australian College of Neonatal Nurses (ACNN): www.acnn.org.au
Canadian Association of Neonatal Nurses (CANN): nna.org.uk
Caring for Hawai'i Neonates (C4HN): https://malamaonakeiki.org
Council of International Neonatal Nurses, Inc. (COINN): www.coinnurses.org
Finnish Neonatal Nurses Association: website
Innovation & Research Neonatal Nurses Netherlands: no website
Japanese Neonatal Nurses Association: www.jann.gr.jp
National Association of Neonatal Nurses (NANN): www.nann.org
Nederlandse Vereniging voor Kindergeneeskunde: (Denmark): www.nvk.nl
Neonatal Nurses Association of Southern Africa: nnasa.org.za
Neonatal Nurses Association (NNA) of the United Kingdom: nna.org.uk
Neonatal Nurses College Aotearoa: (New Zealand): www.nzno.org.nz/groups/colleges_sections/colleges/neonatal_nurses_college
Neonatal Nurses for Healthy Lebanese Preterms: no website
Neonatoloji Hemsireligi Dernegi (Turkey): no website
Russian Nurses Association (RNA): medsestre.ru/
Rwanda Association of Neonatal Nurses (RANN): no website
Sociedad Espanola de Enfermeria Neonatal (no website)
Scottish Neonatal Nurses Group (no website)
*Associations without websites can be contacted through COINN at www.coinnurses.org

RESPIRATORY

American Cleft Palate-Craniofacial Association: acpa-cpf.org/acpa-members
Children's Choanal Atresia Foundation: Choanalatresia.org/aboutccaf.html
MedCalc: Acid-Base Calculator: www.medcalc.com/acidbase.html
MEDNA: Center for Research, Education, Quality & Safety: mednax.cloud-cme.com/default.aspx

MEDNAX: www.pediatrix.com/PediatrixUniversity
Neonatal Educational Resources.org: neonatalgoldenhours.org/
NICUniversity for many respiratory neonatal topics: www.nicuniversity.org

RESUSCITATION

American Academy of Pediatrics (AAP): Neonatal Resuscitation Program:
www.aap.org/nrp
Croop, S. E. W., Thoyre, S. M., Aliaga, S., McCaffrey, M. J., & Peter-Wohl, S.
(2020). The golden hour: A quality improvement initiative for extremely
premature infants in the neonatal intensive care unit. *Journal of
Perinatology, 40*(3), 530–539. www.ncbi.nlm.nih.gov/pmc/articles/
PMC7222905
The S.T.A.B.L.E® Program (Park City, Utah): stableprogram.org

SKIN CARE

Lund, C., & Kuller, J. (2019) The integumentary system. In C. Kenner,
L. Altimier, & M. Boykova (Eds.), *Comprehensive neonatal nursing care*
(6th ed.). Springer Publishing Company.

TRACHEOESOPHAGEAL FISTULA/ESOPHAGEAL ATRESIA

Boston Children's Hospital: Tracheoesophageal Fistula: www.childrens
hospital.org/conditions-and-treatments/conditions/t/
tracheoesophageal-fistula
Children's Hospital of Philadelphia (CHOP): Esophageal Atresia and
Tracheoesophageal Fistula (EA/TEF): www.chop.edu/conditions
-diseases/esophageal-atresia-and-tracheoesophageal-fistula
-eatef
TOFS, a U.K.-based charity providing emotional support to families of children born with tracheo-oesophageal fistula (TOF), esophageal atresia, and
associated conditions. The site also links to a range of European TOF
groups in other languages: www.tofs.org.uk/what-is-tof-oa.aspx

WHOLE-BODY COOLING

Longo, D., Bottino, F., Luignani, G., Scarciolla, L., Pasquini, L., Espagnet, M.
C., Polito, C., Figà-Talamanca, L., Calbi, G., Savarese, I., Giliberti, P., &
Napolitano, A. (2020). DTI parameters in neonates with hypoxic ischemic
encephalopathy after total body hypothermia. *The Journal of Maternal-Fetal
& Neonatal Medicine*. doi.org/10.1080/14767058.2020.1846180

Oliveira, V., Kumutha, J. R., Narayanan, E., Somanna, J., Benkappa, N., Bandya, P., Chandrasekeran, M., Swamy, R., Mondkar, J., Dewang, K., Manerkar, S., Sundaram, M., Chinathambi, K., Bharadwaj, S., Bhat, V., Madhava, V., Nair, M., Lally, P. J., Montaldo, P., . . ., on behalf of HELIX consortium. (2018). Hypothermia for encephalopathy in low-income and middle-income countries: Feasibility of whole-body cooling using a low-cost servo-controlled device. *BMJ Paediatr Open, 2*(1), 3000245. www.ncbi.nlm.nih.gov/pmc/articles/PMC5887762

Index